P9-CEN-099

OCCUPATIONAL *and* ENVIRONMENTAL HEALTH NURSING

CONCEPTS AND PRACTICE

OCCUPATIONAL *and* ENVIRONMENTAL HEALTH NURSING

C O N C E P T S   A N D   P R A C T I C E

2nd Edition

Bonnie Rogers, DrPH, COHN-S, LNCC, FAAN

Associate Professor
Director, North Carolina Occupational Safety and Health Education and Research
 Center
Director, Occupational Health Nursing Program
Director, Public Health Nursing
School of Public Health
University of North Carolina at Chapel Hill
Chapel Hill, North Carolina

SAUNDERS
An Imprint of Elsevier Science

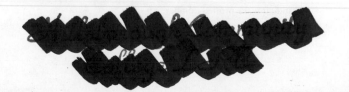

SAUNDERS
An Imprint of Elsevier Science

The Curtis Center
Independence Square West
Philadelphia, Pennsylvania 19106

Occupational and Environmental Health Nursing: Concepts and Practice, second edition   ISBN 0-7216-8511-0

Copyright © 2003, Elsevier Science (USA). All rights reserved.   .

No part of this publication may be reproduced or transmitted in any form or by any means, electronic or mechanical, including photocopying, recording, or any information storage and retrieval system, without permission in writing from the publisher. Permissions may be sought directly from Elsevier's Health Sciences Rights Department in Philadelphia, PA, USA: phone: (+1) 215 238 7869, fax: (+1) 215 238 2239, e-mail: healthpermissions@elsevier.com. You may also complete your request on-line via the Elsevier Science homepage (http://www.elsevier.com), by selecting 'Customer Support' and then 'Obtaining Permissions'.

NOTICE

Nursing is an ever-changing field. Standard safety precautions must be followed, but as new research and clinical experience broaden our knowledge, changes in treatment and drug therapy may become necessary or appropriate. Readers are advised to check the most current product information provided by the manufacturer of each drug to be administered to verify the recommended dose, the method and duration of administration, and contraindications. It is the responsibility of the licensed prescriber, relying on experience and knowledge of the patient, to determine dosages and the best treatment for each individual patient. Neither the publisher nor the author assumes any liability for any injury and/or damage to person or property arising from this publication.

Previous edition copyrighted 1994

Library of Congress Cataloging-in-Publication Data
Rogers, Bonnie.
  Occupational and environmental health nursing: concepts and practice / Bonnie Rogers.—
2nd ed.
    p. cm.
Includes bibliographical references and index.
ISBN 0-7216-8511-0
1. Industrial nursing. I. Title.

RC966.R64 2003
610.73'46—dc21

2002044516

Executive Editor: Loren Wilson
Managing Editor: Linda Thomas
Publishing Services Manager: John Rogers
Project Manager: Doug Turner
Senior Designer: Kathi Gosche
Cover Art: Kathi Gosche

Printed in United States of America

Last digit is the printed number: 9   8   7   6   5   4   3   2   1

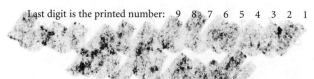

About the Author

Bonnie Rogers is an Associate Professor of Nursing and Public Health and is Director of the North Carolina Occupational Safety and Health Education and Research Center, the Occupational Health Nursing Program, and the Health Services Research in Occupational Safety and Health Program at the University of North Carolina, School of Public Health, Chapel Hill, North Carolina. Dr. Rogers is also Director of the Public Health Nursing Program. Dr. Rogers received her diploma in nursing from the Washington Hospital Center School of Nursing, Washington, DC; her baccalaureate in nursing from George Mason University, School of Nursing, Fairfax, Virginia; and her master of public health degree and doctorate in public health, with a major in environmental health sciences and occupational health nursing, from Johns Hopkins University, School of Public Health, Baltimore, Maryland. She holds a postgraduate certificate as an adult health clinical nurse specialist and is a fellow at the American Academy of Nursing and the American Association of Occupational Health Nurses. Dr. Rogers is certified in occupational health nursing, as a legal nurse consultant, and as an MBTI practitioner.

In addition to managerial, consultant, and educator/researcher positions, Dr. Rogers also has practiced for many years as a public health nurse, occupational health nurse, and occupational health nurse practitioner. She has published more than 150 articles and book chapters and two books, including *Occupational Health Nursing Guidelines for Primary Clinical Conditions* and the first edition of this book, *Occupational Health Nursing: Concepts and Practice*. She is a member of several editorial panels and has given more than 350 presentations nationally and internationally on occupational health and safety issues, environmental health, and ethics. Dr. Rogers has had several funded research grants on clinical issues in occupational health, research priorities, hazards to health care workers, and ethical issues in occupational health. She was invited to study ethics as a visiting scholar at the Hastings Center in New York and was granted a NIOSH Career Award to study ethical issues in occupational health.

Dr. Rogers is a strong advocate of occupational health research and serves as Chairperson of the NIOSH National Occupational Research Agenda Liaison Committee. She has served on numerous Institute of Medicine committees, including both the Nursing, Health, and Environment Committee and the Committee to Assess Training Needs for Occupational Safety and Health Personnel in the United States. Dr. Rogers is a past president of the American Association of Occupational Health Nurses and is an appointed member of the National Advisory Committee on Occupational Safety and Health. She is a consultant in occupational health and ethics.

DM B&T #69.95 B7032-12 06/03/03

Contributor

Susan A. Randolph, RN, MSN, COHN-S,
  FAAOHN
Clinical Instructor
School of Public Health
Occupational Health Nursing Program
University of North Carolina at Chapel Hill
Chapel Hill, North Carolina
*Chapter 4, Roles of the Occupational and
  Environmental Health Nurse*

Reviewer

Grace Rome Schnakenberg, BSN, MA, COHN-S,
  CCM
Occupational Health Nurse Consultant
Texas Instruments
Tucson, Arizona

To my family

My husband, Jon Klein, who always shares his enthusiasm for life, health, and
his passion, swimming, and our beautiful, exhuberant daughter, Lara, now 9 years old,
who prides me with her caring and spontaneous love for being Lara.

My dad, in his memory, and my mom, who at age 81
still works as a worker and a mom, and who both always valued
and instilled in me a good work ethic.

My sister, Barbara Ann, who is a colleague but more my best friend, and my
brother-in-law, Rob, who is always sharing his entrepreneurial spirit.

Preface

Occupational and environmental health nursing is a dynamic nursing specialty practice that continues to evolve in autonomy, knowledge, and expertise. Occupational and environmental health nurses continue to provide traditional occupational health services emphasizing health promotion and prevention of illnesses and injuries in worker populations; at the same time, expansion into case management, independent practice, environmental health, travel health, research, and family services is increasing the scope of the practice.

Occupational and Environmental Health Nursing: Concepts and Practice, second edition, provides a framework for and conceptual approach to occupational and environmental health nursing practice, with practical application of the concepts. The reader is exposed to the complexity and rich diversity of occupational and environmental health nursing practice and is stimulated to think critically about the challenges and opportunities that exist for role and knowledge expansion in the specialty. This text

- Provides a conceptual framework for the development and delivery of a comprehensive occupational health service
- Addresses skill and expertise needed in managing occupational health programs within the context of legal-ethical parameters and external influences
- Discusses challenges affecting occupational and environmental health nursing, including international health, genetics, work organization, and workplace terrorism

This text provides a discussion of the meaning and relevance of work, important occupational health status indicators of the working population, and general health status issues of the U.S. population that set the stage for occupational health and safety prevention and intervention strategies. The history and the nature and scope of occupational health nursing practice are thoroughly discussed within the context of philosophical and public health underpinnings and the application of health promotion and prevention principles.

Exposure to toxins in the workplace can produce significant stress for the worker and family. The occupational and environmental health nurse must possess relevant epidemiologic knowledge and skills to assess and monitor work-related health hazards, evaluate health status indicators, and analyze and interpret data regarding illness and injury trends. Multidisciplinary approaches to problem solving cannot be overemphasized, and knowledge and application related to concepts of industrial hygiene, toxicology, safety, and ergonomics are discussed.

A conceptual model for practice is presented that emphasizes the relationship of internal and external influences on workers' health and the work environment. The model challenges the occupational and environmental health nurse to consider a variety of parameters in establishing a comprehensive approach to service delivery. Useful practical guides to help assess both the organization and the work setting related to organizational culture and comprehensive worksite assessments are provided. Health assessment, monitoring, surveillance, and clinical management, which are important components of the nurse's practice, as well as an in-depth discussion of and model for health promotion and health protection and levels of prevention are presented.

Occupational and environmental health nurses are assuming a much greater role in management, and this topic is addressed from both leadership and administrative perspectives. Managerial functions, quality, and change are discussed. Legal parameters for practice are addressed, and several examples of recent occupational health and safety legislation are discussed along with general content related to workers' compensation. The ethical practice of occupational and environmental health nursing is critical; is presented within the framework of ethical theories, principles, and a model for ethical decision making; and is threaded throughout the text.

The occupational and environmental health nurse will need to become more skilled and involved in research, which provides the foundation for practice. A general overview of the research process and critical areas needing occupational and environmental nursing research is presented.

New chapters on case management, international health, environmental health, and profes-

sionalism have been added to this edition to reflect the expanding practice base of the specialty. Future issues important to occupational and environmental health nursing practice, including increased expansion in primary care, genetics, work organization effects, workplace terrorism, and more emphasis on environmental health, are critical to address as we proceed into the twenty-first century.

Bonnie Rogers

Acknowledgments

A special appreciation is given to the many occupational and environmental health nurses I continue to have the privilege to work with as students and as colleagues. In particular, Kathleen Buckheit, Liz Lawhorn, Judy Ostendorf, Susan Randolph, and Grace Rome Schnakenberg have provided consistent and extraordinary professionalism and role modeling . . . and friendship.

A sincere thank you is given to Lynette Roesch for her expert professional assistance through all the revisions of the manuscript.

Contents

1 Work and Health: Trends and Challenges

THE MEANING OF WORK

Work, work ethic, and related productivity have been integral to the nation's culture since its beginning. Most adults spend approximately one fourth to one third of their time at work and often perceive their work as part of their identity. In addition, most men and women who are employed indicate they would work even if it was financially unnecessary.

Kahn (1981) points out that work involves an exchange between the employee and employer wherein a contractual relationship exists (written or unwritten) in which the worker agrees to perform certain tasks in exchange for a monetary commitment by the employer. However, for many the value of work is characterized not solely by extrinsic rewards such as compensation, benefits, and status, but often, and more important, by intrinsic rewards such as self-satisfaction, achievement, pride, joy, self-enhancement, socialization, and improved self-esteem (Bezold et al., 1986; Public Broadcasting System, 1992, U.S. Department of Labor [USDOL], 1999). What workers like most about work is the opportunity to make a meaningful contribution to society, guide and manage their own work, display creativity and innovation, and maintain some control in decision making (Levenstein, 2000). Organizations and management should assume some responsibility in fostering opportunities.

The quality of the work environment can be viewed in terms of the organization's willingness to meet the needs and abilities of the employees (Graham, 1991). Significant changes in the characteristics of the workforce population (e.g., older, more diverse) have caused the employer to reexamine the fit between the employee and the job. More emphasis is being placed on developing worker potential and work task demands, enhancing health and safety standards at the worksite, increasing organizational flexibility in terms of job design, demands, and home-based work, and addressing critical issues such as child and elder care, family stressors, disability, and family friendly work policies. To this end work influences all aspects of the employee's well-being (i.e., physical, psychological, emotional, social) and extends beyond the working walls to affect one's overall quality of life. The occupational and environmental health nurse needs to be cognizant of changing population and workforce demographics; the changing relationship between workplace landscape and work performance (e.g., telecommuting); employee and employer perceptions of work, health, and work-related health hazards; and other influences (e.g., family) in order to be an effective and knowledgeable team member in the design of programs and services that promote and protect the health of all workers.

This chapter will discuss the changing face of the U.S. workforce and workplace, health of the workforce as reflected by national health status indicators, work-related illness and injury trends, factors influencing worker health and safety, and issues related to health care costs. In addition, *Healthy People 2010: Occupational Safety and Health Objectives* is presented along with related occupational safety and health objectives that provide national guidance for worker health and safety and hazard reduction.

CHANGING POPULATION AND WORKFORCE CHARACTERISTICS

The population of the United States is expected to increase nearly 50% from 275 million in 2000 to an estimated 394 million people by 2050. In 1995 33.5 million people were at least 65 years of age, and by 2050 this group is expected to more than double, representing 20% of the population (U.S. Census Bureau, 1996). In addition, the number of youths (under 17) is expected to increase from 70 million in 2000 to over 96 million in 2050.

The composition of U.S. racial and ethnic populations is changing. Estimates show that the white population, not including Hispanic Americans, will decline from 73.6% in 1995 to 52.8% in 2050. In the same period the fastest growing population group will be Hispanic Americans, increasing from 10.2% to 24.5% of the population. The black population will increase slightly from 12% to 13.5%; and native and Asian-Americans will increase from 3.3% to 8.2%. By 2010 Hispanics will make up the largest minority group. Economic expansion will create approximately 18 million new jobs, and racial/ethnic populations will enter the workforce at higher rates than whites, reflective of the population changes (U.S. Department of Health and Human Services [USDHHS], 2000).

Workforce changes also include a shift in the proportion of men and women in the workplace and the types of jobs available to and occupied by each group. According to the Current Population Survey (CPS) (Bureau of Labor Statistics [BLS], 1999), in 1998 54% of the approximately 131 million people employed in the United States were male. By race 84% of these workers were white, and 11% were black; by ethnicity 10% were Hispanic (of any race). Distributions between genders vary by industry division (Table 1-1) and occupation (Table 1-2). From 1983 to 1998 the largest increases in employment occurred in the service occupations, executive, administrative and managerial occupations, and professional specialty occupations. Based on employment trends from 1983 to 1998, by 2008 20 occupations (of 500 listed by the Bureau of Labor Statistics, or BLS) are projected to gain the largest number of jobs—about 8 million, or 39% of growth (Figure 1-1). The four fastest growing occupations from this list are computer engineers, computer support specialists, computer systems analysts, and personal care and home health aides.

The distribution of the labor force is projected to change by age, with workers age 45 and older

TABLE 1-1   Persons 16 Years or Older Employed in the United States in 1998, by Major Industry and Gender

INDUSTRY DIVISION	NUMBER EMPLOYED (THOUSANDS)	MALE (%)	FEMALE (%)
All industries	131,464	53.8	46.2
Agriculture	3,378	75.6	24.4
Mining	620	86.3	13.7
Construction	8,518	90.6	9.4
Manufacturing—durable goods	12,566	72.7	27.3
Manufacturing—nondurable goods	8,168	61.2	38.8
Transportation and public utilities	9,307	70.9	29.1
Wholesale and retail trade	27,203	52.8	47.2
Finance, insurance, and real estate	8,605	41.3	58.7
Service	47,212	37.9	62.1
Public administration	5,887	56.4	43.6

From *Current Population Survey,* by Bureau of Labor Statistics, Washington, DC: U.S. Department of Labor, Bureau of Labor Statistics. 1999.

increasing from 33% to 40% (Figure 1-2). From 1998 to 2008 the number of women in the labor force will increase by 15%, compared with 10% for men and 12% overall. Women's total share of the workforce is projected to increase from 46% in 1998 to 48% in 2008. The number of working women with children has been increasing. Once, women were well-represented in the labor force only before they had children or after their children had completed school. However, this trend has dramatically shifted (Table 1-3). The share of labor force by race/ethnicity is also projected to shift, with decreases for whites, little or no change for blacks, and increases for Hispanics, Asians, and other races.

HEALTH STATUS OF THE NATION AND WORKFORCE

The health of the U.S. workforce can best be improved through health promotion and preventive and risk reduction strategies. The occupational and environmental health nurse must be familiar with current literature describing relevant health status indicators in addition to occupational health and safety problems. One important document, *Healthy People 2010: Understanding and Improving Health* (USDHHS,

2000), provides a thorough discussion of the nation's health, including occupational health and safety issues, and sets forth national health objectives to enhance health and reduce disease. The two overarching goals of *Healthy People 2010* are as follows:

1. Increase the quality and years of healthy life.
2. Eliminate health disparities.

Clearly, workplace health promotion efforts can contribute to this mission. A very brief presentation of health status indicators relative to the U.S. workforce is presented (from *Healthy People 2010*). Health professionals are encouraged to obtain this document as an important reference and resource.

THE NATION'S HEALTH

The leading causes of death, which have changed dramatically over the past 100 years, are frequently used to describe the health status of the nation (USDHHS, 2000). At the beginning of the twentieth century, infectious diseases topped the list of leading causes of death, but by the end of the century these diseases were replaced by chronic diseases (Figure 1-3). The leading causes of death in the United States generally result from (1) a mix of behaviors, (2) injury, violence, and other factors in the environment, and (3) the inability to gain access to quality health services (USDHHS, 2000).

TABLE 1-2 Persons 16 Years or Older Employed in the United States in 1998, by Major Occupation and Gender

Occupation	Number employed (thousands)	Male (%)	Female (%)
All occupations	131,463	53.8	46.2
Executive, administrative, and managerial	19,054	55.6	44.4
Professional specialty	19,883	46.7	53.3
Technicians and related support	4,261	46.4	53.6
Sales occupations	15,850	49.7	50.3
Administrative support, including clerical	18,410	21.4	78.6
Service occupations	17,836	40.5	59.5
Precision production, craft and repair	14,411	91.7	8.3
Operators, fabricators, and laborers	18,256	75.4	24.6
Farming, forestry, and fishing	3,502	81.0	19.1

From *Current Population Survey,* by Bureau of Labor Statistics, Washington, DC: U.S. Department of Labor, Bureau of Labor Statistics. 1999.

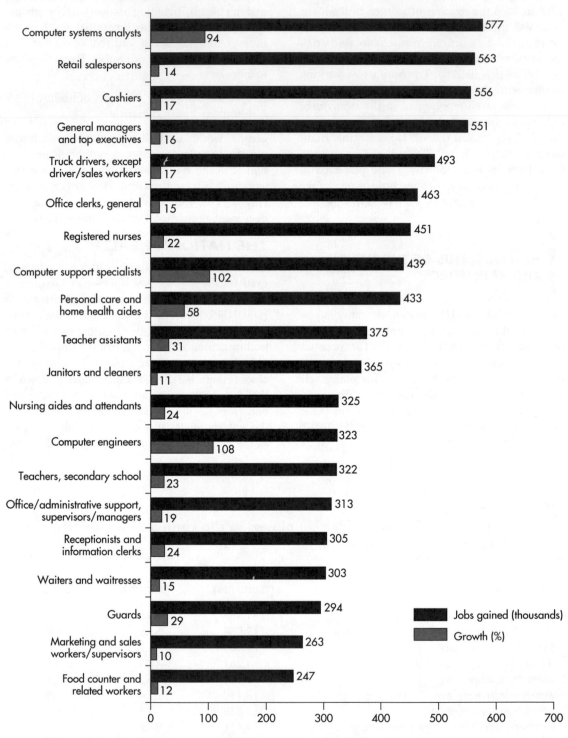

Figure 1-1 Employment growth in occupations gaining the largest number of jobs, projected for 1998-2008. *(From* Current Population Survey, *by Bureau of Labor Statistics, 1999, Washington, DC: U.S. Department of Labor, Bureau of Labor Statistics)*

Among the many problems apparent in the nation's health are musculoskeletal disorders, cancer, diabetes, heart disease and hypertension, nutritional deficiency, substance abuse, and other chronic and debilitating diseases (many of which are tobacco related) which are mirrored in the

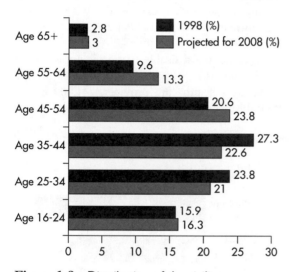

Figure 1-2 Distribution of the civilian labor force by age group, 1998 and projected for 2008. *(From* Worker Health Chartbook, 2000 *[Publication No. 2000-127], by U.S. Department of Health and Human Services, National Institute for Occupational Safety and Health, 2000, Cincinnati, OH: National Institute for Occupational Health and Safety).*

workforce and affect productivity. To better understand the health of the nation and its relationship to the health of the workforce, some of these factors must be examined.

The current and projected growth in the number of people age 65 and older in the United States has focused attention on preserving both quality and length of life. Chief among the factors concerning quality of life are the prevention and treatment of musculoskeletal conditions—the major causes of disability in the United States (USDHHS, 2000). Among musculoskeletal conditions arthritis (and other rheumatic disorders) and chronic back conditions have the greatest impact on public health, quality of life, and work life. Demographic trends suggest that people will continue working at older ages (i.e., older than age 65), and this will only increase the social and economic consequences of the high rates of activity limitation and disability associated with musculoskeletal conditions.

Arthritis

Various forms of arthritis affect more than 15% of the U.S. population—over 43 million people—and more than 20% of the adult population, making arthritis one of the most common conditions in the United States (Lawrence et al., 1998).

The significant effect of arthritis on public health is reflected in a variety of measures (Centers for Disease Control and Prevention

TABLE 1-3   Percentage of Mothers in Labor Force 1975-1998 by Age of Youngest Child in March 1973

YEAR	ALL MOTHERS	CHILD AGE 6-17	CHILD AGE 3-5	CHILD AGE <3
1975	47.3	54.8	44.9	34.1
1980	56.6	64.3	46.8	41.9
1985	62.1	69.9	59.5	49.5
1990	66.7	74.7	65.3	53.6
1995	69.7	76.4	67.1	58.7
1996	70.2	77.2	66.9	59.0
1997	72.1	78.1	69.3	61.8
1998	72.3	78.4	69.3	62.2

From *Current Population Survey,* by Bureau of Labor Statistics, Washington, DC: U.S. Department of Labor, Bureau of Labor Statistics. 1999.

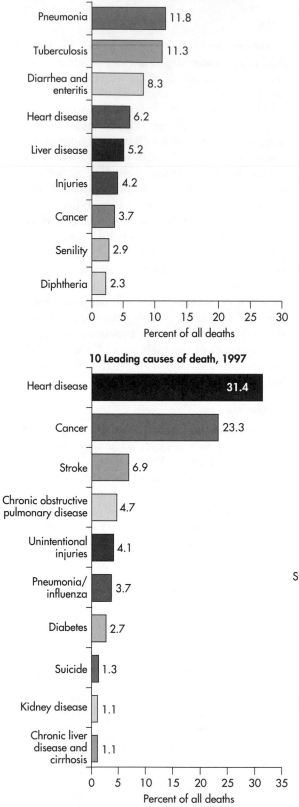

9 Leading causes of death, 1900

Cause	Percent of all deaths
Pneumonia	11.8
Tuberculosis	11.3
Diarrhea and enteritis	8.3
Heart disease	6.2
Liver disease	5.2
Injuries	4.2
Cancer	3.7
Senility	2.9
Diphtheria	2.3

[CDC], 1994a). First, arthritis is the leading cause of disability (Figure 1-4). Arthritis limits the major activities (e.g., working, housekeeping, and school) of nearly 3% of the population (7 million), including nearly one out of every five people with arthritis. Arthritis trails only heart disease as a cause of work disability. As a consequence arthritis can limit the independence of affected persons and disrupt the lives of family members and other care givers (CDC, 1999a; Helmick et al., 1995; LaPlante, 1988; Lawrence et al., 1998).

Arthritis has a sizable economic impact. Each year, arthritis is the source of at least 44 million visits to a health care provider, 744,000 hospitalizations, and 4 million days of hospital care

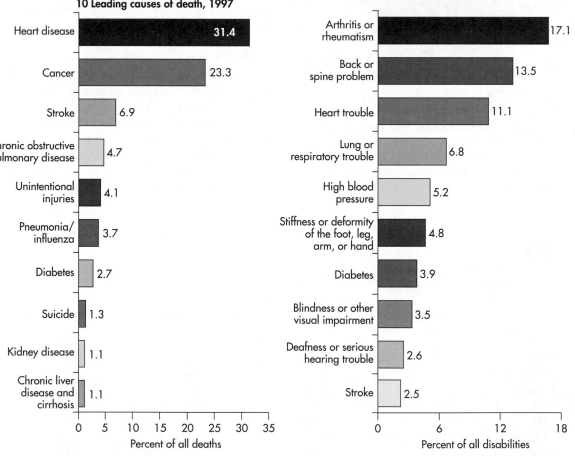

10 Leading causes of death, 1997

Cause	Percent of all deaths
Heart disease	**31.4**
Cancer	23.3
Stroke	6.9
Chronic obstructive pulmonary disease	4.7
Unintentional injuries	4.1
Pneumonia/influenza	3.7
Diabetes	2.7
Suicide	1.3
Kidney disease	1.1
Chronic liver disease and cirrhosis	1.1

Cause	Percent of all disabilities
Arthritis or rheumatism	17.1
Back or spine problem	13.5
Heart trouble	11.1
Lung or respiratory trouble	6.8
High blood pressure	5.2
Stiffness or deformity of the foot, leg, arm, or hand	4.8
Diabetes	3.9
Blindness or other visual impairment	3.5
Deafness or serious hearing trouble	2.6
Stroke	2.5

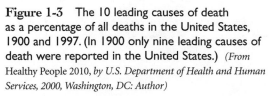

Figure 1-3 The 10 leading causes of death as a percentage of all deaths in the United States, 1900 and 1997. (In 1900 only nine leading causes of death were reported in the United States.) *(From* Healthy People 2010, *by U.S. Department of Health and Human Services, 2000, Washington, DC: Author)*

Figure 1-4 Leading causes of disability (persons age 15 years and older, United States, 1991-92). *(From* Prevalence of Disabilities and Associated Health Conditions—United States, 1991-92, *by Centers for Disease Control and Prevention, 1994, Atlanta, GA: Author.)*

(CDC, 1999a). In 1992 estimated medical care costs for people with arthritis were $15 billion, and total costs (medical care plus lost productivity) were $65 billion, an amount equal to 1.1% of the gross domestic product (GDP) (CDC, 1998a; Yellin et al., 1995). Nearly 60% of people with arthritis are in the working-age population and have a low rate of labor force participation (CDC, 1994, 1999a; Helmick et al., 1995; Lawrence et al., 1998; Trupin et al., 1997).

Demographic trends indicate that the impact of arthritis will only increase. Given current population projections, arthritis will affect more than 18% of the population (nearly 60 million) in the year 2020 and will limit the major activities of nearly 4% (11.6 million) (Boult et al., 1996; CDC, 1994b; Helmick, 1995; Lawrence et al., 1998). Direct and indirect costs are expected to increase proportionately.

Chronic Back Conditions

Chronic back conditions are both common and debilitating. Back pain occurs in 15% to 45% of the U.S. population each year, and 70% to 85% have back pain some time in their lives (Anderson, 1997; Biering-Sorensen, 1984; Frymoyer, 1988; Frymoyer et al., 1983; Svenson & Anderson, 1983). Back pain is the most frequent cause of activity limitation in people younger than age 45, the second most frequent reason for physician visits, the fifth-ranking reason for hospitalization, and the third most common reason for surgical procedures (Praemer et al., 1992).

Work-related risk factors such as heavy physical work, lifting and forceful movements, awkward postures, and whole body vibration account for 28% to 50% of low back problems in an adult population (Wegman & Fine, 1996). Personal factors may be risk factors for low back pain and include nonmodifiable factors such as age and gender, anthropometric characteristics (e.g., height and body build), previous history of low back problems, and spinal abnormalities, as well as modifiable factors such as weight, physical fitness, smoking, and some aspects of lumbar flexibility, trunk muscle strength, and hamstring elasticity. A history of previous low back problems is one of the most reliable predictors of subsequent back problems (Shelerud, 1998).

Cancer

Cancer is the second leading cause of death in the United States. In 1999 an estimated 1,221,800 people in the United States were diagnosed with cancer (Figure 1-5); 563,100 people were expected to die from cancer. These estimates did not include most skin cancers, and new cases of skin cancer are estimated to exceed 1 million per year. Half of the new cases of cancer occur in people age 65 years and older (Ries et al., 1999).

About 491,400 people who get cancer in a given year, or four in ten individuals, are expected to be alive 5 years after diagnosis. When adjusted for normal life expectancy (accounting for other factors such as dying of heart disease, injuries, and diseases of old age), a relative 5-year survival rate of 60% is seen for all cancers (Landis et al., 1999.) (A relative 5-year survival rate means that the chance of a person recently diagnosed with cancer being alive in 5 years is 60% of that of someone not diagnosed with cancer). The relative 5-year survival rate is commonly used to monitor progress in the early detection and treatment of cancer and includes persons who are living 5 years after diagnosis, whether their cancer is in remission, eradicated, or under treatment.

Cancer death rates for all sites combined decreased an average of 0.6% per year from 1990 to 1996 (Wingo et al., 1999). This decrease occurred after rates had increased by 0.4% per year from 1973 to 1996 (Wingo et al., 1998). Death rates for male lung cancer, female breast cancer, prostate cancer, and colorectal cancer decreased significantly from 1990 to 1996 (Wingo et al., 1999). The lung and bronchus, prostate, female breast, colon and rectum were the most common cancer sites for all racial and ethnic populations in the United States and together accounted for approximately 54% of all newly diagnosed cancers (Landis et al., 1999).

Financial costs of cancer are substantial (Brown et al., 1996). Overall annual costs are estimated at $107 billion, with $37 billion for direct medical costs (the total of all health expenditures), $11 billion for costs of illness (the cost of low productivity due to illness), and $59 billion for costs of death (the cost of lost productivity due to death). Treatment for lung cancer, breast cancer, and prostate cancer alone accounts for more than half of the direct medical costs.

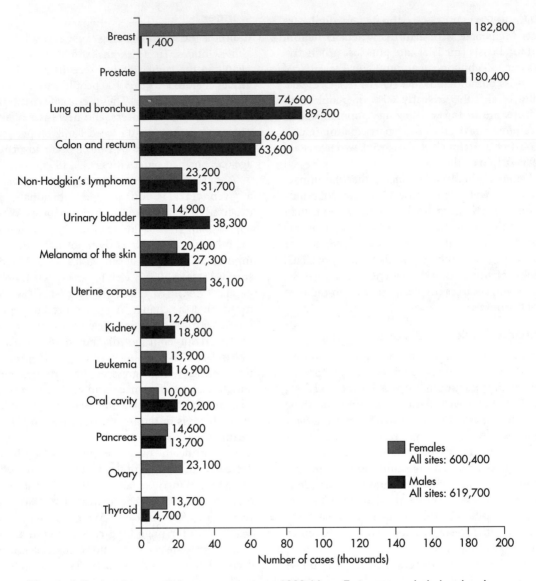

Figure 1-5 Leading sites of new cancer cases, 1999. Note: Estimates exclude basal and squamous cell skin carcinomas in situ except urinary bladder. *(From* Surveillance Research, *by American Cancer Society, 2000, New York: Author.)*

The *Healthy People 2000* objective for total cancer deaths was achieved for the total population by 1995. Lung cancer deaths declined for the first time in 50 years in 1991, declined again in 1992, remained level in 1993, and then dropped again in 1994, 1995, and 1996.

Diabetes

Diabetes remains a significant public health challenge. Some 800,000 new cases are diagnosed each year, or 2,200 per day. Changing demographic patterns point to an increase in the number of people who are at risk for diabetes and who eventually develop the disease.

The occurrence of diabetes, especially type 2 diabetes, as well as associated diabetes complications, is increasing in the United States (Burke et al., 1999; Clark, 1998; King et al., 1997). The number of people with diabetes has increased steadily over the past decade. At present 10.5 million people have been diagnosed with diabetes, while 5.5 million are estimated to have the disease but are undiagnosed. This increase in the number of cases of diabetes has occurred particularly within certain racial and ethnic groups (Flegal et al., 1991). Over the past decade diabetes, primarily from associated cardiovascular disease (CVD), has remained the seventh leading cause of death in the United States. Although premenopausal nondiabetic women usually are at less risk of cardiovascular disease than men, the presence of diabetes in women is associated with a threefold to fourfold increase in coronary heart disease compared with nondiabetic women (American Diabetes Association [ADA], 1996). In the United States diabetes is the leading cause of nontraumatic amputations (approximately 57,000 per year or 150 per day); blindness among working-age adults (approximately 20,000 per year or 60 per day); and end-stage renal disease (ESRD) (approximately 28,000 per year or 70 per day) (CDC, 1999b).

The toll of diabetes on the health of people is expected to worsen before it improves, especially in vulnerable, high-risk populations—blacks, Hispanics, American Indians or Alaska Natives, Asians or other Pacific Islanders, elderly persons, and economically disadvantaged persons. Several factors account for this chronic disease epidemic, including behavioral elements (improper nutrition, decreased physical activity, and obesity); demographic changes (aging and increased growth of at-risk populations); improved ascertainment and surveillance systems that more accurately gauge occurrence of diabetes; and the relative weakness of interventions to change individual, community, or organizational behaviors (CDC, 1997b; Clark, 1998; King et al., 1997). These and other health problems associated with diabetes contribute to an impaired quality of life and substantial disability among people with the disease (CDCb, 1997). Diabetes is costly, with estimates of the total attributable cost close to $90 billion ($43 billion direct, $45 billion indirect) (ADA, 1998; Hodgson & Cohen, 1999).

Activity Limitations

An estimated 54 million people, nearly 20% of the population, currently live with disabilities (McNeil, 1997). Data for the period 1970 to 1994 suggest that the proportion is increasing (National Institute on Disability and Rehabilitation Research [NIDRR], 1998). The increase in disability among all age-groups indicates a growing need for public health programs to serve affected persons.

Disability rates among youths increased from 1990 to 1994. Activity limitations increased 33% among girls, from 4.2% to 5.6%, and 40% among boys, from 5.6% to 7.9% (NIDRR, 1998).

Activity limitations among adults 18 to 44 years old increased 16% in the same period, from 8.8% to 10.3%. This increase suggests that 3.1 million more people in this age-group were limited in 1994 than in 1990 (NIDRR, 1998).

The number of adults age 65 and older with disabilities increased from 26.9 million in 1982 to 34.1 million in 1996. Because the total number of adults in this age-group increased even faster, the proportion of those with disabilities declined from 24.9% in 1982 to 21.3% in 1994. However, the increase in numbers indicates a growing need for programs and services to serve this population (NIDRR, 1998).

People who have activity limitations report having had more days of pain, depression, anxiety, and sleeplessness and fewer days of vitality during the previous month than people not reporting activity limitations (CDC, 1998b). However, increased emotional distress does not arise directly from a person's limitations. The distress is likely to stem from encounters with environmental barriers that reduce the individual's ability to participate in life activities and that undermine physical and emotional health. It is particularly important to target activities and services that address all aspects of health and well-being, including those that promote health, prevent secondary conditions, remove environmental barriers, and provide access to medical care.

The direct medical and indirect annual costs associated with disability are more than $300 billion, or 4% of the GDP. This total cost includes $160 billion in medical care expenditures (1994 dollars) and lost productivity costs approaching $155 billion (Institute of Medicine [IOM], 1997).

Heart Disease, Stroke, and Hypertension

Heart disease is the leading cause of death in the United States. Stroke is the third leading cause of death. Heart disease and stroke continue to be major causes of disability and significant contributors to increases in health care costs (National Heart, Lung, and Blood Institute [NHLBI], 1998).

At 12 million cases coronary heart disease (CHD) accounts for the largest proportion of heart disease. The CHD death rate peaked in the mid-1960s and has declined in the general population over the past 35 years. This decline began in females in the 1950s and in males in the 1960s. During this time period absolute declines (reduction in the total number of cases) and rates of decline (decrease in the number of cases over a given period of time) have been greater in males than in females. However, in recent years both the rates of decline and absolute declines have been greater in females (NHLBI, 1998).

High blood cholesterol is a major risk factor for CHD, but one that can be modified. More than 50 million adults have blood cholesterol levels that require medical advice and treatment. More than 90 million adults have cholesterol levels that are higher than desirable (Sempos et al., 1993). All adults age 20 years and older should have their cholesterol levels checked at least once every 5 years to prevent or lower their risk of CHD. Lifestyle changes that prevent or lower high blood cholesterol include eating a diet low in saturated fat and cholesterol, increasing physical activity, and reducing excess weight (Expert Panel, 1994).

About 4 million people have cerebrovascular disease, a major form of which is stroke. About 600,000 strokes occur each year in the United States, resulting in about 158,000 deaths. Death rates for stroke are highest in the southeastern United States. Like CHD death rates, stroke death rates have declined over the past 30 years. The overall decline has occurred mainly because of improvements in the detection and treatment of high blood pressure (hypertension) (Psaty et al., 1997; NHLBI, 1998).

High blood pressure, known as "the silent killer," remains a major risk factor for CHD, stroke, and heart failure. About 50 million adults have high blood pressure (Burt et al., 1995). High blood pressure also is more common in older people. Comparing the 1976-1980 National Health and Nutrition Examination Survey (NHANES II) and the 1988-1991 survey (NHANES III, phase 1) reveals an increase from 51% to 73% in those who were aware that they had high blood pressure (Sixth Report, 1997). Nevertheless, a large proportion of the population with high blood pressure still is unaware that they have this disorder (Joint National Committee on Detection, Evaluation, and Treatment of High Blood Pressure, 1998).

Heart disease and stroke share several risk factors, including high blood pressure, cigarette smoking, high blood cholesterol, and overweight. Physical inactivity and diabetes are additional risk factors for heart disease. The lifetime risk for developing CHD is very high in the United States: one of every two males and one of every three females age 40 and younger will develop CHD sometime in their lives. Primary prevention, specifically through lifestyle interventions that promote heart-healthy behaviors, is a major strategy to reduce the development of heart disease or stroke.

Progress on smoking cessation will play a critical role in achieving the national goal for heart disease reduction. Smoking cessation has major and immediate health benefits. For example, people who quit smoking before age 50 have half the risk of dying in the next 15 years, compared with people who continue smoking (USDHHS, 1990).

Screening for CHD and stroke risk factors, particularly high blood pressure and high blood cholesterol, is an important step in identifying individuals who may be at risk so they can be referred for ongoing care. A host of studies have shown that dietary and pharmacologic therapy can reduce CHD and stroke risk factors. These interventions, coupled with other lifestyle changes, such as stopping smoking, increasing physical activity, and maintaining a healthy weight, can reduce even more the risk of heart attack or stroke (Blair, et al., 1995; O'Connor et al., 1995; Willett et al., 1999).

Each year in the United States about 1.1 million people experience heart attacks (myocardial infarction). In 1996 476,000 persons died from heart attacks—about 51% were males and 49% were females. More than half of these deaths occurred suddenly, within 1 hour of symptom onset, outside the hospital. For those patients who survive, delay in treatment can mean increased damage to the heart muscle and poorer outcomes (Expert Panel, 1994; NHLBI, 1998; Sixth Report, 1997).

Patients with CHD, atherosclerotic disease of the aorta or peripheral arteries, or carotid artery disease are at high risk for heart attack and CHD death (Criqui et al., 1992; Salonen & Salonen,

1991). About 50% of all heart attacks and at least 70% of CHD deaths occur in individuals with prior symptoms of CVD (Kannel & Schatzkin, 1985; Kuller et al., 1975). The risk of heart attack and death among people with established CHD (or other atherosclerotic disease) is five to seven times greater than among the general population.

Risk factor control can greatly reduce the chance of subsequent cardiovascular problems in patients with CHD. For example, lowering LDL cholesterol levels in CHD patients dramatically reduces heart attacks, CHD and CVD deaths, and total deaths. In addition, lowering blood pressure in these patients reduces CVD endpoints and deaths from all causes (Long-Term Study Group, 1998; MacMahon & Rodgers, 1993; Psaty et al., 1997; Sacks et al., 1996; Scandinavian Survival Study, 1994; Sixth Report, 1997).

Dietary factors are associated with four of the ten leading causes of death: coronary heart disease (CHD), some types of cancer, stroke, and type 2 diabetes (Frazao, 1999). These health conditions are estimated to cost society over $200 billion each year in medical expenses and lost productivity (Frazao, 1996). Dietary factors also are associated with osteoporosis, which affects more than 25 million people in the United States and is the major underlying cause of bone fractures in postmenopausal women and elderly people (National Institutes of Health [NIH], 1994). Many dietary components are involved in the relationship between nutrition and health. A primary concern is the consumption of too much saturated fat and too few vegetables, fruits, and grain products that are high in complex carbohydrates, dietary fiber, vitamins, and minerals.

Obesity

There has been an alarming increase in the number of overweight and obese people. When a body mass index (BMI) cut-point of 25 was used, nearly 55% of the U.S. adult population was defined as overweight or obese in 1988-1994, compared with 46% in 1976-1980 (Flegal et al., 1998; Kuczmarski et al., 1997; NHLBI, 1998). In particular, the proportion of adults defined as obese by a BMI of 30 or greater increased from 14.5% to 22.5%. A similar increase in overweight and obesity also was observed in children older than age 6 in both genders and in all population groups (Troiano & Flegal, 1998).

Many diseases are associated with overweight and obesity. People who are overweight or obese are at increased risk for high blood pressure, type 2 diabetes, coronary heart disease, stroke, gallbladder disease, osteoarthritis, sleep apnea, respiratory problems, and some types of cancer. The health outcomes related to these diseases, however, often can be improved through weight loss or, at a minimum, no further weight gain (World Health Organization, 1998). Total costs (medical costs and lost productivity) attributable to obesity alone amounted to an estimated $99 billion in 1995 (Wolf & Colditz, 1998).

Substance Abuse

Substance abuse and its related problems are among society's most pervasive health and social concerns. Each year about 100,000 deaths in the United States are related to alcohol consumption (McGinnis & Foege, 1993). Illicit drug abuse and related acquired immunodeficiency syndrome (AIDS) deaths account for at least another 12,000 deaths.

A substantial proportion of the population drinks alcohol. Of adults age 18 years and older, 44% (more than 82 million) report having consumed 12 or more alcoholic drinks in the past year (Dawson et al., 1995). Among these current drinkers 46% report having been intoxicated at least once in the past year; nearly 4% report having been intoxicated weekly. More than 55% of current drinkers report having consumed five or more drinks on a single day at least once in the past year; more than 12% did so at least once a week (National Institute on Alcohol Abuse and Alcoholism [NIAAA], 1999).

Alcohol use has been linked with a substantial proportion of injuries and deaths from traffic crashes, falls, fires, and drownings (NIAAA, 1997). It also is a factor in homicide, suicide, marital violence, child abuse, and high-risk sexual behavior. People who drink even relatively small amounts of alcohol may contribute to alcohol-related death and injury in occupational incidents or vehicular accident (NIAAA, 1997; Strunin & Hingson, 1992). In 1996 alcohol use was associated with 41% of all motor vehicle crash fatalities, a significantly lower percentage than in the 1980s.

Although there has been a long-term drop in overall use, many Americans still use illicit drugs. In 1997 users age 12 and older of any illicit drug totaled 13.9 million, representing 6.4% of the U.S. population (USDHHS & SAMHSA, 1997). Marijuana is the most commonly used illicit drug, and 60% of drug abusers use marijuana only. Of people age 12 and older, 36% have used an illegal drug in their lifetimes. More than 90% of these people used marijuana or hashish, and approximately 30% tried cocaine. Relatively rare in 1996, methamphetamine use began spreading in 1997 (Community Epidemiology Work Group, 1998).

Estimated rates of chronic drug use also are significant. Of the estimated 4.4 million chronic drug users in the United States in 1995, 3.6 million used cocaine (primarily crack cocaine), and 810,000 used heroin (Office of National Drug Control Policy, [ONDCP], 1997).

In 1995 the economic cost of alcohol and drug abuse was $276 billion. This represents more than $1,000 for every man, woman, and child in the United States to cover the costs of health care, motor vehicle crashes, crime, lost productivity, and other adverse outcomes of alcohol and drug abuse (Harword et al., 1998).

Scientific knowledge about the health effects of tobacco use has increased greatly since the first Surgeon General's report on tobacco was released in 1964 (USDHHS, 1989, 1990). Cigarette smoking causes heart disease, several kinds of cancer (lung, larynx, esophagus, pharynx, mouth, and bladder), and chronic lung disease. Cigarette smoking also contributes to cancers of the pancreas, kidney, and cervix. Smoking during pregnancy causes spontaneous abortions, low birth weight, and sudden infant death syndrome (DiFranza & Lew, 1995).

Tobacco use is responsible for more than 430,000 deaths per year among adults in the United States, representing more than 5 million years of potential life lost (CDC, 1997a). If current tobacco use patterns persist, an estimated 5 million people under age 18 will die prematurely from a smoking-related disease (CDC, 1996). Evidence is accumulating that shows smoking during pregnancy is associated with mental retardation and birth defects such as oral clefts (California Environmental Protection Agency [CEPA], 1997; United States Environmental Protection Agency [USEPA], 1992). Exposure to secondhand smoke has serious health effects. Researchers have identified more than 4000 chemicals in tobacco smoke, at least 43 of which cause cancer in humans and animals (USEPA, 1992). Each year, because of exposure to secondhand smoke, an estimated 3,000 nonsmokers die of lung cancer, and 150,000 to 300,000 infants and children under age 18 months experience lower respiratory tract infections (CEPA, 1997; USEPA, 1992). Asthma and other respiratory conditions often are triggered or worsened by tobacco smoke.

Studies also have found that secondhand smoke exposure causes heart disease among adults (Glantz & Parmley, 1995; Howard et al., 1998). Data reported from a study of the U.S. population age 4 years and older (Glants & Parmley, 1995) indicate that 88% of people who do not use tobacco had detectable levels of serum cotinine, a biological marker for exposure to secondhand smoke. Both home and workplace environments contributed to the widespread exposure to secondhand smoke. Data from a 1996 study indicate that 22% of U.S. children and adolescents under aged 18 years (approximately 15 million) were exposed to secondhand smoke in their homes (CDC, 1997b). Smoking among adults declined steadily from the mid-1960s through the 1980s (USDHHS, 1991). However, smoking among adults appeared to have leveled off in the 1990s. The rate of smoking among adults in 1997 was 25% (CDC, 1997b). Direct medical costs related to smoking total at least $50 billion per year; direct medical costs related to smoking during pregnancy are approximately $1.4 billion per year (CDC, 1997).

WORKER HEALTH

Premature deaths, diseases, disabilities, injuries, and other unhealthful conditions resulting from occupational exposures pose important problems. Current occupational safety and health surveillance systems indicate that approximately 6.1 million injuries and illnesses were recorded in 1997 in private sector establishments in the United States. Several pieces of legislation have been enacted to provide protection for the worker and the environment. However, in terms of occupational health, the strongest legislation enacted was the William-Steiger Act, better known as the Occupational Safety and Health Act of 1970. The purpose of the act is "to assure so far as possible every working man and woman in the nation safe and healthful working conditions." This is accomplished through the establishment and enforcement of health and safety standards. The act created the National Institute for Occupational Safety and Health (NIOSH), which was charged with focusing on education and research in order to identify work-related health hazards and develop interventions and prevention strategies that help eliminate or minimize workplace hazards (Millar, 1988; National Institute for Occupational Safety and Health [NIOSH], 2000).

Injuries

Injuries are generally easier than illnesses to categorize as occupationally related because their occurrence at the workplace or during work activities is usually obvious. Designating illnesses as occupational in origin is not as straightforward because illnesses often take a long time to develop and may be influenced by nonoccupational factors such as age, family history, or lifestyle habits (e.g., tobacco use or avocational noise exposure).

According to the Census of Fatal Occupational Injuries (CFOI) (1999), about 17 workers were fatally injured each day in 1997, resulting in 6,238 deaths that year, a number that was roughly unchanged from 1992 (NIOSH, 2000) (Figure 1-6). Data from National Traumatic Occupational Fatalities Surveillance System (NTOF) suggest that the overall rate of traumatic occupational fatalities declined during the 1980s and was sta-

ble in the early 1990s. CFOI fatality estimates exceeded those of NTOF by 1,000 or more for years reported in both surveillance systems (1992-1997).

Transportation incidents accounted for 42% of all fatal occupational injuries in 1997 (Figure 1-7), with highway crashes being the most frequent cause of death (NIOSH, 2000). Other frequent transportation incidents included roadside crashes, jackknives, and overturns (U.S. Department of Transportation, National Highway Traffic Administration, 1996). Assaults and other violent acts, including suicide, were the second most common fatal occupational events, accounting for 18% of total cases. Most violent acts were homicides, the second single leading type of fatality. Shootings were the cause of 80% of homicides (CFOI, 1999), and 85% of these occurred during a robbery or another crime.

NTOF classifies a fatality by the industry and occupation in which the worker was usually employed. By industry division, mining had the highest fatal occupational injury rates recorded in NTOF from 1980 to 1995. Following mining were agriculture, forestry, and fishing; construction; and transportation and public utilities. The most deaths occurred in construction, transportation and public utilities, and manufacturing (Figure 1-8).

According to CFOI, the largest number of fatalities occurred among truck drivers, farm occupations, sales occupations, and construction laborers (Figure 1-9). The leading causes of death for these groups were highway crashes and jackknives for truck drivers, tractor-related injuries for farmers, homicides for sales occupations, and falls for construction laborers. The occupations with fatal occupational injury rates at least 10 times the national average of 4.8 per 100,000 workers included timber cutters, fishers, water transportation occupations, aircraft pilots, and extractive occupations (Figure 1-10).

The number of deaths among truck drivers increased fairly steadily from 699 in 1992 to 862 in 1997. More than 50% of the fatalities occurred in trailer-type trucks or semitrailers.

Homicides, the second leading cause of fatal occupational injuries, declined by 7% from 1996 to 1997. Taxi drivers experienced the highest rate of homicide; the highest number of homicides occurred in retail trade in grocery stores and eating and drinking establishments.

Figure 1-6 Number of fatal work injuries, 1992-1997. *(From* Census of Fatal Occupational Injuries, *1992-1997, 1999, Washington, DC: U.S. Department of Labor, Bureau of Labor Statistics.)*

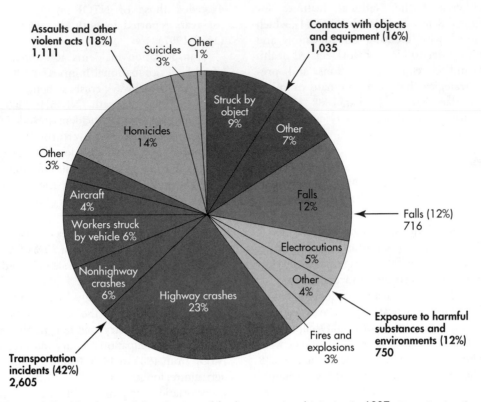

Figure 1-7 Number and distribution of fatal occupational injuries in 1997. (*From* Census of Fatal Occupational Injuries, 1992-1997, *1999, Washington, DC: U.S. Department of Labor, Bureau of Labor Statistics.*)

Falls accounted for more than 12% (*n* = 716) of all fatal injuries. More than half of these fatal falls occurred in the construction industry (BLS, 1999a).

Work-related Illnesses

Illnesses are generally more difficult to link with work than are injuries, because many diseases related to occupational exposures (e.g., tuberculosis, cancers, central nervous system disorders, and asthma) are encountered in the absence of occupational exposures. However, the pneumoconioses are a class of respiratory diseases attributed solely to workplace factors. From 1968 through 1996 pneumoconiosis was an underlying or contributing cause of 114,557 deaths in the United States. The largest number of pneumoconiosis deaths were attributed to coal worker's pneumoconiosis (CWP), but deaths from this disease have declined over the years. From 1968 to 1996 silicosis deaths decreased, byssinosis deaths varied substantially each year from 1979 to 1996, and other

types of pneumoconioses decreased. By contrast, asbestosis deaths increased from fewer than 100 in 1968 to nearly 1200 in 1996.

Characeristic information regarding nonfatal occupational injuries is provided by three surveillance systems: the Survey of Occupational Injuries and Illnesses (SOII), the National Electronic Injury Surveillance System (NEISS), and the National Hospital Ambulatory Medical Care Survey (NHAMCS). SOII is based on employer-generated workplace incident logs, and NEISS and NHAMCS are based on visits to hospital emergency departments. NEISS and NHAMCS collect data on occupational injuries by different methods.

Nonfatal occupational injuries constitute more than 90% of the events recorded by SOII. In 1997 more than 5.7 million nonfatal occupational injuries were estimated to have occurred in the United States, resulting in a rate of 6.6 cases per 100 full-time, private sector workers. Among industry

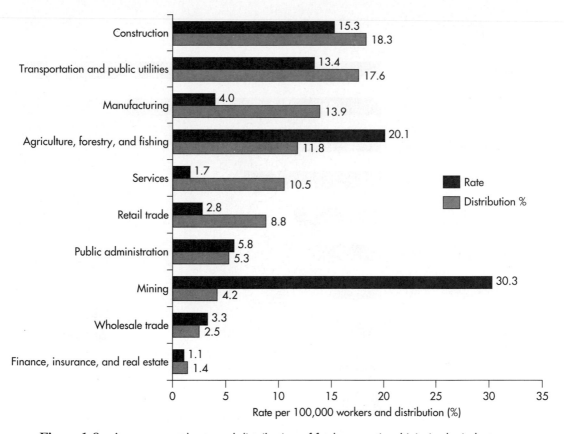

Figure 1-8   Average annual rate and distribution of fatal occupational injuries by industry division, 1980-1995. *(From* National Traumatic Occupational Fatalities Surveillance System, *1999, Morgantown, WV: U.S. Department of Health and Human Services, Public Health Service, Centers for Disease Control and Prevention, National Institute for Occupational Safety and Health.)*

divisions, incidence rates for the total number of nonfatal injuries ranged from a low of 2 cases per 100 full-time workers in finance, insurance, and real estate to a high of 9.3 cases per 100 full-time workers in construction (Figure 1-11). Rates for four of the eight industry divisions are above the average for all industries.

Injuries treated in emergency departments are usually more urgent or severe than those treated in physicians' offices or walk-in clinics. NEISS estimates that approximately 3.6 million nonfatal occupational injuries were treated in hospital emergency departments in 1998. The average rate for all nonfatal occupational injuries treated in emergency departments that year was 2.8 per 100 full-time workers. The rate for men (3.4 per 100 full-time workers) was nearly twice the rate for women (2 per 100 full-time workers). While rates were higher in younger workers (age 16 to

19), there were steady declines in the rates for male and female workers age 20 and older (Figure 1-12). Hands and fingers were the most commonly injured parts of the body, accounting for 30% of the total (Figure 1-13). Lacerations and punctures (26%), sprains and strains (25%), and contusions, abrasions, and hematomas (19%) were the most frequent types of injuries recorded in NEISS in 1998.

New nonfatal occupational illness cases recorded in SOII totaled 429,800 in 1997—the third year of decline in reported illnesses after a high of more than 500,000 cases in 1994. Disorders associated with repeated trauma accounted for most of the decrease from 1994 to 1997. Of nonfatal occupational illnesses reported in 1997, manufacturing accounted for 60%, the highest rate by industry division. The overall incidence rate that year was 49.8 illnesses per 10,000

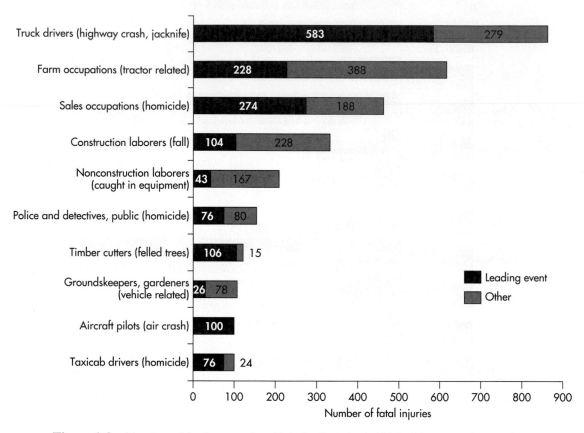

Figure 1-9 Number of fatal occupational injuries by selected high-risk occupations and leading event, 1997. *(From* Census of Fatal Occupational Injuries, 1992-1997, *1999, Washington, DC: U.S. Department of Labor, Bureau of Labor Statistics.)*

full-time workers, with the highest rates reported by establishments with 1,000 or more workers.

Repeated trauma disorders accounted for 64%, (276,600) of all nonfatal occupational illness cases recorded in SOII in 1997. Included in this category are carpal tunnel syndrome (CTS), tendinitis, and noise-induced hearing loss. Repeated trauma disorders accounted for most of the increases in nonfatal occupational illnesses recorded in SOII from 1976 through 1994. Manufacturing accounted for 72% of the cases in private industry in 1997. Industries associated with the highest rates of nonfatal occupational disorders involving repeated trauma were meat-packing (1,192 cases per 10,000 workers), motor vehicles and car bodies (741 cases per 10,000 workers), and poultry slaughtering and processing (523 cases per 10,000 workers).

Ten occupations accounted for nearly one third of the 1.8 million injuries and illness involving days away from work in 1997 (Figure 1-14). Truck drivers, nonconstruction laborers, and nursing aid orderlies each accounted for more than 90,000 job-related injuries and illnesses involving days away from work and, when combined, accounted for almost 19% of these cases.

CTS accounted for more than 29,000 nonfatal occupational illness cases with days away from work recorded in SOII in 1997. Women represented 70% of these cases, and more than half of all CTS cases required 25 or more days away from work (Figure 1-15). Most CTS cases occurred in the manufacturing (42%) and service (21%) industries among operators, fabricators, and laborers (39%) and technical, sales, and administrative support personnel (30%).

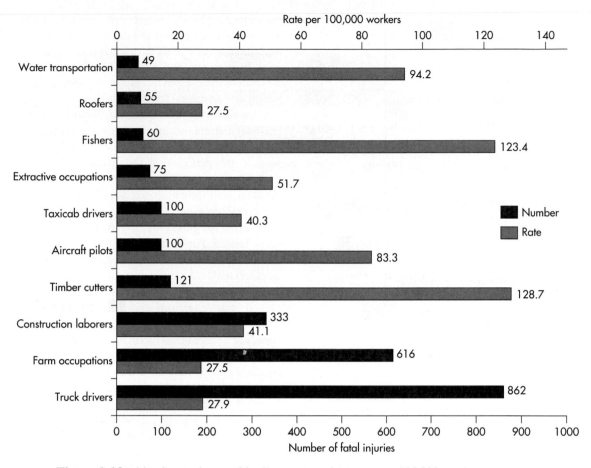

Figure 1-10 Number and rate of fatal occupational injuries per 100,000 workers in high-risk occupations, 1997. *(From* Census of Fatal Occupational Injuries, 1992-1997, *1999, Washington, DC: U.S. Department of Labor, Bureau of Labor Statistics.)*

Nearly 18,000 tendinitis cases recorded in SOII in 1997 required days away from work. Women accounted for more than 60% of those cases, and the upper extremities were affected in more than 70% of cases. Most occurred in the manufacturing (45%) and service (20%) industries among operators, fabricators, and laborers (47%) and technical, sales, and administrative personnel (17%). Worker motion or position was the event or exposure accounting for 73% of cases.

From 1992 to 1998 13,177 cases of noise-induced hearing loss were reported by companies, audiologists, otolaryngologists, the Bureau of Workers' Compensation, and hospitals. Companies accounted for 85.2% of these cases; in 1998 most were associated with manufacturing. Within the manufacturing sector 60% of cases were associated with transportation manufacturing, which includes automobile manufacturing. According to patient interviews, 25% to 76% of companies in major industry divisions did not test hearing at the time the worker was exposed to noise. Patients with hearing loss reported by companies tended to be younger than patients whose hearing loss was reported by health professionals.

Skin diseases or disorders accounted for 13% (57,900) of all illness cases reported in SOII in 1997. These disorders include allergic and irritant dermatitis, skin cancer, and other conditions. Manufacturing accounted for 45% of the skin diseases or disorders in private industry. Dermatitis, a subcategory of skin diseases and disorders, was associated with nearly 6,600 cases involving time away from work. A median number of 3 days away from work was associated with dermatitis. Exposures to chemicals and chemical products

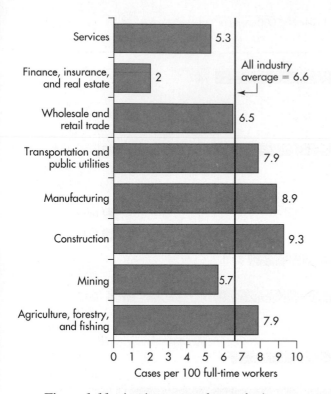

Figure 1-11   Incidence rates for nonfatal occupational injuries in private industry by major industry division, 1997. *(From* Annual Log and Summary of Occupational Illnesses and Injuries, *by Survey of Occupational Injuries and Illnesses, 1999, Washington, DC: Bureau of Labor Statistics.)*

accounted for 53% of job-related dermatitis cases. The manufacturing and service industry divisions accounted for the most dermatitis cases with days away from work (29% each).

Under the SENSOR program several state health departments have developed surveillance systems for work-related asthma, including occupational asthma, occupationally induced reactive airways dysfunction syndrome (RADS), and work-aggravated asthma. Occupational asthma is now the most common disease reported in occupational respiratory disease surveillance systems in several developed countries. However, most cases either are not recognized or not reported as work-related. Population-based estimates suggest that about 20% of new-onset asthma in adults is work-related.

The 10 million health care workers in the United States constitute approximately 8% of the workforce. Health care workers can be exposed to a variety of occupational hazards, including repeated trauma, toxins, and a broad range of infectious agents. Between June 1995 and October 1999, 60 participating National Surveillance System for Hospital Health Care Workers (NaSH) hospitals reported 6,983 cases of exposure to blood or body fluids. Most of these cases involved nurses (43%) and physicians (29%). The largest number of exposures to blood or body fluids occurred in

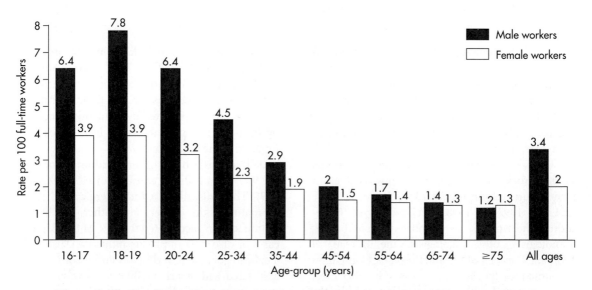

Figure 1-12   Rate of nonfatal occupational injuries treated in emergency departments, by age and gender, 1998. *(Source:* National Electronic Injury Surveillance System, *1999, Washington, DC: U.S. Consumer Product Safety Commision, Division of Hazards and Injuries.)*

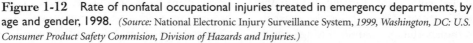

inpatient settings (30%) and operating/procedure rooms (29%). The major route of exposure was percutaneous (Figure 1-16).

Disorders attributable to physical agents represented 4% (16,600) of all nonfatal occupational illness cases recorded in SOII in 1997. These disorders include heat-stroke, sunstroke, heat exhaustion, and other effects of environmental heat; freezing and frostbite; effects of ionizing radiation (isotopes, x-rays, radium); and effects of nonionizing radiation (welding flash, ultraviolet rays, microwaves, and sunburn). Illnesses from toxic exposures are excluded. Among industry divisions manufacturing accounted for 55% of disorders attributable to physical agents in private industry in 1997.

Nearly 5300 cases of anxiety, stress, or neurotic disorders with time away from work were recorded in SOII in 1997. These represent 1% of all reported nonfatal occupational illness cases. Women accounted for more than 60% of all occupational anxiety, stress, and neurotic disorder cases with time away from work. Half of all such disorder cases required 23 or more days away from work, and more than 40% of workers with these disorders required more than 31 days away from work. The industry divisions accounting for most cases were service (35%), wholesale and retail trade (20%), and manufacturing (20%). The occupational groups most frequently experiencing these disorders were technical, sales, and administrative personnel (47%) and operators, fabricators, and laborers (18%). The exposures most frequently associated with anxiety, stress, or neurotic disorders were harmful substances (30%) and assaults or violent acts (13%).

In 1997 new workers (i.e., workers having less than 1 year of service with their employer) accounted for 31% of nonfatal injuries and illnesses involving days away from work. The percentages for new workers were even higher in mining (44%), agriculture, forestry, and fishing (43%), construction (41%), and wholesale and retail trade (34%). Nearly two thirds of these cases occurred among workers with 5 or fewer years of service with their employer.

Sprains and strains were by far the most frequent disabling conditions, accounting for 799,012 cases (43.6%) with days away from work. Bruises accounted for 165,800 cases (9.0%), and cuts and punctures accounted for another 156,700 cases (8.5%). The back was the part of the body most often affected by disabling work incidents. Bodily reaction and exertion, contact with objects and equipment, and falls were the most frequent events or exposures leading to work injury or illness that involved days away from work.

There are a vast number of data sources regarding work-related injury and illness. Selected data system sources to occupational health can be found in Chapter 5 (see Table 5-14).

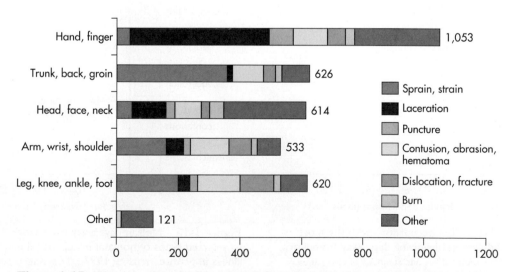

Figure 1-13 Number of nonfatal occupational injuries treated in emergency departments, by anatomic site and type of injury, 1998. *(From* National Electronic Injury Surveillance System, *1999, Washington, DC: U.S. Consumer Product Safety Commision, Division of Hazards and Injuries.)*

HEALTH CARE COSTS

In 1997 health care costs in the United States totaled $1.092 trillion representing 13.5% of GDP (Levit et al., 1998). Although the rate of growth spending has declined during the past 5 years by only 4.8%—the slowest rate of growth in 35 years (Inglehart, 1999)—the Health Care Financing Administration predicts national spending on health care to increase at a faster rate than the rate of growth of the economy as a whole and that by 2002 it will total $2.1 trillion, or 16.6% of GDP (Smith, 1998).

An increasing number of Americans are either uninsured or underinsured, equaling 44.2 million in 1998 or 16.8% of the population (U.S. Census Bureau, 1998). These increases seem to be more

closely related to a decrease in employer-based coverage than to unemployment (Figure 1-17), because unemployment was declining (U.S. Census Bureau, 1998). According to the U.S. Census Bureau (1998), 69% of those younger than age 65 had employer-based health insurance coverage in 1987 compared with 64% in 1997. Findlay (1999) reports that small employers are decreasing health care insurance coverage to employees because of the increased cost of premiums. A study conducted at the Center for Survey Research showed that employees in firms with fewer than 200 workers paid an average of 49% of the premium for family coverage in 1998, up from 44% in 1996 and 34% in 1988 (Findlay, 1999). By comparison, employees in larger firms paid an average of 30% of the premium for family coverage in 1996, the

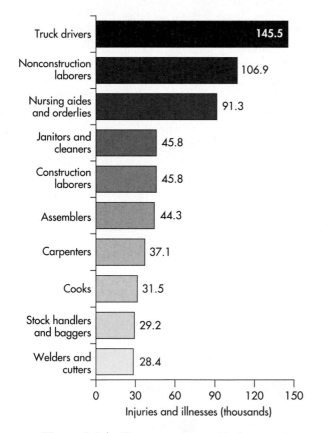

Figure 1-14   Ten occupations with the most injuries and illnesses involving days away from work, 1997. *(From* Annual Log and Summary of Occupational Illnesses and Injuries, *by Survey of Occupational Injuries and Illnesses, 1999, Washington, DC: Bureau of Labor Statistics.)*

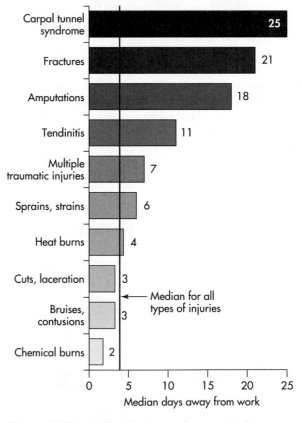

Figure 1-15   Median days away from work due to selected types of nonfatal occupational injury or illness in private industry, 1997. *(From* Annual Log and Summary of Occupational Illnesses and Injuries, *by Survey of Occupational Injuries and Illnesses, 1999, Washington, DC: U.S. Bureau of Labor Statistics.)*

same as in 1988. Sixty percent of businesses with fewer than 10 workers, employing about eight million people nationwide, offer no health insurance coverage. More than 80% cite cost as the major reason for not offering health insurance, which has risen to an average of $5,400 a year for family coverage. As a result of this cost shift, about 6 million fewer people benefited from employer-based health insurance.

Trends toward part-time or temporary employment, self-employment, and contractual work have left many workers and their families with inadequate coverage or no coverage at all. In addition, the costs of health care insurance were predicted to rise by as much as 10% in 1999 (Findlay, 1999). Furthermore, if workers forgo health insurance coverage, they might choose not to see a health care provider when illness occurs. This, in turn, could increase absenteeism rates and related indirect costs such as reduced productivity, worker replacement costs, and decreased morale.

As reported by the Institute of Medicine in *Safe Work in the 21st Century* (2000), efforts to reduce costs and improve health have fueled a renewed emphasis on population medicine, health promotion, disease prevention, and greater integration of the health care disciplines with public health. There is little controversy about the relationship between lifestyle risk factors (e.g., sedentary lifestyle, tobacco use, poor nutrition, obesity, and high lipid levels) and outcomes that increase morbidity and mortality. The economic effects of these health risks are substantial (Goetzel et al., 1998; Pelletier, 1996). Furthermore, these risk factors can be modified, and workplace health promotion programs

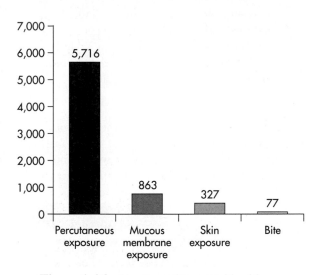

Figure 1-16 Number of reported health care worker exposures to blood or body fluids in 60 participating hospitals by exposure type, June 1995 to October 1999. (*Source:* National Surveillance System for Hospital Health Care Workers, *1999, Atlanta, GA: National Center for Infectious Diseases.*)

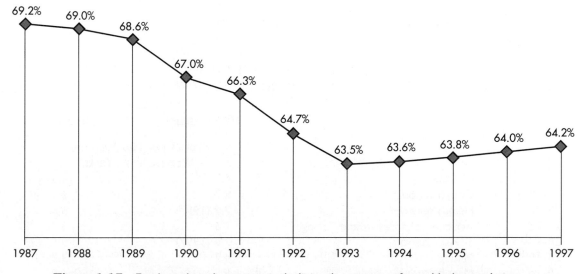

Figure 1-17 Employer-based coverage is declining (percentage of nonelderly population covered through job). (*From* Health Insurance Coverage: 1998, *U.S. Census Bureau, Employee Benefits Research Institute, 1999, Washington, DC: U.S. Government Printing Office.*)

can exert a long-term positive influence on health and lifestyle practices (Heaney & Goetzel, 1997). Consequently, worksite counseling efforts and health promotion and disease prevention programs must be further increased to offer strategies for modification of risky health behaviors and cost containment (Kosinski, 1998; Rogers, 1994).

NATION'S HEALTH OBJECTIVES: OCCUPATIONAL SAFETY AND HEALTH

Within the framework of *Healthy People 2010* are 28 focus area objectives, each stipulating specific targeted objectives for improving the nation's health. The goal for the Occupational Safety and Health focus area (area number 20) is to "promote the health and safety of people at work through prevention and early intervention"

(USDHHS, 2000). This will be accomplished by preventing occupational health hazards through changes in work practices, engineering controls, use of protective devices, and monitoring of workforce and workplace surveillance for health risks, and through increased education of the working population. This focus area has 11 occupational safety and health objectives, which include baseline and target measures (Table 1-4). (Occupational safety and health-related objectives in other focus areas are shown in Table 1-5; baseline and target data for these related objectives can be found in *Healthy People 2010*.)

Summary

Much has been accomplished in the control of work-related injuries and illnesses, particularly during the past three decades; however, much more needs to be done. Implementation of what

---

TABLE 1-4 *Healthy People 2010* Objectives for Occupational Safety and Health

OBJECTIVE 20-1 REDUCE DEATHS FROM WORK-RELATED INJURIES.

		1998 BASELINE	2010 TARGET
		DEATHS PER 100,000 WORKERS ≥16 YEARS	
20-1a	All industry	4.5	3.2
20-1b	Mining	23.6	16.5
20-1c	Construction	14.6	10.2
20-1d	Transportation	11.8	8.3
20-1e	Agriculture	24.1	16.9

Target setting method: 29% improvement.

OBJECTIVE 20-2 REDUCE WORK-RELATED INJURIES RESULTING IN MEDICAL TREATMENT, LOST TIME FROM WORK, OR RESTRICTED WORK ACTIVITY.

		1998 BASELINE	2010 TARGET
		INJURIES PER 100 FULL-TIME WORKERS ≥16 YEARS	
20-2a	All industry	6.2	4.3
20-2b	Construction	8.7	6.1
20-2c	Health services	7.9 (1997)	5.5
20-2d	Agricultural, forestry, and fishing	7.6	5.3
20-2e	Transportation	7.9 (1997)	5.5
20-2f	Mining	4.7	3.3
20-2g	Manufacturing	8.5	6.0
20-2h	Adolescent workers	4.8 (1997)	3.4

Target setting method: 30% improvement.

Modified from *Healthy People 2010,* by U.S. Department of Health and Human Services, Washington, DC: Author. 2000.

TABLE 1-4	*Healthy People 2010* Objectives for Occupational Safety and Health—cont'd

OBJECTIVE 20-3 REDUCE THE RATE OF INJURY AND ILLNESS CASES INVOLVING DAYS AWAY FROM WORK DUE TO OVEREXERTION OR REPETITIVE MOTION.

1997 BASELINE	2010 TARGET
INJURIES PER 100,000 FULL-TIME WORKERS ≥16 YEARS	
675	338

Target setting method: 50% improvement.

OBJECTIVE 20-4 REDUCE PNEUMOCONIOSIS DEATHS.

1997 BASELINE	2010 TARGET
DEATHS FOR THOSE ≥15 YEARS	
2,928	1,900

Target setting method: 10% fewer than the number of pneumoconiosis deaths projected for 2010 based on a 15-year trend (1982-1997).

OBJECTIVE 20-5 REDUCE DEATHS FROM WORK-RELATED HOMICIDES.

1997 BASELINE	2010 TARGET
DEATHS PER 100,000 WORKERS ≥16 YEARS	
0.50	0.40

Target setting method: 20% improvement.

OBJECTIVE 20-6 REDUCE WORK-RELATED ASSAULT.

1987-1992 BASELINE	2010 TARGET
ASSAULTS PER 100 WORKERS ≥16 YEARS	
0.85	0.60

Target setting method: 29% improvement.

OBJECTIVE 20-7 REDUCE NUMBER OF PERSONS WHO HAVE ELEVATED LEAD CONCENTRATIONS IN BLOOD FROM WORK EXPOSURES.

1998 BASELINE	2010 Target
BLOOD CONCENTRATIONS ≥25 μG/DL PER MILLION PEOPLE ≥16 YEARS	
93	0

Target setting method: total elimination.

OBJECTIVE 20-8 REDUCE OCCUPATIONAL SKIN DISEASES OR DISORDERS AMONG FULL-TIME WORKERS.

1997 BASELINE	2010 TARGET
SKIN DISORDERS PER 100,000 FULL-TIME WORKERS ≥16 YEARS	
67 new cases	47 new cases

Target setting method: 30% improvement.

Continued

TABLE 1-4	*Healthy People 2010* Objectives for Occupational Safety and Health — cont'd

OBJECTIVE 20-9 INCREASE THE PROPORTION OF WORKSITES EMPLOYING 50 OR MORE PERSONS THAT PROVIDE PROGRAMS TO PREVENT OR REDUCE EMPLOYEE STRESS.

1992 BASELINE	2010 TARGET
STRESS REDUCTION PROGRAMS PER WORKSITES WITH ≥50 EMPLOYEES	
37%	50%

Target setting method: 35% improvement.

OBJECTIVE 20-10 REDUCE OCCUPATIONAL NEEDLESTICK INJURIES AMONG HEALTH CARE WORKERS.

1996 BASELINE	2010 TARGET
ANNUAL NEEDLESTICK EXPOSURES	
600,000	420,000

Target setting method: 30% improvement.

OBJECTIVE 20-11 REDUCE NEW CASES OF WORK-RELATED, NOISE-INDUCED HEARING LOSS.

No data—developmental

Modified from *Healthy People 2010*, by U.S. Department of Health and Human Services, Washington, DC: Author. 2000.

TABLE 1-5	Occupational Safety and Health Related Objectives in Other Focus Areas

FOCUS OBJECTIVE AREA	OBJECTIVE	RELATED OBJECTIVE
Arthritis, Osteoporosis, and Chronic Back Conditions	2-5	Increase the employment rate among adults with arthritis in the working-age population
Disability and Secondary Conditions	6-8	Eliminate disparities in employment rates between working-aged adults with and without disabilities
	6-12	Reduce the proportion of people with disabilities reporting environmental barriers to participation in home, school, work, or community activities
Educational and Community-Based Programs	7-5	Increase the proportion of worksites that offer a comprehensive employee health promotion program to their employees
	7-6	Increase the proportion of employees who participate in employer-sponsored health promotion activities

From *Healthy People 2010*, by U.S. Department of Health and Human Services, Washington, DC: Author. 2000.

TABLE 1-5	Occupational Safety and Health Related Objectives in Other Focus Areas—cont'd		
FOCUS OBJECTIVE AREA	**OBJECTIVE**	**RELATED OBJECTIVE**	
Environmental Health	8-24	Reduce exposure to pesticides as measured by blood and urine concentrations of metabolites	
Heart Disease and Stroke	12-2	Increase the proportion of adults aged 20 years and older who are aware of the early warning symptoms and signs of a heart attack and the importance of accessing rapid emergency care by calling 911 (developmental)	
	12-4	Increase the proportion of adults aged 20 years and older who call 911 and administer cardiopulmonary resuscitation (CPR) when they witness an out-of-hospital cardiac arrest (developmental)	
	12-8	Increase the proportion of adults who are aware of the early warning symptoms and signs of a stroke (developmental)	
	12-11	Increase the proportion of adults with high blood pressure who are taking action (for example, losing weight, increasing physical activity, and reducing sodium intake) to help control their blood pressure	
Immunization and Infectious Diseases	14-3	Reduce hepatitis B	
	14-6	Reduce hepatitis A	
	14-15	Increase the proportion of international travelers who receive recommended preventive services when traveling in areas of risk for select infectious diseases: hepatitis A, malaria, typhoid (developmental)	
	14-28	Increase hepatitis B vaccine coverage among high-risk groups	
	14-29	Increase the proportion of adults who are vaccinated annually against influenza and ever vaccinated against pneumococcal disease	
Mental Health and Mental Disorders	18-4	Increase the proportion of persons with serious mental illnesses who are employed	
Nutrition and Overweight	19-6	Increase the proportion of worksites that offer nutrition or weight management classes or counseling	

Continued

TABLE
1-5   Occupational Safety and Health Related Objectives in Other Focus Areas—cont'd

Focus Objective Area	Objective	Related Objective
Physical Activity and Fitness	22-13	Increase the proportion of worksites offering employer-sponsored physical activity and fitness programs
Respiratory Diseases	24-5	Reduce the number of school or work days missed by persons with asthma due to asthma (developmental)
	24-8	Establish in at least 15 states a surveillance system for tracking asthma death, illness, disability, impact of occupational and environmental factors on asthma, access to medical care, and asthma management (developmental)
Substance Abuse	26-8	Reduce the cost of lost productivity in the workplace due to alcohol and drug use (developmental)
Tobacco Use	27-12	Increase the proportion of worksites with formal smoking policies that prohibit smoking or limit it to separately ventilated areas
Vision and Hearing	28-8	Reduce occupational eye injury (developmental)
	28-16	Increase the use of appropriate ear protection devices, equipment, and practices (developmental)

From *Healthy People 2010,* by U.S. Department of Health and Human Services, Washington, DC: Author. 2000.

is already known about promoting health and preventing disease is the challenge health care professionals face, not only in terms of saving lives and dollars but also in reducing unnecessary suffering, illness, and disability and improving working and environmental conditions. Efforts guided by an appropriate cost-containment conscience must focus not only on health enhancement and protection in the workplace but also on improvement of the overall health and quality of life of the nation's workers.

References

American Diabetes Association. (1996). *Diabetes 1996: Vital statistics.* Alexandria, VA: Author.

American Diabetes Association. (1998). Economic consequences of diabetes mellitus in the U.S. in 1997. *Diabetes Care, 21,* 296-306.

Anderson, G. B. J. (1997). The epidemiology of spinal disorders. In J. W. Frymoyern (Ed.), *The adult spine: Principles and practice* (2nd ed., pp. 305-314). Philadelphia: Lippincott-Raven.

Bezold, C., Carlson, R. J., & Peck, J. C. (1986). *The future of work and health.* Dover, MA: Auburn House.

Biering-Sorensen, F. (1984). Physical measurements as risk indicators for low-back trouble over a one year period. *Spine, 9,* 106-119.

Blair, S. N., Kohl, H. W., III, Barlow, C. E., Paffenbarger, R. S., Jr., Gibbons, L. W., & Macera, C. A. (1995). Changes in physical fitness and all cause mortality: A prospective study of healthy and unhealthy men. *Journal of the American Medical Association, 273,* 1093-1098.

Boult, C., Altmann, M., Gilbertson, D., Yu, C., & Kane, R. L. (1996). Decreasing disability in the 21st century: The future effects of controlling six fatal and non-fatal conditions. *American Journal of Public Health, 86,* 1388-1393.

Brown, M. L., Hodgson, T. A., & Rice, D. P. (1996). Economic impact of cancer in the United States. In D. Schottenfeld & J. R. Fraumen, Jr. (Eds.) *Cancer epidemiology and prevention* (2nd ed., pp. 269-292). New York: Oxford University Press.

Bureau of Labor Statistics. *Census of fatal occupational injuries, 1992-1997.* (1999a). stats.bls.gov/iif.

Bureau of Labor Statistics. (1999b). *Current population survey.* Washington, DC: Author.

Burke, J., Williams, K., Gaskill, S., Hazuda, H., Haffner, S., & Stern, M. (1999). Rapid rise in the incidence of type 2 diabetes from 1987 to 1996: Results from the San Antonio Heart Study. *Archives of Internal Medicine, 159,* 1450-1457.

Burt, V. L., Culter, J. A., Higgins, M. (1995). Trends in the prevalence, awareness, treatment, and control of hypertension in the adult U.S. population. *Hypertension, 26,* 60-69.

California Environmental Protection Agency. (1997). *Health effects of exposure to environmental tobacco smoke* (Final Report). Sacramento, CA: California Environmental Protection Agency, Office of Environmental Health Hazard Assessment.

Centers for Disease Control and Prevention. (1994a). Arthritis prevalence and activity limitations—United States, 1990. *Morbidity and Mortality Weekly Report, 43,* 433-438.

Centers for Disease Control and Prevention. (1994b). Leading causes of disability. *Morbidity and Mortality Weekly Report, 43,* 730-736.

Centers For Disease Control and Prevention. (1996). Projected smoking-related deaths among youth—United States. *Morbidity and Mortality Weekly Report 45,* 971-974.

Centers For Disease Control and Prevention. (1997a). Cigarette smoking-attributable mortality and years of potential life lost—United States, 1984. *Morbidity and Mortality Weekly Report, 46,* 444-451.

Centers for Disease Control and Prevention. (1997b). *Diabetes surveillance, 1997.* Atlanta, GA: Author.

Centers for Disease Control and Prevention. (1998a). Health related quality of life and activity limitation: Eight states, 1995. *Morbidity and Mortality Weekly Report, 47,* 134-140.

Centers For Disease Control and Prevention. (1998b). *Targeting arthritis: The nation's leading cause of disability (At-a-Glance).* Atlanta, GA: Technical Information and Editorial Services Branch, National Center for Chronic Disease Prevention and Health Promotion.

Centers For Disease Control and Prevention. (1999a). Impact of arthritis and other rheumatic conditions on the health-care system. *Morbidity and Mortality Weekly Report, 48,* 349-353.

Centers for Disease Control and Prevention. (1999b). *National diabetes fact sheet: National estimates and general information on diabetes in the United States.* Atlanta, GA: Author.

Clark, C. (1998). How should we respond to the world-wide diabetes epidemic? *Diabetes Care, 21,* 475-476.

Community Epidemiology Work Group. (1998, December). *Epidemiological trends in drug abuse: Advance report.* Rockville, MD: National Institute on Drug Abuse.

Criqui, M. H., Langer, R. D., Fronek, A., Feigelson, H. S., Klauber, M. R., & McCann, T. J. (1992). Mortality over a period of 10 years in patients with peripheral arterial disease. *New England Journal of Medicine, 326,* 381-386.

Dawson, D. A., Grant, B. F., Chou, S. P., & Pickering, R. P. (1995). Subgroup variation in U.S. drinking patterns: Results of the 1992 National Longitudinal Alcohol Epidemiologic Study. *Journal of Substance Abuse, 7,* 331-344.

DiFranza, J. R., & Lew, R. A. (1995). Effect of maternal cigarette smoking on pregnancy complications and sudden infant death syndrome. *Journal of Family Practice, 40,* 385-394.

Expert Panel on Detection, Evaluation, and Treatment of High Blood Cholesterol in Adults. (1994). National Cholesterol Education Program: Second report of the Expert Panel on Detection, Evaluation, and Treatment of High Blood Cholesterol in Adults (Adult Treatment Panel II). *Circulation, 89,* 1333-1445.

Findlay, S. (1999). Business & health special report: Affordable coverage. *State of health care in America, 17* (6, Suppl. A), 27-32.

Flegal, K., Ezzati, T., Harris, M., Haynes, S., Juarex, R., Knowler, W., Perez-Stable, E., & Stern, M. (1991). Prevalence of diabetes in Mexican Americans, Cubans and Puerto Ricans from the Hispanic Health and Nutritional Examination Survey, 1982-1984. *Diabetes Care, 14,* 628-638.

Flegal, K. M., Carroll, M. D., Kuczmarski, R. J., & Johnson, C. L. (1998). Overweight and obesity in the United States: Prevalence and trends, 1960-1994. *International Journal of Obesity, 22* (1), 39-47.

Frazao, E. (1996, January-April). The American diet: A costly problem. *Food Review, 19,* 2-6.

Frazao, E. (1999). The high costs of poor eating patterns in the United States. In E. Frazao (Ed.), *America's eating habits: Changes and consequences* (Publication No. AIB-750, April). Washington, DC: Economic Research Service, U.S. Department of Agriculture.

Frymoyer, J. W. (1988). Back pain and sciatica. *New England Journal of Medicine, 318,* 291-300.

Frymoyer, J. W., Pope, M. H., & Clements, J. H. (1983). Risk factors in low-back pain: An epidemiological survey. *Journal of Bone and Joint Surgery, 65,* 213-218.

Glantz, S. A., & Parmley, W. W. (1995). Passive smoking and heart disease: Mechanism and risk. *Journal of the American Medical Association, 273,* 1047-1053.

Goetzel, R., Anderson, D., Whitmer, W., Ozminkowski, R. J., Dunn, R. L., Wasserman, J., & Health Enhancement Research Organization Research Committee. (1998). The relationship between modifiable health risks and health care expenditures: An analysis of the multi-employer HERO health risk and cost database. *Journal of Occupational and Environmental Medicine, 40,* 500-510.

Graham, K. J. (1991). Quality of life in the working environment. *Public Health Nursing, 8,* 67.

Harwood, H., Fountain, D., & Livermore, G. (1998). *The economic costs of alcohol and drug abuse in the United States, 1992* (NIH Publication No. 98-43327). Rockville, MD: National Institutes of Health.

Heaney, C. A., & Goetzel, R. Z. (1997). A review of health-related outcomes of multi-component worksite health promotion programs. *American Journal of Health Promotion, 11,* 290-307.

Helmick, C. G., Lawrence, R. C., & Pollard, R. A. (1995). Arthritis and other rheumatic conditions: Who is affected now, who will be affected later? *National Arthritis Data Workgroup Arthritis Care and Research, 8,* 203-211.

Hodgson, T., and Cohen, A. (1999). Medical care expenditures for diabetes, its chronic complications and its comorbidities. *Preventive Medicine, 29,* 173-186.

Howard, G., Wagenknech, L. E., Burke, G. E. (1998). Cigarette smoking and progression of atherosclerosis. *Journal of the American Medical Association, 279,* 119-124.

Inglehart, J. (1999). The American health care system: Expenditures. *New England Journal of Medicine, 340,* 70-76.

Institute of Medicine. (1997). *Enabling America: Assessing the role of rehabilitation science and engineering.* Washington, DC: National Academy Press.

Institute of Medicine. (2000). *Safe Work in the 21st Century.* Washington, DC: National Academy Press.

Joint National Committee on Detection, Evaluation, and Treatment of High Blood Pressure. (1998 November 24-25). *The sixth report of the Joint National Committee on Detection, Evaluation, and Treatment of High Blood Pressure* (NIH Publication No. 98-4080). Bethesda, MD: National High Blood Pressure Education Program, National Institutes of Health, National Heart, Lung, and Blood Institute.

Kahn, R. L. (1981). *Work and health.* New York: John Wiley & Sons.

Kannel, W. B., & Schatzkin, A. (1985) Sudden death: Lessons from subsets in population studies. *Journal of the American College of Cardiology, 5*(6 Suppl.), 141B-149B.

King, H., Aubert, R., & Herman, H. (1997). Global burden of diabetes, 1995-2025: Prevalence, numerical estimates, and projections. *Diabetes Care, 21,*1414-1431.

Kosinski, M. (1998). Effective outcomes management in occupational and environmental health. *AAOHN Journal, 46,* 500-509.

Kuczmarski, R. J., Carroll, M. D., Flegal, K. M., & Troiano, R. P. (1997). Varying body mass index cutoff points to describe overweight prevalence among U.S. adults: NHANES III (1988-1994). *Obesity Research, 5,* 542-548.

Kuller, L., Perper, J., & Cooper, M. (1975). Demographic characteristics and trends in arteriosclerotic heart disease mortality: Sudden death and myocardial infarction. *Circulation, 51*(1 Suppl.), 111-115.

Landis, S. H., Murray, T., Bolden, S., & Wingo, P. A. (1999). Cancer statistics, 1999. *CA: A Cancer Journal for Clinicians, 49*(1), 8-31.

LaPlante, M. P. (1988). *Data on disability from the National Health Interview Survey, 1983-1985.* Washington, DC: U.S. National Institute on Disability and Rehabilitation Research, U.S. Department of Education.

Lawrence, R. C., Helmick, C. G., & Arnett, F. C. (1998). Estimates of the prevalence of arthritis and selected musculoskeletal disorders in the United States. *Arthritis & Rheumatism, 41*(5), 778-799.

Levenstein, C. (2000) *The social context of occupational health in recognizing and preventing work-related disease.* Boston: Little, Brown & Company.

Levit, K., Cowan, C., Braden, B., Stiller, J., Sensenig, A., & Lazenby, H. (1998). National health expenditures in 1997: More slow growth. *Health Affairs, 17,* 99-110.

Long-Term Intervention with Pravastatin in Ischaemic Disease (LIPID) Study Group. (1998). Prevention of cardiovascular events and death with pravastatin in patients with coronary heart disease and a broad range of initial cholesterol levels. *New England Journal of Medicine, 339,* 1349-1357.

MacMahon, S., & Rodgers, A. (1993). The effect of blood pressure reduction in older patients: An overview of five randomized controlled trials in elderly hypertensives. *Clinical and Experimental Hypertension, 15,* 15967-15978.

McGinnis, J. M., & Foege, W. H. (1993). Actual causes of death in the United States. *Journal of the American Medical Association, 270,* 2207-2212.

McNeil, J. M. (1997, August). Americans with disabilities 1994-95. *Current Populations Report* (Publication No. 70-61), 3-6.

Millar, J. D. (1988). Summary of proposed national strategies for the prevention of leading work-related diseases and injuries, Part I. *American Journal of Industrial Medicine 13,* 223-240.

National Heart, Lung, and Blood Institute. (1998, October). *Morbidity and mortality: 1998 chartbook on cardiovascular, lung, and blood diseases.* Bethesda, MD: National Institutes of Health, Public Health Service, National Heart, Lung, and Blood Institute.

National Institute for Occupational Safety and Health. (2000). *Worker health chartbook, 2000* (Publication No. 2000-127). Cincinnati, OH: Author.

National Institute on Alcohol Abuse and Alcoholism. (1997, June). *Ninth special report to the U.S. Congress on alcohol and health* (NIH Publication No. 97-4017). Rockville, MD: National Institutes of Health.

National Institute on Alcohol Abuse and Alcoholism. (1999). Unpublished raw data.

National Institute on Disability and Rehabilitation Research. (1998). Trends in disability prevalence and their causes. *Proceedings of the Fourth National Disability Statistics and Policy Forum, May 16, 1997, Washington, DC.* San Francisco: Disability Statistics Rehabilitation Research and Training Center.

National Institutes of Health. (1994, June 6-8). NIH consensus statement: Optimal calcium intake. 12 (4).

National Traumatic Occupational Fatalities Surveillance System. (Database). (1999). Morgantown, WV: U.S. Department of Health and Human Services, Public Health Service, Centers for Disease Control and Prevention, National Institute for Occupational Safety and Health [Producers and Distributors].

O'Connor, G. T., Hennekens, C. H., Willett, W. H., Goldhaber, S. Z., Paffenbarger, R. S., Jr., Breslow, J. L., & Buring, J. E. (1995). Physical exercise and reduced risk of nonfatal myocardial infarction. *American Journal of Epidemiology, 142,* 1147-1156.

Office of National Drug Control Policy, Rhodes, W., Layne, M., Johnston, P., & Hozik, L. (2000). *What America's users spend on illegal drugs, 1988-1998.* Washington, DC: U.S. Government Printing Office.

Pelletier, K. R. (1996). A review and analysis of the health case cost-effective outcome studies of comprehensive health promotion and disease prevention programs at the worksite: 1993-1995 update. *American Journal of Health Promotion, 10,* 380-388.

Praemer, A., Furner, S., & Rice, D. P. (1992). *Musculoskeletal conditions in the United States.* Park Ridge, IL: American Academy of Orthoscopic Surgery.

Psaty, B. M., Smith, N. L., & Siscovick, D. S. (1997). Health outcomes associated with antihypertensive therapies used as first-line agents: A systematic review and meta-analysis. *Journal of the American Medical Association, 277,* 739-745.

Public Broadcasting Service. (1992). *The Deming of America.*

Ries, L. A. G.; Kosary, C. L.; Hankey, B. F., SEER (1999). *Cancer statistics review, 1973-1996,* Bethesda, MD: National Cancer Institute.

Rogers, B. (1994). *Occupational health nursing: Concepts and practice.* Philadelphia: W. B. Saunders.

Sacks, F. M., Pfeffer, M. A., Moye, L. A., Rouleau, J. L., Rutherford, J. D., Cole, T. G., Brown, L., Warnica, J. W., Arnold, M. O., Wun, C. C., Davis, B. R., Braunwald, E, the Cholesterol and Recurrent Events Trial Investigators (1996). The effect of pravastatin on coronary events after myocardial infarction in patients with average cholesterol levels. *New England Journal of Medicine, 335,* 1001-1009.

Salonen, J. T., & Salonen, R. (1991). Ultrasonographically assessed carotid morphology and the risk of coronary heart disease. *Arteriosclerosis and Thrombosis, 11* (5), 1245-1249.

Scandinavian Simvastatin Survival Study Group. (1994). Randomized trial of cholesterol lowering in 4444 patients with coronary heart disease: The Scandinavian Simvastatin Survival Study (4S). *Lancet, 334,* 1383-1389.

Sempos, C. T., Cleeman, J. I., & Carroll, M. K. (1993). Prevalence of high blood cholesterol among U.S. adults: An update based on guidelines from the second report of the National Cholesterol Education Program Adult Treatment Panel. *Journal of the American Medical Association, 269,* 3009-3014.

Shelerud, R. (1998). Epidemiology of occupational low back pain. *Occupational Medicine: State of the Art Reviews, 13,* 1-22.

Sixth report of the Joint National Committee on Prevention, Detection, Evaluation, and Treatment of High Blood Pressure (1997). *Archives of Internal Medicine, 157,* 2413-2446.

Strunin, L., & Hingson, R. (1992). Alcohol, drugs, and adolescent sexual behavior. *International Journal of the Addictions, 27,* 129-146.

Svensson, H. O., & Anderson, G. B. J. (1983). Low-back pain in 40- to 47-year old men: Work history and work environment factors. *Spine, 8,* 272-276.

Troiano, R. P., & Flegal, K. M. (1998). Overweight children and adolescents: Description, epidemiology, and demographics. *Pediatrics, 101,* 497-504.

Trupin, L., Sebesta, D. S., Yelin, E., & LaPlante, M. P. (1997). *Trends in laborforce participation among persons with disability, 1983-1994: Disability Statistics Report 10.* Washington, DC: U.S. Department of Education, National Institute on Disability and Rehabilitation Research.

U.S. Census Bureau. (1996, March) *Resident population projections of the United States: Middle, low, and high series, 1996 to 2050.* Washington DC: U.S. Government Printing Office.

U.S. Census Bureau. (1998). *Health insurance coverage: 1998.* Washington, DC: U.S. Government Printing Office.

U.S. Department of Health and Human Services. (1989). *Reducing the health consequences of smoking: 25 years of progress (A report of the Surgeon General)* (HHS Publication No. [CDC] 89-8411). Atlanta, GA: U.S. Department of Health and Human Services, Public Health Service, Centers for Disease Control and Prevention, National Center for Chronic Disease Prevention and Health Promotion, Office on Smoking and Health.

U.S. Department of Health and Human Services. (1990). *The health benefits of smoking cessation: A report of the Surgeon General* (HHS Publication No. [CDC] 90-8416). Atlanta, GA: U.S. Department of Health and Human Services, Public Health Service, Centers for Disease Control and Prevention, National Center for Chronic Disease Prevention and Health Promotion, Office on Smoking and Health.

U.S. Department of Health and Human Services. (1991). *Healthy people 2000: National health promotion & disease prevention objectives* (DHHS Publication

No 91-50212, pp. 94-110). Washington, DC: U.S. Government Printing Office.

U.S. Department of Health and Human Services & Substance Abuse and Mental Health Services Administration. (1997). *1997 National Household Survey on Drug Abuse.* Rockville, MD: Author.

U.S. Department of Health and Human Services. (2000). *Healthy People 2010.* Washington, DC: Author.

U.S. Department of Labor. (1999). *Futurework.* Washington, DC: JIST.

U.S. Department of Transportation, National Highway Traffic Safety Administration. (1996). *Traffic Safety Facts.* Washington, DC: Author.

U.S. Environmental Protection Agency. (1992). *Respiratory health effects of passive smoking: Lung cancer and other disorders* (EPA Publication No. EPA/600/6-90/006F). Washington, DC: Author.

Wegman, D. H., & Fine, L. J. (1996). Occupational and environmental medicine. *Journal of the American Medical Association, 275,* 1831-1832.

Wingo, P. A., Ries, L. A. G., & Giovino, G. A. (1999). Annual report to the nation on the status of cancer, 1973-1996, with a special section on lung cancer and tobacco smoking. *Journal of the National Cancer Institute, 91,* 675-690.

Wingo, P. A., Ries, L. A. G., Rosenberg, H. M., Miller, D. S., & Edwards, B. K. (1998). Cancer incidence and mortality 1973-1995: A report card for the U.S. *Cancer, 82,* 1197-1207.

Willett, W. H., Dietz, W. H., & Colditz, G. A. (1999). Primary care: Guidelines for healthy weight. *New England Journal of Medicine, 341,* 427-434.

Wolf, A. M., & Colditz, G. A. (1998). Current estimates of the economic cost of obesity in the United States. *Obesity Research, 6,* 97-106.

World Health Organization. (1998). *Obesity: Preventing and managing the global epidemic: Report of a WHO consultation on obesity, Geneva, 3-5 June 1997.* Geneva, Switzerland: Author.

Yellin, E., & Callahan, L. F. for the National Arthritis Data Workgroup (1995). The economic cost and social and psychological impact of musculoskeletal conditions. *Arthritis & Rheumatism, 38,* 1351-1362.

2 Historical Perspectives in Occupational Health Nursing

THE SPIRIT

Give of yourself this day, my nurse
to those along your path;
give them the care that brims your heart,
share yet the hope you hath.
Lend them a bit of comfort for
their hurt and pain within;
let them rest in your spirit calm
so they may heal again.
For you are blessed each day with a
reward greater than wealth—
'tis you who have the privilege
of helping them to health. . .

Wynona M. Bice-Stephens, 1992

Nursing is older than civilization. Whenever and wherever people first cared for the injured, the sick, and the wounded, then nursing began. Medicine and nursing have often been represented in language by the same person; however, in more recent years a distinction has been made between the two. The emergence of modern nursing has brought with it a thirst and quest for knowledge in a practice-based discipline with a strong emphasis on research as the foundation for practice. However, the importance of historical events cannot be understated as they provide evidence of advancement, change, and stability. This chapter will present an overview of key events that have influenced occupational health and occupational and environmental health nursing practice.

Nursing in the Middle Ages was primarily conducted by religious orders. From the sixteenth to the eighteenth centuries nursing had largely deteriorated to a job of housework, laundry, and scrubbing (Dock & Stewart, 1938). Women were subjugated and deprived of education in a deliberate attempt to keep them in an inferior status. However, in the 1600s the work of St. Vincent de Paul and the Sisters of Charity brought a fresh enthusiasm into nursing. These nurses performed both hospital and visiting nursing, were considered earnest and dedicated by the society they served, treated the sick with respect and humility, and gave medicines according to the prescriptions of the physician (Bullough & Bullough, 1964).

Modern nursing began with reforms initiated at the end of the eighteenth century and developed in conjunction with the First Industrial Revolution (1760-1830). Centered in England in the 1700s and to a lesser degree in France, the Industrial Revolution gradually spread to Germany, the United States, and the rest of the world in nineteenth and twentieth centuries. This parallel development of nursing and industry provided a natural link to offer nursing services to workers and their families at the worksite.

In England during the Industrial Revolution mechanically powered and paced machinery was substituted for manual labor. This gave rise to many problems that affected workers' health. The factory system developed to house new and expensive machines, which had to be located near sources of power, primarily water. Families were disrupted by having to move away from their farms, which had been sources of income and pride, to be near the factories. The primary motive for the factory owners was profit, and employees were not only required to work 14-hour days but also were often laid off when product demand declined. In addition, employers

Milestones in Occupational Health and Occupational Health Nursing

1700	Bernardino Ramazzini, widely considered the Father of Industrial Medicine, publishes *Treatises on the Diseases of Workmen.*
1867	Phillipa Flowerday is hired by the firm of J & J Colman in Norwich, England. Her employment at this mustard company is considered the earliest recorded evidence of a company specifically hiring an industrial nurse.
1884	Bureau of Labor, which later becomes the Department of Commerce and Labor (1903) and then the U.S. Department of Labor (1913), is established.
1888	Betty Moulder (nurse) of Pennsylvania works with coal miners.
1895	Vermont Marble Company initiates industrial nursing services with Ada Mayo Stewart as the industrial nurse.
1897	Great Britain passes a workmen's compensation act for occupational injuries. English legislators later (1906) extend the aegis of the act to encompass occupational diseases. John Wanamaker Company (New York City) hires Anna B. Duncan as its industrial nurse.
1899-1906	Several U.S. businesses hire industrial nurses: • Frederick Loeser Department Store (New York City) • The Emporium (San Francisco) • Plymouth Cordage Company (Massachusetts) • Anaconda Mining (Montana) • Broadway Store (Los Angeles) • Macy's Department Store (New York City) • Filene's (Boston) • Carson, Pirie, Scott (Chicago) • Fulton Cotton Mills (Georgia) • Bullock's (Los Angeles)
1902	The state of Maryland passes the first workers' compensation law. The first attempt by a state government to force employers to compensate their employees for on-the-job injuries is overturned when the U.S. Supreme Court declares Maryland's workers' compensation law to be unconstitutional.
1903	First nurse practice acts are passed into law.
1908	Alice Hamilton, M.D., the first physician to devote herself to research in industrial medicine, publishes her first article about occupational diseases in the United States.
1909	Metropolitan Life Insurance provides nursing services for workers through the efforts of Lillian Wald.
1911	Workers' compensation laws are enacted. National Organization for Public Health Nursing is formed. Fire at the Triangle Shirt Waist Factory in New York City results in 146 worker deaths.
1912	38 nurses are employed by business firms. National Council for Industrial Safety, which becomes the National Safety Council in 1913, is established.
1913	Industrial nurses registry is established in Boston.
1914	World War I begins. The U.S. Public Health Service establishes the Office of Industrial Hygiene and Sanitation. Its primary function is research in occupational health. After several name changes it becomes the National Institute for Occupational Safety and Health (NIOSH) in 1970.
1915	Boston Industrial Nurses Club, which expands into the New England Association of Industrial Nurses (NEAIN), is founded.

Milestones in Occupational Health and Occupational Health Nursing—cont'd

1916	Factory Nurses Conference is established (later calls itself the American Association of Industrial Nurses (AAIN) and then merges with the New England Association of Industrial Nurses (NEAIN) in 1933).
	American Association of Industrial Physicians and Surgeons formed, later called the American Occupational Medicine Association, then the American College of Occupational Medicine, and the American College of Occupational and Environmental Medicine in 1991.
1917	First industrial nursing course is offered at Boston University, College of Business Administration.
1918	1,213 nurses are employed in 871 business firms.
	The American Standards Association is founded with responsibility for the development of many voluntary safety standards, some of which are put into law; today it is known as the American National Standards Institute.
1919	*Industrial Nursing,* which is the first book on industrial nursing and was written by Florence Wright, is published.
1929	Stock market crashes and Great Depression begins.
1930	3,189 nurses are employed by industry.
1935	National Labor Relations Act (Wagner Act) and Social Security Act are passed.
1936	Walsh-Healey Public Contracts Act for worker health and safety standards is enacted and applies to employers receiving federal contracts over $10,000.
1937	2,200 nurses are employed by industry.
1938	Regional annual industrial nurses conferences begin.
	Fair Labor Standards Act (Wage and Hour Act) is passed.
	American Conference of Governmental Industrial Hygienists is formed.
1939	American Industrial Hygiene Association is formed.
1941	World War II begins with 6,000 nurses working in industry.
	The federal government employs its first industrial nurse, Olive Whitlock.
1942	American Association of Industrial Nurses (AAIN), the national association, is founded, and Catherine Dempsey is elected its first president.
	An estimated 11,000 nurses are working in industry.
1943	Army directives are created for the establishment of industrial medical programs in all Army-owned and operated plants, arsenals, depots, and ports of embarkation.
1947	Taft-Hartley Act is passed.
1948	All states (48 at that time) have workers' compensation laws.
1953	The first issue of *Industrial Nursing Journal,* which later becomes *Occupational Health Nursing Journal* and then *AAOHN Journal,* is published.
1955	American Board on Preventative Medicine recognizes occupational medicine as a subspecialty with its own certification requirements.
1956	*Occupational Health Nursing,* a textbook by Mary Louise Brown, is published.
1960	Specific safety standards are promulgated for the Walsh-Healey Act.
1964	Civil Rights Act is passed.
	Journal of Safety Research begins publication.
1966	Federal Metal and Non-Metalic Safety Act is passed.
1969	Federal Coal Mine and Safety Act is enacted.
	Construction Safety Act is passed into law.
	Board of Certified Safety Professionals, which certifies practitioners in the safety profession, is established.

Continued

Milestones in Occupational Health and Occupational Health Nursing—cont'd

1970	Occupational Safety and Health Act is passed, establishing: • Occupational Safety and Health Administration (OSHA) • National Institute for Occupational Safety and Health (NIOSH) • Occupational Safety and Health Review Commission Occupational Safety and Health Education and Resource Centers, now called Occupational Safety and Health Education and Research Centers, are established. Environmental Protection Agency is established.
1970s	Graduate programs in occupational health nursing are offered, with University of North Carolina at Chapel Hill, Yale, and New York University being the forerunners.
1972	Equal Employment Opportunity Act is passed into law. Noise Control Act is passed. Black Lung Benefits Act is passed. Clean Water Act is passed into law. American Board for Occupational Health Nurses is established.
1973	Health Maintenance Organization Act is passed into law. Rehabilitation Act is passed.
1976	Toxic Substances Control Act is passed.
1977	AAIN is renamed the American Association of Occupational Health Nurses (AAOHN). Mine Safety and Health Administration is established to administer the provisions of the Mine Safety and Health Act of 1977.
1978	Federal Lead Standard is established.
1980	OSHA Generic Carcinogen Standard is established.
1983	AAOHN establishes research awards. Hazard Communication Standard is enacted.
1986	National Center for Nursing Research is established at the National Institutes for Health. Revised OSHA Asbestos Standard is established.
1988	OSHA hires its first occupational health nurse. The American Academy of Occupational Medicine and the American Occupational Medicine Medical Association merge to become the American College of Occupational Medicine. *Role of the Primary Care Physician in Occupational and Environmental Medicine* is published by the Institute of Medicine.
1990	Americans with Disabilities Act is passed.
1991	Bloodborne Pathogens Standard is enacted.
1993	National Center for Nursing Research becomes the National Institute of Nursing Research, the seventeenth institute at NIH. Office of Occupational Health Nursing is established at OSHA.
1995	*Nursing, Health, and Environment* is published by the Institute of Medicine.
1998	AAOHN adopts *environmental* as a key descriptor of its practice and incorporates the term into its governance documents and publications so they read *occupational and environmental health nursing.* American Association of Occupational Health Nurses Foundation is established.
2000	*Safe Work in the 21st Century* is published by the Institute of Medicine.
2001	Needlestick Safety and Prevention Act is established.

began to replace male employees with women and children, who would work for less money. With the lack of farm revenue previously enjoyed, the result was not only a decline in living conditions and overall income but also an increase in family tension. Reforms were demanded, and laws were enacted that regulated working conditions in factories, including the length of the work day for women and children. Eventually British law prohibited child labor under a certain age (Bullough & Bullough, 1964; Hunter, 1978).

Nursing reform began in England under the direction of Florence Nightingale, whose determination and vision laid the foundation for the profession and discipline of nursing as we view and practice it today (Bullough & Bullough, 1964; Dock, 1938). Many events influenced her thinking and modern approach to nursing science. Born in 1820, Nightingale came from a well-to-do English family and had all the benefits and comforts of genteel privilege. Though intense in her desire to enter nursing and help the helpless, she encountered stern opposition from her family. Much of her nursing knowledge was self-taught, gained from care of her relatives.

Through friends she learned of the work of the Fliedners, who had established a deaconess house at Kaiserwerth, Germany, in 1836. The intention of the Fliedners was to organize an order of deaconesses to care for the sick. Qualified physicians and pharmacists instructed nurse deaconesses in both medicine and pharmacy. These nurses bathed patients, gave them medications, fed the weaker ones, and did the necessary mending, darning, and ward work (Bullough & Bullough, 1964). Deaconesses were trained in four areas, including hospital and private nursing, relief of the poor, care of children, and work with unfortunate women; their primary thrust, however, was religious (Dock, 1938). Hearing of the work of the Fliedners, Nightingale visited Kaiserwerth against her family's wishes and stayed for 3 months in 1851. In later writings she described the nursing there as poor and crude.

After her return to England she was even more determined to become a nurse. In 1853, after she spent 1 month of study with the Sisters of Charity in Paris, she returned home to care for a dying grandmother. Nightingale subsequently became the superintendent of a hospital system in London, where she was widely known for her quality of patient care, executive abilities, and visionary ideas in the practice of nursing.

Nightingale is probably best known, however, for her reform methods in the provision of nursing care to soldiers in the British Army during the Crimean War (Woodham-Smith, 1950). In 1854 she was asked by Sidney Herbert, the secretary of war, to command a party of nurses to provide care to the ill and injured soldiers. It was reported that hospital conditions were horrid (Nightingale, 1946). There were no medical supplies, the men were devoured by vermin, and the mortality rate was approximately 50% (Cohen, 1984). Nightingale and her nurses systematized a nursing service for the first time for the British Army, brought about extensive sanitary and engineering controls, and provided humanistic and rigorous care that decreased the death rate at the hospital in Scutari from 42.7% of the cases treated to 2.2% (Cohen, 1984). However, Nightingale was reportedly dictatorial in her methods with both nurses and physicians, causing moderate dissension. Despite these difficulties, the mission was successful. Her sanitary reform methods improved the environmental/occupational work conditions for the soldiers, which drastically reduced the mortality that occurred primarily from disease rather than battlefield wounds.

After the Crimean War the popular image of the nurse had been transformed. In gratitude to Nightingale, the British nation established the Nightingale Fund, which the now-acclaimed nursing leader used to start a nurse training school at St. Thomas' Hospital in 1860. As a result of this revolutionary process in nursing education, Nightingale nurses were educated nurses. This model was soon emulated in many other countries, including the United States (Nightingale, 1946).

Nursing in the United States during colonial times was provided primarily by religious orders. However, ties with England had always been close, and the English example was very influential. By 1731 Bellevue Hospital in New York and Philadelphia General Hospital (formerly called Blockley) were established. Almshouses were prevalent in many cities, but the nursing care, which required no special training, was poor. Both religious and secular groups were interested in reforms, and in 1861 the Women's Hospital in Philadelphia opened a school for nurses under the direction of the medical staff, who were all women. However, the teaching was considered too elementary and the educational standards had to be revised. Another "first school" in the United States was organized at the New England Hospital for Women and Children by Marie Zakrzewska, a physician who reportedly began teaching nurses as early as 1860. However, when the Civil War broke out in 1861, there were practically no trained nurses, and most war nurses were self-taught volunteers. After the war these experiences helped focus attention on the weaknesses of the nursing system and the need for reform. Three nursing schools in the United States to be organized along the lines of the Nightingale system, each with a nurse superintendent, opened in 1873. The first school was at Bellevue Hospital in New York City, followed by the Connecticut Training School in New Haven, and Massachusetts General Hospital in Boston. Soon thereafter, nursing schools in the United States proliferated. The women who brought nursing reform to the forefront in this country were dedicated, strong, and determined not only in the training and education of nurses but also in the development of sound nursing practice and a strong nursing profession (Bullough & Bullough, 1964).

OCCUPATIONAL HEALTH AND DISEASE

Occupational diseases have been studied for more than 2000 years (Hunter, 1978). As early as 400 B.C. Hippocrates wrote of occupational diseases experienced by tradesmen and craftsmen, including metallurgists and fillers, and the earliest record of the use of protective masks for miners is found in the writings of Pliny the Elder (ca, A.D. 23-79). This apparatus consisted of a bladder tied over the mouth to prevent inhalation of poisonous dusts and vapors. Until the sixteenth century little was known about occupational disease and even less about occupational health. Georg Bauer, known as Georgius Agricola (1494-1555), a physician and mineralogist, and Theophrastus Phillippus Aureolus Bombastus von Hohenheim, known as Paracelsus (1493-1541), were leaders in what was to become the field of occupational medicine. They spent many years studying the effects of mining, smelting, and the toxicology of certain metals.

Agricola, who wrote *De Re Metallica,* reported on the hazards of dust exposure, poor ventilation, mercurialism, occupational trauma, and environmental contamination, and the resultant harmful effects, including asthma, silicosis, and tuberculosis. Agricola stated that

> *If the dust has corrosive qualities, it eats away the lungs and implants consumption in the body. In the mines of the Carpathian Mountains women are found who have married seven husbands, all of whom this terrible consumption has carried off to a premature death (Hunter, 1978, p. 27-28).*

Paracelsus also wrote about miner's ailments and published his major contribution, titled (in English) *On Miners' Sickness and Other Miners' Diseases,* in 1567.

Bernardino Ramazzini (1633-1714) of Italy published the first complete, systematic, and classic book on occupational diseases, *De Morbis Artificum Diatriba (Treatises on the Diseases of Workmen)* in 1700, which earned him the title "the Father of Occupational Medicine." This book, which has also been published in German, French, English, and Dutch, covers more than 100 occupations and associated hazards as well as the significance of faulty posture, insufficient ventilation, unsuitable temperatures, personal cleanliness, and protective clothing. Regarding exposure of miners to metals, Ramazzini wrote

> *The first and most potent is the harmful character of the materials that they handle, for these emit noxious vapors and very fine particles inimical to human beings and induce particular diseases; the second cause I ascribe to certain violent and irregular motions and unnatural postures of the body, by reason of which the natural structure of the vital machine is so impaired that serious diseases gradually develop therefrom (Ramazzini, 1700, trans. 1993, p. 43).*

Ramazzini was clearly aware of the discipline now called ergonomics. In addition to his classic work on occupational diseases, Ramazzini counseled that when obtaining information concerning illness from a patient, particularly one from the working class, it is vital to ask about the nature of the patient's occupation and to consider this a potential cause for the illness or condition at hand (Goldwater, 1985).

The introduction of machinery into the textile industries of England began not with cotton but silk, with the first silk factory being built in 1718 (Hunter, 1978). The machinery was complicated, yet the operational processes were relatively simple. Again, the First Industrial Revolution (1760-1830) transformed the face of England. Many inventions and innovations were introduced, including the spinning wheel, the power loom, the advent of steam power into mill factories, the improvement of the steam engine, and the development of a railway system. The rapidity of these developments left Great Britain unprepared and disorganized. With the sudden and rapid population growth in urban areas, epidemics of cholera broke out; however, social reform and regulation of public hygiene in the early nineteenth century made town life healthy and tolerable. With the advent of steam power it became possible to build many factories near population centers.

Social consequences of the Industrial Revolution fell with particular severity on women and children. Orphaned or unwanted children were often virtually sold into slavery to the mill owners for cheap labor. Children were often abused and made to work up to 18 hours per day, and there was no legal provision for their welfare. Gradually, public opinion began to regard the excessive toil of children in the factory system as a monstrous exploitation. In 1819 the Factory Act was passed, which stipulated 9 years as the minimum age for child employment and limited the number of working hours. Later the Factory Act of 1833 forbade night work for those under age 18 and restricted their hours to 12 per day, not to exceed 69 per week; factory schools were established, and children under 13 were required to attend school at least 2 hours a day. This Act applied to all textile factories, whereas the previous Act (1819) did not (Hunter, 1978).

Mining was not affected by The Factory Act of 1833. The employment of women and girls was confined to certain mining districts, where they were paid lower wages than men. Women were often harnessed, like horses, to coal trucks for hauling coal or carried it in baskets on their backs up steep ladders and work passages. In some cases 6-year-old girls carried 50 pounds of coal on their backs up ladders. In 1842 the Mines Act was passed, which forbade the employment of girls and women and boys under age 10 in underground mining.

Reforms were also advanced in the United States with the passage of the first child labor law in Massachusetts in 1836. This law stipulated that children under age 15 were to receive at least 3 months of school during the work year. Six years later an amendment to the law mandated that children under age 12 could not work more than 10 hours per day in manufacturing establishments.

The first paper on occupational medicine that related to society's concerns about child labor and occupational safety was produced by Benjamin McCready in 1837. Titled "On the Influence of Trades, Professions, and Occupations in the United States, in the Production of Disease," it warned about the dangers of child labor, long working hours, and improper ventilation (McCready, 1943). However, it was not until 1868 that the first federal legislation was passed regarding the 8-hour workday for certain groups of workers.

In the late nineteenth century several companies and associations, including the Northern Pacific Railway Beneficial Association; the Macy Mutual Aid Association; the Domestake Mining Company of Lead, South Dakota; and the Pennsylvania Steel Company established programs for industrial medical services through hiring or contracting with physicians and surgeons (Felton, 1990). With nearly 200 members in 1916 the American Association of Industrial Physicians and Surgeons was formed. It was later renamed the American Occupational Medicine Association, still later the American College of Occupational Medicine, and in 1991 it became the American College of Occupational and Environmental Medicine.

As industry continued to flourish in the United States, the concern for the health and safety of the workforce increased. In most countries the process of industrialization resulted in the creation of a factory system that changed people's experience of work. Workers encountered a whole new set of conditions, working in large plants and using the new technology of modern industry. Powerless and tied to the speed of the machines they served, facing the ever-present dangers of physical injury from conveyor belts and speeding looms, and exposed to a range of dyes, bleaches, and gases—workers found that the workplace had become a source of injury, disease, disability, and death (Levenstein, 2000).

Massachusetts, the first state to study occupational safety, created the first factory inspection department in the United States in 1867, and required the reporting of industrial accidents in 1886. Several states followed the example of Massachusetts and formed their own state bureaus of labor statistics between 1872 and 1884. In 1884 the federal government established the Bureau of Labor, which later became the Department of Commerce and Labor (1903), and then the U.S. Department of Labor (1913) (Grossman, 1973).

Working conditions in many factories were deplorable and deteriorated even further in the face of an industrial ethic that placed property rights above human rights. The proponents of this ethic maintained that industrial accidents were inevitable and were simply the cost of progress (LaDou, 1981). One of the major industrial catastrophes of this time was a fire that caused the deaths of 146 workers at the Triangle Shirt Waist Factory in New York City in 1911 (Stein, 1962).

The United States lagged far behind Europe in protecting its workers. By 1897 Great Britain and several other countries had instituted worker safeguards and workers' compensation systems. However, workers' compensation was not instituted in the United States until 1911, and then only as a result of a continual increase in industrial injuries. By 1920 40 states had workers' compensation laws, which were usually inadequate and rarely enforced. The Depression of the 1930s contributed to worker injuries; however, workers often overlooked the hazards of the workplace in order to keep their jobs (LaDou, 1981). In 1912 the National Council for Industrial Safety, which became the National Safety Council in 1913, was organized to collect data and promote accident prevention programs.

In the early 1900s Dr. Alice Hamilton, a pioneer in the field of occupational health, began studying toxic industrial exposures, particularly lead. Her work on lead received a great deal of attention and resulted in her appointment, as the first woman, to the faculty of the Harvard School of Medicine.

Little activity in occupational health was seen during World War I. However, delayed effects of cancer among radium watch dial painters (who dipped their brushes in radium and then to their lips, with subsequent absorption) were brought to the public eye (Levy & Wegman, 2000). In addition, silicosis was becoming a more visible problem as a result of work in the "dusty trades," which brought to the forefront job-related lung disease.

In 1936 Congress passed the Walsh-Healey Public Contracts Act, which set worker safety and health standards for employers receiving federal contracts over $10,000. Before World War II, most industrial enterprises were designed to exploit mineral resources (e.g., diamonds, oils, chrome, copper), as well as conduct agricultural operations (e.g., coffee, tea, rubber, cotton) (Herstein et al., 1998). The need for workers in defense plants and other manufacturing operations grew during the Second World War, and this brought with it occupational hazards related to repetitive motion disorders and effects of hazardous chemical exposures. However, worker health was viewed as important to furthering the war effort. In addition, increasing numbers of physicians, nurses, and other health professionals became engaged in the field of occupational health (Klein, 1950). After World War II and into the 1950s and early 1960s, occupational health received little attention, excepting the establishment of radiation safety standards under the Atomic Energy Act of 1954 (Levy & Wegman, 2000). The role of unions, stated as improving working conditions and standards, waxed and waned over the course of the Industrial Revolution and well into the twentieth century. However, in the 1960s organized labor regained some political clout under the Democratic administrations of Presidents Kennedy and Johnson (Levinstein, 2000).

From the mid-1960s to the early 1970s several laws were enacted to protect worker health and safety. The Federal Metal and Non-Metalic Safety Act of 1966 and the Federal Coal Mine Safety and Health Act of 1969 were passed as a result of fatal accidents in those industries, including the deaths of 78 miners in a 1968 coal mine explosion in Farmington, West Virginia. Shortly thereafter the Black Lung Benefits Act was passed in 1972.

The comprehensive Occupational Safety and Health Act (OSH Act) of 1970 was the first law to mandate a safe and healthful work environment for all employees. The OSH Act created three bodies: the Occupational Safety and Health Administration (OSHA) within the Department of Labor to set and enforce standards; the

National Institute for Occupational Safety and Health (NIOSH) in the Department of Health and Human Services for research and education; and the Occupational Safety and Health Review Commission (OSHRC) to arbitrate disputes (Occupational Safety and Health Act 1970; Goldstein, 1971). OSHA's responsibilities, which will be discussed in closer detail in a later chapter, include the promulgation and enforcement of occupational health and safety standards, and the agency requires most employers to maintain records of work-related illnesses and injuries to be reported. Also in 1970 the Environmental Protection Agency (EPA) was formed to protect and provide for clean air and water.

The chemical industry proliferated with the development of new dyes, synthetic dyestuffs, explosives, perfumes, plastics, and soaps, which brought with them new work processes and hazards that society was unprepared to handle. In 1976 the Toxic Substances Control Act (TSCA) was passed to require the testing of certain chemicals and enable the EPA to regulate or ban those found harmful, thereby providing individual and environmental protection from their effects.

In the 1980s federal budget cuts and deregulation weakened OSHA. However, community and activist concern for the workplace and environment resulted in the passage of several OSHA standards such as the Hazard Communication Standard in 1983. The standard requires manufacturers and importers to determine if hazards are associated with products they produce or import, evaluate those hazards, and develop a written hazard communication program, including hazardous substance labeling and employee training. This standard was later expanded to include all industries (Babbitz, 1986).

The entrance of HIV/AIDS into society created more awareness about the health and safety of at-risk individuals such as health care workers who may be exposed to blood and other body fluids. This resulted in the Bloodborne Pathogens Standard in 1991, designed to protect workers from potential and actual exposures to contaminated body fluids. This standard, along with other relevant examples, will be discussed in a later chapter.

In 1990 the Americans With Disabilities Act (ADA) was passed and became effective in 1992. ADA is designed to protect disabled individuals from discrimination, and Title I of the Act specifically addresses employment discrimination. The act requires that employers treat disabled individuals fairly and equally with respect to employment practices. Health care professionals play major roles within these provisions in such areas as understanding job functions, recommending reasonable accommodations, and job placement activities.

In 2000 and after an arduous controversy, OSHA established the final Ergonomic Standard, which was repealed by Congress the following year.

OCCUPATIONAL HEALTH NURSING

The emergence of occupational health nursing, formerly called industrial nursing, was gradual. The current practice of occupational and environmental health nursing is the result of an evolutionary process that began late in the nineteenth century. Health hazards related to workplace exposures and working conditions resulted in illnesses and injuries that were largely preventable. This gave rise to a new field of nursing practice. The first nurses in industry based their practice on a prevention/public health nursing model; they provided family and community health services, as well as industrial health services, that focused on prevention and treatment of work-related illness and injury. Today the occupational and environmental health nurse's role has expanded considerably in scope to include such practice areas as health promotion, management, research, and policy development; this role also has been influenced by and is a reflection of the growth and type of industry in contemporary society. However, the historical underpinnings of the practice remain grounded in preventive health care efforts and public health principles.

The earliest recorded evidence of industrial nursing was the employment of Phillipa Flowerday by the firm of J & J Colman of Norwich, England, in 1878 (Slaney, 1984). Flowerday, who had trained for more than a year at the Norfolk and Norwich Hospital, was engaged at the mustard company by Mrs. Colman to assist the doctor in the dispensary and visit sick employees and their families in their homes (Godfrey, 1978). Flowerday made work-related home visits until her marriage in 1888.

J & J Colman continued to employ nurses to provide health service to employees, established three shelters for those suffering from tuberculosis, and provided an ambulance service for transporting ill or injured employees to the hospital. The company espoused prevention as being better than cure; it provided employees with a recreational club house and made rental houses available to ensure good, clean living conditions. Soon other companies appointed nurses to care for the ill and injured at work. During World War I the prevention of illness gained great impetus because it was thought that workers in ammunition factories were dying as a result of exposure to and absorption of toxic materials used in the work processes (Slaney, 1984). In addition, tuberculosis was rampant, and industrial nurses provided a large measure of health education with respect to sanitation and hygiene.

Occupational health nursing in the United States dates back to the late nineteenth century. In 1888 a group of coal mining companies in Pennsylvania reportedly hired a nurse named Betty Moulder, a graduate of Philadelphia's Blockley Hospital, to care for ailing miners and their families (AAIN, 1976; Markolf, 1945; McGrath, 1945; Wright, 1919). The Vermont Marble Company is often credited with the first employment of an industrial health nurse, Ada Mayo Stewart in 1895 (Felton, 1985; Markolf, 1945).

Felton (1985) gives an interesting description of the industrial operations in Vermont from the eighteenth century to the twentieth century. During the 1700s Vermont, a state with promising economic potential in agriculture and lumber, became the site of a major marble industry after important deposits were discovered. The first commercial quarry opened in Dorset around 1784, and the quarry at Sutherland Falls opened in 1836. The Sutherland Falls Marble Company did not prosper and eventually dissolved; however, Colonel Redfield Proctor, who saw great promise in quarrying, acquired the company in 1869 and reorganized it into a viable business enterprise in 1870. In the early 1880s the rival Rutland Marble Company merged with the Sutherland Falls Company to become the Vermont Marble Company, with Proctor as its president.

In 1889 Proctor, then governor of Vermont, became the secretary of war and followed that with a tenure as a U.S. senator in 1891. He was succeeded at the Vermont Marble Company by his son, Fletcher Proctor in 1889. The company continued to acquire other quarry properties and focused on the sale of sawed marble for monument use; finishing processes were added later. The Proctors were concerned about the welfare of their employees and their families, and Fletcher Proctor, who later also became governor of Vermont, had become familiar with the work of district nurses in several cities. In 1895 he persuaded the board of directors to employ Stewart, a graduate of the Waltham School of Nursing in Massachusetts and a district nurse who was skilled in surgical and dispensary nursing. Waltham School was unique in its training in visiting nursing.

Safety devices were nearly nonexistent in the quarrying process, resulting in what would now be considered preventable injuries such as lacerations, contusions, and fractures. The worker population was ethnically varied, which made communication challenging. Stewart, whose primary mode of transportation was a bicycle, visited sick employees in their homes, provided emergency care, taught habits for healthy living, and instructed mothers on child care. She learned much about the customs and methods used to care for the sick in the native countries of the workers and their families. Stewart also gave talks on health and hygiene to school children, initially at the request of the school teacher, a personal friend.

A second nurse, Harriet Stewart, sister of Ada M. Stewart, was hired by the Vermont Marble Company in late 1895 to provide nursing services primarily to employees in the West Rutland and Center Rutland areas. With the success of its nursing service, the Vermont Marble Company opened a company hospital in August 1896 for the employees and their families. Community residents also could be admitted as pay patients. Ada M. Stewart, who served as the first matron for 2 years, and Katherine Feld constituted the entire nursing staff and provided hospital and home care services. Ada Stewart left Rutland and worked in several states as a private duty nurse, office nurse, massage therapist, and teacher of student nurses. She married in 1918 after returning to Rutland; however, little more is known of her activities. She died in the Eastern Star nursing home in Randolph, Vermont, in 1945.

In the nineteenth century only two other accounts of nurses employed by industries in the United States were recorded. In 1897 Anna B. Duncan was hired by the Benefit Association of the John Wanamaker Company, New York City, to visit sick employees, distribute funds fairly, provide emergency care, make referrals for ill and injured employees, conduct follow-up visits and carry out a communicable disease program aimed at prevention and rehabilitation (AAIN, 1976; Cahall, 1981). In 1899 Frederick Loeser established a nursing service for employees of his department store in Brooklyn, New York (AAIN, 1976; McGrath, 1945).

In the early 1900s employee health services proliferated throughout the country. Industrial products reflected their geographical areas; for example, in 1905 a Georgia nurse was employed by Fulton Cotton Mills, and in Maine nursing services were offered to employees of Great Northern Paper Company in 1913 (Obuchowski, 1963). By this time several employers in New England had hired industrial nurses, recognizing that the provision of organized, comprehensive, and well-managed health services to employees resulted in a more productive workforce and decreased absenteeism. In 1909 Metropolitan Life Insurance Company of New York City began offering a home visiting service to industrial workers insured through company policies. This type of service was extremely successful and spread to other regions of the country and Canada (AAIN, 1976; McGrath, 1946).

The growth of industrial nursing from 1910 to 1920 was accelerated by the advent of workers' compensation laws, World War I, and the emphasis on prevention of communicable diseases, especially tuberculosis (McGrath, 1945). The first organized movement in U.S. industrial health nursing began in New England with the establishment of the first industrial nurses registry in 1913. In 1915 the Boston Industrial Nurses Club was organized under the leadership of Anna Stabler and gave nurses working in industry an opportunity to study and discuss common problems. This group soon evolved into the Massachusetts Industrial Nurses' Association and then merged with adjoining state associations that soon developed to form the New England Association of Industrial Nurses in 1918 (McGrath, 1946).

Another organization, the Factory Nurses Conference, composed of graduate, state-registered nurses affiliated with the American Nurses' Association (ANA), was founded in Boston in 1916. Meetings of this group resulted in an identified need for specialty education in industrial nursing in addition to that of customary hospital training. As a result arrangements were made with the Boston University College of Business Administration to offer a course, "Industrial Service for Nurses," which began in 1917 and continued annually for 5 years (McGrath, 1945). The course consisted of 4 hours of lecture per week for 16 weeks and a 2-week practice experience. Course content seemed to focus on industrial health issues and economics. In 1919 Florence Wright's *Industrial Nursing,* the first book in its field, was published.

During this period several prominent organizations that affected industrial nursing came into existence, including the American Nurses' Association (ANA) in 1911 (formerly organized as the Association Alumni, 1908), the National Organization for Public Health Nursing (NOPHN) in 1912, and the National League of Nursing Education (NLNE) in 1913 (formerly the Society of Superintendents, 1890) (Best, 1940). NOPHN and ANA established Industrial Nursing Sections in 1920 and 1944, respectively. By 1922 several branches of the Factory Nurses Conference had formed in the United States and Canada, and the organization changed its name to the American Association of Industrial Nurses (AAIN), although its activities were never national in scope (McGrath, 1946).

During the 1920s several colleges and universities offered short courses in principles of industrial hygiene to industrial nurses (Heimann, 1964). NOPHN was instrumental in the development of quality education in nursing and undertook, through a survey, an examination of the state of nursing. The study resulted in the *Winslow-Goldmark Report* (1923), which in part emphasized the need for reform in industrial nursing education and recommended that all nursing education be conducted in colleges or universities. NLNE disagreed with the recommendation to close diploma schools and instead developed revised curricula for these schools; however, industrial nursing was not given much emphasis (Rood, 1941).

During the Great Depression, industrial growth ceased, unemployment increased, and worker health and safety programs became less important.

As a result, the need for industrial nurses decreased. This reduction in force also had its impact on association memberships, and AAIN merged with the more viable New England Association of Industrial Nurses in 1933 (McGrath, 1946).

In the late 1930s the American Public Health Association and the National Organization of Public Health Nursing conducted a study of the duties and functions of 85 nurses working in 42 companies. The results of the study indicated a lack of (1) uniformity in industrial nursing practices, (2) awareness of the importance of community resources on the part of industrial nurses, (3) public health standards in this area, and (4) training courses in industrial nursing (National Organization for Public Health Nursing [NOPHN], 1940).

The report emphasized that the responsibility for the status, image, education, professionalism, and setting of standards for practice rested with nursing and encouraged nursing to meet the challenge and accept the responsibility. However, nursing leaders both in service and education were slow to respond.

By 1928 there was a sufficient number of nurses employed by industry to support an independent specialty nursing association, and the First Joint Conference of the New England, New Jersey, New York, and Philadelphia Industrial Nurses Associations was held in New York City (AAIN, 1976). Industries grew during World War II, and the demand for nurses increased dramatically. State nurse consultants were used to help meet the needs of new nurses in industry, with the first industrial health nurse consultant, Ruth Scott, employed in Indiana in 1939 (McGrath, 1945). The Industrial Hygiene Division of the U.S. Public Health Service added nurse consultants to their staff to expand their advisory services (Roberts, 1964). Annual conferences continued, with more regional and local associations joining as members, and it was soon recognized that a broader based organizational structure was needed. In 1942 at the Fourth Joint Conference, members voted to create a national association, the American Association of Industrial Nurses (AAIN), with Catherine Dempsey as its first president; annual dues were set at 50 cents (AAIN, 1976). The purposes of AAIN were to improve industrial nursing practice and education, increase interdisciplinary collaboration, and act as

the professional voice for industrial health nurses. Bylaws were adopted in 1943. (Note that the national organization, AAIN, was not the same organization previously identified as AAIN as an outgrowth of the Factory Nurses' Conference.)

Well into the 1940s industrial nurses worked in isolation with no standardized practice approaches and limited course and field work available in industrial nursing in university settings. NOPHN sought to correct the situation through development of a staff training course in industrial nursing (NOPHN, 1942). In 1944 AAIN published an "Outline of Basic College Courses for Industrial Nurses," which was circulated for use among interested colleges and universities. In addition, five universities—Columbia, Harvard, Johns Hopkins, University of Michigan, and Yale—offered graduate programs in industrial hygiene to nurses.

In 1945 at least 15 colleges and universities offered industrial nursing courses at the baccalaureate level (Roberts, 1964). The NOPHN Industrial Nursing Section, AAIN, and NLNE established an advisory committee to study the issue of preparing nurses at the baccalaureate level for industrial nursing positions (American Nurses' Association, 1945). The committee concluded that this was a specialty area that should be taught at the graduate level. The report of the Advisory Committee on Industrial Nursing resulted in the discontinuance of the industrial nursing courses in baccalaureate schools of nursing, excepting the University of Pittsburgh (Roberts, 1964). Schools that offered additional specialties at the baccalaureate level were not accredited by NLNE. During the same year AAIN opened its first headquarters in New York City and published its "Qualifications of Nurses in Industry," which it distributed to corporate managers (AAIN, 1976).

In 1946 AAIN began participation in a structure study of the six existing national nursing organizations. (In addition to AAIN were the American Nurses' Association, National League for Nursing Education, Association of Collegiate Schools of Nursing, National Association of Colored Graduate Nurses, and the National Organization of Public Health Nursing.) The purpose of the study was to explore the possibility of incorporating all six groups into one national nursing organization, and during the next six years the directors of each of these groups met and considered the proposal. In 1952, at the annual AAIN conference in Cincinnati, members voted to remain an independent and autonomous voice for the nation's industrial nurses. (As a result of that study, three associations—the National League for Nursing Education, the Association of Collegiate Schools of Nursing, and the National Organization of Public Health Nursing—merged to form the National League of Nurses, and the National Association of Colored Graduate Nurses merged with the American Nurses' Association.)

The decision by AAIN to remain independent was perhaps the most carefully considered decision in the Association's entire history. This decision was based on the belief that the interest of the nation's industrial nurses would best be served if AAIN focused its power, thought, and effort as a single group organized by and for industrial nurses. At the same time, however, AAIN reaffirmed its intention of working closely with other nursing organizations, a practice that continues today.

AAIN was incorporated in 1953, the same year that the first issue of its *Industrial Nurses Journal* was published. During the 1950s AAIN, NLN, ANA, and the Public Health Service (PHS) formed a committee that established the functions of industrial health nurses and identified the educational needs of nurses in the specialty. During this period several separate studies on the role, function, and educational preparation of the industrial health nurse were conducted. Recommendations included increasing industrial health nursing content in nursing curricula and encouraging industrial managers to employ qualified industrial health nurses. In 1958 the ANA Industrial Nursing Section voted to change its section name to Occupational Health Nursing, the rationale being that the term was broader, more inclusive, and more descriptive of the role of the nurse in the specialty (1958 Convention, 1958).

In the 1960s occupational health and safety became a public issue via the media and environmental and civil rights movements. Of particular concern were mining accidents, cave-ins, and black lung disease. The importance of adequate education and training for professional disciplines was gaining congressional support. In 1962 AAIN appointed a committee to study the possibility of establishing the American Board for Certification of Industrial Nurses, which was later established in 1972 (AAIN, 1976). However, education for occupational health nurses in the 1960s continued to wax and wane, and additional studies were conducted to examine occupational health nursing content in baccalaureate programs and make recommendations for additional content to be included. In 1965 ANA recommended that all nursing education be taught in colleges and universities and that diploma schools be closed. NLN again opposed this idea and reversed its position for approval of public health nursing in both baccalaureate and master's programs (ANA, 1965).

By the beginning of the 1970s nursing education and practice were in a transitional state and more emphasis was placed on the expanded clinical role of the nurse. The landmark Occupational Health and Safety Act of 1970 provided a new stimulus and interest among both the practice and academic communities to prepare occupational health nurses and nurse practitioners at the graduate level to work in occupational health settings. Under the auspices of NIOSH, Occupational Safety and Health Educational Resource Centers, now called Occupational Safety and Health Education and Research Centers (Apendix 2-1), were established to provide education and research opportunities in the field of occupational health and safety for nurses, physicians, engineers, and industrial hygienists. Undergraduate, graduate (master's and doctoral level), and continuing education are provided for within the mission of the act; however, much more emphasis is placed on graduate level training and continuing education courses.

In 1977 AAIN changed its name to the American Association of Occupational Health Nurses (AAOHN). The term *occupational health nurse* replaced *industrial nurse* to reflect the broad scope of practice of the occupational health nurse. In 1994 AAOHN membership exceeded 12,000, representing more than 50% of the estimated number of practicing occupational health nurses.

During the 1980s the role of the occupational health nurse expanded with more involvement in health promotion, management and policy development, cost containment, research, and regulatory issues affecting practice (Babbitz, 1983; Rogers, 1988). As mentioned previously, the

Hazard Communication Standard was promulgated in 1983. In order to protect the trade secret of a chemical, the original standard stated that the identity of a chemical would be disclosed to a health care professional only in emergency situations or in nonemergency situations, to a health care professional upon written need to know. The definition of health care professional was limited to physician, epidemiologist, toxicologist, and industrial hygienist. Occupational health nurses were blatantly excluded. Through intense negotiations with OSHA and lobbying activities by AAOHN and occupational health nurses nationwide, access to trade secret chemical identity was extended to occupational and environmental health nurses. In addition, employees and their designated representatives who could demonstrate a need to know were granted access with the provision that confidentiality be maintained. The importance of this standard is not only reflected by its notification to workers and others concerning hazards related to chemical trade secrets but also in the rightful recognition of registered nurses as health care professionals.

Efforts by AAOHN contributed to the hiring of the first occupational health nurse consultant by OSHA in 1988 to give technical assistance in occupational health standards development and field consultation regarding OSHA regulatory statutes. This provided further recognition of the importance of the nurse's contribution to the health of the workforce and ultimately resulted in the establishment of the Office of Occupational Health Nursing at OSHA in 1993.

As with other fields of nursing practice, research in occupational and environmental health nursing has become more important. In 1983 AAOHN established the first research award, named for Mary Louise Brown, an occupational health nurse consultant, educator, and author of the textbook *Occupational Health Nursing* (published in 1956). This award is given to recognize research that advances occupational and environmental health nursing practice. In 1986 Congress acknowledged the important role nurses play in health care and the contributions of nursing research to the delivery of more effective, efficient, and humane health care; hence, the National Center for Nursing Research (NCNR), which was designated the National Institute for Nursing Research (NINR) in 1993, was established to promote the growth and quality of research related to nursing and patient care and to help focus the nation's nursing research activities (Rogers, 1986). In 1989 the first AAOHN research priorities in occupational health nursing (see Chapter 14), which have now been updated, were established and published in order to identify the most pertinent areas needing investigation and to encourage private and public sources, such as NINR and NIOSH, to recognize the need for funding occupational and environmental health nursing research (Rogers, 1989).

Occupational health nursing has continued to expand in both knowledge and skill. Recognizing this, OSHA changed the language in several of its standards, indicating that qualified licensed health care professionals could perform certain health/medical surveillance or screening activities previously designated as physician only or physician supervised. In addition, in 1998 AAOHN adopted the concept of environmental health as a significant component of the practice field. To this end AAOHN has incorporated the term *environmental* (as in *occupational and environmental health nursing*) in its documents and publications.

In 1998 AAOHN published its first set of competencies in occupational and environmental health nursing (White et al., 1999) and also established the AAOHN Foundation to support education, research, and leadership activities in occupational and environmental health nursing.

Summary

For approximately a century, occupational and environmental health nurses have been providing health care at the worksite in order to promote, protect, and preserve the health of America's workforce. During this time occupational and environmental health nursing practice has expanded considerably, and nurses have embraced new areas of health promotion, research, and policy making. The history of occupational and environmental health nursing is rich and provides the underpinnings for our practice, which is sound and continues to evolve.

References

American Association of Industrial Nurses. (1976). *The nurse in industry.* New York: Author.

American Nurses' Association. (1945). Industrial nursing in the basic curriculum. *American Journal of Nursing, 45,* 478.

American Nurses' Association. (1965). *A position paper.* New York: Author.

Babbitz, M. (1983). The practice of occupational health nursing in the U.S. *Occupational Health Nursing, 31,* 23-25.

Babbitz, M. (1986). Hazard communication: Workers' right to know, nurses' need to know. *AAOHN Journal, 34,* 260-263.

Best, E. (1940). *Brief historical review and information about current activities of the American Nurses' Association including certain facts relative to the National League for Nursing Education.* New York: American Nurses' Association.

Bice-Stephens, W. (1992). *The art of nursing.* (p. 6). Pittsburgh, PA: Dorrance Publishing Co.

Bullough, B., & Bullough, V. L. (1964). *The emergence of modern nursing.* New York: Macmillan.

Cahall, J. B. (1981). The history of occupational health nursing. *Occupational Health Nursing, 29,* 11-13.

Cohen, B. (1984). Florence Nightingale. *Scientific American, 250,* 128-137.

Dock, L. L., & Stewart, I. M. (1938). *A short history of nursing.* New York: G. P. Putnam's Sons.

Felton, J. S. (1985). The genesis of American occupational health nursing: Pan I. *Occupational Health Nursing, 33,* 615-621.

Felton, J. S. (1990). *Occupational medical management.* Boston: Little, Brown & Company.

Godfrey, H. (1978). One hundred years of industrial nursing. *Nursing Times,* pp. 1966-1969.

Goldstein, D. H. (1971). The occupational safety and health act of 1970. *American Journal of Nursing, 71,* 1535-1538.

Goldwater, L. (1985). Historical highlights in occupational medicine. *Readings and Perspectives in Medicine, 9,* 1-42.

Grossman, J. (1973). *The Department of Labor,* New York: Praeger.

Heimann, H. (1964). Occupational health 1914-1964. *Public Health Reports, 79,* 941-947.

Herstein, J., Bunn, B., Fleming, L., Harrington, M., Jeyaratnam, J., Gardner, I. (1998). *International occupational and environmental medicine.* New York: Mosby.

Hunter, D. (1978). *The diseases of occupations* (6th ed.). London: Hodder & Stroughton.

Klein, M. (1950). *Industrial health and medical programs.* Washington, DC: U.S. Government Printing Office.

LaDou, J. (1981). *Occupational health law.* New York: Marcel Dekker.

Levenstein, C. (2000). The social context of occupational health. In B. Levy & D. Wegman (Eds.), *Occupational health: Recognizing and preventing work-related disease.* Boston: Little, Brown & Company.

Levy, B. & Wegman, D. (2000). *Occupational health: Recognizing and preventing work-related disease.* Boston: Little, Brown & Company.

Markolf, A. S. (1945). Industrial nursing begins in Vermont. *Public Health Nursing, 37,* 125-129.

McCready, B. (1943). *On the influence of trades, professions and occupations in the United States in the production of disease, 1837.* Baltimore: Johns Hopkins Press.

McGrath, B. J. (1945). Fifty years of industrial nursing. *Public Health Nurse, 37,* 119-124.

McGrath, B. J. (1946). *Nursing in commerce and industry.* New York: The Commonwealth Fund.

National Organization for Public Health Nursing. (1940). A study of industrial nursing services. *Public Health Nursing, 32,* 631-636.

National Organization for Public Health Nursing. (1942). A program for staff education. *Public Health Nursing, 34,* 39-47.

Nightingale, F. (1946). *Notes on nursing: What it is and what it is not.* New York: Appleton-Century-Crofts.

The 1958 Convention. (1958). *American Journal of Nursing, 58,* 980.

Obuchowski, M. (1963). *The industrial nurse in New England.* New England Association of Industrial Nursing.

Occupational Safety and Health Act of 1970. (1987). *Public Law 91-596.* Washington, DC: U.S. Government Printing Office.

Ramazzini, B. (1993). *Treatises on the Diseases of Workmen* (W. C. Wright, Trans.) Thunder Bay, Canada: OH&S Press. (Original work published in 1576).

Roberts, M. M. (1964). *American nursing: History and interpretation.* New York: Macmillan.

Rogers, B. (1986). National Center for Nursing Research. *AAOHN Journal, 34,* 196-197.

Rogers, B. (1988). Perspectives in occupational health nursing. *AAOHN Journal, 36,* 151-155.

Rogers, B. (1989). Establishing research priorities in occupational health nursing. *AAOHN Journal, 37,* 493-500.

Rood, D. (1941). The university and the industrial nurse. *American Journal of Nursing, 41,* 201-205.

Slaney, B. (1984). The development of occupational health nursing. *Nursing (Lond.), 2,* 1-3.

Stein, L. (1962). *The Triangle Fire.* Philadelphia: Lippincott.

White, K., Cox, A. R., & Williamson, G. C. (1999). Competencies in occupational and environmental health nursing: Practice in the new millennium. *AAOHN Journal, 47,* 552-568.

Woodham-Smith, C. (1950). *Florence Nightingale.* London: Constable.

Wright, F. S. (1919). *Industrial nursing.* New York: Macmillan.

2-1 National Institute for Occupational Safety and Health Education and Research Centers (ERCs)

ALABAMA EDUCATION
AND RESEARCH CENTER
University of Alabama at Birmingham
School of Public Health
1665 University Blvd.
Birmingham, AL 35294-0022
(205) 934-6208
Fax: (205) 975-5444

CALIFORNIA EDUCATION
AND RESEARCH CENTER—NORTHERN
University of California at Berkeley
School of Public Health
140 Warren
Berkeley, CA 94720-7360
(510) 642-0761
Fax: (510) 642-5815

CALIFORNIA EDUCATION
AND RESEARCH CENTER—SOUTHERN
University of California
School of Public Health
650 Young Dr. South
Los Angeles, CA 90095-1772
(310) 825-7152
Fax: (310) 206-9903

CINCINNATI EDUCATION
AND RESEARCH CENTER
University of Cincinnati
Department of Environmental Health
P.O. Box 670056
Cincinnati, OH 45267-0056
(513) 558-1749
Fax: (513) 558-2772 or 4397

HARVARD EDUCATION
AND RESEARCH CENTER
Harvard School of Public Health
Department of Environmental Health
665 Huntington Ave.
Boston, MA 02115
(617) 432-3323
Fax: (617) 432-0219

ILLINOIS EDUCATION
AND RESEARCH CENTER
University of Illinois at Chicago
School of Public Health
2121 West Taylor St., Rm. 215
Chicago, IL 60612-7260
(312) 996-7469
Fax: (312) 413-9898

IOWA EDUCATION AND RESEARCH CENTER
Heartland Center for Occupational Health
    and Safety
Department of Occupational
    and Environmental Health
100 Oakdale Campus—108 IREH
Iowa City, IA 52242-5000
(319) 335-4415
Fax: (319) 335-4225

JOHNS HOPKINS EDUCATION
AND RESEARCH CENTER
Johns Hopkins University
School of Hygiene and Public Health
615 North Wolfe St.
Baltimore, MD 21205
(410) 955-4037
Fax: (410) 955-1811

MICHIGAN EDUCATION
AND RESEARCH CENTER
University of Michigan
School of Public Health
1420 Washington Heights
Ann Arbor, MI 48109
(734) 936-0758
Fax: (313) 763-8095

MINNESOTA EDUCATION
AND RESEARCH CENTER
University of Minnesota
School of Public Health
Box 807 Mayo Memorial Building
Minneapolis, MN 55455
(612) 626-4855
Fax: (612) 626-0650

NEW YORK/NEW JERSEY EDUCATION
AND RESEARCH CENTER
Mount Sinai School of Medicine
Department of Community
  and Preventive Medicine
P.O. Box 1057
One Gustave L. Levy Pl.
New York, NY 10029-6574
(212) 241-4804
Fax: (212) 996-0407

NORTH CAROLINA EDUCATION
AND RESEARCH CENTER
University of North Carolina
School of Public Health
Rosenau Hall, CB# 7400
Chapel Hill, NC 27599-7410
(919) 966-1765
Fax: (919) 966-9081

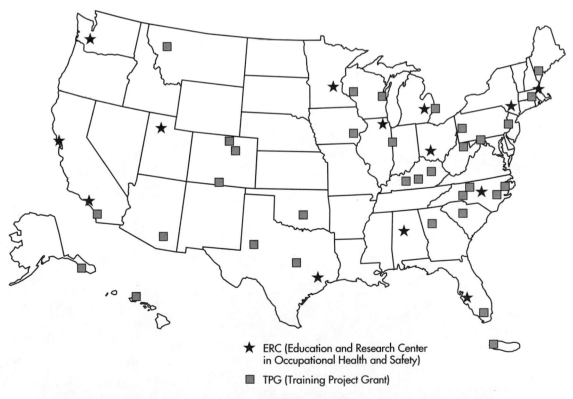

★ ERC (Education and Research Center
   in Occupational Health and Safety)

■ TPG (Training Project Grant)

Locations of Occupational Safety and Health Education and Research Centers funded by NIOSH.

SOUTH FLORIDA EDUCATION
AND RESEARCH CENTER
University of South Florida
College of Public Health
13201 Bruce B. Downs Blvd.,
    MDC Box 56
Tampa, FL 33612-3805
(813) 974-6626
Fax: (813) 974-4986

TEXAS EDUCATION
AND RESEARCH CENTER
University of Texas Health Science Center
    at Houston
School of Public Health
P.O. Box 20186
Houston, TX 77225-0186
(713) 500-9459
Fax: (713) 500-9442

UTAH EDUCATION AND RESEARCH CENTER
University of Utah
Rocky Mountain Center for Occupational
    and Environmental Health
75 South 2000 East
Salt Lake City, UT 84112
(801) 581-8719
Fax: (801) 581-7224

WASHINGTON EDUCATION
AND RESEARCH CENTER
University of Washington
Department of Environmental Health
P.O. Box 357234
Seattle, WA 98195-7234
(206) 685-3221
Fax: (206) 543-9616

3 The Nature and Practice of Occupational and Environmental Health Nursing

Occupational and environmental health nursing has expanded considerably in recent decades. The basic philosophy of occupational and environmental health nursing has not changed; it still is a population-focused (i.e., workforce) approach to health care delivery whose goals are to maintain a health orientation, protect worker health, prevent disease, keep workers healthy, and provide a safe and healthful work environment. However, contemporary occupational and environmental health nursing philosophy incorporates increased emphasis on health promotion, health surveillance, research-based practice, interdisciplinary collaboration, improved quality of life in general and work life in specific, and program and policy development. In addition, environmental health, which is deeply rooted in nursing's heritage, is recognized by the professional association AAOHN as integral to the specialty practice and by the Institute of Medicine (1995), recommending the integration of nursing, health, and environment (described in a later chapter). The term *environment* has been integrated into the AAOHN governance structure (AAOHN Bylaws, 1998) and association documents, which now reflect occupational and environmental health nursing (still known by the acronym OHN) as the practice. The integration of environmental health is recognition of both the foundation and expansion of occupational and environmental health nursing practice.

This is a crucial time for occupational and environmental health nursing, a time of both opportunity and challenge. With the changing demography of the United States, such as the aging population and increased ethnic diversity, more

demands will be made on health care professionals to provide a wider array of health care services and occupational health resources. Occupational and environmental health nursing is in a position in both traditional and nontraditional practice settings to provide and influence the types and comprehensiveness of occupational health services offered.

The occupational and environmental health nurse functions in many roles (see Chapter 4). Within the scope of these roles the nurse acts as an employee advocate and as a liaison with management to influence the concept of health and delivery of health care at the worksite. These underpinnings of practice provide the foundations upon which occupational and environmental health nursing practice builds.

This chapter focuses on a discussion of the nature and scope of practice in occupational and environmental health nursing. Practice philosophy, public health, foundational underpinnings, and prevention concepts will be explored as major contributors to the practice base.

PRACTICE UNDERPINNINGS

From its beginnings in the nineteenth century occupational and environmental health nursing practice, then called industrial nursing, has been grounded in the concepts and principles of public health practice and has focused on prevention, health teaching, health maintenance, and control and elimination of health hazards in the workplace and community. For example, early occupational and environmental health nurses provided health-oriented nursing services not only to employees at the worksite but also to workers and families in the community. Community surveillance observations and school-based health talks to children were also part of the industrial nurse's activities in the late nineteenth century (Felton, 1985). The industrial nurse worked to provide industries with public health agency-sponsored nursing services aimed particularly at controlling communicable diseases (Felton, 1985; Lee, 1978; McGrath, 1946; Wright, 1919). In addition, in 1909 the first home nursing service program, established by Lillian Wald, was offered through the Metropolitan Life Insurance Company to provide public health nursing services to holders of industrial policies (ANA, 2000; Christy, 1970). Parker-Conrad (1988) states that "out of the home nursing services provided by early occupational and environmental health nurses, employers recognized that nurses could save them money by teaching good health habits, monitoring and following up on medical care, and assuring that employees were following medical advice and that they returned for necessary care" (p. 157).

The specialty of occupational and environmental health nursing has always been closely linked to community health/public health nursing, which provides the underpinnings for the practice base. The community and public health nurse utilizes knowledge synthesized from public health and nursing fields to improve the health of the population through prevention and health promotion strategies (ANA, 1999). All nurses in a given community, including those working in hospitals, physicians' offices, and health clinics, contribute positively to the health of the community. However, the special contributions of the public health nursing specialist includes examining the community population as a whole; raising questions about its overall health status and factors associated with that status, including environmental factors (physical, biologic, and social-cultural); and working with the community to improve the population's health status.

Consistent with historical and contemporary public health philosophy, Williams (2000) describes public health nursing as aggregate or population-focused, which distinguishes it from other nursing specialties (e.g., medical-surgical, oncological). A population focus is historically consistent with public health philosophy, and while such practice is built on basic clinical nursing practice, it is different from clinical nursing practice. It may be helpful to define the term *population* and to comment on what is meant by population-focused practice. A population, or aggregate, is a collection of individuals who have one or more personal or environmental characteristics in common. Those who are members of a community are defined either in terms of geography (e.g., a county, group of counties, or state) or a special interest (e.g., children attending a particular school or a workforce) and can be seen as constituting a population. In addition, the following factors distinguish public health nursing as a specialty (Williams, 2000):

- *Population focus.* Primary emphasis on populations that are free-living in the community, as opposed to those that are institutionalized
- *Community orientation.* (1) Concern for the connection between the health status of the population and the environment in which the population lives (physical, biological, sociocultural), and (2) an imperative to work with members of the community to carry out core public health functions
- *Health and preventive focus.* Predominant emphasis on strategies for health promotion, health maintenance, and disease prevention, particularly primary and secondary prevention
- *Interventions at the community and/or population level.* The use of political processes to affect public policy as a major intervention strategy for achieving goals
- *Health concern.* Concern for the health of all members of the population/community, particularly vulnerable subpopulations

When viewed from the perspective of a public health and prevention foundation, the purpose of occupational and environmental health nursing is consistent with the mission of public health.

The occupational and environmental health nurse utilizes nursing, public health, and medical knowledge as cornerstones for practice in addition to more specific knowledge areas such as the occupational health sciences, social/behavioral sciences, and business and legal/ethical fields. The occupational and environmental health nurse practices with a large degree of legal autonomy and through evolutionary change that is complemented by an interdependent role with other disciplines to effect health and safety at the worksite (Rogers & Livsey, 2000). Knowledge and understanding about complex work processes and related hazards, mechanisms of exposure, and control strategies to minimize or abate risks are essential to occupational and environmental health nursing practice. Expertise in this area is grounded in a multidisciplinary knowledge framework guided by nursing science (Figure 3-1).

Nursing science provides the context for health care delivery by recognizing the needs of individuals, groups, and populations within the framework of prevention, health promotion, and illness and injury care management, including risk assessment, risk management, and risk communication; nursing science incorporates the following:

1. Medical science specific to the treatment and management of occupational health illness and injury, integrated with nursing health surveillance activities
2. Occupational health sciences
   a. Toxicology to recognize routes of exposure, examine relationships between chemical exposures in the workplace and acute and latent health effects, such as cancer, and understand dose-response relationships
   b. Industrial hygiene to identify and evaluate workplace hazards so control mechanisms can be implemented for exposure reduction
   c. Safety to identify and control workplace injuries through active safeguards and worker training and education programs
   d. Ergonomics to match the job to the worker while emphasizing capabilities and minimizing limitations
3. Epidemiology to study health and illness trends and characteristics in the worker population, investigate work-related illness and injury episodes, apply epidemiologic methods to analyze and interpret risk data in order to determine causal relationships and participate in epidemiologic research
4. Environmental health to systematically examine interrelationships between the worker and the extended environment as a basis for development of prevention and control strategies
5. Social and behavioral sciences to explore influences of various environments (e.g. work, home), relationships, and lifestyle factors on worker health and determine which interactions affect worker health
6. Business and economic theories, concepts, and principles for strategic and operational plan-

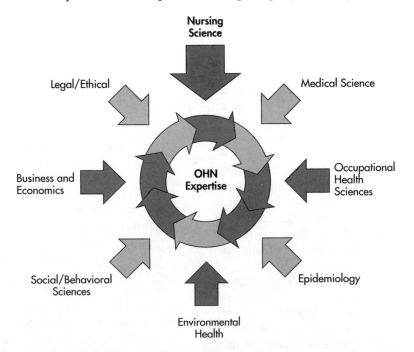

Figure 3-1   Occupational health nursing knowledge. *(Copyright Bonnie Rogers, 1997.)*

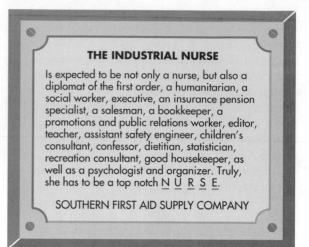

Figure 3-2 The Industrial Nurse. *(From Southern First Aid Supply Company.)*

ning, valuing quality and cost-effective services, and for management of occupational health and safety programs

7. Legal and ethical issues to assure compliance with regulatory mandates and contend with ethical concerns that may arise in a competitive environment

OCCUPATIONAL AND ENVIRONMENTAL HEALTH NURSING PRACTICE

In the 1950s Southern First Aid Supply Company developed a classic definition of the industrial nurse (Figure 3-2), a definition that provides a historical view of the nurse's work activities. The definition of industrial nursing has evolved over time to reflect the changing role of the occupational and environmental health nurse, with more emphasis on autonomous decision making, independent functioning, health promotion, prevention, analytical and investigative skills, education and teaching, management of health care services, and policy setting. Many factors have influenced the evolution of occupational and environmental health nursing practice, such as the changing population and workforce; work and organizational factors such as downsizing, increased work demands, and stress; and introduction of new work processes and chemicals into the work environment with a concomitant increase in work-related hazards. Other influences include technological

advances, increased regulatory mandates, and increased interest in health promotion, illness/injury prevention, and integrated health care. The growth in complex health issues at the worksite coupled with increasing health care costs and workers' compensation claims also has influenced the practice (Vernarac, 1997). Because of the nature of occupational and environmental health nursing, the nurse must utilize multidisciplinary approaches to address the health problems of the workforce.

Adapted from the scope of practice of the American Association of Occupational Health Nurses (1999b) and embodied within the standards for practice, the following definition of occupational and environmental health nursing practice is provided

> *Occupational and environmental health nursing is the specialty practice that focuses on the promotion, prevention, and restoration of health within the context of a safe and healthy environment. It includes the prevention of adverse health effects from occupational and environmental hazards. It provides for and delivers occupational and environmental health and safety services to workers, worker populations, and community groups. Occupational and environmental health nursing is an autonomous specialty and nurses make independent nursing judgements in providing health care services (p. 2).*

Occupational and Environmental Health Nursing Context

Community-Oriented Nursing Practice is a philosophy of nursing service delivery that involves the generalist or specialist public health and community health nurse. The nurse provides "health care" through community diagnosis and investigation of major health and environmental problems, health surveillance, and monitoring and evaluation of community and population health status for purposes of preventing disease and disability and promoting, protecting, and maintaining "health" in order to create conditions in which people can be healthy.

Public Health Nursing Practice is the synthesis of nursing theory and public health theory applied to promoting and preserving the health of populations. The focus of public health nursing practice is the community as a whole and the effect of the community's health status (resources) on the health of individuals, families, and groups. Care is provided within the context of preventing disease and disability and promoting and protecting the health of the community as a whole.

Community Health Nursing Practice is the synthesis of nursing theory and public health theory applied to promoting, preserving, and maintaining the health of populations through the delivery of personal health care services to individuals, families, and groups and the effect of their health status on the health of the community as a whole.

Community-Based Nursing Practice is a setting-specific practice whereby care is provided for "sick" individuals and families where they live, work, and attend school. The emphasis of community-based nursing practice is acute and chronic care and the provision of comprehensive, coordinated, and continuous services. Nurses who deliver community-based care are generalists or specialists in maternal-infant, pediatric, adult, or psychiatric-mental health nursing.

Figure 3-3 Definitions of the four key nursing areas in the community. *(Modified from "Community-Oriented Population Focused Practice," by C. A. Williams, in M. Stanhope and J. Lancaster (eds.)* Community and Public Health Nursing, *5th ed., St. Louis, MO: Mosby, 2000. OHN modification by Bonnie Rogers, 2001.)*

As previously discussed, occupational and environmental health nursing is closely linked to community health and public health nursing through their philosophies and theoretical and practice applications. In 1998 the Quad Council of Public Health Nursing (American Nurses Association, Council of Community, Primary, and Long Term Care; the American Public Health Association, Section of Public Health Nursing; the Association of Community Health Nursing Educators; and the Association of State and Territorial Directors of Nursing) developed a statement on the scope of public health practice in an attempt to clarify differences between public health nursing and community-based nursing. Discussions indicate that occupational and environmental health nursing practice falls in the domains of public health nursing and community health nursing. Thus, the occupational and environmental health nurse will want to be familiar with these definitions (Figure 3-3).

PREVENTION FOUNDATION

Developed by the Core Functions Project, a working group within the U.S. Public Health Service, the Health Services Pyramid (Figure 3-4) depicts five levels of population-focused public health programs, such as with occupational health, with

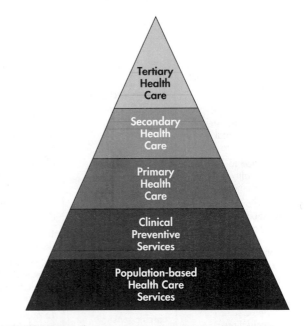

Figure 3-4 Health Services Pyramid. *(From* The Core Functions Project, *by U.S. Public Health Service, Washington, DC: Office of Disease Prevention and Health Promotion, 1993.)*

the goals of disease prevention, health protection, and health promotion that provide a foundation for primary, secondary, and tertiary health care services. Service emphasis placed at the lower levels of the tiers to prevent morbidity and health risk factors reduces the need for greater services at the upper levels (U.S. Public Health Service, 1993).

Consistent with public health philosophy, prevention marks the foundation for occupational and environmental health nursing practice. Within this health-orientation framework of prevention are the following primary goals of occupational and environmental health nursing practice:

• Prevent and reduce the threat of disease and illness;
• Promote, maintain, and restore the physical and psychosocial well-being of the worker in order to enhance optimal functioning;
• Protect the worker from work-related hazards;

• Encourage and participate in a company culture supportive of health, which may include family work health if a component of the company mission;
• Collaborate with workers, management, other disciplines, and health care professionals to ensure a safe work environment.

Health promotion and protection and disease and injury prevention are discussed in much greater detail in Chapter 13; conceptual definitions as they apply to the occupational and environmental health nurse's scope of practice will be discussed here.

Leavell and Clark (1965) first classified prevention in three levels: primary, secondary, and tertiary (Figure 3-5). Primary prevention may be ac-

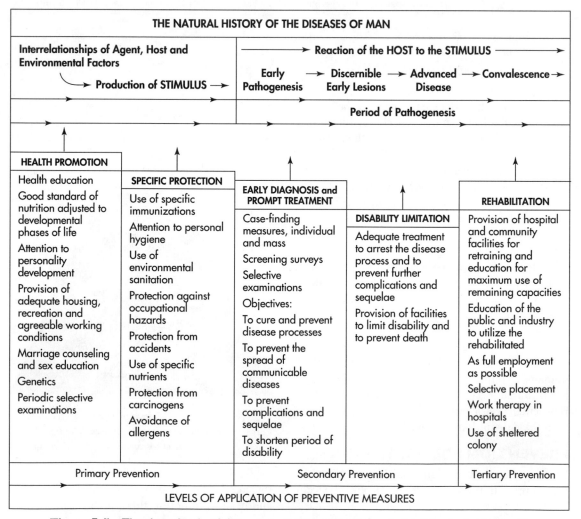

Figure 3-5 **The three levels of disease prevention.** (*From* Preventive Medicine for the Doctor and His Community, *3rd ed., by H. R. Leavall and E. G. Clark, New York: McGraw-Hill, 1965.*)

complished in the prepathogenesis period by measures designed to promote general optimum health, protect against disease agents, or establish barriers against agents in the environment. As soon as the disease is detectable—early in pathogenesis—secondary prevention may be achieved by early diagnosis and prompt and adequate treatment. When the process of pathogenesis has progressed and the disease has advanced beyond its early stages, secondary prevention also may be achieved by means of adequate treatment to prevent sequelae and limit disability. Later, when defect and disability have been fixed, tertiary prevention may be accomplished by rehabilitation (Leavell & Clark, 1965).

Within this framework primary prevention incorporates both health promotion and protection; secondary prevention is aimed at early detection, treatment, and disability limitation; and rehabilitation is the main strategy for tertiary prevention. This model has provided a useful guide for public health professionals in recognizing health intervention strategies prior to disease development or during different stages of a disease's development.

The occupational and environmental health nurse practices at all levels of prevention (Blix, 1999). Using the Leavell and Clark framework, Wachs and Parker-Conrad (1990) present programmatic activities that relate to prevention strategies in the occupational health setting (Table 3-1). Delivery of primary prevention services to the employee is directed toward promoting health and averting a problem. In the occupational health setting the purpose of health promotion is to maintain or enhance the well-being of individuals or groups of employees and the company in general. Activities are designed to bring about changes in understanding, attitudes, and behaviors of workers and management regarding health and safety practices at work and, in the larger sense, lifestyle patterns. This may include programs designed to enhance coping skills, good nutrition, or knowledge about potential health hazards both inside and outside the workplace.

Health protection measures are designed to eliminate or reduce the risk of disease in order to prevent the development of an illness or injury. Walk-throughs by the occupational and environmental health nurse and/or other team members to identify workplace hazards are aimed at health protection. Environmental engineering strategies to contain and control toxic substances in the workplace so workers are not harmed are health protection strategies.

Specific protection programs or interventions often require active participation on the part of the

TABLE 3-1	Examples of Comprehensive Occupational Health Program Elements		
PRIMARY PREVENTION		**SECONDARY PREVENTION**	**TERTIARY PREVENTION**
HEALTH PROMOTION	DISEASE PREVENTION		
Nutrition	Injury prevention	Preplacement and periodic exams	Early back to work
Fitness/exercise	Accident investigation	Health surveillance	Modified duty
Coping enhancement	Disease prevention	Triage system	Work hardening
Recreation	Health risk appraisal	Employee record system	Onsite therapy
Parenting skills	Smoking cessation	Accident reporting	Chronic illness monitoring
Health education	Weight control	Injury diagnosis and treatment	
	Stress management		

From "Occupational Health Nursing in 1990 and the Coming Decade," by J. Wachs and J. Parker-Conrad, *Applied Occupational and Environmental Hygiene, 5,* 200-203. 1990.

employee. Participation in an immunization program, utilization of personal protective equipment such as respirators or gloves, or use of puncture-resistant needle containers are examples of specific health protection measures.

Secondary prevention occurs after a disease process has already begun and is aimed at early detection, prompt treatment, and prevention of further limitations. For employees with potential work-related exposures, early detection utilizes preplacement examinations and health surveillance and periodic screening activities to identify illness at the earliest possible moment in its course and eliminate or modify hazard-producing agents or conditions (Rogers & Livsey, 2000). The provision of screening services, such as high blood pressure monitoring or periodic breast screening/examinations, and the reporting and analysis of injury trend data are examples of early detection measures. Interventions aimed at disability limitation are intended to prevent further harm or deterioration. For example, referral for counseling and treatment of an employee who has an emotional/mental health problem and whose work performance has deteriorated or removal of workers who manifest neurologic symptoms from heavy metal exposure—these interventions would provide avenues for prevention of potentially harmful or serious disorders.

Tertiary prevention is intended to restore health as fully as possible and help individuals achieve their maximum level of functioning. Rehabilitation strategies, such as return to work programs after a heart attack or traumatic injury, or transitional duty programs after a cumulative trauma injury are examples of tertiary prevention. Continued rehabilitation of an employee with a substance abuse problem through hospitalization or outpatient treatment, counseling of an employee with chronic obstructive lung disease regarding smoking cessation, or chronic disease monitoring also constitute tertiary preventive measures.

Pender (1996) distinguishes health promotion from prevention. Health promotion increases one's level of well-being toward a state of optimal health and includes activities such as regular exercise and good nutrition. Prevention and health protection activities are directed toward risk avoidance (e.g., smoking cessation), disease detection and disability limitation (e.g., screening and periodic examinations), and health rehabilitation or restoration (e.g., chronic disease monitoring). Pender's model and the occupational and environmental health nurse's role in health promotion and protection and disease and injury prevention will be described more in-depth in Chapter 13.

SCOPE OF PRACTICE

The scope of practice in occupational and environmental health nursing (Figure 3-6) is broad and comprehensive and is directed toward improving and promoting worker health. As the figure depicts, the practice is interwoven and integrated, encompassing several areas.

WORKER/WORKPLACE ASSESSMENT AND SURVEILLANCE

Assessment and surveillance of the worker and workplace is critical to identifying potential health problems and determining the state of health of the worker and overall workforce population (Rogers, 1998). Knowledge of the demographics and characteristics of the worker population, such as smoking habits or age, is essential for consideration of factors that may interact with workplace agent exposures. The occupational and environmental health nurse may perform several types of assessments, examinations, monitoring, and surveillance activities. For example, the preplacement assessment helps identify health problems or conditions that may be aggravated by job duties for which appropriate accommodations may be recommended. In addition, preplacement assessments help establish baseline data indexes for future health monitoring. Knowledge of all jobs and their demands is necessary in order to match the job to the capabilities of the worker, monitor work-relatedness and health, and effect job transfers if adverse health effects occur as a result of working conditions and exposures. Expert occupational health history taking is required so that all previous jobs and exposures can be properly examined.

Periodic health assessments are performed to determine if adverse health effects have occurred as a result of work conditions and hazards in order to recommend appropriate corrective measures and for early identification of chronic health

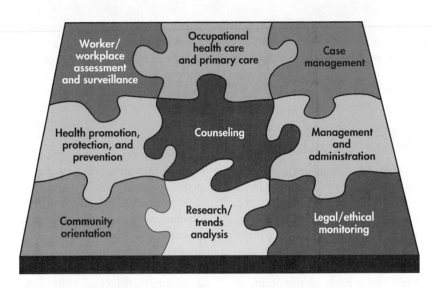

Figure 3-6 Occupational health nursing practice expertise. *(Copyright Bonnie Rogers, 1997.)*

conditions. The periodic evaluation may be part of the medical/health surveillance program to monitor employees who may be at risk of exposure to toxic substances. The occupational and environmental health nurse critically analyzes each job task to detect task situations that place employees at risk and notes work-related risk factors, such as bending or twisting that may additionally compromise the worker. The occupational and environmental health nurse is usually the first person to receive such a complaint and must be prepared to recognize potential exposures and initiate exposure monitoring (typically performed by an industrial hygienist). Other types of assessments may include return to work, fitness for duty, preretirement, or termination from employment.

Workplace assessment, monitoring, and surveillance is done to identify potential hazards harmful to workers' health. By conducting walkthroughs, the occupational and environmental health nurse becomes familiar with the work environment, production processes and methods, and equipment handling and work practices. The walk-through assessment of the workplace provides an opportunity for the occupational and environmental health nurse to observe employees' work practices and habits, use of personal protective equipment, health characteristics (smoking habits and social interaction), and morale and productivity. The walk-through also helps to identify actual and potential workplace health

and safety hazards. The nurse's conduct of walkthroughs and participation on health and safety committees will enhance the overall health mission (Travers, 1987).

If a hazard is identified, the industrial hygienist or safety specialist will probably be needed to measure levels of exposure to specific substances or help with job task analyses, respectively. In collaboration with the physician and other health care professionals, the occupational and environmental health nurse reviews the data obtained in order to recommend health surveillance activities and participate in control recommendations and implementation strategies. Multidisciplinary collaboration is key to development and implementation of a successful workplace surveillance and hazard control program. Noise level reduction, job rotation, or substitution of a toxic substance with a nontoxic substance are examples of appropriate, feasible, and effective workplace control strategies that must be implemented and discussed with all involved parties.

In addition, during assessment and surveillance activities preventive and corrective strategies such as engineering, work practice, administrative, and personal protection controls can be discussed as approaches to reduce risk and minimize health problems. Knowing the magnitude and distribution of occupational health illness and injury events provides a picture of the overall health of the workforce and potential links to morbidity and premature mortality. This can lead to targeting high risk jobs and exposures, which is integral to any assessment and surveillance program, in specifically focusing on risk reduction control mechanisms. This means taking steps to eliminate or substantially reduce risky working conditions (Rogers, 1998).

OCCUPATIONAL HEALTH CARE AND PRIMARY CARE

Health care given at the worksite is primarily for work-related illnesses and injuries and includes treatment, follow-up, referral for medical care, and emergency care. Examples include urgent illness and injury care for severe burns, head injuries, eye injuries, fractures, amputations, or shock and care for work-related acute injuries and illnesses such as back pain, sprain/strain, or animal bites.

Many occupational and environmental health nurses also provide nonoccupational health care for minor health problems such as headaches, lacerations, or contusions, and stable chronic injury/illness treatment and monitoring of conditions such as musculoskeletal disorders, high blood pressure, and diabetes. The emphasis is on comprehensive care, early investigation, and wellness strategies to improve health and lower costs. Written medical and nursing protocols or guidelines (collaboratively developed as appropriate) should be in place in accordance with state legal requirements. In addition, special or mandated programs such as travel health, hearing conservation, or drug and alcohol testing can be part of the occupational health service, depending on worker and company needs. In some work settings nurse practitioner-managed primary care services, including diagnosis and treatment of minor health problems, referral, and counseling, are offered to family members (Touger & Butts, 1989).

CASE MANAGEMENT

Case management services may be offered to provide coordinated health care for early intervention and to help foster the worker's return to work. Case management is a complex set of activities designed to coordinate and manage services and resources pertinent to the outcome of the individual's health problem (Childre, 1999). Services depend on worker needs (Jones, 1996); however, intensive case management is indicated for a severe illness or injury, a chronic physical or mental health condition likely to result in lost time or permanent change in employee status, or any condition that leads to an extended work absence.

Case management is often focused on high cost, catastrophic cases. However, it is also beneficial to apply case management practices to monitor the outcomes of every case. Early intervention is a key component of case management services because it provides for immediate problem identification, engages the worker in care planning from the beginning of the illness/injury to recovery, and helps to prevent fragmented and delayed care through early coordinated health care at the beginning of care (rather than later after complications may have developed) (Rogers, 1998). Evaluation of case management services—to determine not only their effectiveness, achievement of outcomes, and cost savings, but also worker satisfaction—is essential.

HEALTH PROMOTION, HEALTH PROTECTION, AND PREVENTION

A major component of occupational and environmental health nursing practice includes activities related to health promotion, health protection, and prevention for both individuals and groups of workers. Health promotion activities are directed toward enhancing existing levels of health and increasing the level of well-being in order to move toward optimal health and gain control over health determinants (Rogers & Lawhorn, 2000). Activities are implemented at individual, group, and population levels through educational, behavioral, and environmental strategies. Health protection is best described as preventive health behaviors designed to guard or defend an individual or group against specific illness or injury (Rogers, 1998; Sorenson et al., 1998).

Primary prevention approaches, which include health promotion and protection, are aimed at eliminating or reducing disease risk through specific protective actions. These might include developing strategies or programs to increase employees' awareness and knowledge related to toxic and hazardous exposures and their mitigation; discussing the meaning and application of results from personal and group health risk appraisals; promoting positive lifestyle interventions such as smoking cessation, improved exercise and nutrition, and immunizations (Dille, 1999); designing strategies to help alter attitudes and behaviors that improve health; and encouraging individual responsibility for utilization of personal and organizational health resources. In addition, information obtained from workers' needs assessments may help target health promotion programs or activities, such as diabetes or cardiovascular risk factor screening, so early counseling can be provided so disease onset can be avoided. The occupational and environmental health nurse also may initiate special health activities or programs that are based on regulatory mandates and/or hazards related to the work environment; these activities and programs, cover health issues such as hearing conservation, respiratory protection, or ergonomic workstation designs.

Secondary prevention is aimed at early detection and diagnosis of individuals with disease so prompt interventions to halt disease progression and limit disability can be implemented. Preplacement and periodic examinations, medical/health surveillance activities, and screening activities, such as mammography or diabetes screening, are examples of secondary prevention.

Tertiary prevention is directed at restoration and rehabilitation of individuals to an optimal level of health within the limits of the disabling condition. This includes returning the ill or injured worker to a preinjury state of health or to a productive worklife through, for example, cardiac rehabilitation. This begins at the time that the injury occurs or when the health care provider learns of the health problem (e.g., chronic disease). The rehabilitation plan should address the physical and/or psychosocial needs of the affected worker and include a work adaptation plan, handling of coworkers' concerns, and encouragement of active participation of management in the process. In collaboration with the physician or other health care professionals, the occupational and environmental health nurse will seek to prevent further disability, identify barriers to health restoration early, and, as part of the treatment plan, recommend job restructuring, modified work schedules, and worker retraining.

Helping workers understand the concept of health in order to reduce morbidity and premature mortality and improve one's quality of life, and encouraging workers to utilize health protec-

tion strategies designed to reduce risks in the work environment (e.g., recognizing toxic substances and appropriately using protective equipment)—both of these are integral to enhancing the health state of the workers.

Within the context of a concept of health personal responsibility is essential and includes activities designed to make proactive and progressive behavioral changes regarding lifestyle factors affecting health; this includes such areas as smoking cessation, weight reduction, or enhanced nutrition. In addition, environmental actions fostering a supportive work or living environment promote health. These could include a healthy physical and emotional setting that supports healthy food offerings in the cafeteria and vending machines, the availability and opportunities for use of exercise facilities, and an organizational workforce committed to health and wellness (Rogers, 1998).

COUNSELING

Counseling is designed to help employees clarify problems and make informed decisions and choices and to give positive reinforcement. The occupational and environmental health nurse, being the health care provider most available to the employee, is in the best position to provide counseling services to the worker. The occupational and environmental health nurse provides counseling with respect to such issues as prevention and management of occupational and nonoccupational illnesses and injuries, work-related stress, productivity, family, and interpersonal relationships. Some issues may interfere with the employee's ability to work or perform the job, and the employee would probably benefit from some form of intervention such as listening, support, or referral. Health issues including nutrition, exercise, stress, breast cancer symptoms, chronic disease, or substance abuse often require counseling, which provides strategic interventions and appropriate referrals to deal with a crisis situation as well as time to reflect on impending decisions and evaluate actions taken.

The occupational and environmental health nurse may also be involved in counseling managers regarding problems of the workforce, such as substance abuse. Employees may be initially referred to the occupational and environmental health nurse by the supervisor for problems that affect performance. These might involve behavioral, marital, social, financial, or work-related events that may result in absenteeism, accidents, or stress-related illnesses. Employees may be referred to in-house or externally offered employee assistance programs designed to identify troubled employees early, help them seek appropriate assistance to manage the problem and remain productive, and help management recognize and appropriately deal with workers' problems.

The occupational and environmental health nurse may be directly involved in managing the employee assistance program or may be the referral liaison. The occupational and environmental health nurse needs to have specific counseling knowledge and skills such as problem recognition; ability to build a supportive, trusting, and confidential relationship; crisis intervention approaches; and knowledge about community resources for referral to effectively assist the employee and in some cases the family. In addition, the nurse will want to demonstrate a sensitive, nonjudgmental, caring attitude and a respect for the employee and the problem.

MANAGEMENT AND ADMINISTRATION

The occupational and environmental health nurse assumes a major role in the management and administration of the occupational health unit. In order to effectively manage the occupational health unit and contribute to the company's overall health goals, the nurse must be fully aware of the corporate mission, culture, and business goals; characteristics of the workforce and related health and safety priorities and needs; and occupational health and safety laws and regulations. The scope of management responsibilities at the occupational health unit level includes program planning and goal development; budget planning and management; organization, staffing, and coordination of activities, including the development of policy, procedure, and protocol manuals; and unit performance evaluation, based on achievement of goals and objectives.

The occupational and environmental health nurse should be involved in quality improvement and assurance, which require specific activities such as satisfaction determinations, audits, and record reviews. Quality performance should take into consideration the match between effectiveness and efficiency. Cost-effectiveness and cost containment of health care services must be a health management imperative.

The nurse is increasingly becoming a key figure in the development of policies that affect the health and safety of the workforce. Strategic planning—setting the vision, mission, and long-term goals—is key for the long-term success of the organization. Noting the needs and capabilities of departmental units such as occupational health service, strategic planning shapes the future of the total organization. With employee input policy development should be a collaborative effort among company management, the occupational health nurse manager, the physician (if one is employed), and other appropriate health care professionals. At the very least the occupational and environmental health nurse should have input into strategic and operational policy decisions affecting the occupational health program and should have managerial responsibility for operation of the occupational and environmental health nursing service.

COMMUNITY ORIENTATION

Company collaboration and partnerships with community agencies and groups can be vital and mutually satisfying experiences, enabling the occupational and environmental health nurse to develop a network of resources to more efficiently and effectively provide services to employees and the company. Voluntary or governmental agency services, such as parenting programs, cardiac, drug rehabilitation, or home health care services, can be beneficial in terms of cost to both the employee and employer. In addition, using occupational health and safety consultants from governmental agencies also can help address problems and issues.

The nurse also can help the industry focus on health in its relationship with the community through modeling environmental health awareness and providing or sponsoring health-related activities to workers' families and the community at large. Providing or sponsoring health fairs for workers, their families, and the community is another example of a successful partnership. The community/industry relationship should be mutually beneficial. In addition, the nurse will be involved in disaster preparedness of the workforce, and these preparations may entail consulation with environmental, emergency, and other public agencies.

RESEARCH AND TREND ANALYSIS

Research in occupational health and occupational and environmental health nursing is vital to improvement in occupational health practice. The role that the occupational and environmental health nurse plays in research related to worker health conditions cannot be overstated. The provision of a safe and healthful work environment is contingent upon knowledge of the relationship between the worker and elements in the work environment. For example, understanding the effects of toxic exposures, designing strategies to prevent work-related accidents/injuries or illnesses, evaluating the cost-effectiveness of health interventions, or understanding human behavior and motivation related to health promotion activities are important avenues of occupational and environmental health nursing investigation.

After the research is completed, the findings should be disseminated so the information can be used to improve clinical outcomes and practice procedures. Knowledge used then can be built upon to advance the practice and the profession. Research and practice go hand in hand with the mission to improve and foster the health and well-being of the worker and workforce and improve working conditions by eliminating or minimizing potential or actual hazards.

The occupational and environmental health nurse is always in a position to collect data through accurate and detailed recordkeeping, which can be an invaluable source for identifying trends in illness and injury patterns and other events in the workforce. As part of the research team the occupational and environmental health nurse can participate in the design of research studies and collection of data about occupational health and related problems. Data can be used to determine which types of programs or interventions are most effective in promoting health and minimizing risk.

LEGAL/ETHICAL MANAGEMENT

Company management has the responsibility to ensure a safe and healthful work environment for all employees through implementation of programs to support this effort. The occupational and environmental health nurse must know the laws and regulations that cover the occupational health and safety of workers (e.g., OSH Act, Hazard Communication Standard) and recommend and implement programs responsive to mandated health and safety requirements. The importance of good recordkeeping cannot be overemphasized with respect to legal documentation.

Occupational and environmental health nursing practice is regulated by state nurse practice acts and guided by standards of occupational and environmental health nursing practice. The occupational and environmental health nurse should have copies of and be familiar with these documents to ensure adequate and appropriate nursing care.

Many issues in the work environment such as confidentiality of employee health records, hazardous exposures to vulnerable populations, and threats to worker health, can create ethical conflicts. The nurse needs to recognize and understand both personal and corporate values related to occupational health and safety and that these values may sometimes compete. The nurse is obligated to act always in the best interest of the worker and provide effective leadership skills in ethical health care. The nurse as a moral agent is concerned with values, choices, and duties related to the good of individuals and larger societies and upholding and advancing the standards of the profession (Videbeck, 1997). In this role the occupational and environmental health nurse not only brings an expertise to occupational health dilemmas but also structures the issues so sound and deliberate decisions are made using a reasoned approach. The occupational and environmental health nurse's framework for practice is guided by the ethical treatment of workers as expressed in the AAOHN Code of Ethics (AAOHN, 1999a); ethical decision making is integral to the nurse's practice and is discussed in Chapter 17.

COMPETENCIES IN OCCUPATIONAL AND ENVIRONMENTAL HEALTH NURSING

As health care continues to evolve, the need for high quality, cost-effective care by health care professionals is critical. One responsibility of the professional society is to determine what constitutes competent behavior practices in the specialty and offer ways to measure this performance (Chamberlin & Rogers, 1997). As past president of the American Association of Occupational Health Nurses, this author recognized the need for and importance of establishing competencies in the specialty field. To this end two consecutive committees spanning 4 years (1995-1999) were established to develop the work and determine essential competencies in nine identified areas for professional occupational and environmental health nurses practicing the specialty (Appendix 3-1) (White et al., 1999). Using a framework developed by Benner (1984), these competencies are identified at the following three levels:

- *Competent.* Nurse whose confidence has increased and whose perception of the role is one of mastery and an ability to cope with specific situations. The nurse's reliance on the judgments of peers and other professionals is decreased. Work habits tend to stress consistency rather than routinely tailoring care to encompass individual differences (Benner, 1984).

  Example: The competent occupational and environmental health nurse has sufficient knowledge and experience to recognize a range of clinical problems and manage/refer appropriately. The occupational and environmental health nurse acts as a case manager and program or service manager, utilizing policies, procedures, and protocols to effect desired outcomes.

- *Proficient.* Nurse who has an increased ability to perceive client situations as a whole based on past experiences and focuses on the relevant aspects of the situation. The nurse can predict the events to expect in a particular situation and can recognize that protocols sometimes must be altered to meet the needs of the client (Benner, 1984).

  Example: The proficient occupational and environmental health nurse quickly assesses and analyzes multiple problems and places them in priority order of need and concern. Higher levels of clinical and managerial skills are evident and include policy and protocol initiation and development.

- *Expert.* Nurse who has extensive experience and a broad knowledge base and can grasp a situation quickly and initiate appropriate action. The nurse has a sense of salience that is grounded in practice and guides actions and priorities (Benner, 1984).

  Example: The expert occupational and environmental health nurse provides leadership in developing occupational health policies within an organization. The occupational and environmental health nurse functions in executive level positions and in consulting and governmental roles and helps develop theory and knowledge relevant to advancing the specialty.

Each practitioner is at different levels of competency depending on past experiences, education, and skills developed. For example, a nurse may have achieved a proficient level of competency in clinical care or case management but only a beginning competency level in research, which will need to be developed. Therefore, the nurse's level of competency should be characterized in relation to each specific competency and move to at least the competent level in occupational and environmental health nursing practice as a whole. The competent level is considered to reflect core competencies for the specialty, with movement to the proficient and expert levels with increasing knowledge, skills, and abilities.

PHILOSOPHY

A philosophy helps clarify and establish beliefs and values about one's orientation to and direction in life, including such aspects as relationships with other people and the society and environment in which one lives and works; it assists in understanding why certain decisions and choices are made. Personal philosophical beliefs extend to and are integrated in a philosophy of professional nursing practice.

The heritage of occupational and environmental health nursing is reflected in a degree of independence in practice not often shared by other nursing colleagues in acute care settings. This independence is complemented by an interdependent role with other professionals and groups and is not only integral to occupational and environmental health nursing practice but also enhances the health care provided at the worksite. In the delivery of occupational and environmental health nursing services, comprehensive professional health care must be provided to individuals, groups, and workforces with respect to human dignity and self-worth while promoting accountability. The occupational and environmental health nurse has the primary responsibility for the management of worker health and safety with consideration to ethical, cultural, spiritual, and corporate beliefs.

The worksite is a community with health needs requiring attention to health promotion and protection, prevention of disease and disability, and treatment of illness and injury. However, in many industries health services may be considered of secondary importance because they cost the company money rather than generate income. The nurse helps management recognize the economic and human benefits of occupational health programs and helps maximize productivity by promoting employee mental and physical well-being while ensuring cost-effectiveness.

Within a values framework the occupational and environmental health nurse functions autonomously, maintains personal and professional integrity, and demonstrates leadership in decision making. Uustal (1978) defines values as general guides to behavior and standards of conduct that one endorses and tries to live up to or maintain. Values provide a basic frame of reference to guide individuals as they deal with issues and make decisions, and for the occupational and environmental health nurse values frame and guide how decisions regarding the types and delivery of health care services to worker clients are made. The occupational and environmental health nurse will be involved in many workplace issues that will have a direct effect on the health and well-being of the individual worker and the workforce. For example, issues related to access of health records may present problems or conflicts if the premise of confidentiality is not shared by others. When conflicts arise, the occupational and environmental health nurse will need to make decisions that involve some risk taking (Rogers, 1988). Management, occupational and environmental health nurses, and other health care professionals must strive to understand and respect each others' roles and confront issues that threaten worker health and safety.

Brown (1981) stated that the smooth administration of the occupational health unit is in part contingent upon the occupational and environmental health nurse's commitment to a philosophy of providing quality services to workers and that this philosophy should be in writing. A philosophy of occupational and environmental health nursing service should be a clear, concise statement that reflects the nurse's fundamental beliefs and forms the basis for practice and professional activities. A philosophy of occupational and environmental health nursing practice and service should emphasize the conviction that the health and safety of the worker and workforce is the primary concern of the occupational and environmental health nurse and should reflect statements of beliefs and values about the following:

1. Respect for worker rights and treatment related to principles of self-determination and nondiscrimination and the provision of quality health care while protecting employee confidentiality
2. The promotion and protection of health and prevention of disease throughout the work community
3. A commitment to a concept of quality health as reflected in the goals and objectives of the occupational health service, including resource appropriation and utilization
4. The dynamics of the work environment and diversity of the worker population
5. Employer and employee responsibility for health and safety
6. The benefits of the occupational health service to the worker population and company
7. The competence and continuing professional development of the staff, including recognition of legal and ethical considerations and accountability for practice
8. Collaborative multidisciplinary relationships that support and enhance worker health and safety and the relationship of the occupational health service to the community

Knowledge of the company and workers, including the history, culture, policies, programs, workplace hazards, and workforce trends will be helpful because this may provide information regarding congruence between the occupational and environmental health nurse's philosophy and the organization's philosophy of health and safety. If there are differences, they will need to be discussed and resolved with management. The Code of Ethics of the American Association of Occupational Health Nurses (AAOHN, 1999a) can serve as a guide for developing a philosophy statement for the occupational and environmental health nursing service. An example of a philosophy statement is shown in Box 3-1.

In the work environment a philosophy statement can aid in the orientation of employees to the corporate and health unit missions and

---

Box 3-1 *Philosophy of Occupational Health Nursing Service*

The occupational health service contributes to a safe and healthful work environment through programs aimed at reducing and eliminating work-related hazards and enhancing health promotion. Occupational health services are provided to individual workers and the collective workforce within an environment that considers and meets the needs of a diverse workforce.

The occupational health nursing service is central and integral to an effective occupational health program. The occupational and environmental health nurse professional is an advocate for the worker and often manages the occupational health service. As such the nurse is concerned not only with how the worker's health is affected or influenced by the worksite and organization but also with how the worker, her or his family, the community, and the environment interact to affect worker health and productivity.

To protect worker rights, workers are given information regarding work-related hazards so that informed decisions can be made. In addition, confidentiality of health records and information is safeguarded.

The occupational and environmental health nurse professional is part of a collaborative team that has the responsibility to inform the employer of unsafe and unhealthful working conditions and practices and of the need for workplace controls. The employer has the responsibility to provide a safe and healthful work environment and to recognize and support the nurse as a professional with specialized knowledge and skills.

The occupational and environmental health nurse professional has an obligation to maintain and improve knowledge and skills relative to her or his position and to keep current with research and legislation affecting occupational health and nursing practice. The occupational and environmental health nurse professional is accountable for interventions, judgments, and decisions made according to practice standards.

The occupational health nursing service encourages a mutually supportive relationship with the community through referrals and utilization of resources and by being a productive part of the larger ecosystem that enhances the environment. High quality occupational health care is provided in a cost-effective manner that promotes productivity through good health.

---

provide a foundation for the delivery of quality services (Brown, 1984). The formulation of a written philosophy will help to establish the beliefs about the health care of the workforce, provide the foundation for putting those beliefs into practice, and guide the activities of the occupational and environmental health nurse. Over time an individual's philosophy will evolve through new experiences, and those the nurse considers meaningful will be integrated into her or his belief system.

OCCUPATIONAL AND ENVIRONMENTAL HEALTH NURSING PROFILE AND PRACTICE SETTINGS

As reported by AAOHN membership surveys (AAOHN, 1999b), approximately 40% of occupational and environmental health nurses work in single-nurse occupational health units. More than 20% of occupational and environmental health nurses work at worksites with at least 3,000 workers, and more than 50% are employed where there are more than 1,000 workers. The largest number of AAOHN members are 45-54 years old (47%) and have an average occupational health work experience of 13 years. Forty-four percent hold either a diploma or associate degree in nursing; 56% hold a baccalaureate or higher degree, which reflects a substantial increase. Nearly 25% of AAOHN members report working primarily as a clinician or nurse practitioner, 20% as an occupational health service coordinator, 16% as a case manager, and 20% as a manager or corporate director of occupational health services.

Occupational and environmental health nursing services are provided in a variety of workplace settings, with the largest percentage employed at manufacturing sites (74%). Occupational and environmental health nurses can be found in pharmaceutical companies, furniture factories, banks, department stores, food processing plants, oil refineries, cosmetic and meat packing companies, construction sites, government and insurance agencies, automotive and telephone industries, hospitals, airline industries, apparel finishing factories, and wherever a workforce is in need of occupational health services. Often the workforce and work processes at a worksite are quite diverse, thereby requiring the nurse to have broad and substantive knowledge related to hazards, populations, health care, and service management and delivery.

The types of services and programs provided will depend on the characteristics and size of the workforce, actual and potential health hazards, available resources, company culture, and worker and management attitudes about health and safety and regulatory mandates. For example, hazard reduction programs in a textile mill will in part focus on cotton dust exposure and hearing conservation, whereas programs for office environment hazards will focus primarily on ergonomics and stress.

Occupational health services at a construction site or area will vary depending on factors such as location of a jobsite, availability of equipment and health facilities (which by necessity may be a mobile unit), and the make-up and needs of the workforce population. Construction work is one of the most dangerous types of employment, with hazards such as noise from blasting and heavy machinery; exposure to whole body vibration, solar radiation, and cold; dermatitis from irritants such as rubber, epoxy fixatives, and degreasing agents; lacerations, contusions, and amputations; and exposure to potential carcinogens such as paints, plastics, resins, and a variety of chemicals (Felton, 1990).

Even with all these hazards, health services for construction workers, including surveillance, job placement, and care for traumatic injuries, have not been provided consistently, to say nothing of health promotion, education, and restoration activities. However, contractual services with occupational medicine clinics and outreach hospital services recently have been of some aid.

A growing number of hospitals and related health care facilities sometimes employ occupational and environmental health nurses to provide and manage health care services to employees. The hospital environment is abundant with hazard risks of all types, including exposure to infectious diseases, chemical and physical agents, and ergonomic and psychosocial stressors.

The risks are numerous and ubiquitous and affect all occupational groups; yet employee health services are provided to only a small segment of the hospital/health care facility community, and the types of services provided vary greatly (Rogers & Haynes, 1991). Hospital settings may employ thousands of workers who are at risk every day from serious health threats, and many of these workers have minimal or no occupational health services, monitoring, or surveillance activities. Occupational or employee health nurses are the health care professionals most frequently employed to deliver these services, and many more are needed.

Summary

The bulk of health care services provided at the worksite are delivered by the occupational and environmental health nurse, who is the primary health care manager at the worksite and works with management to provide cost-effective health services. In recent decades the scope of practice has expanded, with more emphasis on health promotion. The nurse utilizes a prevention framework with a philosophy of practice aimed at promoting and protecting the health of the workforce and maintaining a healthy work environment through interdisciplinary collaboration.

References

American Association of Occupational Health Nurses. (1999a). *Code of ethics.* Atlanta, GA: Author.

American Association of Occupational Health Nurses (1999b). *Compensation and benefits study.* Atlanta, GA: Author.

American Association of Occupational Health Nurses. (1999c). *Standards of occupational and environmental health nursing practice.* Atlanta, GA: Author.

American Association of Occupational Health Nurses Bylaws. (1998). Atlanta, GA: American Association of Occupational Health Nurses.

American Nurses Association. (1999). *Scope and standards of public health nursing practice.* Washington, DC: Author.

American Nurses Association. (2000). *Public health nursing: A partnership for healthy populations.* Washington, DC: Author.

Benner, P. (1984). *From novice to expert: Excellence and power in clinical nursing practice.* Menlo Park, CA: Addison-Wesley.

Blix, A. (1999). Integrating occupational health protection and health promotion: Theory and program application. *AAOHN Journal, 47,* 168-174.

Brown, K. (1984). Development of philosophy, policies, and procedures for an organizational health nursing service. *AAOHN Update Series, 1*(1), 1-8.

Brown, M. L. (1981). *Occupational health nursing.* New York: MacMillan.

Chamberlin, E., & Rogers, B. (1997). Credentialing study: An AAOHN report. *AAOHN Journal, 45*(9), 431-437.

Childre, F. (1997). Nurse managed occupational health services. *AAOHN Journal, 45,* 484-490.

Christy, T. (1970). Portrait of a leader: Lillian Wald. *Nursing Outlook, 18,* 50-54.

Dille, J. H. (1999). A worksite influenza immunization program: Impact on lost work days, health care utilization, and health care spending. *AAOHN Journal, 47,* 301-309.

Felton, J. S. (1985). The genesis of American occupational health nursing. *Occupational Health Nursing, 33,* 615-621.

Felton, J. S. (1990). *Occupational medical management.* Boston: Little, Brown & Company.

Jones, M., & Sanford, J. (1996, October). Disability demographics – how are they changing? *Team Rehab Report, 10,* 36-44.

Leavell, H. R., & Clark, E. G. (1965). *Preventive medicine for the doctor and his community* (3rd ed.). New York: McGraw-Hill.

Lee, J. (1978). *The new nurse in industry.* Cincinnati, OH: U.S. Department of Health, Education & Welfare, National Institute for Occupational Safety and Health.

McGrath, B. J. (1946). *Nursing in commerce and industry.* New York: Commonwealth Fund.

Parker-Conrad, J. (1988). A century of practice in occupational health nursing. *AAOHN Journal, 36*(4), 156-161.

Pender, N. J. (1996). *Health promotion in nursing practice.* Stamford, CT: Appleton & Lange.

Rogers, B. (1988). Ethical dilemmas in occupational health nursing. *AAOHN Journal, 378,* 100-105.

Rogers, B. (1998). Occupational health nursing expertise. *AAOHN Journal, 46,* 477-483.

Rogers, B., & Haynes, C. (1991). A study of hospital employee health programs. *AAOHN Journal, 39*(4), 157-166.

Rogers, B., & Lawhorn, E. (2000). Advanced practice nursing. In J. Hickey, R. Ouimette, & S. Venegoni (Eds.), *Occupational health nursing strategies for health promotion* (pp. 348-355). Philadelphia: Lippincott.

Rogers, B., & Livsey, K. (2000). Occupational health nursing practice in health surveillance, screening, and prevention activities. *AAOHN Journal, 48,* 92-99.

Sorenson, G., Stoddard, A., Hunt, M. K., Herbert J. R., Ockene, J. K., Avrunin, J. S., Himmelstein, J., & Hammond, S. K. (1998). The effects of a health promotion-health protection intervention on behavior change: The WellWorks study. *American Journal of Public Health, 88,* 1685-1690.

Southern First Aid Supply Company. *The industrial nurse.* Greensboro, NC: Author.

Touger, G. N., & Butts, J. (1989). The workplace: An innovative and cost-effective practice site. *The Nurse Practitioner, 14*(1), 35-42.

Travers, P. H. (1987). In A. R. Cox & P. Ryan (Eds.), A comprehensive guide for establishing an occupational health service. Atlanta, GA: American Association of Occupational Health Nurses.

U.S. Public Health Service. (1993). *The Core Functions Project.* Washington, DC: Office of Disease Prevention and Health Promotion.

Uustal, D. B. (1978). Values clarification in nursing: Application to practice. *American Journal of Nursing, 78,* 2058-2063.

Vernarac, E. (1997). The consumer as healthcare manager: The state of health care in America 1997. *Special Report, Business & Health, 15,* 51-56.

Videbeck, S. L. (1997). Critical thinking: A model. *Journal of Nursing, 36,* 23-28.

Wachs, J., & Parker-Conrad, J. (1990). Occupational health nursing in 1990 and the coming decade. *Applied Occupational and Environmental Hygiene, 5,* 200-203.

White K., Cox, A. R., & Williamson, G. C. (1999). Competencies in occupational and environmental health nursing: Practice in the new millennium. *AAOHN Journal, 47*(12), 552-568.

Williams, C. A. (2000). Community-oriented population focused practice. In J. Lancaster & M. Stanhope (Eds.), *Community and public health nursing* (5th ed. pp. 2-19). St. Louis, MO: Mosby.

Wright, F. S. (1919). *Industrial nursing.* New York: MacMillan.

3-1 Competencies and Performance Criteria in Occupational and Environmental Health Nursing*

CATEGORY 1: CLINICAL AND PRIMARY CARE

Competent

1. Utilizes and documents the nursing process in care management
   a. Acquires general, occupational, and environmental health histories
   b. Assesses and diagnoses occupational and nonoccupational injuries and illnesses
   c. Develops a plan of care
   d. Implements direct care and treatment
   e. Maintains current knowledge of treatment modalities
   f. Evaluates care effectiveness
   g. Documents all aspects of assessment and care management
   h. Communicates findings to client and other appropriate individuals
   i. Educates clients with consideration for literacy and culture to enhance compliance with treatment plan
   j. Follows up with client to ensure compliance with treatment plan and modifies plan as needed
   k. Refers client to health care provider(s) as indicated
   l. Provides consultation when appropriate
2. Assesses, diagnoses, and treats client consistent with appropriate standards and laws
   a. Functions within the scope of state nursing practice regulations
   b. Functions within the scope and standards of occupational and environmental health nursing practice
   c. Distinguishes between the scope of nursing practice and the scope of practice for both paraprofessionals and other professionals providing care and consultation at the site
   d. Identifies components of other practice acts (e.g., medicine, pharmacy) that impact nursing practice

3. Counsels clients on reduction of risks associated with occupational and environmental health and safety hazards
   a. Assesses the client's knowledge regarding work-related hazards, as well as potential exposures in the client's home and community
   b. Advises the client regarding exposures, risk reduction, and measures available to protect employee health and safety
   c. Fosters client responsibility for use of preventative and protective measures within the context of the organization's duty to provide a safe and healthful work environment
4. Uses and maintains an accurate, complete recordkeeping system, while maintaining confidentiality
   a. Utilizes a recordkeeping system that documents health information in the client health record
   b. Utilizes policies and procedures to maintain confidentiality
   c. Maintains and abides by the legal parameters governing documentation and recordkeeping

Proficient

1. Develops and evaluates clinical protocols and practice guidelines
   a. Identifies and evaluates current resources (e.g., published texts, research literature, Internet searches) for development and modification of clinical guidelines and protocols
   b. Utilizes knowledge of disease entities and advances in research and practice in developing protocols and guidelines
   c. Collaborates with other occupational and environmental heath professionals in the development of guidelines and protocols
   d. Evaluates the effectiveness of protocols and guidelines

---

*These competencies as printed are under revision. New competencies are to be accepted by the AAOHN Board of Directors in May 2003 and published after that date.

Expert

1. Facilitates the clinical professional development of other occupational and environmental health care providers
   a. Provides clinical teaching and preceptorship to students and other providers
   b. Provides clinical mentoring

CATEGORY 2: CASE MANAGEMENT

Competent

1. Identifies the need for case management intervention
   a. Establishes criteria and uses case finding/screening to identify workers who are appropriate candidates for case management
   b. Identifies cases for early intervention
   c. Identifies gaps existing in the service continuum
2. Conducts a thorough and objective assessment of the client's current status and case management needs
   a. Assesses and documents a broad spectrum of client needs, including physical and psychosocial, using data from clients and families, other health care providers, health records, environmental exposure data, etc.
   b. Maintains awareness of cultural issues that may impact health
   c. Documents the client's health status and case management needs
   d. Assesses informal and formal support systems
   e. Assesses workplace, community, and vendor resources
   f. Assesses essential functions of job (e.g., physical and mental demands) to facilitate hiring, proper placement, and return to work activities
   g. Periodically reassesses the health status of the worker
   h. Assesses disability plan, policies, procedures, and communication links
   i. Monitors the worker's decision making abilities in relation to choices, utilization, and consequences
3. Provides workers' compensation case management consistent with state workers' compensation laws
   a. Identifies applicable components of workers' compensation statutes
   b. Completes appropriate documentation (e.g., workers' compensation, short-term disability, long-term disability)
4. Collaborates with the client and other health care providers to utilize a multidisciplinary approach to achieve desired outcome(s)
   a. Establishes communication plans involving internal and external parties appropriate to the case management plan
   b. Develops a comprehensive case management plan including client goals, objectives, and actions to achieve desired outcomes (e.g., return to work or optimal alternative)
   c. Identifies community resources and coordinates referrals as appropriate
   d. Engages in multidisciplinary consultation for complex cases
   e. Utilizes primary, secondary, and tertiary prevention and health promotion strategies in planning to optimize each client's health status
   f. Documents the plan and current status of the client in the health record
   g. Communicates status and plan to others involved in the case
5. Utilizes and evaluates available health care resources to achieve an optimal health care outcome
   a. Identifies and evaluates applicable components of health care, benefit programs, and workers' compensation processes
   b. Facilitates the participation of the client in designated plans for desired outcomes
   c. Coordinates administration of case management among benefit plans utilizing legal, labor, and regulatory guidelines
   d. Implements early return to work and modified duty programs
   e. Facilitates rehabilitation and job accommodation for workers' compensation and nonoccupational disabilities
   f. Evaluates and monitors the plan of care to ensure its quality, efficiency, timeliness, and effectiveness
6. Uses and maintains an accurate, complete recordkeeping system, while maintaining confidentiality
   a. Utilizes a recordkeeping system that documents case management activity
   b. Maintains and safeguards client's case management records in keeping with established

codes of ethics and legal or regulatory requirements to ensure confidentiality of health information

c. Obtains written client permission to release health information for a specific health condition

7. Monitors and documents the quality and effectiveness of care, services, and products provided to the client(s)

a. Monitors, documents, and evaluates the quality of individual client outcomes and makes adjustments as indicated

b. Monitors, evaluates, and revises agreements with vendor and provider services on a continual basis to ensure the quality of care, services, and products provided to the client

8. Identifies changes in case management practice and treatment plans to bring about appropriate care and cost-effective outcomes

a. Identifies an effective treatment modality and makes appropriate recommendations

b. Utilizes current and relevant research findings in developing and evaluating case management plan of care

c. Provides appropriate education for the worker, family, and community, and other resource providers

d. Identifies challenges to successful outcomes

Proficient

1. Develops case management policies, procedures, and guidelines

a. Conducts review of current research and other literature in case management

b. Utilizes appropriate research findings in the development of policies, procedures, and guidelines

c. Defines jointly with management the goals and scope of the organization's case management program

2. Manages the case management program

a. Reviews case management process annually

b. Conducts comprehensive assessment of all disability-related expenses and benefit utilization

c. Assesses workplace policies on return to work and job accommodations and modifies as needed

d. Determines and communicates role and responsibility of the worker, supervisor/

manager, case manager, benefits/risk manger, health care providers, third party administrators/insurers, and others in the case management process

e. Prepares analysis and synthesis of all data to formulate appropriate plan of care

f. Designs quality monitoring and improvement program

g. Analyzes trends and outcomes for success of case management activities (e.g., reduced accidents, reduced severity, reduced cost, efficiency of process, customer satisfaction)

h. Evaluates disability-related expenses and programs for program and benefit enhancement and refinement, as well as for areas of duplication

i. Modifies the program and program protocols accordingly

j. Establishes policies and procedures for appeal of case management recommendations, to include a grievance committee

k. Participates with interagency groups and community agencies to support or represent the case management program

Expert

1. Functions as a case management expert to management and business

a. Serves as a consultant to business and management

b. Develops and conducts educational programs to enhance the use of case management by health care providers, management, and employees

c. Manages data and information systems for the purposes of research, trend analysis, program modification, and continuous quality improvement

d. Participates in marketing and research related to case management services and the programs provided

2. Designs integrated disability case management systems for employers

a. Acts as a resource for the organization in the design, implementation, and evaluation of the case management system

b. Develops disability case management systems and plans that consider client satisfaction; client, employer, and vendor desired outcome(s); and cost-effectiveness measures

c. Conducts outcomes research aimed at identifying best practices

CATEGORY 3: WORKFORCE, WORKPLACE, AND ENVIRONMENTAL ISSUES

Competent

1. Coordinates employee health screening and surveillance programs
   a. Conducts health screening and surveillance activities including occupational and environmental health histories and health assessments
   b. Identifies the scope and distribution of occupational and environmental disease and injury occurrences using individual history health assessments and other aggregate data
   c. Collaborates with others to implement prevention and control strategies designed to maintain employee health and safety
   d. Maintains appropriate documentation of health information (e.g., health records, Occupational Safety and Health Administration [OSHA] logs) according to regulatory requirements and company policies and procedures
   e. Serves as a member of health and safety committees
2. Monitors the work environment to ensure the health and safety of employees
   a. Collaborates with other professionals (e.g., safety, environmental, industrial hygienists, physicians) to identify potential for employee exposures
   b. Conducts periodic worksite walk-throughs, focused inspections, records reviews, job hazard analyses, and incident investigations
   c. Identifies exposure monitoring techniques (e.g., area sampling, personal monitoring)
   d. Reviews exposure monitoring data and determines appropriate action, if any
   e. Anticipates and assesses health effects of hazards including review of resources such as Material Safety Data Sheets
   f. Ensures availability and maintenance of appropriate control measures

3. Ensures compliance with current laws and regulations governing work force and worksite safety, health, and environmental issues
   a. Identifies compliance issues consistent with local, state, and federal laws and regulations for environmental health and employee health and safety (e.g., OSH Act and OSHA standards, workers' compensation, Americans With Disabilities Act (ADA), Department of Transportation [DOT])
   b. Implements mechanisms to address compliance requirements
   c. Utilizes data from exposure monitoring to take action based on protocols
   d. Evaluates compliance activities
   e. Participates in providing employee training to ensure compliance
4. Interacts with organizations that provide community health and safety resources
   a. Identifies community resources available to assist with the company's occupational and environmental health and safety program
   b. Develops relationships with community organizations to further occupational and environmental health and safety objectives
   c. Participates in community and organizational functions relevant to occupational and environmental health and safety

Proficient

1. Analyzes the risks associated with worksite hazards
   a. Reviews records concerning production and quality control problems, workers' compensation claims, OSHA recordkeeping logs, safety surveys, inspection reports, accident reports, exposure monitoring reports, and relevant data from job hazard analyses to determine sources of risk
   b. Performs risk assessments
   c. Conducts trend analysis
   d. Determines aggregate health risk patterns by reviewing scientific data and other informational sources (e.g., National Institute for Occupational Safety and Health [NIOSH] criteria documents, other NIOSH publications, Agency for Toxic Substances and Disease Registry toxicological profiles, National Library of Medicine's hazardous substance databases)

e. Serves as risk communicator to corporations, labor, and government

2. Develops, manages, and evaluates population risk reduction and health surveillance programs
   a. Develops collaborative recommendations for prevention and control of occupational injuries and illnesses based on hazard identification and trend analysis
   b. Develops site-specific control strategies based on hazard identification and trend analysis
   c. Develops strategies of hazard abatement and methods to evaluate current strategies
   d. Designs methods to evaluate program effectiveness and implement quality improvement efforts

Expert

1. Serves as an occupational and environmental health and safety expert to corporations, government agencies, the community, and other outside groups
   a. Provides expert consultation on occupational and environmental health and safety issues
   b. Offers expert testimony to governmental agencies and others on occupational and environmental health and safety issues
   c. Advances the knowledge base in risk management and health surveillance (e.g., publications, research)

2. Influences policy relating to occupational and environmental health risk reduction surveillance
   a. Provides leadership within the organization to develop and revise occupational and environmental health policy
   b. Serves on national committees, boards, or agencies that address occupational and environmental health policy

CATEGORY 4: REGULATORY/LEGISLATIVE

Competent

1. Demonstrates compliance with state laws and regulations governing nursing practice
   a. Maintains current license(s) to practice as a registered nurse
   b. Provides care within the scope of state nurse practice act(s)

2. Utilizes knowledge of current laws, regulations, and standards governing employee, worksite, and environmental safety and health to achieve compliance
   a. Identifies applicable regulations (e.g., OSH Act, DOT, ADA, Family and Medical Leave Act, Clean Air Act, Safe Drinking Water Act)
   b. Monitors legislative activities that may impact the employee, worksite, and environment
   c. Provides occupational health tests (e.g., pulmonary function, audiometric, vision, laboratory) according to established standards and procedures
   d. Participates in the formulation of programs and services that support occupational and environmental health and safety programs and services that promote compliance
   e. Complies with recordkeeping requirements consistent with laws and regulations
   f. Serves as a member of interdisciplinary occupational and environmental health and safety committees

3. Maintains and safeguards confidentiality of health information consistent with nurse practice acts and other laws and regulations
   a. Applies security measures to ensure confidentiality of all health information
   b. Releases health information only as required or permitted by law after establishing "need to know" or upon written consent of employee

Proficient

1. Engages actively in efforts to affect policy making and practices governing employee, worksite, and environmental safety and health issues
   a. Serves as a spokesperson for occupational and environmental health and safety issues to local community and regulatory agencies
   b. Assesses the needs of the employee population, worksite, and community in relation to regulatory compliance
   c. Plans, implements, and evaluates compliance programs and services
   d. Acts to influence regulatory and legal processes in relation to occupational and environmental health and safety issues through individual and collective action

e. Collaborates with external agencies, organizations, and communities to influence regulatory and legal processes

f. Serves as a mentor and resource to others (e.g., occupational and environmental health nurses, other occupational and environmental health professionals, employees, management) concerning legislative issues

g. Provides written comment on proposed regulation

Expert

1. Influences occupational and environmental health legislative and regulatory public policy
   a Serves on national committees, boards, or agencies addressing policy
   b. Serves as an expert or spokesperson in providing written comment or testimony

2. Advances occupational and environmental health and safety by influencing related policy
   a. Serves as an expert or spokesperson in providing written comment or testimony
   b. Initiates efforts to gain national support for occupational and environmental health and safety policy

CATEGORY 5: MANAGEMENT

Competent

1. Coordinates the provision of occupational health services and programs
   a. Identifies the organization's structure, culture, and climate
   b. Organizes and implements occupational health programs
   c. Utilizes professional and regulatory standards to promote efficient, effective, and safe care delivery as well as safe working conditions
   d. Participates in the formulation of goals, plans, and decisions related to services
   e. Contributes to the development of the budget for the clinic or service
   f. Participates in the design and implementation of methods for quality improvement/quality assurance
   g. Collaborates with other disciplines to ensure appropriate services
   h. Identifies and utilizes community resources
   i. Determines and acquires support services, equipment, and supplies to facilitate occupational and environmental health nursing practice
   j. Participates in decisions related to acquisition, allocation, and utilization of occupational health unit resources
   k. Maintains knowledge of current technology, laws, trends, risk assessment, and cost-benefit analysis
   l. Maintains knowledge or occupational and environmental health structures and systems
   m. Participates in strategic and long-range planning

2. Monitors the quality and effectiveness of vendor services
   a. Reviews and evaluates vendor services
   b. Utilizes quality improvement methods to identify quality and effectiveness of vendor services
   c. Recommends changes to improve quality of services

3. Collaborates with the multidisciplinary team to foster the provision of effective health, safety, and environmental services
   a. Engages all appropriate staff and other health care professionals in developing occupational health and environmental services
   b. Engages team members in problem solving activities and in evaluating services
   c. Participates in health and safety committees, team meetings, and workplace walk-throughs
   d. Recommends changes in services to the multidisciplinary team

4. Uses an ethical decision making framework in all activities
   a. Maintains client confidentiality
   b. Advocates accessible, equitable, and quality health care services, including a safe and healthful work environment
   c. Involves clients in decisions that impact their well-being
   d. Establishes mechanisms for identifying and resolving ethical dilemmas and participates in decision making process

Proficient

1. Designs and manages health, safety, and environmental services consistent with corporate culture, business objectives, and the needs of employee and community populations
   a. Develops position descriptions for occupational health services personnel

b. Determines hiring, staffing, and orientation requirements of occupational health services personnel

c. Assesses job functions and develops job analyses for employees

d. Evaluates potential hazards of new technologies and work processes and their respective occupational health surveillance and prevention needs

e. Develops program assessment tools to identify areas of need, value, and importance for health programs and topics

f. Collects and analyzes data, and identifies trends to establish priorities and manage programs

g. Collaborates with management to provide resources that support an occupational and environmental health and safety program that meets the needs of the employee population and work environment

h. Identifies resources for program activities

i. Develops goals and objectives consistent with the organizational philosophy and culture

j. Uses knowledge of organizational theory, business principles, and dimensions of professional practice in management role

k. Manages human, operational, and financial resources to adequately implement health, safety, and environmental programs

l. Establishes standards of performance and conducts performance appraisals

m. Develops policies and procedures related to health and safety

n. Collaborates with internal and external multidisciplinary teams to facilitate change

o. Critically evaluates reported research and applies findings to practice

p. Develops methods to control the cost of occupational injuries and illnesses while monitoring quality care and effectiveness

q. Conducts and documents program evaluation, which includes measurement of outcomes, quality of interventions, and cost-benefit analysis

r. Determines appropriate information management systems and coordinates resources to facilitate use

s. Coordinates elements of strategic, long-range planning within the organization

2. Develops and manages a budget to meet assessed needs

a. Develops, monitors, and recommends a budget that provides for efficient and cost-effective services, including human, operating, and financial resources

b. Provides adequate resources for ongoing staff education and professional development

c. Demonstrates effective use of resources, including cost benefits

3. Develops or coordinates the company's health and corporate disability management programs

a. Maintains knowledge of current technology, laws, and trends

b. Identifies, reviews, and recommends alternative approaches to improve efficiency of health care systems

c. Collaborates with management and employees to develop and administer an integrated and cost-effective disability case management program

d. Develops policies and procedures for disability management and treatment guidelines

e. Acts as liaison with employer benefit plans, health care providers, and managed care organizations

4. Negotiates vendor and provider contracts and evaluates effectiveness of services

a. Participates in decisions regarding acquisition, allocation, and utilization of services

b. Develops cost-effective contractual relationships with vendors and providers

c. Monitors and evaluates services provided and outcomes achieved

5. Designs and implements quality improvement methods to measure health outcomes

a. Identifies appropriate standards, guidelines, or protocols indicative of quality processes and outcomes

b. Develops procedures for the evaluation of health outcomes

c. Conducts audits or reviews

d. Conducts or participates in benchmarking

6. Communicates with senior management on health service initiatives, outcomes, and cost-effectiveness

a. Documents and submits plans to meet developed goals and objectives, target outcomes, and other measures

b. Submits periodic reports that document budget projections versus actual expenditures, quality activities and measures, staff development activities, outcomes such as participation in programs and services, staff participation in interdepartmental and interdisciplinary activities, and trends related to injuries and illnesses

c. Submits periodic reports that summarize accomplishments and assesses progress toward goal attainment

7. Conducts activities and mentors occupational and environmental health personnel to enhance level of performance

a. Provides an environment for occupational and environmental health nursing staff to participate in decision making related to practice and human and material resources

b. Coordinates orientation of new occupational and environmental health nurses and other health services personnel

c. Coordinates opportunities for inservice education, staff development, and continuing professional education

d. Creates learning opportunities for students in the occupational and environmental health setting

Expert

1. Functions as an expert and leader in a consultative or senior management role, both internally and externally, to business, academia, government, and the community

a. Advises clients on the recommended scope and content of occupational and environmental health and safety services

b. Presents options for the structure and delivery of occupational and environmental health and safety systems

c. Implements options for the structure and delivery of occupational and environmental health and safety services

d. Conducts research studies and synthesizes results to enhance occupational and environmental health and safety services

e. Plans and directs marketing and visibility of occupational and environmental health and safety services' value within the organization

2. Provides leadership in the establishment of the vision and mission statements

a. Establishes the vision and mission of corporate occupational and environmental health services

b. Contributes to the development of the vision and mission of the corporation, community agency, or other organization

CATEGORY 6: HEALTH PROMOTION AND DISEASE PREVENTION

Competent

1. Assesses the health needs of employees and employee populations

a. Performs needs assessment

b. Reviews the needs assessment results for program planning

2. Plans, implements, and evaluates health promotion and disease prevention strategies and programs

a. Defines goals and objectives utilizing needs assessment data and the principles of the levels of prevention

b. Collaborates with other disciplines and community organizations to target and plan programs

c. Provides programs such as health fairs and health education seminars that increase awareness of health issues and choices

d. Implements prevention, follow-up, and referral programs as needed

e. Assists employees, dependents, and communities to modify health risk behaviors (e.g., support groups, smoking cessation, stress management)

f. Collaborates with management to provide a healthy work environment (e.g., fitness facility, healthy food choices, indoor air quality, work organizational changes)

g. Evaluates program effectiveness

3. Utilizes adult learning approaches in health education programs

a. Selects teaching methods with consideration of levels of prevention, readiness to change, and learning abilities

b. Provides health education using multiple teaching methods and strategies designed to enhance motivation

c. Includes techniques that promote personal and community wide responsibility for health by fostering empowerment

Proficient

1. Develops health promotion and disease prevention programs
   a. Assesses the psychosocial and physical environment, the organization of work, and the community to determine impact on health risks
   b. Analyzes benefit and other health data to assess and target health promotion programs needs for the employee population and the community
   c. Develops primary prevention interventions to reduce the risk of disease (e.g., immunizations, lead based paint reduction activities)
   d. Develops secondary prevention strategies to encourage early identification and diagnosis of employee and community disease conditions (e.g., health surveillance, lead screening)
   e. Develops tertiary prevention programs designed to restore health and productivity (e.g., disability case management, chronic illness monitoring)
   f. Collaborates with other business and community health promotion personnel in planning and implementing programs
   g. Implements strategies based on findings from assessment of health risks
   h. Designs programs utilizing health behavior change models
   i. Critically evaluates and applies research findings to practice
2. Manages health promotion and disease prevention programs
   a. Provides operational direction for health promotion programs for planning, staffing, organizing, and directing consistent with organizational philosophy and culture
   b. Identifies resources for program activities
   c. Selects, manages, and evaluates vendor contracts to ensure quality of health promotion services
   d. Plans and directs marketing of the health promotion program to increase employee participation
3. Evaluates the health outcomes and costs of health promotion and disease prevention programs
   a. Develops evaluation methodologies to detect changes in employee health behaviors and other health indicators following implementation of health promotion programs
   b. Designs processes for evaluation of the cost-effectiveness and cost-benefit analysis of specific health promotion activities and the comprehensive health promotion program
   c. Conducts trend analysis targeting health promotion and disease prevention programs
4. Communicates with senior management on health promotion and disease prevention initiatives, outcomes, and effectiveness
   a. Submits periodic reports that document productivity, quality of services, and progress toward goal attainment
   b. Submits periodic budget reports documenting budget projections versus actual expenditures, quality activities and measures, staff development activities, outcomes such as participation in programs and services, staff participation in interdepartmental and interdisciplinary activities, trends related to injuries and illnesses, and projected methods
   c. Submits annual reports to provide an overview of goal achievement and program performance

Expert

1. Serves as an expert in health promotion and disease prevention to corporations, government agencies, the community, and other outside groups
   a. Develops organizational policies to facilitate and support healthy employee and community behaviors and environments
   b. Provides consultation to senior management, other occupational and environmental health staff, and employees on health promotion issues
   c. Advises clients on the recommended scope and content of health promotion services including resources and staff
   d. Presents options for the structure and delivery of health promotion services, including managed care
   e. Develops comprehensive, cost-effective, long-range plans for health promotion services
   f. Conducts research studies and synthesizes results to enhance health promotion services

g. Provides information to facilitate understanding of issues related to health promotion and disease prevention programming and effectiveness
2. Designs systems for integration of health promotion strategies
   a. Develops mechanisms to integrate vision, goals, and strategies across health-related program areas and departments (e.g., direct care, case/disability management, workers' compensation, employee assistance program, benefits)
   b. Develops mechanisms to incorporate primary, secondary, and tertiary prevention services or strategies throughout the company or community

CATEGORY 7: OCCUPATIONAL AND ENVIRONMENTAL HEALTH AND SAFETY EDUCATION AND TRAINING

Competent

1. Implements occupational and environmental health and safety education and training to recognize and control hazardous exposures
   a. Identifies training goals and objectives based on employee needs assessment, company practices, and regulatory requirements
   b. Develops training programs incorporating knowledge of current laws and regulations governing employee, worksite, and community health and safety
   c. Collaborates with other disciplines regarding education and training programs
   d. Provides training to employees or community
   e. Evaluates effectiveness of training programs
   f. Maintains training records according to regulatory and other requirements
2. Utilizes adult learning approaches in education and training programs
   a. Provides education and training using multiple teaching methods and strategies that are culturally sensitive and designed to enhance comprehension and compliance
   b. Provides training related to knowledge, skills, and directions needed for employee and community empowerment and for employees to perform jobs in a safe and healthy manner

Proficient

1. Develops, manages, and evaluates occupational and environmental health and safety education and training programs
   a. Designs and manages a program that considers the objectives, outcomes, characteristics of the learner, size of the group, available time, equipment, facilities, and budget
   b. Evaluates program effectiveness
   c. Facilitates community action through education and outreach activities
2. Communicates with senior management on education and training initiatives, outcomes, and effectiveness
   a. Submits periodic reports that document productivity, quality of services, and progress toward goal attainment
   b. Submits periodic budget reports documenting budget projections versus actual expenditures, quality activities and measures, staff development activities, outcomes such as participation in programs and services, staff participation in interdepartmental and interdisciplinary activities, trends related to injuries and illnesses, and projected needs
   c. Submits annual reports to provide an overview of goal achievement and program performance

Expert

1. Serves as an expert in occupational and environmental health and safety education and training to corporations, government agencies, the community, and other outside groups
   a. Develops organizational policies
   b. Provides consultation
   c. Provides options for the structure and delivery of education and training programs
   d. Develops comprehensive, cost-effective long-range plans for education and training
   e. Conducts research studies and synthesizes results to enhance education and training
2. Educates occupational and environmental health and other professionals (e.g., academic or continuing education setting)
   a. Develops, implements, and evaluates curricula appropriate to various levels of educational preparation
   b. Synthesizes research findings in curriculum development
   c. Contributes to the peer reviewed literature

d. Mentors and encourages others to contribute to the peer reviewed literature

CATEGORY 8: RESEARCH

Competent

1. Identifies resources that describe relevant research findings and applies them to practice
   a. Reviews periodicals and other publications featuring research related to the field of occupational and environmental health and safety
   b. Conducts search of the literature and other resources to address specific occupational and environmental health issues
   c. Applies research supported interventions to practice in cooperation with the occupational and environmental health and safety team
2. Assists in identifying researchable problems
   a. Contributes to identification of problems observed in practice setting
   b. Works with community to identify environmental health research issues or questions based on community concerns and interests

Proficient

1. Enhances research skills utilizing mentoring and preceptorship opportunities
   a. Identifies experienced researchers in the practice or academic setting
   b. Seeks assistance as necessary to identify researchable problems, conduct research investigation, and interpret and evaluate research findings
2. Identifies need for and initiates or participates in research on practice issues or problems
   a. Evaluates research studies to determine quality of study, reliability and validity of methodology, and relevance to occupational and environmental health
   b. Identifies researchable problems with consideration of current research priorities and other needs
   c. Evaluates feasibility of conducting research
   d. Protects rights of research study participants
   e. Identifies potential sources of funding, if applicable
   f. Prepares or assists in preparing proposal(s) for peer review and potential funding

g. Conducts or assist in conducting research utilizing all components of the research process
h. Analyzes and interprets data to form sound conclusions, seeking assistance as needed
i. Communicates research findings through reports, articles, or presentations
j. Promotes application of findings to occupational and environmental health and safety practice

3. Collaborates with researchers, other occupational and environmental health nurses, and members of the occupational and environmental health and safety team in participating in research
   a. Identifies expertise and other resources needed to plan and conduct research and analyze findings
   b. Serves as a peer reviewer for professional publications

Expert

1. Builds and validates the scientific knowledge base and conceptual models of occupational and environmental health and safety
   a. Develops a program of research building on previous knowledge and findings
   b. Utilizes, tests, and expands specific theoretical models in research studies
2. Performs independent research and disseminates results
   a. Serves as principal investigator for the research conducted
   b. Disseminates findings through presentations, published articles in professional journals, and other media
3. Serves as a mentor for nurses and other occupational and environmental health and safety professionals in the research process
   a. Acts as a resource for identifying researchable problems, conducting research investigating, and interpreting and evaluating research findings
   b. Facilitates involvement of other occupational and environmental health and safety professionals in the clinical research process
   c. Seeks opportunities to share expertise and encourage the novice researcher
4. Influences occupational and environmental health public policy and research related decisions
   a. Serves as a peer reviewer for research grants

b. Serves on national committees, boards, or agencies addressing occupational and environmental health research policy

CATEGORY 9: PROFESSIONALISM

Competent

1. Develops and implements a lifelong learning plan, including strategies for academic education, continuing professional education, and certifications as appropriate
   a. Develops a plan for maintaining and expanding knowledge in nursing and occupational and environmental health and safety, based on self-assessment
   b. Participates in regular continuing education activities to meet knowledge and skill needs
   c. Obtains academic qualifications and certifications commensurate with job and performance responsibilities
   d. Reviews plan and adjusts as needed
2. Maintains scientific and regulatory knowledge appropriate to the nursing profession and to the specialty
   a. Maintains current state based licensure requirements
   b. Uses standards and practice guidelines and other relevant professional and regulatory documents as a framework for practice
   c. Reads publications and attends scientific meetings to obtain updated information
   d. Implements scientific findings in practice and decision making
   e. Monitors laws and regulations affecting practice
   f. Maintains professional behavior guided by laws, regulations, practice standards, and ethical codes
3. Implements an ethical framework for practice
   a. Recognizes ethical dilemmas in practice
   b. Maintains confidentiality of health information and records in accordance with professional codes, laws, and regulations
   c. Uses *AAOHN Code of Ethics* (1996) to guide practice
   d. Seeks consultation as needed for ethical decision making and develops resolution
   e. Evaluates resolutions to ethical conflicts
4. Establishes and maintains communication with employees, employers, and colleagues to accomplish occupational and environmental health and safety goals
   a. Works with employees, employers, and colleagues to develop occupational and environmental health and safety goals and objectives
   b. Meets regularly with employees, employers, and colleagues to identify progress toward goal achievement using an interdisciplinary framework
   c. Evaluates goal accomplishment
5. Evaluates own performance using appropriate documents
   a. Establishes annual goals and objectives for work performance
   b. Uses performance appraisal and self-assessment techniques to measure goal accomplishment, areas of strength, and need for improvement
6. Supports a research based discipline
   a. Uses research based finding to improve practice
   b. Participates in research activities appropriate to skill
7. Supports professional society(ies)
   a. Maintains current membership(s) in relevant professional organization(s)
   b. Participates in association governance and other related volunteer activities

Proficient

1. Acts as a role model and student mentor
   a. Fosters excellence in practice
   b. Acts as a preceptor to students
   c. Provides support and directions to nurses new to the specialty
2. Assumes leadership roles in advancing the profession
   a. Assumes a leadership role within the work environment
   b. Participates in leadership activities (i.e., committee work or chairmanships in the work environment and professional organization structures)
   c. Participates in election to leadership positions in the professional organization at all levels

Expert

1. Advances the scope and science of the specialty
   a. Develops new knowledge or theory to expand the specialty

b. Advances occupational and environmental health nursing standards commensurate with role expansion

c. Disseminates information through scholarly publications and presentations at scientific meetings

2. Participates in or guides the development of policy initiatives that impact occupational health and safety at all levels

a. Develops policy for occupational health and safety programming and directives

b. Influences legislative policy at all levels

Reprinted by permission of the American Association of Occupational Health Nurses, *AAOHN Journal 47*(12).

4 Roles of the Occupational and Environmental Health Nurse

SUSAN A. RANDOLPH

Since the early nineteenth century the scope of occupational and environmental health nursing practice has been gradually evolving and expanding while maintaining a public health model of prevention (Rogers, 1998) and an environmental health focus as an important component of the practice role. Occupational and environmental health nurses no longer only provide health care for work-related injuries and illnesses or focus solely on a worker's illness; they are committed to the total well-being of the worker and workforce and integrate health promotion, disease and injury prevention, health education and counseling, safety, and case management into their practice. At the same time occupational and environmental health nurses recognize environmental health risks facing employee populations at work, at home, and in the community and examine ways to reduce these risks. This continual focus on prevention has been partially responsible for the advancement of occupational and environmental health nursing roles. More important, the growth of graduate and doctoral programs in occupational and environmental health nursing has contributed to the development of advanced practice roles. As mentioned in Chapter 2, the term *occupational and environmental health nurse* has been adopted by the American Association of Occupational Health Nurses (AAOHN) in its governance and publication documents to reflect the emphasis on environmental health in the nurses' practice. While recognizing the importance and validity of this concept, the term *occupational and environmental health nurse* will be used in this text for consistency and standardization.

Occupational and environmental health nurses function in a variety of roles and work in diverse settings such as industry, hospital employee health units, occupational health clinics, government facilities, and independent practice (Randolph & Migliozzi, 1993). However, occupational and environmental health nurses must adapt to a changing workforce population that may be based internationally, in nonfixed worksites, like those found in construction and agriculture, and in virtual workplaces through telecommuting. As a result occupational and environmental health nurses must be aware of continual changes in the work environment and adjust the necessary health services accordingly. Theory and research are increasingly integrated with occupational and environmental health nursing practice. A sound theoretical base for practice contributes to clear role definition and scope of practice. In addition, occupational and environmental health nurses must remain competent in their practice through a variety of ways, including academic study, professional experience, and continuing education (White et al., 1999). This chapter will examine and define the seven major roles of the occupational and environmental health nurse. The purpose and function of each role will be described in detail by utilizing a theoretical base for practice.

ROLE DEVELOPMENT

A role is defined as a set of expected behaviors that are associated with a particular position (Gillies, 1994) and refers to both the expected and actual behaviors associated with a job either by the person doing the job or by someone else (Hardy & Conway, 1988). A role is shaped by the person's intentions and understandings (Fein, 1990) and through creativity and expertise. Whenever a person changes an existing role or takes on a new role, she or he goes through phases of role development or career stages. In the role development process common themes are evident: the nurse must clearly identify the purpose and function of the role, implement the role through goal-directed interactions, and achieve positive recognition and support of the role (Oda, 1977). Factors affecting progression through career stages of entry, mastery, and disengagement may be related to time on the job, skill development, and attitude (McNeese-Smith, 2000). Congruence between individual and organizational values greatly helps nurses remain in the mastery stage of the job and out of the disengagement stage. Active goal setting, self-evaluation, and continuous, challenging growth opportunities are ways to keep nurses engaged in their jobs. Role definition can assist the occupational and environmental health nurse in examining and clarifying a role and then communicating that role to peers, workers, management, and society.

Several factors influence the role or roles the occupational and environmental health nurse will develop in the workplace. These factors include the commitment of the company's management, skill level or expertise of the occupational and environmental health nurse, role perception, and worksite size and type. The first, commitment of management to the occupational health and safety service, is of major importance. To ascertain the degree of management's commitment, the philosophy of management toward health must be examined. The philosophy will determine the scope of the occupational health and safety service and, to some extent, the role of the occupational and environmental health nurse. Is the company's emphasis on health episodic in that only emergency care and first aid services are provided, or is the philosophy of health more comprehensive, encompassing all levels of prevention? Will only occupationally related injuries and illnesses be treated, or will nonoccupational health problems be managed to create an integrated approach to health care delivery? If the fo-

cus is only on occupational injury and illness, the occupational and environmental health nurse will have a difficult time implementing worker health promotion and disease prevention programs, thus limiting the nurse's role. In addition to the company health philosophy, the goals and objectives of the occupational health and safety service will further clarify the scope of services to be provided.

A second factor that influences the occupational and environmental health nurse's role is the position for which the nurse is hired. Ideally, the most qualified occupational and environmental health nurse will be selected for the position. The occupational and environmental health nurse should meet the requirements of the position based on the philosophy of health, the mission, and the goals and objectives of the occupational health and safety service. There should be congruence among the goals and objectives of the company, the needs of the employees, and the knowledge base and abilities of the occupational and environmental health nurse. Some occupational and environmental health nursing positions, such as an occupational and environmental health nurse practitioner or an occupational and environmental health nurse educator, require specific educational preparation and skills. If a nurse manager is needed to administer an occupational health service, then a person with that knowledge base and those skills and abilities should be hired. Generally, a nurse is hired for one primary role, with the position title reflecting specific functions and responsibilities. However, in actual practice the nurse functions in a more comprehensive, multifaceted manner by encompassing more than one role. For instance, an occupational and environmental health nurse consultant provides consultation to other occupational and environmental health nurses and management in various worksites. The same consultant also functions as an educator when lecturing to nursing students and as a researcher when conducting research.

The third factor is the perception of the role by the nurse and the company. The occupational and environmental health nurse has certain expectations about the role, and management may have some different opinions about that same role. This discrepancy may lead to role conflict. For example, a nurse was hired by a company to develop a health promotion program for employees but once on the job discovered that management really wanted an occupational health program to meet the first aid and safety health needs of the employees. Consequently, the health promotion program was delayed until the employees' needs could be met. Another source of potential conflict in role expectations is management's prior experience with an occupational and environmental health nurse. Has the experience been positive or negative? How might that affect management's perception of the nurse? One occupational and environmental health nurse was having difficulty maintaining the confidentiality of employee health records because management was demanding access to these records. The nurse later determined that the previous nurses at the company allowed management access to employee health records. Because the nurse refused management this option, the occupational and environmental health nurse was reprimanded by management as insubordinate. The nurse is now educating management about the profession, the *Code of Ethics* (AAOHN, 1996), and the responsibility to safeguard the employee's right to privacy and maintain the employee's trust. Both examples illustrate the need for clarification of the occupational and environmental health nurse's functions and accurate communication between the nurse and management.

A well-written position description helps delineate clear position functions and responsibilities as well as clarify role expectations. Role clarity allows nurses to know what is expected of them, to whom they report, and to whom they should go for help (Tomey, 2000). However, the job description should not be so detailed that creativity is discouraged. Basic elements of a position description include title, job summary, functions, organizational placement, and personal requirements (AAOHN, 1997). The title should accurately reflect the skills and responsibilities required and importance of the position in the organization. The job title should correspond to other titles with similar ranges of responsibility and accountability in the organization. The job summary outlines the key purposes or intentions of the position. The functions describe the specific responsibilities and duties of the job, including the breadth and depth of the work involved. Organizational placement is essential to

determine the lines of communication and authority; it also describes to whom the nurse is accountable and for whom the nurse is responsible, thus reducing role ambiguity. Personal requirements describe the knowledge and skills, educational preparation, experience, special requirements, and physical and mental energy required to perform the work. For example, a job description may specify that the nurse should have a bachelor's degree in nursing with at least 2 years of occupational and environmental health nursing experience. Special requirements would include a valid license to practice nursing or certification in occupational health nursing. Essential functions of the position should be indicated to comply with the Americans With Disabilities Act (ADA). The challenge is matching the needs of the position to human capacities and resources available.

The size of the company or agency is the fourth factor. As the size of the company increases, so does the need for nursing staff. The number of nursing staff needed also depends on the type of industry and the nature of the hazards. A steel mill or chemical industry with 300 employees is more likely to employ one or more nurses than is an insurance company with 1,200 employees. In addition, the roles and functions of the occupational and environmental health nurse will vary based on the size of the nursing staff. The occupational and environmental health nurse who works in a one-nurse unit (solo practice) has different roles, functions, and responsibilities than an occupational and environmental health nurse who works in a multinurse unit. The occupational and environmental health nurse who works alone typically takes on many roles: manager of the occupational health service; clinician in providing direct care for workers' injuries; educator in planning, implementing, and evaluating health education programs; case manager in coordinating health care services after illness and injury; and consultant in sharing pertinent information with managers, supervisors, and other members of the occupational health team. The nurse must possess skills in decision making, problem solving, and communication and be able to exercise independent nursing judgment. In essence, the nurse is responsible for the operation of the occupational health service. On the other hand, an occupational and environmental health nurse who works in a multinurse unit may have more distinct role responsibilities. She or he may be hired as a clinician to treat workers' injuries; as a health promotion coordinator to plan, implement, and evaluate disease prevention programs; or as a case manager to coordinate health care services.

ROLE DEFINITION

Regardless of position or worksetting, the occupational and environmental health nurse must know the scope of nursing practice from three distinct perspectives: legal, professional, and organizational (Figure 4-1). Every state administers a nursing practice act and related rules that define and set the legal practice of nursing. Other related laws, such as the state pharmacy acts and medical practice acts, may have language that affects nursing practice. As companies become increasingly global and multistate licensure becomes more widespread, the occupational and environmental health nurse must be aware of nursing regulations and other relevant practice boundaries in other states.

The scope of occupational and environmental health nursing practice is defined professionally through standards of practice (AAOHN, 1999b). Implementation of the practice scope is applied through codes of ethics, competency levels, certification in a specialty field such as occupational health nursing, advanced nursing practice, case management, and educational preparation and growth. The organization helps implement the scope of practice through position descriptions, organizational charts, policies and procedures, and mission and vision statements. All of these provide direction for occupational and environmental health nurse practice in the roles encountered in occupational health settings.

Theory and research influence role definition, scope of practice, and nursing's knowledge base. Nursing theories as well as other theories, such as those found in business and behavioral sciences, assist the nurse in using relevant knowledge to guide actions. This knowledge enables the nurse to interpret and apply the research findings to day-to-day practice (Moss, 1999). Several nursing theories apply to the occupational health setting and have been utilized in nursing research. Roy's Adaptation Model (Doyle & Rajacich, 1991; Phillips & Brown, 1992), Orem's Theory of Self-Care (Javid & Lester, 1983), and Newman's Health Care Systems Model (Koku, 1992) are some examples. Nonnursing theories such as General Systems Theory (Putt, 1978; von Bertalanffy, 1968), the epidemiologic framework (Levin et al., 1996; Nelson & Olson, 1996), change theory (Foran & Campanelli, 1995), Donabedian's quality assessment (Mannon et al., 1994), and the health belief model (Parrish & Allred, 1995; Sass et al., 1995) have also been tested successfully in the work setting.

ROLES

Seven major practice roles exist in occupational and environmental health nursing: clinician/practitioner, case manager, health promotion specialist, manager, consultant, educator, and researcher. Each of these roles will be discussed separately.

CLINICIAN/PRACTITIONER

The occupational and environmental health nurse clinician/practitioner is an essential role, encompassing the application of the nursing process to direct care for occupational and nonoccupational injuries and illnesses. In addition, the clinician/practitioner collaborates with other members of the occupational health team to maintain a safe and healthful work environment.

Although a closer examination of the role can reveal a distinction between the clinician

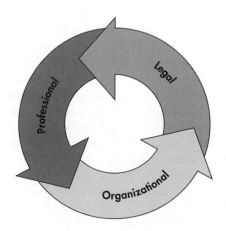

Figure 4-1 Scope of nursing practice.

and the practitioner, commonalties exist. As the commonalties between the clinician and practitioner roles increase due to changes in the health care delivery system, a future merger of the two roles may become apparent (Kitzman, 1989). For purposes of this chapter an occupational health clinician is defined as a registered professional nurse who provides care to employees. An occupational and environmental health nurse practitioner is an advanced practice nurse who provides workers with primary care services with an emphasis on the diagnosis and management of common acute illnesses/injuries and stable chronic diseases. The nurse practitioner practices autonomously and in collaboration with other health care professionals to deliver health care services (American Academy of Nurse Practitioners, 1998). The practitioner has completed formal education through postbasic or advanced education, increasingly at the master's level, with emphasis on occupational health if that is the specialty area of design. Both the clinician and practitioner use expert clinical knowledge, critical thinking, and judgment in assessing and evaluating the worker. They maintain high degrees of professionalism through continuing education, certification, and adherence to a code of ethics when providing health care services.

The theoretical base for the clinician/practitioner is the nursing process. This systematic approach to nursing care provides the framework for care management and decision making. The main steps of the nursing process are assessment, diagnosis, planning, implementation, and evaluation.

The clinician/practitioner assesses the individual's health problem by gathering general and occupational-health–specific data about the worker and the work environment. What does the worker state about the chief complaint? What signs and symptoms does the worker exhibit? Could the health problem be related to the job? What actual or potential health hazards are present in the work environment? Is a program needed to reduce the exposure to a health hazard? Answering these questions requires appropriate interdisciplinary collaboration. Other members of the occupational health team can contribute additional information about the worker and the work environment. The occupational physician offers medical information about the worker; the industrial hygienist provides area or personal sampling data (or both) about actual or potential health hazards in the work environment; and the safety professional provides information about the work environment related to hazards and poor or potentially unsafe working conditions.

Once all the relevant data are collected and analyzed, diagnoses are formed and serve as the basis for planning and managing employee health care through the development of a care plan or health program. The occupational and environmental health nurse and the worker mutually identify goals and objectives, as well as actions/methods to achieve them.

The care plan is implemented through direct nursing care, worker (and perhaps family) education, communication, or program development. Appropriate referral and follow-up are initiated to ensure continuity of care. To accomplish this effectively, the clinician communicates with community and health services resources, health care providers, and members of the occupational health team. Information about complementary and alternative therapies should be provided because an increasing number of people are interested in and want these options.

Finally, the goals and objectives are evaluated. Were they met? Why or why not? What could be improved? Were the desired behaviors, actions, or outcomes achieved? Reassessment occurs and the nursing process continues, illustrating its cyclic and dynamic nature.

Illness and injury data from sources such as daily logs, workers' compensation claims, health care cost expenditures, and studies of leading causes of death—coupled with trends influencing healthcare—must be analyzed to identify and develop potential programs. For example, after reviewing the daily log of visits to the health facility, an occupational and environmental health nurse in a furniture plant noticed an increase in the number of workers in one department being seen for foreign bodies in the eye from wood dust. The nurse conducted an assessment of the specific work area and observed that a machine was missing a guard and that no safety glasses were required (assessment/diagnosis). Based on that information, the nurse developed a plan to reduce the number of eye injuries: meet with the supervisor and the safety professional about the missing guard to have it replaced and establish a vision safety program (planning). With management's support the occupational and environmental health nurse implemented the plan. Safety glasses are now required in that area, and workers were educated on vision safety (implementation). A reduction in the number of eye injuries in that department was seen after the program was implemented (evaluation). Periodic walk-throughs are also conducted to ensure that the guard remains in place and that workers are wearing eye protection.

Cost-effectiveness for on-site occupational and environmental health nursing services should be documented and monitored (Davidson et al., 1992a, 1992b). A worker with a simple respiratory infection can be treated in the occupational health facility and receive follow-up care for less cost compared with having to go to an off-site provider, such as a physician's office or clinic-based medical group practice, for evaluation and treatment. In addition, cost savings are generated from no lost work time because the worker was treated on-site (Davidson et al., 1992a, 1992b; Zentner et al., 1995).

Specific functions of the occupational and environmental health nurse clinician/practitioner include, but are not limited to, the following activities:

1. Monitors the work environment for actual or potential health and safety hazards
2. Assesses the health status of workers
   a. Health history
   b. Occupational health history
   c. Lifestyle-health risk appraisal
3. Performs physical examinations
   a. Job placement
   b. Periodic
   c. Return to work
   d. Health surveillance
   e. Termination/retirement
4. Conducts appropriate laboratory tests
5. Provides direct nursing care for occupational and nonoccupational injuries and illnesses
6. Provides primary care for workers and perhaps insured family members
7. Conducts health education and counseling on reduction of risks associated with occupational and environmental health and safety hazards
8. Establishes mutual goals and objectives with the worker for the health care plan

9. Collaborates, communicates, and consults with other members of the occupational health team
10. Maintains accurate and complete health records of the workers while maintaining and safeguarding confidentiality
11. Analyzes data for illness and injury trends
12. Develops and implements programs designed to correct or minimize the identified health and safety hazards
13. Identifies, implements, and evaluates a plan of care, including pharmacological, nonpharmacological, and nursing interventions
14. Institutes appropriate personal protection programs
    a. Safety glasses
    b. Safety shoes
    c. Hearing protection
    d. Respiratory protection
    e. Personal protective clothing
15. Initiates referrals to other health care professionals and community agencies
16. Conducts preventive screening procedures based on worker age, history, and exposure
    a. Hearing
    b. Vision
    c. Respiratory
    d. Cancer
    e. Cholesterol
17. Develops and implements a health promotion program or a disease prevention program or both
18. Conducts health education and counseling on reduction of health risks associated with occupational and environmental health and safety hazards
19. Evaluates the various programs
20. Develops and maintains rapport with workers and management
21. Collaborates and communicates with other health care providers in the community
22. Researches and prepares clinical protocols, as appropriate, with necessary collaboration
23. Manages workers' compensation claims and provides workers' compensation case management
24. Conducts training for cardiopulmonary resuscitation and first aid
25. Documents cost savings of treating workers on-site compared with treatment received in the community

26. Serves as a preceptor for nursing students
27. Functions as a mentor to colleagues
28. Provides clinical education to others as appropriate
29. Maintains competency, professionalism, and ethical conduct

CASE MANAGER

The occupational and environmental health nurse case manager has continued to evolve as an important role over the past decade, primarily because of concerns about rising health care costs and quality of health care services (Salazar et al., 1999). An occupational and environmental health nurse working in a single nurse unit may have case management as one of several job responsibilities, or an occupational and environmental health nurse working in a multinurse setting or employed by a case management firm may have case management as the primary job function. Regardless of the setting, the goal is the timely coordination of quality health services to meet an individual's specific health care needs in a cost-effective manner (Case Management Society of America, 1995). The case manager establishes a provider network, recommends treatment plans that assure quality and efficacy while controlling costs, monitors outcomes, and maintains communication among all involved (AAOHN, 1994). Case management services may be limited to occupational injury or illness or can include nonoccupational injury or illness. Services typically begin at the onset of injury or illness and continue until the individual returns to work or achieves an optimum level of functioning. Regardless, the health outcomes must be measurable. The case management framework follows the nursing process (Table 4-1) (Cohen & Cesta, 2001; Salazar, 1997).

For case management to be successful, the occupational and environmental health nurse needs to identify those workers who would benefit from case management interventions. Do certain diagnostic codes indicate a need for case management? What about chronic disease cases or catastrophic injuries, such as head injury or trauma? Work-related illnesses or injuries that have the potential for high annual claims expenditures, extended length of hospital stay, or multiple admissions (e.g., AIDS or a spinal cord injury) are also good indicators for case management (Shrey &

TABLE 4-1	Common Phases of the Case Management Process Paralleled With the Nursing Process	
NURSING PROCESS	**CASE MANAGEMENT PROCESS**
Assessment	Client identification and outreach
Diagnosis	Individual assessment and diagnosis
Planning	Service planning and resource identification
	Linking clients to needed services
Implementation	Service implementation and coordination
	Monitoring service delivery
	Advocacy
Evaluation	Evaluation

Lacerte, 1995). For example, a 48-year-old white male sustains a spinal cord injury from a motor vehicle crash. Because of the nature of the injury, the occupational and environmental health nurse case manager initiates the case management process immediately. The key is early intervention.

The case manager then conducts a thorough assessment of the injured worker and identifies the physical and functional status. Based on this assessment, diagnoses are formulated and determine the level of functioning and service needs. This aids in the coordination and monitoring of case management services. In the spinal cord injury example, the case manager conducts this assessment after the worker is stabilized and able to enter the rehabilitative phase of recovery. Is a spinal cord rehabilitation unit located close by? Are necessary services, like physical therapy and occupational therapy, available on an outpatient basis? What support systems are in place for the family? Is the home wheelchair accessible? What is the worker's mental outlook? Based on the worker's level of functioning, when would he be able to return to work? These assessments and considerations form the basis for planning and coordinating services and identifying necessary resources, and all of this involves coordination and communication with the physician, therapists, family, human resources, and others.

Service planning and resource identification refer to the development of care plans and determination of resources and networking systems. These are collaborative activities involving the worker, family members, health care providers, and other members of the multidisciplinary team. Clients are then linked to needed services. Getting back to the example, a return to work plan is developed with input from the injured worker, his family, the company's human resource department, and others involved in his care. It is determined that he could work part-time from home while continuing therapy sessions. Transportation is arranged using community services. The employer provides the equipment and supplies for basing the worker at home.

The case manager ensures that services are being provided and coordinated and are meeting the client's needs. Extensive records are kept, documenting the appropriateness, efficiency, and effectiveness of the care services. The worker's progress is periodically evaluated. In the example, the worker is gaining strength and endurance from the therapy and works about 15 hours per week from home. He hopes to increase his work hours soon and starts going into the office at least 1 day per week.

The evaluation process involves ongoing monitoring and analysis of the client's needs and the services being provided. If problems are identified, then changes are made accordingly. The worker continues to make progress. He is now working full-time, primarily from home.

The occupational and environmental health nurse case manager is a registered professional nurse who assists ill and injured workers to reach maximum health and productivity. The nurse assesses, plans, implements, coordinates, monitors, and evaluates care for workers and must know and understand pertinent laws and regulations, such as workers' compensation laws, Americans With Disabilities Act, Family and Medical Leave Act, and the Occupational Safety and Health Act. Experience in coordinating health care services, independent thinking and decision making, and expert communication skills are musts. Certification as a case manager documents expertise in this area.

Specific functions of the occupational and environmental health nurse case manager include, but are not limited to, the following activities:

1. Determines the need for case management intervention
2. Establishes criteria to identify workers who would benefit from case management services
3. Establishes communication plans involving internal and external parties
4. Uses data from various sources to assess worker needs
5. Identifies goals, objectives, and actions as part of a comprehensive case management plan
6. Implements interventions to achieve worker goals and objectives
7. Collaborates with the worker and other health care providers
8. Consults with a multidisciplinary team for complex cases
9. Utilizes community resources and coordinates referrals as indicated
10. Implements early return to work and modified duty programs
11. Develops and conducts an evaluation process for the case management program
12. Facilitates claims processing with insurance and third party representatives
13. Provides workers' compensation case management consistent with state workers' compensation laws
14. Monitors, documents, and evaluates the quality of individual worker outcomes and makes adjustments as necessary
15. Monitors benefit systems and conducts cost-benefit analysis
16. Maintains accurate and complete health records while maintaining and safeguarding confidentiality
17. Serves as a preceptor for nursing students
18. Functions as a mentor to colleagues
19. Maintains competency, professionalism, and ethical conduct

HEALTH PROMOTION SPECIALIST

The health promotion specialist is a key role in occupational and environmental health nursing. The occupational and environmental health nurse designs, implements, and evaluates worksite health promotion programs with a goal of improving the overall health status and productivity of the workforce and reducing health care costs (Slagle et al., 1998). The nurse manages multilevel, wide-ranging health promotion programs that are integrated into the corporate business objectives (Arendasky et al., 1997). The programs may do one or more of the following: address an awareness level, focus on lifestyle or behavior change programs, or encompass environments that encourage healthy lifestyles. Because wellness is multidimensional, programs can encompass social, occupational, spiritual, physical, intellectual, or emotional dimensions.

A systematic approach is needed to develop, plan, and implement successful health promotion programs. First, the corporate culture needs to be assessed. Is health promotion valued within the organization? What is the commitment of management to health promotion? Are there other issues that affect which programs can be offered? For instance, an occupational and environmental health nurse working for a paper company wanted to offer a smoking cessation program. Because the company made cartons for a tobacco manufacturer, approval was not given to offer a formal program, but one-on-one educational sessions with interested workers were provided.

Assessing employee involvement is also critical for success. What programs would they like to have offered and when? An interest survey for health promotion programs is one way to determine employee interests. For example, programs on health issues, such as fitness, weight control, nutrition, smoking cessation, stress management, and back care, could be included on a survey tool. Employee involvement is critical for success of the program.

Existing health care data are critical to justify the need for programs. One occupational and environmental health nurse wanted to develop a health promotion program in the company. The nurse examined available data and learned that the workforce primarily comprised women in childbearing ages. After examining health insurance cost data, the nurse determined that the top three health care expenditures were pregnancy, neoplasms, and cardiovascular disorders. This information was used to convince management to establish prenatal education, breast self-examination and mammography, and nutrition/exercise programs.

After all information is gathered, the planning and designing of health promotion and disease prevention programs begins. A wellness committee with employee representation can assist with program planning and contribute to program success. Goals and objectives are established along with a budget and an evaluation plan. What resources are available for the program? Where and when will the program be held? Who is the target audience? What supplies are needed? Who will conduct the program? Is this something that the occupational and environmental health nurse can do, or should the program be done by someone else in the community or company? Various voluntary community agencies, such as the American Cancer Society, American Lung Association, American Heart Association, March of Dimes, and American Red Cross, are willing to provide programs free of charge or at a minimal cost. Other health professionals in the community, including health profession students, may be willing to present programs. The program needs to be advertised at key locations in the worksite, which could include break areas, cafeteria, bulletin boards, or company newsletter. Incentives may be offered to increase attendance at the program. After the program is completed, it must be evaluated. An evaluation of the program serves many important functions, including assessment of the achievement of objectives, identification of the strengths and weaknesses of the program, and analysis of its outcomes.

The health promotion specialist is a registered professional nurse with expertise in health promotion, illness and injury prevention, risk reduction, and adult learning principles. Specific functions of the occupational and environmental health nurse health promotion specialist include, but are not limited to, the following activities:

1. Uses appropriate data sources to assess and target health promotion program needs for the workforce
2. Develops and monitors the goals and strategies for the health promotion program
3. Implements prevention, follow-up, and referral programs as needed
4. Develops primary, secondary, and tertiary prevention programs
5. Provides programs, such as health fairs and health education seminars, that increase awareness of health issues and choices
6. Helps employees, dependents, and communities modify health risk behaviors

7. Collaborates with management to provide a healthy work environment
8. Selects, directs, and monitors vendor contracts
9. Conducts ongoing evaluation of the specific activities, as well as the overall health promotion program, and integrates cost-containment and cost-effectiveness aspects
10. Plans and directs marketing of health promotion programs
11. Plans and directs the evaluation process
12. Collaborates with other business and community health promotion personnel
13. Supervises and trains staff as needed
14. Maintains accurate and complete health records while maintaining and safeguarding confidentiality
15. Serves as a preceptor for nursing students
16. Functions as a mentor to colleagues
17. Maintains competency, professionalism, and ethical conduct

MANAGER

The occupational and environmental health nurse manager serves an important function in the total operation of the occupational health service by providing the structure and direction for the development, implementation, and evaluation of an effective, high quality nursing program. Furthermore, the occupational and environmental health nurse manager communicates and interprets the occupational health program to management and other members of the occupational health team.

While functioning in a comprehensive executive role, the manager sets goals, formulates policy, and manages the health service. The ability to reach a decision and then act on it is essential. All of these activities refer to the basic functions of the management framework: data gathering, planning, organizing, staffing, leading, and evaluating (Gillies, 1994).

Data gathering consists of accumulating information about the worksite and workforce. Key worksite information includes the company mission, vision, and value statements; major goals and objectives; organizational culture; management's views toward health; known health hazards and control measures; and illness and injury trends. Information about workers, which includes demographic characteristics and health needs, is used for planning purposes.

Planning can be defined as using assessed data for future operations and providing for implementation of the plan, which is the most important but most difficult function to accomplish. Planning also involves considering problems or unmet needs, determining solutions or ways to meet those needs, and providing for resources and budget control to support the plan. Strategic planning is another tool used to define the actions necessary to achieve an outcome (Amann, 2000). An example is the development of a modified duty/return to work program for injured workers (Randolph & Dalton, 1989). The occupational and environmental health nurse manager plans for both long-range and short-term goals. Long-range goals are necessary to anticipate and meet the needs of the organization or industry as well as those of the employees. For instance, based on knowledge of an upcoming merger of the company, a manager anticipates that different health services may be offered as new company goals and objectives are defined, the number of employees changes, environmental exposures alter, and stress levels increase. Perhaps health services will be subject to outsourcing. Short-term goals reflect more ongoing or current needs and result in such decisions as plans for stress management programs or other specific programs (e.g., an early retirement seminar for workers and their spouses).

Organizing involves developing a framework so that people relate to each other and their surroundings in such a manner as to reach an objective. It can also be necessary in defining the tasks and time frames necessary to achieve the solution. The occupational and environmental health nurse manager organizes the occupational health service through use of all available resources to meet the defined program objectives. This involves appropriate utilization of the occupational health staff, training of staff to maintain or acquire new skills or abilities, as well as delegation of tasks—along with the authority to get the job done—to personnel. Besides people, the manager organizes the budget, equipment, supplies, facilities, and anything else related to the efficient operation of the program. In the early retirement seminar example, staff define the goals and objectives along with a tentative timetable, such as 1 session per week for 6 weeks. Resources for successful implementation of the program also must be identified.

Another management function is staffing, which is defined as having the right people to do the work in order to accomplish the goals of the organization. Staffing includes recruiting, interviewing, hiring, and placing people in appropriate positions throughout their tenure in the organization.

Leading/directing refers to any harmonizing activities aimed at achieving the desired outcome and includes supervising, guiding, and structuring responsibilities through direct assignment or delegation of activities. To be able to direct effectively, the manager must have excellent communication skills, both oral and written, and for any program the occupational and environmental health nurse manager must coordinate resources and activities, including management's approval and support. For instance, at this point the nurse manager delegates the responsibility for the early retirement seminar implementation to one of the staff. Then the occupational and environmental health nurse must determine and coordinate the number of workers close to retirement age and their spouses; the budget allocated for the seminar; the community resource people and company representatives, such as personnel, needed to participate; and the handout materials and equipment. The preretirement seminar represents the goal.

Evaluating, the last managerial function, is defined as verifying whether everything occurred in conformity with the plan, objectives, and budget allocation. Evaluating implies a monitoring and controlling process. The occupational and environmental health nurse manager has the ability to monitor and adjust the occupational health work according to standards, such as the standards for occupational and environmental health nursing as well as company-established benchmarks. Evaluation is another mechanism to determine if the plan, program, or occupational health service was successful. Were the objectives of the preretirement seminar met? How did the workers like it? Did it meet their needs or answer their questions? What could be done to improve the seminar when it is offered again? Quality assurance uses peer review, audit criteria, and performance appraisal; all are tools that the occupational and environmental health nurse manager may use to evaluate the program as well as the staff.

The occupational and environmental health nurse manager improves interpersonal relations with staff and workers, along with work conditions, through planning, organizing, staffing, leading/directing, and evaluating. With everyone working toward a common goal, anything is possible. To function efficiently and effectively, the manager is a registered professional nurse who has education in occupational and environmental health nursing, safety, management or nursing administration or both, communications, and group dynamics. Ideally, the person has had administrative experience.

Specific functions of the occupational and environmental health nurse manager follow the managerial functions or the nursing process. They include, but are not limited to, the following activities:

1. Establishes goals (long-range and short-term) and objectives of the occupational health service
2. Designs, implements, and evaluates the occupational health services and programs
3. Formulates policies and procedures
4. Develops and manages a budget to meet program needs
5. Plans, develops, and promotes the necessary facilities, equipment, supplies, and record-keeping system needed to operate the employee health service
6. Monitors the quality and effectiveness of vendor services
7. Determines the nursing staff required and minimum qualifications and functions for various positions and participates in staff selection
8. Coordinates in-service education and professional growth opportunities for staff
9. Assesses program needs in consultation with other members of the occupational health team
10. Implements new programs and program changes and manages ongoing programs consistent with goals and objectives
11. Develops or coordinates the company's health and corporate disability management program
12. Evaluates quantitative outcomes of employee health and safety programs
13. Assumes responsibility for adequate data collection that allows for quantitative evaluation of program outcomes of worker health and safety while maintaining confidentiality

14. Initiates quality assurance, audits, and peer review of the occupational health staff
15. Participates as an active member of the central management team
16. Uses community resources appropriately
17. Keeps abreast of technological, legal, and professional changes associated with occupational health and safety
18. Serves as a preceptor for nursing students
19. Functions as a mentor to colleagues
20. Maintains competency, professionalism, and ethical conduct

EDUCATOR

With the development of undergraduate, graduate, and doctoral programs in occupational and environmental health nursing, the role of occupational and environmental health nurse educator has emerged with growing importance. This nurse educator teaches and prepares nursing students to function as expert clinicians/practitioners, administrators, educators, researchers, or consultants at the worksite. The responsibility parallels the educator's goal, which is to prepare occupational and environmental health nurses to assume leadership positions in order to improve, maintain, and account for quality health outcomes for workers.

In order to serve as faculty in a school of nursing or school of public health—occupational and environmental health nursing programs are found in both—the nurse educator for these programs must be a registered professional nurse who is academically and professionally prepared to teach occupational and environmental health nursing. In addition, the occupational and environmental health nurse educator must be familiar with concepts in industrial hygiene, safety, loss prevention, toxicology, epidemiology, management, case management, occupational health, health promotion, human behavior and motivation, research, and statistics. At least two years experience in occupational health and safety is helpful. Experience in occupational and environmental health nursing is important so that the educator can integrate theory with practice. Most baccalaureate and master's level nursing programs require that nursing faculty have a doctoral degree or be in the process of obtaining such a degree. The educator must also know various worksites in the geographic area for appropriate practicum placement of students with

nursing preceptors who will serve as expert role models. Furthermore, the occupational and environmental health nurse educator designs curriculum content and learning strategies to ensure that graduates can develop and implement new roles (Snyder, 1989) in occupational and environmental health nursing.

Changes in nursing education generally reflect changes in nursing practice. The educator must keep current on issues affecting both nursing practice in general and occupational and environmental health nursing practice in particular. Areas such as politics, legal and ethical concerns, health care delivery systems, malpractice and liability issues, company mergers and closings, and violence should be considered topics of interest because they relate to worker health care. Information about these topics can be obtained from research reports, journal articles, key informants, and other sources. In addition, the occupational and environmental health nurse educator is encouraged to maintain a service or practice base, thus blending education and service; the educator can then illustrate how theory-based practice is applied in real world situations.

In some schools of nursing limited content on the role of the occupational and environmental health nurse and general concepts of occupational and environmental health nursing practice are integrated within a basic community health nursing course. However, occupational and environmental health nursing is considered a specialty area and should therefore be taught at the graduate level; thus most occupational and environmental health nurses learn about the field through on-the-job training and continuing education programs.

Continuing education is another fundamental area in which the occupational and environmental health nurse educator plays an invaluable role. By conducting continuing education programs, the educator has the opportunity to expand and/or update occupational and environmental health nurses' knowledge and skills in delivering quality nursing care to workers. In addition, continuing education courses taught by qualified educators are needed to help occupational and environmental health nurses qualify for or maintain certification in occupational and environmental health nursing or in another area of nursing practice. The educator should have adult education/adult learning expertise in order to teach occupational and environmental health nurses who have varied educational levels, career goals, and experiences.

Specific functions of the occupational and environmental health nurse educator include, but are not limited to, the following activities:

1. Develops, implements, and evaluates curricula appropriate to various levels of educational preparation
2. Promotes integration of occupational and environmental health nursing content into undergraduate nursing education
3. Uses research findings and conducts research relevant to occupational and environmental health nursing and occupational health and safety
4. Disseminates research findings to other nurses, health care professionals, and occupational health specialists by publication or presentation or both
5. Promotes occupational and environmental health nursing as a challenging area of nursing practice
6. Uses experts in occupational health and safety in planning and coordinating relevant education programs
7. Plans and conducts continuing education programs relevant to occupational and environmental health nursing and occupational safety and environmental health
8. Maintains occupational and environmental health nursing practice expertise
9. Collaborates with other occupational and environmental health nurses regarding practice issues and student practice sites
10. Serves as a role model for students
11. Functions as a mentor to colleagues
12. Maintains competency, professionalism, and ethical conduct

RESEARCHER

The role of the occupational and environmental health nurse researcher is rapidly growing, with the focus on improving the health and safety of the nation's workforce and preventing occupational illness and injuries. Occupational and environmental health nursing research is necessary to support and expand the knowledge base that provides the foundation for practice (Rogers, 1994); it will also help bridge the gap between the development and implementation of theory and its application to practice.

A researcher develops researchable questions, conducts research, and communicates the research findings to occupational and environmental health nurses, other researchers, and the public. The importance of identifying answerable research questions to which appropriate statistical techniques are applied cannot be overemphasized because this will make the conduct of the research easier and more meaningful (Rogers, 1991). As occupational and environmental health nurses become aware of research findings and their implications, these nurses will start to apply them in their own practice at the worksite. The intent, then, of research-based practice is to promote, maintain, protect, and restore the health of the workers as well as improve the work environment.

Two examples of research studies that have made a significant contribution to occupational and environmental health nursing follow. Dille (1999) conducted a retrospective case control survey to measure and evaluate the outcomes of a comprehensive worksite influenza immunization program, comparing vaccinated and unvaccinated workers. A self-administered questionnaire was used to collect data on demographic variables; motivating factors for obtaining influenza vaccine; factors that contributed to not getting the immunization; existing chronic diseases; symptoms of an influenza-like illness; and absenteeism, complications, and medical care that resulted from an episode of influenza-like illness. The results indicated that unvaccinated workers were significantly more likely to have influenza-like symptoms than were vaccinated workers. Unvaccinated workers were also more likely to have more lost workdays and health complications resulting from influenza compared with vaccinated workers. The direct and indirect cost savings from vaccinations were estimated to be $83.84 per person, with a total program cost savings of $531,462. As a result, the findings were used to justify further expansion of the program. In a time of downsizing and emphasis on cost containment, other occupational and environmental health nurses may be able to use these findings to initiate or expand their own immunization programs.

Moore (1998) conducted a primary prevention program aimed at preventing muscle strain.

The investigator used a one group pretest-posttest design to gather physiologic and perception measurements before and after employee participation in a workplace stretching program designed to improve flexibility through conditioning. Physiologic flexibility was measured by a flexibility profile of a sit and reach test, right and left body rotation, and shoulder rotation. The intervention consisted of 36 stretching sessions held at 5 specific times during each of those days, each lasting between 5 and 8 minutes. A statistically significant increase was found in all flexibility measurements at the end of the study for the total group. The participants' perceptions of body attractiveness, physical conditioning, and overall self-worth, as measured by the Fox Physical Self-Perception Profile (PSPP), also showed a significant increase. No musculoskeletal injuries were reported during the 2-month intervention. The results indicated that stretching programs in the workplace might increase flexibility and help prevent muscle strains. This information is important as occupational and environmental health nurses examine ways to offer cost-effective, employee-supported injury prevention programs to reduce costs associated with the treatment of musculoskeletal injuries.

Characteristics of the occupational and environmental health nurse researcher include curiosity, open-mindedness, and tenacity (McKechnie & Rogers, 1985). Instead of accepting things the way they are, the researcher wonders, Why . . . ? What if . . . ? Is there a better way? How can this program or my practice be improved? With this quest for knowledge or improvement in practice, the researcher initiates a study. Open-mindedness means being receptive to new ideas or free from bias. Once the study is completed, the researcher must be able to interpret the data, draw accurate conclusions from the findings, and demonstrate the information through publication or presentation. Rogers (1997) identified factors that enhance beginning research efforts: excite an interest, develop a program of research, conduct meaningful research, collaborate with seasoned researchers, maintain an open mind, keep perspective, and persevere.

The occupational and environmental health nurse researcher, from an academic perspective, is a registered professional nurse with an advanced degree, usually a doctoral degree. Graduates from a master's program in occupational and environmental health nursing generally complete a research study or thesis in partial fulfillment of the requirements for their degree. Doctoral programs have a strong research emphasis that is essential in the development of the researcher/investigator role.

Practicing occupational and environmental health nurses utilize research findings and can identify possible research questions. Basic research techniques that occupational and environmental health nurses can implement are often used to solve occupational health problems (McKechnie & Rogers, 1985). Examples of researchable topics that occupational and environmental health nurses could examine include effectiveness of health promotion nursing intervention strategies, factors that influence workers' return to work, effects of shift work on worker health and safety, and methods of handling ethical issues related to occupational health (AAOHN, 1999a). For more complex problems or answers to research design questions, the beginning researcher is encouraged to contact an experienced researcher for assistance.

Specific functions of the occupational and environmental health nurse researcher include, but are not limited to, the following activities:

1. Identifies resources that describe relevant research findings and applies them to practice
2. Helps to identify researchable problems/questions
3. Participates in the development and implementation of research in occupational and environmental health nursing
4. Analyzes and interprets data
5. Disseminates research findings to others through presentation, publication, and practice
6. Promotes, assists, and collaborates with occupational and environmental health nurses in developing and conducting research
7. Collaborates with other members of the occupational health team in developing and conducting research
8. Protects the participants' (employees' and employers') rights before the research is conducted
9. Develops research proposals for funding
10. Functions as a mentor to colleagues
11. Maintains competency, professionalism, and ethical conduct

CONSULTANT

The last major role of the occupational and environmental health nurse is that of the occupational and environmental health nurse consultant. The consultant serves as a resource person to other occupational and environmental health nurses, management, members of the occupational health team, and related organizations and agencies. The consultant assists in evaluating and developing occupational health services by recommending specific actions and alternatives. Services are often provided in the areas of administration, education, research, and community resources. However, the consultant generally does not have direct responsibility for implementing or enforcing the recommendations.

"For the nurse, a 'position of consultant' is likely to involve not only specific consultative duties, but also some functioning as a teacher, supervisor, administrator, coordinator, etc." (Lange, 1979, p. 31). To obtain the skills necessary for this multifaceted and complex role, the consultant is a registered professional nurse who has knowledge and experience in occupational and environmental health nursing. The consultant must be able to communicate effectively, both orally and in writing, and possess good administrative, consultative, and listening skills.

Nurse consultants in occupational health are either internal or external to the company. The internal consultant is someone within the company who is given the responsibility to plan and implement constructive change, whereas the external consultant is brought into the company from the outside (Lange, 1987; Nail, 1986; Roy, 1997). Examples of an internal consultant could be a regional director of nursing or a corporate director of nursing; both provide consultation to occupational and environmental health nurses within the company. External occupational and environmental health nurse consultants may be self-employed, employed by an insurance company, hired by a private consulting firm, or located in the occupational health section of a governmental agency, such as a state public health agency or department of labor. The place of employment determines the focus of the consultant's services, fee schedule if applicable, and types of services available. An occupational and environmental health nurse consultant in a state public health agency offers free consultative services to occupa-

tional and environmental health nurses and management but does not have the authority to implement or enforce the recommendations. A consultant hired from a consulting firm charges a fee for specified services but is not responsible for carrying out the suggestions. However, a consultant hired by the U.S. Department of Labor (or its equivalent at the state level) may have enforcement as well as consultative responsibilities, which can be a potential source of conflict for the consultant and the client.

The consultation process is the theoretical base for practice. Although different phases or steps of the process have been identified (Oda, 1982; Ulschak & SnowAntle, 1990), commonalties exist that parallel the nursing process. This is illustrated in Table 4-2 as three key questions are addressed: What is the problem? What can be done about it? Was the problem resolved? (Forti, 1981).

For example, a state occupational health consultant was contacted by an occupational and environmental health nurse (entry and initial contact) for assistance regarding confidentiality of employee health records. The consultant gathered the following information (data gathering): the occupational and environmental health nurse's management was demanding access to employee health records without appropriate justification; the occupational and environmental health nurse refused management's request and was reprimanded as being insubordinate; previous occupational and environmental health nurses at the company allowed management access to employee health records; and there was no policy, written or otherwise, addressing confidentiality. After listening to the occupational and environmental health nurse, the consultant determined the occupational and environmental health nurse's areas of stress, which included how to maintain confidentiality of the records and still keep her job, how to maintain her credibility among employees and keep the employees' trust, and how to maintain an effective occupational health service.

The defined problem (diagnosis) was twofold: (1) management's lack of understanding regarding confidentiality of employee health records and (2) lack of a written policy on that issue. Obviously the occupational and environmental health nurse has a responsibility as a registered professional nurse to practice nursing

TABLE 4-2	Common Phases in the Consultative Process Paralleled With the Nursing Process
NURSING PROCESS	**CONSULTATION PROCESS**
Assessment	Entry, Initial Contact, Data Gathering
	Recognize own needs and motives
	Establish relationship
	Define roles/expectations
	Find out where the client is coming from
	Define the client's relationship to the problem
	Define areas for data gathering
	Build support
	Gather data
Diagnosis	Diagnosis, Feedback, and Decision to Risk
	Define areas of stress
	Define the problem
	Define the objectives
	Acknowledge the problem to be explained
	Agree on the next step
	Determine client responsibility
	Initiate a contract
Planning/Action	Planning and Action
	Determine timing and readiness
	Identify resources
	Identify areas of power and legitimacy
	Determine priorities and goals
	Determine types of intervention
	Identify consequences and impacts of the interventions
	Build understanding and proceed
Evaluation	Evaluation and Recycle; Closure and Termination
	Use client criteria for success
	Evaluate outcome
	Complete contract
	Determine if follow-up is needed
	Write report/summary

according to the standards of occupational and environmental health nursing and the profession's *Code of Ethics*. Both the consultant and the occupational and environmental health nurse agreed that the problems were valid and of concern and that prompt action was needed (feedback and decision to risk). The consultant and the occupational and environmental health nurse discussed strategies (planning) to deal with the problems of education, policy development, and continued refusal of access by management to

records. Among the things also discussed were resources such as the professional associations AAOHN and ANA, pertinent articles, and references such as the *Code of Ethics* and the standards of practice. One identified consequence of the intervention was that the occupational and environmental health nurse could lose her job. The implementation of the recommendations is up to the occupational and environmental health nurse, not the consultant, although the consultant will support the occupational and environmental health nurse's decision—assuming legal and ethical consequences are not the issue. The occupational and environmental health nurse is still working with and educating management about the role of the nurse and her or his responsibility in maintaining the confidentiality of employee health records. A policy on confidentiality has yet to be written. The consultant continues to monitor the occupational and environmental health nurse's progress and will visit the nurse on-site as needed.

Consultation may be requested by the client, who may be an occupational and environmental health nurse or management or a hospital, university, or local health department. Sometimes the consultant may initiate contact with the client to learn about the health services offered to employees. Depending on the expertise of the consultant, assistance may be provided in the following areas:

- Planning and development of a new occupational health service
- Facility design, equipment, and supplies
- Policy and procedure manual
- Job descriptions
- Orientation of new occupational and environmental health nurses
- Computerized record and reporting systems
- Environmental programs
- Health surveillance programs
- Safety
- Immunization
- Confidentiality
- Program development
- Certification
- Specific problems that concern the occupational and environmental health nurse or management or both
- Health promotion and health education programs
- Staffing ratios
- Protocols/clinical guidelines
- Budgeting
- Legislation
- Disaster planning
- Job opportunities
- Continuing education
- Community resources
- References and resources
- Publications
- Research and development

Specific functions of the occupational and environmental health nurse consultant include, but are not limited to, the following activities:

1. Advises clients on the scope and content of employee health services recommended based on needs assessment and analysis
2. Consults with management to stimulate the development of new occupational health programs
3. Assists with orienting nurses new to occupational health and safety
4. Encourages and supports opportunities for occupational and environmental health continuing education
5. Keeps current on issues pertinent to nursing, occupational health and safety, and occupational and environmental health nursing
6. Serves as a resource on acceptable occupational and environmental health nursing practice issues
7. Promotes interdisciplinary health management of toxic or hazardous situations in the work environment
8. Stimulates the introduction of some occupational health content into the basic curricula within a school of nursing
9. Participates in research activities and disseminates the research findings
10. Serves as a resource person for matching occupational and environmental health nurses who are looking for employment with employers who have available positions
11. Provides advice concerning statutes affecting occupational health practice
12. Serves as a preceptor for nursing students
13. Functions as a mentor to colleagues
14. Maintains competency, professionalism, and ethical conduct

FUTURE DIRECTIONS

Occupational and environmental health nurses must remain competent and integrate evidence-based practice and best practices into care management (Hickey et al., 2000). Computer skills are essential, as is the ability to analyze data for trends. In addition, occupational and environmental health nurses must also be visionary in their roles and anticipate what may be coming in order to adapt to these changes. Critical thinking is essential to survival and negotiation within the organization. The occupational and environmental health nurse must be a health and productivity management leader in order to influence the success of business operations (Goetzel & Ozminkowski, 2000).

New roles must be forged as opportunities arise. As technology changes at a rapid pace, what implications exist for practice? Telecommuting is a prime example of how work is changing and of the challenges these changes bring in caring for workers. Distance learning assists in reducing barriers to life-long learning opportunities.

The link between environmental and occupational health will continue to strengthen. More emphasis will be placed on trying to identify common bonds among exposures from home, work, community, and lifestyle activities; this will result in the development of prevention strategies.

Graduate and doctoral programs in occupational and environmental health nursing prepare students to function in these roles. In fact, various industries, agencies, municipalities, and universities have successfully recruited many of the graduates from the programs for advanced clinical, administrative, educational, research, and/or consultative positions.

Other roles are inherent in occupational and environmental health nursing. The occupational and environmental health nurse is an agent of change, a role model, an innovator, a risk taker, and a policy maker. In these capacities the ability and the foresight necessary to lead, motivate, and influence others regarding occupational and environmental health nursing, health, wellness, disease prevention, quality health care, and professionalism are important characteristics. Furthermore, the occupational and environmental health nurse strives to promote fellow occupational and environmental health nurses through networking and mentoring.

Nurses are "responsible and accountable for professional behavior that involves application of the nursing process and cooperation with appropriate others, within current legislation affecting the practice of nursing, according to the profession's code of ethics and of practice, within the context of the policies and practices of the employing agency and within the customs and values of the society in which the nursing care is being provided" (Curtin & Flaherty, 1982, p. 74).

This has direct application to occupational and environmental health nursing practice.

Summary

Each of the seven major roles in occupational and environmental health nursing practice (clinician/practitioner, case manager, health promotion specialist, manager, educator, researcher, and consultant) is essential to the further development, refinement, and advancement of occupational and environmental health nursing. Although a nurse is hired for one of these practice roles, certain aspects of the other roles are often intertwined in her or his practice. For this reason occupational and environmental health nurses must clarify and communicate their individual roles to themselves, their peers, the workers, management, and the public. Regardless of role, each occupational and environmental health nurse is committed to wellness of workers, research and education, standards of practice, personal and professional accountability, quality care and health outcomes, and advancement of occupational and environmental health nursing practice (Randolph, 1988).

References

Amann, M. C. (2000). Developing a strategic plan for the new millennium. *AAOHN Journal, 48*(3), 145-147.

American Academy of Nurse Practitioners. (1998). *Scope of Practice.* Austin, TX: Author.

American Association of Occupational Health Nurses. (1994). *Advisory: Case management.* Atlanta, GA: Author.

American Association of Occupational Health Nurses. (1996). *Code of ethics.* Atlanta, GA: Author.

American Association of Occupational Health Nurses. (1997). *Guidelines for developing job descriptions in occupational & environmental health nursing.* Atlanta, GA: Author.

American Association of Occupational Health Nurses. (1999a). *Research priorities in occupational health nursing.* Atlanta, GA: Author.

American Association of Occupational Health Nurses. (1999b). *Standards of occupational and environmental health nursing.* Atlanta, GA: Author.

Arendasky, K., Radford, J. B., & Bayer, F. J. (1997). Occupational health and safety and occupational health nursing: An overview. In M. Salazar (Ed.), *AAOHN Core Curriculum for Occupational Health Nursing* (p. 20). Philadelphia: W.B. Saunders.

Case Management Society of America. (1995). *Standards of practice for case management.* Little Rock, AR: Author.

Cohen, E. L., & Cesta, T. G. (2001). *Nursing Case Management.* St. Louis, MO: Mosby.

Curtin, L., & Flaherty, M. J. (1982). *Nursing ethics: Theories and pragmatics* (p. 74). Bowie, MD: Robert J. Brady.

Davidson, G., Widtfeldt, A., & Bey, J. (1992a). On-site occupational health nursing services: Estimating the net savings—Part I. *AAOHN Journal, 40*(4), 172-181.

Davidson, G., Widtfeldt, A., & Bey, J. (1992b). On-site occupational health nursing services: Estimating the net savings—Part II. *AAOHN Journal, 40*(5), 242-249.

Dille, J. H. (1999). A worksite influenza immunization program: Impact on lost work days, health care utilization, and health care spending. *AAOHN Journal, 47*(7), 301-309.

Doyle, R., & Rajacich, D. (1991). The Roy Adaptation Model: Health teaching about osteoporosis. *AAOHN Journal, 39*(11), 508-512.

Fein, M. L. (1990). *Role change: A resocialization perspective.* New York: Praeger.

Foran, M., & Campanelli, L. C. (1995). Health promotion communications system: A model for a dispersed population. *AAOHN Journal, 43*(11), 564-569.

Forti, T. J. (1981). Advice: A well-intended ineffectual notion. *Nurse Practitioner, 6*(1), 25-27.

Gillies, D. A. (1994). *Nursing management: A systems approach* (3rd ed.). Philadelphia: W. B. Saunders.

Goetzel, R. Z., & Ozminkowski, R. J. (2000). Health and productivity management: Emerging opportunities for health promotion professionals for the 21st century. *American Journal of Health Promotion, 14*(4), 211-217.

Hardy, M. E., & Conway, M. E. (1988). *Role theory: Perspectives for health professionals* (2nd ed.). Norwalk, CT: Appleton and Lange.

Hickey, J. V., Ouimette, R. M., & Venegoni, S. L. (2000). *Advanced practice nursing: Changing roles and clinical applications* (2nd ed.). Philadelphia: Lippincott Williams & Wilkins.

Javid, L. B., & Lester, M. M. (1983). Occupational health nursing: A model for practice. *Occupational Health Nursing, 31*(3), 38-40.

Kitzman, H. J. (1989). The CNS and the nurse practitioner. In A. B. Hamric & J. A. Spross (Eds.), *The clinical nurse specialist in theory and practice* (2nd ed., pp. 379-394). Philadelphia: W. B. Saunders.

Koku, R. V. (1992). Severity of low back pain: A comparison between participants who did and did not receive counseling. *AAOHN Journal, 40*(2), 84-89.

Lange, F. C. (1987). *The nurse as an individual, group, or community consultant.* Norwalk, CT.: Appleton-Century-Crofts.

Lange, F. M. (1979). The multifaceted role of the nurse consultant. *Journal of Nursing Education, 18*(9), 30-34.

Levin, P. F., Hewitt, J. B., & Misner, S. (1996). Workplace violence: Female occupational homicides in metropolitan Chicago. *AAOHN Journal, 44*(7), 326-331.

Mannon, J. A., Conrad, K. M., Blue, C. L., & Muran, S. (1994). A case management tool for occupational health nurses: Development, testing, and application. *AAOHN Journal, 42*(8), 365-373.

McKechnie, M., & Rogers, B. (1985). Developing research skills in occupational health nursing: Where to begin? *Occupational Health Nursing, 33*(10), 515-516.

McNeese-Smith, D. K. (2000). Job stages of entry, mastery, and disengagement among nurses. *Journal of Nursing Administration, 30*(3), 140-147.

Moore, T. M. (1998). A workplace stretching program: Physiologic and perception measurements before and after participation. *AAOHN Journal, 46*(12), 563-568.

Moss, M. T. (1999). Management forecast: Optimizing the use of organizational and individual knowledge. *Journal of Nursing Administration, 29*(1), 57-62.

Nail, F. C., & Singleton, E. K. (1986). The corporate nurse consultant. *Journal of Nursing Administration, 16*(7, 8), 13-20.

Nelson, M. L., & Olson, D. K. (1996). Health care worker incidents reported in a rural health care facility: A descriptive study. *AAOHN Journal, 44*(3), 115-122.

Oda, D. (1977). Specialized rode development: A three phase process. *Nursing Outlook, 25*(6), 374-377.

Oda, D. S. (1982). Consultation: An expectation of leadership. *Nursing Leadership, 5*(1), 7-9.

Parrish, R. S., & Allred, R. H. (1995). Theories and trends in occupational health nursing: Prevention and social change. *AAOHN Journal, 43*(10), 514-521.

Phillips, J. A., & Brown, K. C. (1992). Industrial workers on rotating shift pattern: Adaptation and injury status. *AAOHN Journal, 40*(10), 468-476.

Putt, A. (1978). *General systems theory applied to nursing.* Boston: Little, Brown & Company.

Randolph, S. A. (1988). Occupational health nursing: A commitment to excellence. *AAOHN Journal, 36*(4), 166-169.

Randolph, S. A., & Dalton, P. C. (1989). Limited duty work: An innovative approach to early return to work. *AAOHN Journal, 37*(11) 446-453.

Randolph, S. A., & Migliozzi, A. A. (1993). The role of the agricultural health nurse: Bringing together community and occupational health. *AAOHN Journal, 41*(9), 429-433.

Rogers, B. (1991). The question and the answer, Part II: Planning for data analysis. *AAOHN Journal, 39*(1), 42-44.

Rogers, B. (1994). *Occupational health nursing: Concepts and practice.* Philadelphia: W. B. Saunders.

Rogers, B. (1997). Beginning in research. *AAOHN Journal, 45*(1), 51-52.

Rogers, B. (1998). Occupational health nursing expertise. *AAOHN Journal, 46*(10), 477-483.

Roy, D. R. (1997). Consulting in occupational health nursing: An overview. *AAOHN Journal, 45*(1), 8-14.

Salazar, M. K. (Ed.). (1997). *AAOHN core curriculum for occupational health nursing.* Philadelphia: W. B. Saunders.

Salazar, M. K., Graham, K. Y., & Lantz, B. (1999). Evaluating case management services for injured workers: Use of a quality assessment model. *AAOHN Journal, 47*(8), 348-354.

Sass, J., Bertolone, K., Denton, D., & Logsdon, M. C. (1995). Exposure to blood and body fluid: Factors associated with non-compliance in follow up HIV testing among health care workers. *AAOHN Journal, 43*(10), 507-513.

Shrey, D. E., & Lacerte, M. (1995). *Principles and practices of disability management in industry.* Winter Park, FL: G. R. Press.

Slagle, M. W., Sun, S. M., & Mathis, M. G. (1998). A conceptual model of occupational health nursing: The resource model. *AAOHN Journal, 46*(3), 121-126.

Snyder, M. (1989) Educational preparation of the CNS. In A. B. Hamric & J. A. Spross (Eds.), *The Clinical Nurse Specialist in Theory and Practice,* (2nd ed., pp. 325-342). Philadelphia: W. B. Saunders.

Tomey, A. M. (2000). *Guide to nursing management and leadership* (6th ed.). St. Louis, MO: Mosby.

Ulschak, F. L. & SnowAntle, S. M. (1990). *Consultation skills for health care professionals.* San Francisco: Jossey-Bass.

von Bertalanffy, L. (1968). *General systems theory.* New York: George Braziller.

White, K., Cox, A. R., & Williamson, G. C. (1999). Competencies in occupational and environmental health nursing: Practice in the new millennium. *AAOHN Journal, 47*(12), 552-568.

Zentner, J., Dellinger, C., Adkins, W. E., & Greene, J. (1995). Nurse practitioner provided primary care: Managing health care costs in the workplace. *AAOHN Journal, 43*(1), 52-53.

Diseases and injuries resulting from work are as old as work itself. Early writings over the centuries by such well known occupational authorities including Bernardino Ramazzini, Agricola, and Paracelsus have described the effects of work and working conditions on health, setting the stage for the beginning of quantitative studies in the eighteenth century. Indeed, Florence Nightingale provided descriptive data about the effects of disease and working conditions on the soldiers at Scutari in the 1860s (see Chapter 2).

Epidemiologic investigations further knowledge about the interactions of environmental determinants, exposure sources, and health and disease in order to develop prevention-driven strategies for health maintenance and public health policy. As a health care professional in a work environment the occupational and environmental health nurse needs to be familiar with epidemiologic concepts and principles in order to determine the nature, relevance, and impact of workplace exposures on illness and injury outcomes and design strategies to mitigate exposure risk. For example, employees may come to the occupational health unit with headaches, skin rashes, or any number of complaints, and the occupational and environmental health nurse will need to know how to investigate potential, related exposures. The epidemiologic approach complements clinical diagnostic care in addressing occupational health problems by focusing on group- or population-derived issues, providing evidence for causal associations, estimating dose-response relationships, and determining the effectiveness of preventive methods (Eisen & Wegman, 2000). Here, the nurse will want to examine health and illness trends in the worker population and apply epidemiologic principles to describe and analyze data that may explain an exposure

occurrence. This chapter will provide a review of epidemiologic concepts and principles that are used in assessing and evaluating health-related events so that measures can be instituted to control and prevent health problems and promote health in worker populations. However, the reader is referred to epidemiologic texts such as Gordis (2000) or Rothman and Grunland (1998) for a more in-depth discussion.

DEFINITIONS AND HISTORICAL UNDERPINNINGS

The term *epidemiology* is derived from the Greek language (*epi,* upon; *demos,* people; and *logos,* science); early epidemiologic investigations were concerned primarily with the study of diseases and disease states that were "upon the people." Epidemiology is the study of the distribution and determinants of diseases and injuries in human populations. Tyler and Last (1992) and Wenzel (1992) provide a broader and widely accepted definition of epidemiology as agreed upon by an international panel of epidemiologists: epidemiology is the study of the distribution and determinants of health-related states and events in specified populations and the application of this study to the control of health problems. This definition provides a conceptual expansion to recognize health determinants and prevention.

Until the early 1900s infectious diseases, such as smallpox, tuberculosis, typhoid, cholera, and diphtheria, constituted the primary causes of mortality in populations. The average life expectancy for newborns in 1900 in the United States was about 47.3 years (Gwatkin & Brandel, 1986) compared with an average of nearly 77 years in 2000 (USDHHS, 2000). Much of this increase is attributable to significant improvements in living and working conditions, sanitation, and hygiene; introduction of antibiotics and vaccines that have helped curb the spread of infectious diseases in at-risk groups; prevention-related strategies to decrease lifestyle risk factors, such as smoking and substance abuse; and an increase in health promotion activities, such as improved nutrition and increased exercise.

With the increased control of infectious diseases in the twentieth century, chronic diseases have become the major causes of death in the United States (Table 5-1). Of the nation's 10 leading causes of death in 1997, the top three—heart disease, cancer, and stroke—accounted for nearly 65% of all deaths. By comparison, pneumonia, which was the chief cause of mortality in 1900 (11.8%), accounted for only 3.7% of all U.S. deaths in 1997 (National Center for Health Statistics [NCHS], 1999).

Workplace exposures also contribute to the development of acute and chronic health problems. The concern about the adverse health effects of occupational exposures dates back to Hippocrates, who urged physicians to explore patients' vocational, environmental, and lifestyle influences as potential determinants for disease etiology (Lilienfeld & Lilienfeld, 1980). Occupational epidemiology is concerned with the study of the effects of these workplace exposures on the frequency distribution of diseases and injuries in worker populations.

The recognition of occupational hazards has often begun with anecdotal reports of debilitating conditions or acute traumatic events related to the job; these reports have then led to epidemiologic investigations. For example, Agricola reported premature mortality among miners in the sixteenth century; later mortality surveys described excessive rates of respiratory disease and cancer among underground metal miners (Hunter, 1978; Lorenz, 1944; Peller, 1939; Pirchan & Sikl, 1932).

Percival Pott (1775) described the exposure of chimney sweeps to soot as the cause for scrotal cancer and is credited with providing the first substantiated evidence of chemical carcinogenesis from an occupational exposure (Waldron, 1983). Other classic studies have shown morbidity and mortality patterns, including deaths among asbestos insulation workers due to lung cancer (Selikoff et al., 1964; Selikoff et al., 1979), and bladder cancer among dyestuff factory workers (Case et al., 1954; Goldwater et al., 1965; Wendell et al., 1974).

TABLE 5-1   Leading Causes of Death as a Percentage of All Deaths in the United States 1900 and 1997*

1900		1997	
Pneumonia/influenza	11.8	Heart disease	31.4
Tuberculosis	11.2	Cancer	23.3
Diarrhea/enteritis	8.3	Stroke	6.9
Heart disease	6.2	Chronic obstructive pulmonary disease	4.7
Liver disease	5.2	Unintentional injuries	4.1
Injuries	4.2	Pneumonia/influenza	3.7
Cancer	3.7	Diabetes	2.7
Senility	2.9	Suicide	1.3
Diptheria	2.3	Chronic liver disease and cirrhosis	1.1
		Kidney diseases	1.1

Data from *Vital Statistics of the United States, 1997,* by National Center for Health Statistics, Washington, DC: U.S. Department of Health and Human Services. 1999.

*In 1900 deaths in the United States were reported only by 10 states and only on 9 leading causes.

Studies in occupational health and disease have expanded to examine work practices and behaviors of workers in order to determine associated risks of exposure and identify factors that may contribute to or minimize exposure risk. Behavioral risk factors are important determinants of some diseases that also interact with occupational exposures and therefore require investigation within the framework of occupational epidemiologic research.

The natural history of disease is an evolving, interactive process that occurs over time, and in the case of chronic and many occupational diseases this process occurs in stages that may take years to become apparent. Thus, determining the causes of chronic and many occupational diseases—and thereby the development of preventive strategies to reduce exposure or disease risk—can be particularly difficult. In addition, depending on the specific conditions several factors, including lifestyle and environmental influences, may be collectively involved, and this may result in conflicting or confounding evidence as to the cause of the problem. For example, is smoking or exposure to wool or ceramic fibers the cause of lung cancer, or is there an interactive process involved with smoking related to this disease outcome? The development of new methodologies and refinement of existing ones, including data collection techniques and analyses, provide for improved quantification of (1) the magnitude of the exposure-disease relationship in humans; (2) the alteration of the risk through interventions; and (3) information to serve as the foundation for public health policy decisions.

Observations of workplace conditions and exposures associated with symptom or disease occurrence and the analysis of recorded data about such factors as illness or injury, environment, work practices, and occupational health unit visits provide the basis for designing health protection, health promotion, and surveillance and monitoring programs. The occupational and environmental health nurse must be involved not only in the accurate collection of data but also in the evaluation of outcomes and determination of effective control and prevention procedures to minimize risk exposure. Through increased understanding of epidemiologic concepts and principles, such as the dynamics of health/disease processes and determinates, environmental relationships and interactions, and approaches to

measurement and study design, the occupational and environmental health nurse will be in a position to collaborate more effectively in decisions affecting the health and safety of workers and determine programmatic policy efforts.

EPIDEMIOLOGIC CONCEPTS

The units of concern in the field of epidemiology are the population and its subgroups. Illness and injury conditions are unevenly dispersed throughout the population; therefore, studying the frequency characteristics of disease and injury in groups and trying to tie together related associations between health and illness patterns can help determine if causal relationships exist, can be inferred, or can be predicted.

The basic concept underlying epidemiologic approaches is related to the theory of multiple causation, wherein the development of disease is dependent on the interaction of several factors and cannot be attributed to any single factor alone. Several models have been used to illustrate this interaction, all of which specify a relationship between the host (living species/individual human) and the environment and related elements (external factors that influence the host health state). One model, referred to as the epidemiologic triad, depicts a relationship among three variables, the host, the agent (a factor such as a virus or chemical necessary to produce the condition or disease), and the environment that promotes the exposure (Figure 5-1). Although some diseases are largely genetic in origin, virtually all disease results

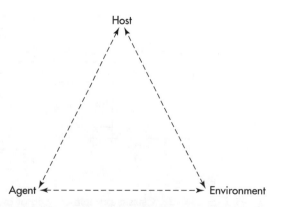

Figure 5-1 Epidemiologic triad depicting dynamic agent-host-environment relationship.

from an interaction of genetic and environmental factors with the exact balance differing for different diseases (Gordis, 2000). This model, still widely used, implies a dynamic relationship among the three variables or factors, with any change in this relationship resulting in either positive or negative influences toward health or illness.

MacMahon and Pugh (1970) offer a classic and conceptually similar model, the web of causation. This model relates multiple factors and linkages involved in a particular health condition or problem (in this example, hepatitis) in which the agent is an integral part of the environment (Figure 5-2). Another example is the development of coronary heart disease, which is influenced by both intrinsic host factors, such as age, genetics, and previous medical history, and extrinsic factors, such as occupation, diet, medication, smoking habits, and exercise. Examples of selected agent, host, and environmental factors adapted in part from Lilienfeld and Lilienfeld (1980) (Table 5-2) are briefly discussed.

AGENT FACTORS

An agent may be thought of as a substance that must be present for a disease or condition to occur (see Table 5-2, I). Transmission of an agent to a host may be accomplished in a variety of ways. For example, toxic chemical agent exposure may occur through toxic vapors inhaled, poisons ingested, or toxins absorbed through the skin. Infectious diseases are spread by infectious agents through direct or indirect contact. For example, direct contact, or person-to-person transmission, may occur through sneezing or sexual intercourse, whereas indirect contact transmission may occur through a contaminated water supply. Exposure to infections/biological agents such as the human immunodeficiency virus, hepatitis B virus, and cytomegalovirus poses threats for disease development in health care and laboratory workers. For example, the agent of hepatitis B is a virus, and the reservoir that perpetuates the agent is an individual infected with the virus. The mode of conveyance of the organism is through contact

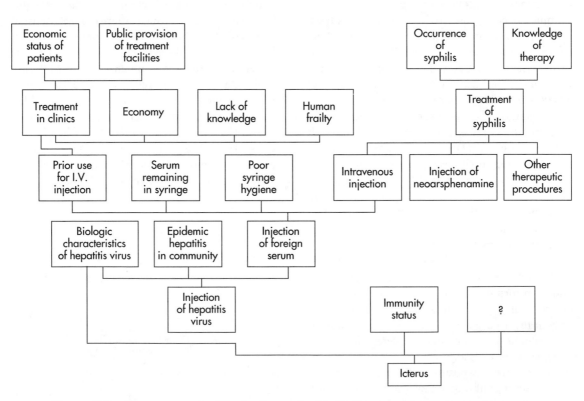

Figure 5-2 Classic example of "web of causation" indicating some components of association between syphilis treatment and serum hepatitis. *(From* Epidemiologic Principles and Methods, *by B. MacMahon and T. F. Pugh, 1970, Boston: Little, Brown & Company.)*

with infected body fluids, and the route or portal of entry is through intimate sexual contact, perinatally, permucosally, or percutaneously via injection with a contaminated needle (e.g., a needlestick injury) or contact with a contaminated sharp (NIOSH, 1998). Routes of entry, including direct contact, inhalation, ingestion, injection, and skin absorption, and modes of transmission, such as airborne droplet spray or contaminated needle, are impor-tant factors related to both the virulence and resultant pathogenicity of the agent.

Chemical agents are well-recognized hazardous substances and take the form of dusts, fumes, gases, liquids, or vapors. Thousands of chemicals

TABLE 5-2 Classification by Selected Agents, Host Factors, and Environmental Factors that Influence the Health and Distribution of Diseases in Human Populations

I. AGENTS OF DISEASE (NECESSARY ETIOLOGIC FACTORS)	EXAMPLES OF RESULTING DISEASE OUTCOMES
A. Biological agents	
Bacteria	Gonorrhea, Lyme disease, pneumonia, staphylococcal/streptococcal infections, syphilis, tuberculosis
Fungi	Candidiasis, dermatophyte infections, histoplasmosis
Rickettsia	Rocky Mountain spotted fever
Viruses	AIDS, hepatitis, herpes, influenza, rabies, rubella, upper respiratory tract infections
B. Chemical agents	
Poisons	Asbestos, arsenic, carbon monoxide, hydrogen sulfide, drugs
Allergens	Medications, poison ivy, ragweed
C. Physical agents	Cold, heat, ionizing radiation, noise
D. Psychosocial	Family stress, personal or work conflicts, work organizational issues
II. HOST FACTORS (INTRINSIC FACTORS)—INFLUENCE EXPOSURE, SUSCEPTIBILITY, OR RESPONSE TO AGENTS	EXAMPLES
A. Genetic profile	Sickle cell disease
B. Age	
C. Gender	
D. Ethnic group	
E. Physiologic state	Fatigue, nutritional state, pregnancy, puberty, resistance, stress
F. Family history	Physiologic profile Health ↔ Disease states
G. Prior immunologic experience	
Active	Hypersensitivity, immunization, prior infection
Passive	Gamma globulin prophylaxis, maternal antibodies
H. Intercurrent or preexisting disease	
I. Human behavior/lifestyle factors	Diet, exercise, food handling, health resources, occupation, personal hygiene, recreation, interpersonal relations, substance abuse, utilization of health resources, marital status, religion

Modified from *Foundations of Epidemiology* by A. Lilienfeld and D. Lilienfeld, New York: Oxford University Press. 1980. *Continued*

TABLE 5-2	Classification by Selected Agents, Host Factors, and Environmental Factors that Influence the Health and Distribution of Diseases in Human Populations — cont'd
III. ENVIRONMENTAL FACTORS (EXTRINSIC FACTORS) — INFLUENCE EXISTENCE OF AGENT, EXPOSURE, OR SUSCEPTIBILITY TO AGENT	**EXAMPLES**
A. Physical environment	Climate, geology wastes, temperature, altitude
Housing	Density
B. Nutrient sources	Food sources (fauna, flora), milk, water
C. Socioeconomic environment	Social support
D. Occupational setting	Exposure to hazardous agents
E. Urbanization and economic development	Urban crowding, literacy, health care access, air pollution
F. Environmental disruption	Disasters, wars, bioterrorism

Modified from *Foundations of Epidemiology by* A. Lilienfeld and D. Lilienfeld, New York: Oxford University Press. 1980.

are prevalent in the workplace, and many of them cause acute, chronic, local, and systemic effects in the human system. Examples include asbestos (asbestosis and lung cancer), benzene (aplastic anemia and leukemia), cotton dust (byssinosis), vinyl chloride (liver cancer), latex (latex allergy), and various contact agents (dermatoses).

Another chemical agent, lead, is commercially produced by mining, smelting, refining, and secondary recovery. Lead is primarily used in the manufacture of storage batteries and in numerous other applications such as paints, plastics, ceramics, electrical cables, and shielding. Workers in these fields are at greatest risk of exposure (Lewis, 1990; WHO, 1986). Lead and its components enter the body through inhalation and ingestion from exposure to lead dust and fumes in operating processes such as grinding, welding, and spray painting and in the manufacture of such products as paints, pigments, and lead batteries. Absorption through the skin is limited to certain organic compounds. Once absorbed, lead is transported through the bloodstream to several organ systems (e.g., brain, kidney, liver, skin, and skeletal muscle); however, the bone constitutes the major site of deposition. Acute and chronic clinical effects may be manifested in disturbances in related body systems, such as the gastrointestinal, hematopoietic, nervous, renal, musculoskeletal, and reproductive systems.

Physical agents may interact with the susceptible host to cause some form of tissue trauma, as, for example, with high levels of noise exposure. The largest number of workers exposed to noise levels potentially damaging to their hearing are in the manufacturing sector. Usually noise-induced hearing loss develops gradually as a result of damage to the sensory hair cells in the cochlea from prolonged loud exposures. The relative hazard to hearing from exposure to continuous or interrupted impact or impulse noise depends on the intensity, duration, and frequency composition of the noise. Metabolic exhaustion and mechanical injury are the presumed mechanisms underlying cochlear damage from noise exposure. In metabolic exhaustion the sensory cells cannot keep pace with the energy demands placed on them. Once the sensory hair cells that respond to a given frequency are destroyed, sounds at that frequency are no longer heard. Destroyed hair cells cannot repair themselves (Levy & Wegman, 2000).

Psychosocial agents (stressors) such as interpersonal conflicts or work organization issues (excessive workloads, time demands, downsizing, depersonalization, and shiftwork) may create highly stressful conditions leading to both physiological and psychological problems (Caplan, 1998; Seigrest, 1996; USDHHS/NIOSH, 1996). For example, shiftwork is associated with the disruption of circadian rhythms and decrement in human performance, which may increase errors and injuries.

HOST FACTORS

Host factors such as age, gender, ethnicity, genetic profile, family history, lifestyle risk factors, and health status (see Table 5-2, II) are intrinsic to the individual. An agent-host interaction occurs once an agent is transmitted to a susceptible host. Susceptibility is dependent on host defenses and inherent resistance, virulence of the agent, and environmental conditions. Immunity is the host's resistance to a specific infectious agent and can be active or passive. Active immunity occurs as an antigen-antibody induced response, generally protects an individual for life, and can be attained naturally by actual infection (e.g., measles, rubella) or artificially by vaccine inoculation designed to stimulate an antibody response (as with pneumococcal or hepatitis B vaccines). Active immunity forms the basis for mass vaccination programs, such as those for influenza virus. Passive immunity is temporary and is provided by an antibody produced in another host. Passive immunity may be acquired naturally through maternal-fetal antibody transfer or artificially by administration of an antibody-containing preparation, such as gamma globulin (Benenson, 2000).

Inherent resistance refers to the host's ability to resist disease unassociated with antibody production and response, and thereby reflects the host's ability to respond not only to infectious agent exposures but also to other types of agent exposures, such as chemical inhalation and stress. Resistance is related to the physiological and health state of the individual. Factors such as good nutrition, regular exercise, proper rest, and activities aimed at general health promotion will probably positively affect resistance to infection or a disease process, even though immunity may or may not be a factor. For example, the relationship between coronary heart disease and the influences of preexisting high blood pressure, smoking, exercise, diet, and occupational stress is well-documented (Doll and Bill, 1964; Goetzel et al., 1998; LIPID Study, 1998; NHLBI, 1998; Olsen & Kristensen, 1991; Psaty et al., 1997; Sempos et al., 1993; Willett et al., 1999). Evidence

regarding the interplay of personality factors have yet to be proven (Sauter et al., 1997).

Two concepts related to the spread of infectious diseases among people or in populations—incubation period and herd immunity—are particularly important. Incubation period refers to the time interval from receipt of infection to onset of clinical illness (Gordis, 2000; Sartwell, 1973). One may become infected today but not develop disease for days, weeks, or longer. However, communicability is usually present during this time. Different diseases have different incubation periods. A classic example is the mumps virus, whose maximum communicability occurs approximately 48 hours before its clinical manifestation. Hepatitis B virus blood infectivity has been shown to occur many weeks before the onset of first symptoms, through the acute clinical course of the disease, and during the carrier state (Benenson, 2000).

The incubation period of infectious diseases has its analog in noninfectious diseases. Thus even when an individual is exposed to a carcinogen or other toxin, the disease is often manifested only after months or years. For example, mesotheliomas resulting from asbestos exposure may occur 20 to 30 years after exposure; this period of time between exposure and onset of symptoms is referred to as the latent period (Gordis, 2000).

Herd immunity is defined as the resistance of a group to an attack by a disease to which a large proportion of the members of the group are immune (Gordis, 2000). This concept is based on the principle that the spread or halt of infection in a particular community or group will be related to the proportion of susceptible or resistant hosts at risk of infection. In other words there must be a relatively large pool of people susceptible to or at risk of acquiring infection for a disease to continue to spread. If a sufficient number of individuals in the population are immune, the spread of disease will be interrupted because of lack of infectious reservoirs or hosts; in other words the likelihood of person-to-person spread decreases. It is generally believed that for most infectious agents 100% population immunity is not needed to prevent an epidemic or control disease spread; however, how much below the 100% level is sufficient to disrupt the spread of disease is unclear. For example, in the case of measles an estimated 94% of the population would need to be immune to break the chain of transmission (Gordis, 2000). In recent years significant outbreaks of measles have occurred in the United States, with approximately 40% of the cases occurring in individuals with a history of previous vaccination. In addition to routine revaccination at school entry, revaccination should also be required of those entering educational institutions beyond high school or workers entering hospital employment, unless measles history or two-dose measles vaccination is documented (Benenson, 2000).

Genetic influences are now thought to play a more prominent role in either increased or decreased host susceptibility to certain diseases. For example, persons with sickle cell trait seem to have a decreased risk of malaria, and individuals with xeroderma pigmentosum have a genetically determined inability to repair ultraviolet light-induced damage, thus placing them at greater risk of skin cancer related to sun exposure. This would pose a potential hazard to workers, such as construction workers, gardeners, and aircraft workers, who have this condition and are occupationally exposed to the sun (Zenz, 1993). In addition, human behavior, in terms of lifestyle practices, is important to consider because this will contribute to the impact of risk factors on health status.

ENVIRONMENTAL FACTORS

Physical and social environments represent external conditions that interact with the host and the agent (see Table 5-2, III). The physical environment involves the geological and atmospheric structures of an area and the source of such elements as water, temperature, and radiation, which may be positive or negative stressors. Humans generally have a great deal of control over the physical environment through the provision of adequate shelter against extremes of weather, purification of drinking water, treatment of sewage, and control of ventilation. However, new environmental problems, such as increases in industrial wastes and toxins and indoor and outdoor environmental pollution, continue to surface as significant health threats to the working and general population.

The social aspects of the environment encompass the economic and political forces affecting society and its health and include factors such as sanitation/hygiene practices, housing conditions, level and delivery of health care services, development and enforcement of health-related standards (e.g., occupational health and safety, pollution), employment conditions, population crowding, lit-

eracy, extent of support for health-related research, and equitable access to health care. Addictive behaviors such as alcohol and substance abuse and various forms of psychosocial stress may be an outgrowth of negative social environments.

The occupational environment comprises the workplace and work setting and their interactive effects on the worker. One must consider the hazards and threats posed by the work environment and the commitment of the employer to providing a safe and healthful workplace through use of preventive strategies and controls (e.g., engineering and substitution).

DESCRIPTIVE EPIDEMIOLOGY

Within an epidemiologic framework investigations generally begin with observations and recording of information related to the condition or event of interest, such as disease or injury. Data are then derived relative to patterns of health and illness and expressed quantitatively in terms such as *frequencies, percentages,* or *rates.* To describe the occurrence of illness or injury in a population, such as a group of workers, certain questions—Who is affected? Where and when do cases occur?—must be answered. These types of questions specify the relationships among person, place, and time and therefore provide descriptive information from which hypotheses about associations or causal relationships can be generated for future analytical epidemiologic investigations.

PERSON

Although numerous variables characterize individuals, the personal variables age, gender, and ethnic/racial group are generally the most important to consider in epidemiologic study. Examination of personal characteristics will help to determine risk factors associated with individuals who get a particular disease. Occupation is increasingly recognized as a variable that has significant impact on the health outcome of exposed populations and provides important data regarding the determinants of health/illness relationships.

Age is probably the most important personal variable and is strongly tied to morbidity (illness/injury) and mortality (death) rates of most conditions. With respect to morbidity acute infectious processes occur most commonly in children, whereas accidents occur more frequently in older children, teenagers, and young adults. Adults may experience conditions related to occupational exposure (e.g., musculoskeletal injuries, respiratory disorders, dermatoses, cancer, and stress), and chronic disease conditions such as arthritis and hypertension increase in frequency with age. Death rates are fairly high in infancy, decrease during childhood, begin to rise gradually until middle age, and then increase sharply with age.

Gender plays a significant role in morbidity and mortality patterns; morbidity rates are generally higher for females than males, but mortality rates are higher for males than females at every age. Coronary heart disease, lung cancer, homicide, cirrhosis of the liver, and chronic obstructive lung disease are more common among men, whereas arthritis and depression are more common in women (USDHHS, 2000). Life expectancy has consistently been higher for females than for males. For 1995 these rates were 78.9 years (females) and 72.5 years (males) (NCHS, 1999).

Racial and ethnic differences exist in both morbidity and mortality and may be related to differences in socioeconomic status, education, and access to health care. Blacks in the United States have higher rates of hypertension, cerebrovascular accidents, homicide, and accidental deaths, while whites have higher rates of death from atherosclerotic heart disease, suicide, and leukemia (NCHS, 1999). Inherited diseases such as sickle cell anemia are primarily restricted to blacks, whereas cystic fibrosis occurs mostly in whites. The nonwhite population in the United States has an average life expectancy of 6 years less than that of the white population (NCHS, 1999).

Because people spend a substantial portion of their lives in the workplace, occupationally related experiences and the work environment itself can contribute significantly to both morbidity and mortality. These influences may occur through a variety of exposures (e.g., chemicals, noise, stress, and infectious agents). Personal work practices and habits play an important role in health maintenance and health protection, particularly as they relate to workplace exposures. Observations of work practice behaviors will contribute to the assessment of workplace exposures, which are further discussed in the next section.

Other influences such as lifestyle behaviors, personality traits, and the degree, quality, and utilization of health care will affect, at least in part, morbidity and mortality rates.

PLACE

Differences exist globally in life expectancy (Table 5-3) and in the most prevalent types of diseases. The occurrence and frequency of disease in individuals often vary by place. Natural boundaries may play a role in the frequency distribution of certain diseases such that certain epidemics may be contained in populations due in part to geographic contours such as mountain ranges. Some cancers show distinct geographic patterns; higher rates of melanoma in the South implicate sun ray exposure as contributing to the pathogenesis of malignant melanoma. Lead poisoning also displays a geographic pattern where airborne lead particulates occur in communities surrounding lead smelters. Multiple sclerosis is much more prevalent in northern latitudes than in southern regions; however, the cause of this is unclear (Hennekens & Buring, 1987). Examining disease rates in groups within specific geographic areas, such as defined population areas, specific industries, and areas surrounding industrial sites, is helpful in etiologic reasoning. For example, Figure 5-3 shows the distribution of Rocky Mountain spotted fever in the United States in 1993, with a clear clustering of cases along the East Coast and south central areas (CDC, 1994).

Health differences are noted between urban and rural populations. People living in urban areas are faced with overcrowding, social problems including homicide, and increasing problems of substance abuse and violence-related crimes. The concentration of industrial worksites has led to increased problems with air pollution and toxic waste dumping. In the past 50 years there has been a significant shift in the population distribution from farms to urban areas (approximately 70% in 1980). For many people remaining in rural areas, illiteracy, lack of job opportunities, malnutrition, and limited access to health care continue. Health problems of the farm community remain largely unrecognized and understudied. Data from the National Safety Council (1998) indicate that injury and death rates in agriculture consistently rank it among the top three hazardous industries. The mortality rate for agricultural workers in 1997 was 20 per 100,000 workers, compared to rates of 13 (construction) and 24 (mining) per 100,000 workers. Farm accidents

TABLE 5-3   Life Expectancy at Birth by Gender and Ranked by Selected Countries, 1995

FEMALE		MALE	
COUNTRY	LIFE EXPECTANCY	COUNTRY	LIFE EXPECTANCY
Japan	82.9	Japan	76.4
France	82.6	Sweden	76.2
Switzerland	81.9	Israel	75.3
Sweden	81.6	Canada	75.2
Spain	81.5	Switzerland	75.1
Canada	81.2	Greece	75.1
Australia	80.9	Australia	75.0
Italy	80.8	Norway	74.9
Norway	80.7	Netherlands	74.6
Netherlands	80.4	Italy	74.4
Greece	80.3	England & Wales	74.3
Finland	80.3	France	74.2
Austria	80.1	Spain	74.2
Germany	79.8	Austria	73.5
Belgium	79.8	Singapore	73.4
England & Wales	79.6	Germany	73.3
Israel	79.3	New Zealand	73.3
Singapore	79.0	Northern Ireland	73.1
United States	**78.9**	Belgium	73.0
		Cuba	73.0
		Costa Rica	73.0
		Finland	72.8
		Denmark	72.8
		Ireland	72.5
		United States	**72.5**

From *Healthy People 2010*, by U.S. Department of Health and Human Services, Washington, DC: Author. 2000.

remain a serious cause of death and disability due to exposure to dangerous equipment, pesticides and other chemicals, and microorganisms.

Migrant workers face difficult living and working conditions, and their health problems remain serious. For these workers cultural and language differences have been shown to be barriers to health care, particularly primary care access. The stresses of the job may vary with the type of crop involved; however, the range of agent exposures is broad and includes pesticide exposure, crop exposure (e.g., tobacco), snake bites, mechanical trauma, sun exposure, and difficult environmental conditions.

Epidemiologic studies have related many disorders and diseases to occupational hazards or exposures: back injury from heavy lifting (Anderson,

1997; Bigos, 1994; Bigos et al., 1992; Chaffin & Park, 1973); reproductive toxicity (Hemminki et al., 1985; Marbury, 1992; Murphy & Graziano., 1990; Scialli, 1993); noise-induced hearing loss (Kryter, 1994; Morata et al., 1993; OSHA, 1983); neurologic and behavioral disorders related to metal and solvent exposure (Baker et al., 1985; Feldman, 1999; WHO & Nordic Council of Ministers, 1985); kidney impairment due to cadmium exposure (Roels et al., 1993; Roels et al., 1997; Thun, 1993); coronary artery disease from carbon monoxide exposure (Stern & Steenland, 1993); and lung and cancer disorders previously described. Carcinogenic occupational substances are listed in Table 5-4.

As a health care professional in an occupational environment, the occupational and environmental

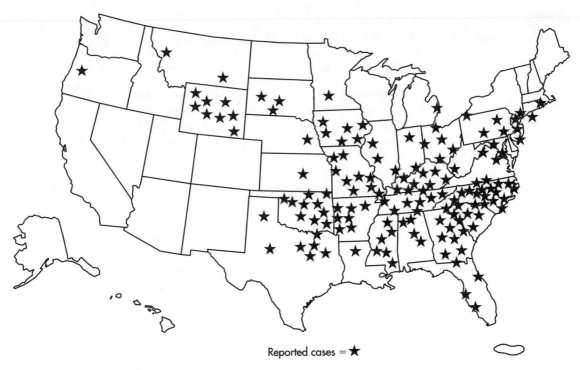

Figure 5-3   Distribution of Rocky Mountain spotted fever by counties reporting cases, U.S., 1993. *(From "Summary of Notifiable Diseases, 1993," by Centers for Disease Control and Prevention, 1994,* Morbidity and Mortality Weekly Report, 42.)

health nurse must be familiar with epidemiologic concepts in order to evaluate workplace exposures. For example, an employee may be concerned about the reproductive effects of job-related chemical exposure. Assessing the nature and scope of workplace exposures, including information about types of jobs, length of employment, potential and specific exposures, (including intensity and duration), and actual agent sampling measurements, are important in quantifying exposure. Variations in exposure due to differences in work performed, work habits and practices, use of personal protective equipment, and general workplace environmental hygiene are important determinants in making risk estimates about disease occurrence.

TIME

The study of disease as related to time of occurrence is basic to epidemiologic investigation. Morbidity and mortality events should be examined not only as a precedent to disease occurrence but also as trends occurring over time. For example, the American Cancer Society's Department of Epidemiology and Surveillance

reports a favorable change in cancer direction, with a reduction in the total number of new cancer cases and in cancer death rates in the United States. In addition, 5-year survival rates continue to improve for most cancer patients (except those with cancer of the lung and bronchus) (Rosenthal, 1998). Specifically, between 1990 and 1994 deaths decreased 1.4% per year for lung cancer among men, 0.5% per year for prostrate cancer, and 1.9% and 1.5% per year among men and women, respectively, for colon and rectal cancer. In addition, breast cancer deaths among women decreased 1.8%, but deaths caused by lung cancer continue to increase among women (Landis et al., 1998).

Time trends of disease patterns may also occur in cycles, such as seasonal epidemics of variant types of influenza virus and other types of infectious diseases (e.g., pneumonia, the common cold, and respiratory infections). However, some of this may be explained by crowding of groups of people into confined spaces in winter months (including the workplace) and other lifestyle habits such as lack of exercise and poor nutrition.

TABLE 5-4	Agents Related to Occupationally Induced Cancer	
AGENT	**SITE OR TYPE OF CANCER**	**OCCUPATION**
Aromatic amines	Bladder	Dye manufacturers, rubber workers, coal gas manufacturers
4-Aminobiphenyl	Bladder	Dye manufacturers
Arsenic	Skin, lung	Copper and cobalt smelters, arsenical pesticide manufacturers, some gold miners
Asbestos	Lung, pleura, peritoneum	Asbestos miners, asbestos textile manufacturers, asbestos insulation workers, certain shipyard workers
Benzene	Marrow, leukemia	Workers with glues and varnishes
Benzidine 2-Naphthylamine	Bladder	Garment, leather, printing, paper workers
Bischloromethyl ether	Lung	Makers of ion-exchange resins, polymer makers
Cadmium	Prostate	Cadmium workers
Chromium	Lung	Manufacturers of chromates from chrome ore, pigment manufacturers
Coke oven emissions	Lung, GI, pancreas, kidney	Coke oven workers
Ionizing radiations	Lung	Uranium and some other miners
	Bone	Luminizers
	Marrow, all sites	Radiologists, radiographers
Isopropyl oil	Nasal sinuses	Isopropyl alcohol manufacturers
Mineral oils, untreated and mildly treated	Skin	Metal working, printing
Mustard gas	Larynx, lung	Poison gas manufacturers
Nickel	Nasal sinuses, lung	Nickel refiners
Polycyclic hydrocarbons in soot, coal tar, oil	Skin, scrotum, lung, bladder	Coal gas manufacturers, roofers, asphalters, aluminum refiners, many groups selectively exposed to certain tars and oils
Talc containing asbestiform fibers	Lung	Miners
UV light	Skin	Farmers, seamen
Vinyl chloride	Liver	PVC manufacturers

Data from *Ninth Report on Carcinogens,* by National Toxicology Program, Washington, DC: U.S. Department of Health and Human Services, U.S. Public Health Service. 1998.

Considerable interest lies in exploring factors related to clustering of events or diseases. For example, the occurrence of dermatitis in a group of workers or increased reproductive insults should be investigated with respect to the relationship of an exposure to time and place and take into consideration the personal variables of those exposed, such as home-based exposures and smoking habits.

MEASURES OF DISEASE FREQUENCY

In order to describe the distribution and patterns of occurrence of illness, injury, or health outcome in a population, the occurrence of the event outcome of interest must be quantified. (For ease of discussion the term *disease* will be used primarily for outcome

TABLE 5-5	Rates Most Frequently Used as Indices of Population Health	
RATES		**USUAL POPULATION FACTOR**
GENERAL MORTALITY		
Crude death rate = Number of deaths in a year/ Average (midyear) population		per 100,000 population
Cause-specific death rate = Number of deaths from a stated cause in a year/Average (midyear) population		per 100,000 population
Age-specific death rate = Number of deaths among persons in given age group in a year/Average (midyear) population in specified age group		per 100,000 population
Proportional mortality rate = Number of deaths from specific percent of deaths/Total deaths in a same time period		percent of deaths
Case-fatality rate = Number cases of specified disease/ Number of deaths due to specified disease		per 100 cases
MORBIDITY		
Incidence = Number of new cases of disease (condition) during a specified time period/Population at risk for same time period		per 100,000 population
Point prevalence = Number of existing cases (conditions) at a point in time/Total population at same time point		per 100,000 population

of interest.) The most basic measure of disease occurrence is the frequency, number, or simple count of affected individuals or events. However, without a reference point the number of health/illness events itself has limited utility in making statements about the determinants and distribution of disease. Yet when the frequency is expressed in relation to the size of the affected or at-risk population and the time frame of occurrence, it is called a rate and is of great value in comparing groups with the disease or the outcome under consideration. A rate is defined as follows:

$$\frac{\text{Number of events (cases or deaths) in a specific period}}{\text{Number of persons (population) at risk of these events (cases or deaths) in a specified period}} \times k \text{ (population constant)}$$

The numerator of the rate includes all those with the disease or event being counted, and the denominator is the population (number of persons) at risk for the disease or event. Rates of disease are called morbidity rates, and rates of death are called mortality rates. For ease of comparing

two rates, a population constant k is used and expressed in terms of multiples of 10, such as 100, 1,000, 10,000, or 100,000. Most vital statistics are reported per 100,000 population. For example, the crude population death rate (NCHS, 2000) for all persons in the United States in 1998 was 867.3 per 100,000 population, which is expressed as follows:

$$\frac{\begin{array}{c}\text{Deaths in U.S residents}\\\text{in 1998 (2,344,303)}\end{array}}{\begin{array}{c}\text{U.S. population}\\\text{in 1998 (270,299,000)}\end{array}} \times 100,000$$

Examples of common rate measures are shown in Table 5-5. The choice of the population constant (i.e., 100, 1,000, 10,000) is arbitrary.

INCIDENCE RATES AND PREVALENCE RATES

Two basic rates are used in epidemiology: incidence rates and prevalence rates.

Incidence Rates

The incidence rate measures the number of new cases of disease occurring during a specified period of time (see Table 5-5). It is a measure of the probability of risk for which new disease develops in previously disease-free individuals. To determine the incidence of a disease, it is necessary to know the actual number of persons or cases with disease (numerator data), the time period of disease occurrence, and the population at-risk of exposure or disease development. The at-risk population must be accurately enumerated and theoretically should not include those who already have disease (or in the case of infectious diseases those who are not susceptible because of immunity). For incidence to be meaningful, any individual who is included in the denominator must have the potential to become part of the group that is counted in the numerator. Thus, if we are calculating incidence for uterine cancer, the denominator must include only women because men would not have the potential to become part of the group that is counted by the numerator—that is, men are not at-risk for developing uterine cancer (Gordis, 2000).

Incidence is measured as follows:

$$\text{Incidence per 1,000} = \frac{\begin{array}{c}\text{Number of \textit{new} cases}\\\text{of a disease (or injury)}\\\text{occurring in the}\\\text{population during a}\\\text{specified period of time}\end{array}}{\begin{array}{c}\text{Number of persons at-risk}\\\text{of developing the disease}\\\text{(or injury) during that}\\\text{period of time}\end{array}} \times 1000$$

In this rate the quotient (result) is multiplied by 1,000 so that the incidence is expressed per 1,000 persons. However, the choice of 1,000 is arbitrary, and 100, 10,000, 100,000 or any other number could be used.

As an example, to determine the incidence of hypertension in a population of workers at a telecommunications company, it is necessary to know the number of workers actually diagnosed with hypertension during a specified time period, usually 1 year (although it may be any length of time), and the total number of workers employed and at-risk, thus excluding those previously diagnosed with hypertension. This means that if the condition is common or if precise information is desired the denominator should only include those at-risk (those without disease) (Nowell, 1995). The number of persons at-risk is likely to change over time; therefore the population at midpoint of the period would be used to represent the average population at-risk. (If the disease frequency is low and the population is large, this correction to the population denominator would make little statistical difference.)

In this example suppose the total population of workers in 1998 was 2,050. A health record review identified 214 individuals with a preexisting diagnosis of hypertension. During 1998 all employees were screened for high blood pressure, and 21 additional employees were diagnosed with hypertension. The incidence rate is calculated to be 11.4 per 1,000 employees ($\frac{21}{2050-214} \times 1000$). Again, note here that the population constant of 1,000 is an arbitrary choice.

As another example, the reporting of 3 cases of infectious hepatitis in Industry A, 9 cases in Industry B, and 10 cases in Industry C might lead to the conclusion that hepatitis is a more common and serious problem in both Industries B and C. However, as shown in Table 5-6, the annual rate of occurrence in Industry A is higher than in either Industries B or C. The populations in both Industries B and C are larger, and to compare the actual incidence in all populations, it is necessary to

TABLE 5-6 Comparison of Incidence Rates

Location	New Cases of Hepatitis	Reporting Period	Industry Population
Industry A	3	1997	10,000
Industry B	9	1997-1999	30,000
Industry C	10	1998-1999	25,000

ANNUAL RATE OF OCCURRENCE

Location			
Industry A	3/10,000/1 year =	3:10,000/year =	30/100,000/year
Industry B	9/30,000/3 years =	3:30,000/year =	10/100,000/year
Industry C	10/25,000/2 years =	5:25,000/year =	20/100,000/year

account for both the difference in population sizes and the lengths of reporting periods. In this example, the annual rate of occurrence of hepatitis is 3 per 10,000 for 1 year in Industry A and 9 per 30,000 for 3 years or 3 per 30,000 for 1 year in Industry B, and the comparable rate for Industry C is 10 per 25,000 for 2 years or 5 per 25,000 for 1 year.

To compare the rates more directly, the same denominator population constant, such as a common unit of 100,000, is used. Hence in Table 5-6, the annual rates of 3 per 10,000, 3 per 30,000, and 5 per 25,000 can be expressed as 30, 10, and 20 per 100,000 in Industries A, B, and C, respectively; thus Industry A has the highest incidence.

Incidence rates are useful in monitoring the occurrence of disease or health-related events in defined populations for a period of time. For example, a sudden increase in spontaneous abortions may reflect the introduction of a new chemical substance or exposure into the work environment. Comparisons over time or with another population can be done to determine any rate increase.

Prevalence Rates

The prevalence rate measures the number of people in a population (cases) who have a disease or an event outcome at a given time. Unspecified prevalence rates usually refer to point prevalence (i.e., a specific point in time) (see Table 5-5). For example, a one-time survey of all workers in the company could determine the prevalence of smoking in the population. Another type of prevalence, period prevalence, includes all cases existing at a point in time, plus any new or recurring cases during a specified time period. Prevalence measures are most useful for planning health care programs and tracking changes in disease patterns over time through a series of cross-sectional surveys. In this way period prevalence is a helpful predictor of workload and program costs.

Prevalence is measured as follows:

$$\frac{\text{Prevalence}}{\text{per 1,000}} = \frac{\begin{array}{c}\text{Number of cases of}\\\text{a disease in the population}\\\text{at a specified time}\end{array}}{\begin{array}{c}\text{Number of persons}\\\text{in the population}\\\text{at that specified time}\end{array}} \times 1,000$$

In this rate the quotient is multiplied by 1,000 so that the prevalence is expressed per 1,000 persons. However, the choice of 1,000 is arbitrary, and 100, 10,000, 100,000 or any other number could be used.

From the hypertension example used to measure an incidence rate, the prevalence rate could also be measured as follows

$$\frac{214 + 21}{2050} \times 1,000 = 114.6 \text{ per 1,000 employees}$$

Crude Rates and Specific Rates

Rates may be expressed as crude or specific. Crude rates represent actual numbers of events during a time period, such as births or deaths in a total population, whereas specific rates are detailed for selected, usually demographic, characteristics such as age, gender, or subgroups of the population. Crude rates require only the number of events being measured in a year and the total population (a crude rate was used earlier to show the crude death rate in the United States in 1998 as 867.3/100,000).

Crude rates are of limited help because they may not show an accurate picture of the risks in population subgroups. For example, crude death rates reflect the probability of dying in the population without consideration for specificity of age. Age is an important consideration because the very young and very old are much more likely to die in a given year than those in other age groups. For example, a geographic region of the country or a state such as Florida, which houses many retirees, is likely to present a biased mortality picture reflected in the crude death rate. Because of the significant effect of age on mortaity, age-specific rates are recommended rather than crude rates when comparing mortality experiences (Hennekens & Buring, 1987) (Tables 5-7 and 5-8).

The data in Table 5-7 represent the number of cancer deaths in the United States in 1998. The crude death rate from cancer equals the total number of cancer deaths divided by the total number of individuals in the population multiplied by 100,000. In this case the crude cancer death rate is calculated as follows:

$$\frac{\text{Cancer}}{\text{death}} = \frac{541,441}{270,299,000} \times 100,000 = \frac{200.3 \text{ per}}{\begin{array}{c}100,000\\\text{population}\end{array}}$$

However, when adjusted for age because of varying population sizes and experiences within age strata groups, the age-adjusted cancer death rate is 123.6 per 100,000 population. Age-specific cancer death rates are measured by the number of cancer deaths occurring among individuals in each age stratum divided by the total number of

individuals in that stratum. Thus the cancer death rate in 1998 for ages 5 to 14 years is calculated as 1031/38,961,537 = 2.6 per 100,000.

Table 5-8 presents data that compares death rates for two industries (Mausner & Kramer, 1985). While the crude death rates differ because of the difference in age distribution in the industry populations (column 6), the age-specific death rates are the same for both industries (column 5), indicating no true difference in the risk of death. Industry A has relatively more older people (i.e., 30% over 45 years in Industry A compared to only 10% in Industry B), and as death rates are higher for older people, the crude death rate for Industry A is higher. However, the true risk of dying in each age group is the same for both populations (column 5). Although of limited utility, crude rates provide at least summary information and are relatively easy to compute.

Specific rates provide valuable and more accurate information about the health of the population than do crude rates because groups may differ with respect to characteristics such as age, race, and gender, which affect the overall rates of disease and death. Notably, males and blacks have higher mortality rates than do females and whites; therefore calculating rates specific to these

TABLE 5-7

Death Rates for Malignant Neoplasms by Age, United States, 1998

Age	1998
All ages, age adjusted	123.6
All ages, crude	200.3
Under 1 year	2.1
1-4 years	2.4
5-14 years	2.6
15-24 years	4.6
25-34 years	11.3
35-44 years	38.2
45-54 years	132.3
55-64 years	383.8
65-74 years	841.3
75-84 years	1,326.3
85 years and older	1,749.4

Data from *Health, United States,* by National Center for Health Statistics, Washington, DC: Author. 2000.

TABLE 5-8

Comparison of Death Rates in Two Industry Populations by Age

Population	Age (Years)	Population Number	Population Prop.	Annual Number of Deaths	Annual Age-specific Death Rate (per 1,000)	Crude Death Rate (per 1,000)
	(1)	(2)	(3)	(4)	(5)	(6)
INDUSTRY A	<15	1,500	0.30	3	2	
	15-44	2,000	0.40	12	6	
	>45	1,500	0.30	30	20	
	All ages	5,000	1.00	45		45/5,000 = 9.0
INDUSTRY B	<15	2,000	0.40	4	2	
	15-44	2,500	0.50	15	6	
	>45	500	0.10	10	20	
	All ages	5,000	1.00	29		29/5,000 = 5.8

Modified from *Epidemiology: An Introductory Text,* by J. Mausner and S. Kramer. Philadelphia: Saunders. 1985.

variables is important. For example, the breast cancer death rate for women for a specified time period would be calculated as follows:

$$\frac{\text{Number of women dying from breast cancer (1999)}}{\text{Number of women in the population midyear (1999)}} \times k \text{ (e.g., 1,000)}$$

An example of disease-specific leading causes of death in 1994 reported from the National Vital Statistics system and expressed as a specific rate is shown in Table 5-9.

EPIDEMIOLOGIC METHODS AND ANALYSIS

Case reports often provide the first clues in the identification of new diseases or adverse effects of exposures and ultimately lead to analytical epidemiologic investigations. Case reports are commonly reported in the medical science journals and describe the experience of a single patient or group with a similar problem or diagnosis. For example, early case reports of *Pneumocystis carinii* pneumonia and Kaposi's sarcoma led the Centers for Disease Control and Prevention to initiate an epidemiologic surveillance program and design analytic studies to identify specific risk factors associated with the development of AIDS (CDC, 1987). The limitation of case reports is that they are based on the experience of one person or a few; however, they do lead the way for further investigative studies.

Occupational epidemiology involves investigating the frequency of occurrence and causal factors for health effects that have nonoccupational as well as potential occupational causes. Lung cancer, for example, can be induced by occupational and nonoccupational exposures. In fact, in all industrialized countries the predominant risk factor for lung cancer is cigarette smoking, not occupational exposures. The practice of occupational epidemiology becomes increasingly complex when the diseases of interest result from delayed effects

---

TABLE 5-9 Fifteen Leading Causes of Death, United States, 1994

RANK	CAUSE OF DEATH	NUMBER OF DEATHS	DEATH RATE PER 100,000 POPULATION*	PERCENT OF TOTAL DEATHS
	All Causes	**2,278,994**	**685.4**	**100.0**
1	Heat diseases	732,409	209.8	32.1
2	Cancer	534,310	171.1	23.4
3	Cerebrovascular diseases	153,306	42.0	6.7
4	Chronic obstructive pulmonary disease	101,628	30.3	4.5
5	Accidents	91,437	31.5	4.0
6	Pneumonia & influenza	81,473	21.6	3.6
7	Diabetes mellitus	56,692	17.4	2.5
8	HIV infection	42,114	13.0	1.8
9	Suicide	31,142	10.8	1.4
10	Diseases of arteries	26,097	7.7	1.1
11	Cirrhosis of liver	25,406	8.8	1.1
12	Homicide	24,926	9.3	1.1
13	Nephritis	22,976	6.5	1.0
14	Septicemia	20,360	5.8	0.9
15	Alzheimer's disease	18,584	4.7	0.8
	Other & ill-defined	316,134		13.9

Data from *Vital Statistics of the United States, 1997*, by National Center for Health Statistics, Washington, DC: U.S. Department of Health and Human Services. 1999.
*Age-adjusted to the 1970 U.S. standard population.

of exposure that become manifest many years after first exposure (latency period) or when the health outcomes are subtle physiologic responses rather than overt diseases.

Once groups have been identified with a specific disease or problem through descriptive studies, analytic studies can be designed to determine associated risk factors and potential reasons for disease occurrence. For example, if a survey was conducted to elucidate respiratory complaints among workers in a certain company department, further studies could be conducted to determine potential exposures that might contribute to the problem. Once such identification has been made, the next step is to determine why the rate is high (or low) in a particular group. Observations of differences in occurrence of disease among populations lead to the formulation of hypotheses (i.e., testable propositions that can be accepted or rejected through investigations). The results of these analytic (i.e., hypothesis-testing) studies generate ideas for additional descriptive studies as well as new hypotheses and contribute to building knowledge about the phenomenon under study. This sequence of events may be schematized as a feedback system in an epidemiologic study cycle (Figure 5-4).

TYPES OF DESIGNS

Four types of epidemiologic designs are commonly used to determine relationships between exposure and disease or health outcome events: cross-sectional studies, case-control studies, prospective studies, and historical prospective/cohort studies (Meininger, 1989) (Table 5-10).

Cross-sectional studies or surveys, also called prevalence studies, provide information about the

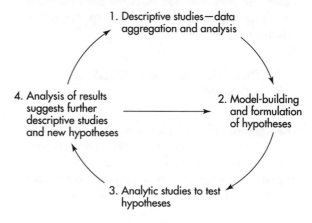

Figure 5-4   Schema for an epidemiologic study cycle. *(From* Epidemiology: An Introductory Text, *by J. Mausner and S. Kramer, 1985, Philadelphia: W.B. Saunders.)*

TABLE 5-10	Types of Epidemiologic Study Designs	
TYPE OF DESIGN	**EQUIVALENT NAME**	**DESCRIPTION**
Cross-Sectional	Prevalence Study Correlational	A group of individuals is studied at a point in time for both the risk factor and the disease or event outcome.
Case-Control	Retrospective	A group of individuals with the study disease and a group without the disease are compared for prior exposure to the study factor under investigation.
Prospective	Cohort	A group of individuals with a known exposure and a similar group without exposure are monitored forward in time and compared with respect to the development of disease or event outcome.
Historical Cohort	Retrospective Cohort Nonconcurrent Cohort	A cohort of workers is enumerated from previous records, and the cohort is traced to the present, and sometimes the future, with analysis of disease rates.

frequency and characteristics of a disease or the health attributes or events in certain groups or occupations at a point in time. For example, the National Health and Nutritional Examination Survey (as previously mentioned) is a cross-sectional survey, conducted by the National Center for Health Statistics, in which data in such areas as health conditions, physiologic measurements, and health utilization patterns are collected from a random sample of the population. Comparisons can then be made between groups (e.g., men and women) about certain attributes, such as blood pressure, diet, lifestyle habits, various diseases, or certain phenomena.

Another example is a cross-sectional study, conducted by Ciesielski et al. (1991), that used verbally administered questionnaires to determine occupational injuries among a random sample of 287 migrant farm workers in 22 migrant camps in eastern North Carolina. Nearly 10% of respondents reported at least one occupational injury. Frequent obstacles to receiving adequate health care were reported by the farm workers and included lack of provision of transportation (legally required) by the employer, earlier return to work than advised by the health care provider, and fear of retribution. In addition, employers covered medical expenses for only 38% of the injured workers and compensated only 20% of the workers for lost time.

Padungtod et al. (2000) reported a cross-sectionally designed study to measure the association between occupational pesticide exposure and semen quality among Chinese workers. Male workers—32 who were exposed to organophosphate pesticides and 43 who were not exposed—were recruited from two nearby factories and interviewed. Following a work shift, semen and urine samples were analyzed for sperm concentration, percentage of mobility, and percentage of normal structure. "Within the exposed group the mean end-of-shift urinary p-nitrophenol levels were 0.22 and 0.15 mg/L for the high- and low-exposure subgroups, respectively. Linear regression analysis of individual semen parameters revealed a significant reduction of sperm concentration ($p < 0.01$) and percentage of motility (47% vs. 57%, $p = 0.03$) but not percentage of sperm with normal structure (57% vs. 61%, $p = 0.13$)."

A study to investigate the relationship of smoking to work absenteeism may be conducted through a survey of groups of workers to determine employee smoking habits and through examination of work employment records of attendance. Although a causal relationship cannot be drawn, data obtained may provide information about the relative impact of smoking on absenteeism. Other examples could include employee attitudinal surveys about occupational health risks or other specific issues, or determination of the most prevalent reasons for visits to the occupational health unit.

Three major analytical design methods available are case-control, prospective, and historical prospective studies (Figure 5-5) (Rogers & Moreland, 1986). The purpose of these kinds of studies (case-control and prospective) is to employ specific statistical comparisons to determine exposure associations and potential causal relationships. Careful evaluation for the strength of the association of the health outcome with a particular risk factor, consistency of the association, time, sequence, dose/response considerations, and concurrence with existing knowledge is necessary.

In a *case-control study*, sometimes called a retrospective study, individuals diagnosed with a disease (cases) are compared with individuals without the disease (controls) for the presence or absence of an antecedent risk factor, such as an exposure, which may have contributed to disease development. For example, to study the relationship between benzene exposure and aplastic anemia, a case-control study would compare a group of individuals with aplastic anemia with a control group of subjects without the diagnosis and determine in each group if benzene exposure had occurred. Statistical calculations are then made by comparing cases and controls with respect to exposure versus nonexposure to the element or factor, in this case benzene, to determine if significant differences are apparent. Selection of a representative sample of cases and controls is important in order to avoid bias, which could lead to false conclusions; that is, selected cases should be representative of the total cases, and controls should be representative of the general population.

An example of a case-control study was reported by Selevan et al. (1985), who examined the relationship between fetal loss and occupational exposure to antineoplastic agents of nurses in Finland. Each nurse with a fetal loss was matched with three

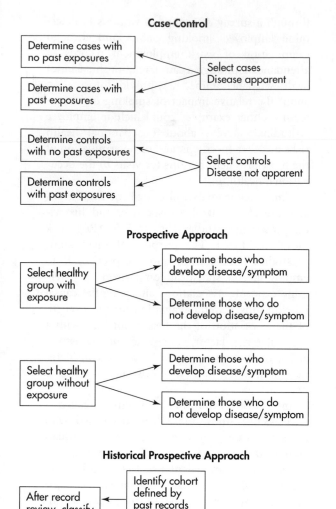

Case-Control

Select cases
Disease apparent
→ Determine cases with no past exposures
→ Determine cases with past exposures

Select controls
Disease not apparent
→ Determine controls with no past exposures
→ Determine controls with past exposures

Prospective Approach

Select healthy group with exposure
→ Determine those who develop disease/symptom
→ Determine those who do not develop disease/symptom

Select healthy group without exposure
→ Determine those who develop disease/symptom
→ Determine those who do not develop disease/symptom

Historical Prospective Approach

Identify cohort defined by past records
→ After record review, classify group as to past exposure to factor
→ Determine if disease/ no disease → Follow forward for disease outcome

Figure 5-5 Comparison of case-control and prospective epidemiological studies.

ence of workers at a dye and resin manufacturing plant in New Jersey (Sathiakumar & Delzel, 2000). The retrospective follow-up study included 3,266 workers employed for at least 6 months at the plant. Plant production areas were South Dyes, where anthraquinone dyes and intermediates were produced; North Dyes, where azo dyes and intermediates were produced; and plastics and additives, where various resins and additives for plastics were made. Analyses used standardized mortality ratios (SMR) to compare the cohort's cause-specific mortality rates from 1952 to 1995 with the rates of the New Jersey population. There were fewer than expected deaths from all causes combined (728 observed vs. 810 expected) and similar numbers of observed and expected cancer deaths (225 vs. 232). Statistically significant work area-specific cancer excesses were limited to white men and included an excess of lung cancer in maintenance workers (40 observed vs. 26 expected) and South Dyes workers (32 observed vs. 19 expected) and an excess of stomach cancer (5 observed vs. 1.3 expected), bladder cancer (4 observed vs. 0.8 expected), and central nervous system cancer (5 observed vs. 1 expected) in North Dye workers. None of these increases was concentrated in work area subgroups with long duration of employment and long potential induction time. It was concluded that the excess of bladder cancer probably was due to exposure to carcinogenic arylamines at another facility, where some employees had worked before coming to the study plant. The other cancer increases may be attributable to chance, to uncontrolled confounding by smoking, or to an unidentified occupational exposure.

In contrast, a *prospective* or *cohort study* starts with a group of people (cohort) considered to be free of disease or health problems but who vary in exposure to a suspected element or factor (i.e., those with differing degrees of exposure and those with no exposure). The cohort is monitored forward in time to determine differences in the rate at which disease develops in relation to the exposure or nonexposure to the suspected agent (Gordis, 2000). Evidence for causal relationships can be obtained because there is a temporal relationship between presumed cause and outcome. For example, data from the classic study by Doll and Hill (1956) on the mortality experience of British physicians (Table 5-11)

nurses who gave birth. Historical data on health and exposure were obtained from study participants through mailed questionnaires. The study found that women who experienced fetal loss were more than twice as likely to have had occupational exposures to antineoplastic drugs during the first trimester as were women who gave birth (odds ratio = 2.30).

Another case-control study example was reported as an evaluation of the mortality experi-

TABLE 5-11

Relative Risk of Mortality From Lung Cancer and Coronary Heart Disease for Heavy Smokers and Nonsmokers Among British Physicians

	ANNUAL DEATH RATES PER 100,000 PERSONS	
	LUNG CANCER	CORONARY HEART DISEASE
EXPOSURE CATEGORY		
Heavy smokers	166	599
Nonsmokers	7	422
MEASURE OF EXCESS RISK		
Relative risk	166/7 = 23.7	599/422 = 1.4

From "Lung Cancer and Other Causes of Death in Relation to Smoking," by R. Doll and A. B. Hill, *British Medical Journal, 2,* 1071-1072. 1956.

show a very high relative risk (23.7) for heavy smokers compared with nonsmokers, which indicates a strong association between heavy smoking and lung cancer. The relative risk (1.4) for coronary heart disease is much lower, which suggests that other attributes, such as diet or stress, may be operating and require alteration.

In another example, data from a community-based 4-year prospective study were used to investigate job characteristics as predictors of neck pain (Eriksen et al., 1999). Of 1,791 working responders who completed a questionnaire in 1990, 1,429 (79.8%) returned a second questionnaire 4 years later (1994). In responders without neck pain during the previous 12 months in 1990, the "little influence on own work situation" factor predicted neck pain during the previous 12 months (odds ratio [OR] = 2.21; 95% confidence interval, 1.18 to 4.14) and previous 7 days in 1994 (OR = 2.85; 95% confidence interval, 1.21 to 6.73) after adjustment for a series of potential confounders. In responders with neck pain in 1990 the "little influence on own work situation factor" was associated with persistent neck pain 4 years later. The study indicates that having little influence on one's own work situation is a predictor of neck pain.

A *historical cohort study* identifies both exposed and unexposed cohorts through previously existing records that permit correct classification of the exposure status of individuals. Study subjects then are traced forward to the present and followed into the future to determine if they have or have not developed the disease or outcome of interest (Gordis, 2000). Statistical calcu-lations are made to determine if associations exist between the risk of disease among those with or without exposure.

EXTRANEOUS VARIABLES

The conduct of any study requires control for extraneous variables—that is, factors known to be associated with the exposure and disease or outcome of interest. For example, if one wants to investigate the relationship between a chemical agent exposure and birth outcomes, factors such as age, parity, cigarette smoking, and drug use would need to be determined and controlled. This can be accomplished in the design stage through restricting participation of study subjects with certain characteristics (e.g., eliminating smokers) or matching cases and controls so they are similar with respect to specific attributes (e.g., matching a case with a control subject on age, parity, and/or smoking status). Another approach to handling extraneous or confounding bias is in the analysis stage through statistical techniques such as stratification on the extraneous variables or other techniques, such as regression analysis, that can adjust for the confounding factors simultaneously (Nowell, 1995). Stratification involves the analysis of data by strata, such as gender, so as to eliminate the potential bias associated with one's sex status. If, for example, gender were a potential confounder, data would be evaluated for men and women separately. Similar strata-specific evaluations can be calculated for other potential extraneous variables, such as race, age, education, smoking status, and parity.

EPIDEMIOLOGIC ANALYSIS

Once data are derived, they must be expressed as a risk estimate in order to evaluate the effects of the exposure. Data are usually presented in a two-by-two table with columns and rows indicating the presence or absence of the disease or exposure (Figure 5-6). Four cells (*a,b,c,* and *d*) are created and represent the following:

a = the number of individuals exposed who have disease
b = the number of individuals exposed who do not have disease
c = the number of individuals unexposed who have disease
d = the number of individuals unexposed who do not have disease

The margins of the table represent the following totals in each column and row:

a + b = the total number of individuals exposed
c + d = the total number of individuals unexposed
a + c = the total number of individuals with disease
b + d = the total number of individuals without disease

The total sample size is represented by the sum of all four cells (*a + b + c + d*).

Two major types of risk estimates are the relative risk for prospective or cohort studies and for case-control studies, the odds ratio (OR), which is an estimate of the relative risk. The relative risk, also called the rate ratio, provides an estimate of the likelihood of developing the disease in the exposed group relative to the unexposed group (i.e., the ratio of the rate in the exposed group to the rate in the unexposed group) and is a measure of the strength of the association between expo-

sure and disease (Hennekens & Buring, 1977). Relative risk is calculated as follows:

$$\frac{\text{Disease rate in the exposed}}{\text{Disease rate in the unexposed}}$$

or

$$\frac{(a/[a + b])}{(c/[c + d])}$$

The data presented in Table 5-11 demonstrate the relative risk for cigarette smokers in developing lung cancer and coronary heart disease.

A relative risk of 1.0 indicates that the disease incidence among the exposed and nonexposed is the same; that is, no association exists between the exposure and disease. A value greater than 1.0 equals an increased risk, whereas a value less than 1.0 indicates a decreased risk among those exposed.

In case-control studies incidence rates cannot be derived directly because participants are selected on the basis of disease status and the total population of those exposed/unexposed and diseased/nondiseased is unknown. Therefore, a relative risk of disease associated with exposure cannot be calculated. However, an estimate of the relative risk, or the odds ratio (OR) (i.e., the odds of having the disease with and without exposure) is a useful measure. From Figure 5-6 it can be seen that $a/(a + b)$ is representative of the disease rate in the exposed group, whereas $c/(c + d)$ represents disease in the unexposed group. Since we assume that *a* is a small portion of $a + b$ and *c* is a small portion of $c + d$, then the odds ratio becomes $([a/b]/[c/d])$ or $(ad)/(bc)$, which yields an approximation or estimate of the relative risk. Table 5-12 presents hypothetical data

Figure 5-6 Presentation format for epidemiologic data for use with prospective or case-control designs.

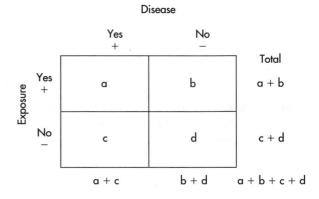

from a case-control study relating cigarette smoking to lung cancer and shows the OR. Because the OR is an estimate of the relative risk, one can conclude that the data show an increased risk of lung cancer in smokers versus nonsmokers.

SOURCES OF DATA

Accurate measures of mortality and morbidity in the nation and in occupational groups are essential for occupational and environmental health nurses to help plan prevention and health promotion and protection programs for workers; however, data are not always readily available. Even notifiable diseases may not always be reported, and for most chronic diseases, such as hypertension, cancer, and coronary heart disease, no nationwide notification system exists. Yet the occupational and environmental health nurse may use many sources of data that provide prevalence estimates of health and illness indices important to worker health. Table 5-13 details selected data systems relevant to occupational injury and illness, and Table 5-14 gives examples of data sources on health statistics relevant to the nation's health.

Census data are necessary for an accurate picture of the health status of the population because these data serve as denominator data for births and deaths. Vital statistics for a variety of events are collected by governmental entities and processed by the National Center for Health Statistics. Of major interest to health care providers are births and deaths in the United States, more than 99% of which are reported. Deaths are classified and recorded according to the International Classification of Diseases, thereby allowing for international comparisons. Epidemiologic studies are often based on mortality data.

The Centers for Disease Control and Prevention (CDC) maintains a system for col-lecting various kinds of data. Examples include demographic, clinical, and laboratory data from state agencies on notifiable diseases, such as AIDS, diphtheria, malaria, sexually transmitted diseases, tetanus, tuberculosis, many childhood infectious diseases, and other conditions that may have a preventable component.

Other sources for morbidity data that may be of interest to the occupational and environmental health nurse include hospital records, health records from private physicians, insurance records, disease registries, and health survey data, such as the National Health and Nutrition Examination Survey (NHANES). The latter is a continuing National Center for Health Statistics survey that is based on a sample of the population and provides information about the health needs of the entire country. Components of the survey include physical examinations, laboratory tests, and household interviews on health and nutrition status.

Occupational disease surveillance is an important measure in efforts to control and prevent work-related illness and injury; however, surveillance efforts in occupationally related diseases and injuries lag far behind those of infectious diseases. The Bureau of Labor Statistics reported that 6.1 million occupational illnesses and injuries were recorded in 1997 along with 6,234 work-related deaths (USDHHS/NIOSH, 2000), which is most likely an underestimate. Reportable occupational illness and injury-related events vary by state; however, only seven states mandate the reporting of any occupational disease (CDC, 1990). Efforts to improve both the recognition of occupational illness and injury events and surveillance activities have been heightened through the establishment of the Sentinel Health Events (Occupational) and the NIOSH-sponsored Sentinel Event Notification

Text continued on p. 128

TABLE 5-12	Odds Ratio (OR) From a Case-Control Study of Cigarette Smoking and Lung Cancer		
	Lung Cancer Cases	**Controls**	**Total**
Smokers	75(a)	425(b)	500
Nonsmokers	25(c)	900(d)	925
Total	100	1,325	1,425
OR = ad/bc =	(75)(900)/(425)(25) = 6.4		

TABLE 5-13   Description of Selected Data Systems in Occupational Injury and Illness

NAME OF SYSTEM	AGENCY	EMPLOYMENT AND OCCUPATION CODING (EXPOSURE SURROGATES)	SAMPLE DERIVATION/ POPULATION DEFINITION	PRIMARY INTEREST OF DATA SYSTEM	FATAL OR NONFATAL OUTCOME	INJURY OR ILLNESS
ABLES	NIOSH	None presently; NAICS and Bureau of the Census occupational codes planned	People (≥16) with blood lead levels ≥25 $\mu g/dL$ from 28 states	Facilitate state lead poisoning intervention; track trend and magnitude of lead exposures, especially in adults	Nonfatal	Illness
CFOI	BLS	BLS Occupational Injury and Illness Classification System, industry and occupations	All injury deaths identified through death certificates, workers' compensation reports, OSHA reports, and news media reports, verified to exclude duplicate counting	Counts of fatalities by various characteristics— worker, employer, and incident	Fatal	Injury
CWXSP	NIOSH	None	Working coal miners employed in underground coal mines	Degree of radiographic opacity	Nonfatal	Illness
HARS	All states report to CDC	Surveillance Branch, Division of HIV/AIDS Prevention (requests occupation and industry information for the health care setting only)	All cases nationwide	Monitoring the HIV epidemic	Nonfatal	Illness
MSHA Mine/ Contractor Address/ Accident/ Injury/Illness Database	MSHA	MSHA classifications for industry (mineral commodity) and occupation	Population of miners whose employment/ injuries/illnesses are required to be reported under 30 CFR Part 50			

					Fatal and Nonfatal	Injury and Illness
Multiple-Cause-of-Death Data	NCHS	Coding available for selected states; coding according to Bureau of the Census occupation and industry codes	Death records include codes for up to 20 conditions cited on death certificates; information from all states in the United States	Cause of death (underlying and contributory), occupation and industry codes where available	Fatal and Nonfatal	Injury and Illness
NaSH	NCID	NCID-generated coding		Incidence and trends of occupationally acquired infections in health care settings	Nonfatal	Illness
NEISS	CPSC for NIOSH (and others)	Bureau of the Census classification	Hospitals (65 of 91 stratified nationally on size) collect occupational identifiers	Injury and illness cases identified as work-related in emergency departments of participating hospitals	Nonfatal	Injury
NHAMCS	NCHS	None	Representative sample of hospital emergency room visits	Type of injury or incident, body part, cause of incident; demographics of individual; work-relatedness by treating professional	Nonfatal	Injury
NHANES	NCHS	Bureau of the Census occupation and industry codes regrouped by NCHS	Cross-sectional household survey interviews, representative sample of U.S. civilian population	Characterizes health and nutritional status of U.S. civilian noninstitutionalized population	Not applicable	Illness
NOMS	NIOSH using NCHS data	Bureau of the Census classification	Death certificates from NCHS	Cause of death, occupation, and industry where available	Fatal	Illness

Data from *Worker Health Chartbook*, by National Institute of Occupational Safety and Health, Washington D.C. Author. 2000.
Abbreviations: *ABLES*, Adult Blood Lead Epidemiology and Surveillance Program; *AIDS*, acquired immune deficiency syndrome; *BLS*, Bureau of Labor Statistics; *CDC*, Centers for Disease Control and Prevention; *CFOI*, Census of Fatal Occupational Injuries; *CPSC*, Consumer Product Safety Commission; *CWXSP*, Coal Workers' X-ray Surveillance Program; *HARS*, HIV/AIDS Reporting System; *HIV*, human immunodeficiency virus; *MSHA*, Mine Safety and Health Administration; *NAICS*, North American Industrial Classification System; *NaSH*, National Surveillance System for Hospital Health Care Workers; *NCHS*, National Center for Health Statistics; *NCID*, National Center for Infectious Diseases; *NEISS*, National Electronic Injury Surveillance System; *NHAMCS*, National Hospital Ambulatory Medical Care Survey; *NHANES*, National Health and Nutrition Examination Survey; *NIOSH*, National Institute for Occupational Safety and Health; *NNIS*, National Nosocomial Infection Surveillance System; *NOMS*, National Occupational Mortality Surveillance System; *OSHA*, Occupational Safety and Health Administration.

Continued

TABLE 5-13 Description of Selected Data Systems in Occupational Injury and Illness—cont'd

NAME OF SYSTEM	AGENCY	EMPLOYMENT AND OCCUPATION CODING (EXPOSURE SURROGATES)	SAMPLE DERIVATION/ POPULATION DEFINITION	PRIMARY INTEREST OF DATA SYSTEM	FATAL OR NONFATAL OUTCOME	INJURY OR ILLNESS
NSSPM	NIOSH using NCHS data	Bureau of the Census classification	Death certificates from NCHS	Cause of death (underlying and contributory), occupation, and industry where available	Fatal	Illness
NTOF	NIOSH	Industry and occupation coding using 1980 and 1990 Bureau of the Census data	Death certificates from 52 U.S. vital statistics reporting units in 50 states for workers ≥16 years old	Represents the minimum number of work-related deaths in the United States for a given period	Fatal	Injury
Sentinel Counties Study of Acute Hepatitis	NCID	None	6 counties in the United States and convenience samples	Provides source data of viral hepatitis infection in the United States	Nonfatal	Illness
SENSOR	NIOSH	Varies by participating state and SENSOR condition	Case-based reporting from a variety of sources, including physicians, agencies, workers' compensation; catchment area varies from geographic area (counties) to entire state	Case-based surveillance directly linked to intervention activities to maximize prevention	Fatal and Nonfatal	Injury and Illness

SOII	BLS	Industry coding using the SIC system; occupation coding using 1990 Bureau of the Census system	Stratified random sample of all private industry employers of one or more workers	The number of work-related injuries and illnesses reported by employers on the OSHA 300 Log	Nonfatal	Injury and Illness
staffTRAK-TB	National Center for HIV, STD, and TB Prevention	1990 Bureau of the Census for population and housing and 1992 Bureau of the Census industry and occupation coding; also includes CDC NNIS coding for occupations	Demonstration project—participating health departments	Tuberculin skin testing targeting health departments	Nonfatal	Illness
VHSP	NCID	NCID-generated coding	All acute cases reported to local health departments	Identifies risk factors for infection	Nonfatal	Illness

Data from *Worker Health Chartbook*, by National Institute of Occupational Safety and Health, Washington D.C. Author. 2000. Abbreviations: *NNIS*, National Nosocomial Infection Surveillance System; *NSSPM*, National Surveillance System for Pneumoconiosis Mortality; *NTOF*, National Traumatic Occupational Fatalities Surveillance System; *SENSOR*, Sentinel Event Notification System for Occupational Risk; *SIC*, standard industrial classification; *SOII*, Survey of Occupational Injuries and Illnesses; *staffTRAK-TB*, Surveillance for Tuberculosis Infection in Health Care Workers; *STD*, sexually transmitted disease; *TB*, tuberculosis; *VHSP*, Viral Hepatitis Surveillance Program.

TABLE 5-14 Selected National Health Data Sources Useful in Occupational Health

AGENCY	DATABASE	PURPOSE
CENSUS DATA		
Bureau of the Census/CDC	Decennial Census	Total enumeration of the U.S. population by demographic characteristics, such as age, race, sex, marital status, education, and employment characteristics
Bureau of the Census/CDC	Current Population Survey	Annual household sample survey of the population for basic demographic variables
VITAL RECORDS		
NCHS	Vital Statistics: Mortality	Underlying cause of death and demographic data for all deaths in the United States: state-specific data, such as age, sex, race, residence, place of death, from death certificates
NCHS	National Death Index	Computerized index of death records from state vital statistics offices for research purposes
NCHS	Vital Statistics: Fetal Mortality	Sample of registered U.S. fetal death certificates and information associated with the deaths and obtained from mothers, physicians, and hospitals
NCHS	Vital Statistics: Natality	Number of registered U.S. live births from birth certificates; includes age, race, education, marital status, and geographic area
FDA	Diet and Health Survey	National probability sample of households; measures public attitudes, knowledge, and practices about food and nutrition relative to chronic disease
FDA	Pesticides, Industrial Chemicals, Toxic Elements	Pesticides, industrial chemicals, and toxic elements in samples of food
FDA	Industrial Chemical Contaminants	Sample analyses of fish to determine the level of industrial chemical contaminants

System for Occupational Risks (SENSOR), which is in place in several states and is designed to establish reporting mechanisms for certain occupational conditions selected by NIOSH, including carpal tunnel syndrome, lead poisoning, noise-induced hearing loss, occupational asthma, pesticide poisoning, and silicosis.

There are many commercially prepared directories for public health data sources as well as federal directories, such as the Health and Human Services Data Inventory (Gable, 1990). Gable has prepared an excellent compendium on public health data sources and accessing information. In addition, the NIOSH *Worker Health Chartbook*

TABLE 5-14 Selected National Health Data Sources Useful in Occupational Health—cont'd

AGENCY	DATABASE	PURPOSE
EPIDEMIOLOGY		
NCHS	National Health Interview Survey	Household interviews of a representative sample of the U.S. population; includes data on illnesses, injuries, chronic conditions, utilization of health resources, and demographic characteristics
NCHS	National Health and Nutrition Examination Survey	National probability sample of the U.S. civilian population to determine prevalence of specific diseases and nutritional deficiencies based on physical exams, medical history, biochemical tests, and dietary intake
CDC	Behavioral Risk Factor Surveillance System	Prevalence of behavioral risk factors such as cigarettes, alcohol, and obesity, contributing to 10 leading causes of premature death and disability
INFANT/MATERNAL		
CDC	Birth Defects Monitoring Program	Hospital discharge on birth defects by county among participating hospitals
CDC	National Infant Mortality Surveillance (NIMS)	U.S. infant deaths from extracts of birth and death records; includes birth weight, maternal age, race, and maternal risk factor
NCHS	National Maternal and Infant Health Survey	National representative data on fetal loss, low birth weight, and infant death
NCHS	National Hospital Discharge Survey	Sample of discharged U.S. hospital inpatients; contains diagnoses, surgical procedures, and characteristics of inpatients

Data from "Surveillance in Occupational Health and Safety," by E. L. Baker, *American Journal of Public Health, 79* (Supplement). 1989; and A Compendium of Public Health Data Sources, by C. Gable, *American Journal of Epidemiology, 131,* 381-394. 1990.

2000 also provides a detailed description of several databases relevant to occupational health. The reader is referred to these sources for further information.

Summary

This chapter has provided a discussion of selected concepts, principles, and methodologies in epidemiology, including agent-host-environmental relationship, descriptive and analytical methods, and approaches to measurement, design, and causal inferences. However, more in-depth information is provided through other sources (see references). The occupational and environmental health nurse will find this information useful in understanding the dynamic processes and interrelationships between health, illness, and injury events in worker populations.

Using epidemiologic tools, the occupational and environmental health nurse will be able to more effectively identify workers at risk of exposure and risk factors that contribute to disease development. Collaborative efforts can then be developed to design preventive and control strategies to minimize risk conditions.

References

Anderson, G. B. J. (1997). The epidemiology of spinal disorders. In J. W. Frymoyer (Ed.), *The adult spine: Principles and practice* (2nd ed., pp. 93-141). Philadelphia: Lippincott-Raven.

Baker, E. L., White, R. F., & Pothier, L. J. (1985). Occupational lead neurotoxicity: Improvement in behavioral effects after exposure reduction. *British Journal of Industrial Medicine, 42,* 507-516.

Benenson, A. S. (Ed.). (2000). *Control of communicable diseases in man* (15th ed.). Washington, DC: American Public Health Association.

Bigos, S. J. (1994). *Acute low back problems in adults. Clinical practice guidelines No. 14.* (Agency for Health Care Policy and Research Publication No. 95-0642, pp. 1-160). Washington, DC: U.S. Department of Health and Human Services, Public Health Service, Agency for Health Care Policy and Research.

Bigos, S. J., & Battie, M. C. (1992). Risk factors for industrial back problems. *Seminars in Spine Surgery, 4,* 2-11.

Caplan, R. (1998). Person-environment fit. In *Encyclopaedia of occupational health* (pp. 34.15-34.17). Geneva, Switzerland: International Labor Office.

Case, R. A. M., Hosker, M. E., McDonald, D. B., & Pearson, J. T. (1954). Tumors of the urinary bladder in workmen engaged in the manufacture and use of certain dyestuff intermediates in the British chemical industry. *British Journal of Industrial Medicine, 11,* 75-104.

Centers for Disease Control and Prevention. (1987). Human immunodeficiency virus infection in the United States: A review of current knowledge. *Morbidity and Mortality Weekly Report, 36*(Suppl.), 148.

Centers for Disease Control and Prevention. (1990). Protection against vital hepatitis. *Morbidity and Mortality Weekly Report, 39,* 1-26.

Centers for Disease Control and Prevention. (1994). Summary of notifiable diseases. *Morbidity and Mortality Weekly, 42,* 48.

Chaffin, D. B., & Park, K. S. (1973). A longitudinal study of low-back pain as associated with occupational weight lifting factors. *Industrial Hygiene Association Journal, 34,* 513-526.

Ciesielski, S., Hall, S. P., & Sweeney, M. (1991). Occupational injuries among North Carolina migrant farmworkers. *American Journal of Public Health, 81,* 926-928.

Doll, R. & Bill, A. B. (1964). Mortality in relation to smoking: Ten years' observations of British doctors. *British Medical Journal, 1,* 1399-1410.

Doll, R., & Hill, A. B. (1956). Lung cancer and other causes of death in relation to smoking. *British Medical Journal, 2,* 1071-1072.

Eisen, E. A., & Wegman, D. H. (2000). Epidemiology. In B. S. Levy & D. H. Wegman (Eds.), *Occupational health.* Philadelphia: Lippincott Williams and Wilkins.

Eriksen, W., Natvig, B., Knardahl, S., & Bruusgaard, D. (1999). Job characteristics as predictors of neck pain. *Journal of Occupational and Environmental Medicine, 41,* 893-902.

Feldman, R. G. (1999). *Occupational and environmental neurotoxicology.* Philadelphia: Lippincott-Raven.

Gable, C. (1990). A compendium of public health data sources. *American Journal of Epidemiology, 131,* 381-394.

Goetzel, R., Anderson, D., Whitmer, W., Ozminkowski, R. J., Dunn, R. L., Wasserman, J., & Health Enhancement Research Organization Research Committee. (1998). The relationship between modifiable health risks and health care expenditures: An analysis of the multi-employer HERO health risk and cost database. *Journal of Occupational and Environmental Medicine 40*(10), 500-510.

Goldwater, L. J., Rosso, A. J., & Kleinfeld, M. (1965). Bladder tumors in a cool tar dye plant. *Archives of Environmental Health, 11,* 814-817.

Gordis, L. (2000). *Epidemiology.* Philadelphia: W. B. Saunders.

Gwatkin, D. R., & Brandel, S. K. (1986). Life expectancy and population growth in the Third World. *Scientific American, 246,* 62.

Harper, A. (1982). *The health of populations.* New York: Springer.

Hemminki, K., Mutanen, P., Saloniemi, I., Niemi, M. L., & Vaino, H. (1982). Spontaneous abortions in hospital staff engaged in sterilization instruments with chemical agents. *British Medical Journal, 285,* 1461-1463.

Hennekens, C. H., & Buring, J. E. (1987). *Epidemiology in medicine.* Boston: Little, Brown & Company.

Hunter, D. (1978). *Diseases of occupations.* London: Hedder & Stoughton.

Kryter, K. D. (1994). *The handbook of hearing and the effects of noise* (pp. 1-15). San Diego, CA: Academic Press.

Landis, S. H., Murray, T., & Bolden, S. (1998). Cancer statistics. *CA: A Cancer Journal for Clinicians, 48,* 6029.

Levy, B., & Wegman, D. (2000). *Occupational health: Recognizing and preventing work-related disease.* Boston: Little, Brown & Company.

Lewis, R. (1990). Metals. In J. LaDou (Ed.), *Occupational Medicine* (pp. 297-326). Norwalk, CT: Appleton & Lange.

Lilienfeld, A., & Lilienfeld, D. (1980). *Foundations of epidemiology.* New York: Oxford University Press.

Long-Term Intervention with Pravastatin in Ischaemic Disease (LIPID) Study Group (1998). Prevention of cardiovascular events and death with pravastatin in patients with coronary heart disease and a broad range of initial cholesterol levels. *New England Journal of Medicine 339,* 1349-1357.

Lorenz, E. (1944). Radioactivity and lung cancer: A critical review of lung cancer in miners of Schneeberg and Joachimisthal. *Journal of the National Cancer Institute, 5,* 1-5.

MacMahon, B., & Pugh, T. F. (1970). *Epidemiologic principles and methods.* Boston: Little, Brown & Company.

Marbury, M. C. (1992). Relationship of ergonomic stressors to birthweight and gestational age. *Scandinavian Journal of Work Environment Health, 18,* 73-83.

Mausner, J., & Kramer, S. (1985). *Epidemiology: An introductory text.* Philadelphia: W. B. Saunders.

Morata, T. C., Dunn, D. E., Kretschmer, L. W., Lemasters, G. K., & Keith, R. W. (1993). Effects of occupational exposure to organic solvents and noise on hearing. *Scandinavian Journal of Work Environment Health, 19,* 245-254.

Murphy, M., & Graziano, J. (1990). Past pregnancy outcomes among women living in the vicinity of a lead smelter in Kosovo, Yugoslavia. *American Journal of Public Health, 80,* 33-35.

National Center for Health Statistics. (1999). *Vital Statistics of the United States, 1997.* Washington, DC: U.S. Department of Health and Human Services.

National Center for Health Statistics. (2000). *Vital Statistics of the United States, 1998.* Washington, DC: U.S. Department of Health and Human Services.

National Heart, Lung, and Blood Institute. (1998). *Morbidity and Mortality 1998 Chartbook on Cardiovascular, Lung, and Blood Diseases.* Bethesda, MD: National Institutes of Health, Public Health Service, National Heart, Lung, and Blood Institute.

National Institute for Occupational Safety and Health. (1999, November). *NIOSH alert: Preventing needlestick injuries in health care workers.* Cincinnati, OH: U.S. Department of Health and Human Services, National Institute for Occupational Safety and Health.

National Institute for Occupational Safety and Health. (2000). *Worker Health Chartbook 2000.* Cincinnati, OH, Author.

National Safety Council. (1998). *Accident facts, 1998.* Chicago: Author.

Nowell, S. E. (1995). *Workbook of epidemiology.* New York: Oxford Press.

Occupational Safety and Health Administration. (1983, March 8). Occupational noise exposure: Hearing conservation final amendment. *Federal Register, 48,* 9738-9785.

Olsen, O., & Kristensen, T. S. (1991). Impact of work environment on cardiovascular diseases in Denmark. *Journal of Epidemiology in Community Health, 45,* 4-10.

Padungtod, C., Savitz, D. A., Overstreet, J. W., Christiani, D. C., Ryan, L. M., & Xu, X. (2000). Occupational pesticide exposure and semen quality among Chinese workers. *Journal of Occupational and Environmental Medicine, 42,* 982-992.

Peller, S. (1939). Lung cancer among miners in Joachimsthal. *Human Biology, 11,* 130-143.

Pirchan, A., & Sikl, H. (1932). Cancer of the lung of miners. *American Journal of Cancer, 15,* 681-722.

Pott, P. (1775). *Chirurgical observations.* London: Hawes, Clark & Collins.

Psaty, B. M., Smith, N. L., & Siscovick, D. S. (1997). Health outcomes associated with antihypertensive therapies used as first-line agents: A systematic review and meta-analysis. *Journal of the American Medical Association 277,* 739-745.

Roels, H. A., Bernard, A. M., & Cardenas, A. (1993). Markers of early renal changes induced by industrial pollutants: Application to workers exposed to cadmium. *British Journal of Industrial Medicine, 50,* 37-48.

Roels, H. A., Van Assche, F. J., & Oversteyns, M. (1997). Reversibility of microproteinuria in cadmium workers with incipient tubular dysfunction after reduction of exposure. *American Journal of Industrial Medicine, 31,* 645-652.

Rogers, B., & Moreland, R. (1986). Principles of epidemiology in occupational health nursing. *Continuing Professional Education Center, 2*(22), 1-7.

Rosenthal, D. S. (1998). Changing trends. *CA: A Cancer Journal for Clinicians, 48,* 3-4.

Rothman, K., & Grunland, S. (1998). *Modern epidemiology.* Philadelphia: Lippincott-Raven.

Sartwell, P. E. (1973). Infectious disease epidemiology. In P. E. Sartwell (Ed.), *Maxcy-Rosenau Preventive Medicine and Public Health* (10th ed.). New York: Appleton-Century Crofts.

Sathiakumar, N., & Delzell, E. (2000). An updated mortality study of workers at a dye and resin manufacturing plant. *Journal of Occupational and Environmental Medicine, 42,* 762-771.

Sauter, S., Hurrell, J., Murphy, L., & Levi, L. (1997). Psychological and organizational factors. In J. Stellman (Ed.), *Encyclopedia of Occupational Health and Safety* (Vol. 1, pp. 34.1-34.77). Geneva, Switzerland: International Labour Office.

Scialli, A. R. (1993). Pregnancy and the workplace. *Seminars in Perinatology, 17,* 1-57.

Selevan, S., Lindbohm, M., Hornung, R., & Hemminki, K. (1985). A study of occupational exposure to antineoplastic drugs and fetal loss in nurses. *New England Journal of Medicine, 313,* 1173-1178.

Selikoff, I. J., Churg, J., & Hammond, E. C. (1964). Asbestos exposure and neoplasia. *Journal of the American Medical Association, 188,* 22-26.

Selikoff, H., Hammond, E. C., & Seidman, H. (1979). Mortality experience of insulation workers in the U.S. and Canada. *Annals of the New York Academy of Sciences, 330,* 91-116.

Sempos, C. T., Cleeman, J. I., & Carroll, M. K. (1993). Prevalence of high blood cholesterol among U.S. adults: An update based on guidelines from the second report of the National Cholesterol Education Program Adult Treatment Panel. *Journal of the American Medical Association, 269,* 3009-3014.

Siegrist, J. (1996). Adverse health effects of high-effort/low-reward conditions. *Journal of Occupational Health Psychology, 1,* 9-26.

Stern, F., & Steenland, K. (1993). Heart disease mortality among workers exposed to carbon monoxide in New York City. In K. Steenland (Ed.), *Case studies in occupational epidemiology* (pp. 21-34). New York: Oxford University Press.

Thun, M. (1993). Kidney dysfunction in cadmium workers. In K. Steenland (Ed.), *Case studies in occupational epidemiology* (pp. 105-126). New York: Oxford University Press.

Tyler, C. W., & Last, J. M. (1992). Epidemiology. In J. Last & R. Wallace (Eds.), *Public Health and Preventive Medicine* (pp. 11-40). Norwalk, CT: Appleton & Lange.

U.S. Department of Health and Human Services. (2000). *Healthy People 2010.* Washington, D.C.: U.S. Government Printing Office.

U.S. Department of Health and Human Services/ National Institute for Occupational Safety and Health. (1996). *National occupational research agenda* (Publication No. 96-115). Cincinnati, OH: Author.

Waldron, H. A. (1983). A brief history of scrotal cancer. *British Journal of Industrial Medicine, 40,* 390-401.

Wendell, R. G., Hoegg, U. R., & Zavon, M. R. (1974). Benzidine: A bladder carcinogen. *Journal of Urology, 2,* 607-610.

Wenzel, P. (1992). Control of communicable disease. In J. Last & R. Wallace (Eds.) *Public Health and Preventive Medicine* (13th. ed., pp. 57-60). Norwalk, CT: Appleton & Lange.

Willett, W. H., Dietz, W. H., & Colditz, G. A. (1999). Primary care: Guidelines for healthy weight. *New England Journal of Medicine 341,* 427-434.

World Health Organization. (1986). *Early detection of occupational diseases* (pp. 85-90). Geneva, Switzerland: Author.

World Health Organization and Nordic Council of Ministers. (1985). *Chronic effects of organic solvents on the central nervous system and diagnostic criteria.* Copenhagen, Denmark: WHO Regional Office for Europe.

Zenz, C. (1993). *Occupational medicine* (pp. 463-464). Chicago: Yearbook Medical Publishers.

6 Developing Occupational Health Services and Programs: A Conceptual Model

Numerous occupational health and safety programs and services are provided in many work settings in order to improve health and reduce work-related health risks. Occupational and environmental health nurses are key managers and providers of occupational health services emphasizing interdisciplinary collaboration in service delivery and cost-effective programming. This chapter presents a conceptual framework or model that can serve as a guide for a systematic approach to occupational health program and services development. This model is predicated on the General Systems Theory and approach developed by von Bertalanffy (1968) and commonly applied in the business sector. However, before discussing the application of this model in the occupational health setting, basic systems theory definitions and conceptual linkages are described so that model elements can be more easily understood.

General Systems Theory provides an approach to examining organizational interactions and relationships in order to achieve desired outcomes or goals. Systems are arranged in hierarchical order, and thus all systems or entities are subsystems of larger entities called suprasystems. In addition, systems may be considered open or closed. All organisms are open systems that enter into an exchange with the environment, which stimulates the internal make-up of the overall system. In contrast, a closed system operates with specific variables that produce predictable outcomes. For example, Putt (1978) describes an individual conceptualized as being composed of a number of cells or body systems, or subsystems, such as the circulatory system or respiratory system. At the same time an individual is part of a number of larger systems, such as a family, work or school group, community, and society. In both cases the individual is an open system interacting with the environment. In like manner the occupational health unit can be considered a subsystem within the business, industry, or institutional system, which may also be part of a complex organizational or corporate structure, or suprasystem, and is influenced by the external environment. Changes in one system are likely to affect another system. Hall and Weaver (1985) point out that all systems, because of their interrelated hierarchical arrangement, may also be viewed as subsystems or suprasystems, depending on one's focus or location within the hierarchy. Thus, it is important to specify which system is the system of analysis or focus—that is, which system is the target system.

SYSTEMS APPROACH AND COMPONENTS

The basic elements of a system (Figure 6-1) can be applied to any organizational setting. In General Systems Theory a system is defined as a set of components or units interacting with each other (Hazard, 1978; von Bertalanffy, 1968). All living systems are open systems, and as depicted in Figure 6-1, there is a continual exchange of information and energy from the interactions of the system with the environment through a semipermeable boundary (dotted line). This boundary allows for the filtering of information into and out of the system (Griffith-Kenney & Christensen, 1986). For example, many occupational health and safety activities are affected by regulatory agencies, such as the Occupational Safety and Health Administration (OSHA). Thus, the employer needs to develop mechanisms to meet regulatory requirements and provide data through accurate recordkeeping to ensure compliance with these requirements.

Components of all systems have inputs, throughput processes, outputs, and feedback mechanisms and function within the context of the environment. The environment of the system includes all factors that affect and are affected by the system, and these include economic and legislative influences. For a system to survive, it must have adaptive capabilities within the environment, integration of system or subsystem components, and effective decision making about the allocation of resources to achieve organizational and system goals.

From a systems perspective inputs are supports, demands, or some form of energy or information that is taken into the system and then processed through into the system's outputs (Hazard, 1978). For example, in the simplest form the employee enters the company system and processes work to achieve the desired output— that is, the product or service of the industry or organization. From the occupational health perspective the occupational health unit as a subsystem of the company is influenced by external entities such as OSHA (environment). The inputs or energy into the occupational health unit (sub)system include the corporate culture, workers, work processes and related hazards, resources, and goals that interact together. Outputs of the occupational health unit system are healthy workers with a good quality of life. This is

accomplished through integration of throughput processes creating both alterations to reduce and eliminate hazards and support for programs and services aimed at health promotion and health protection efforts that reduce illness and injury. The feedback mechanism allows the system to use output information as a measure of the effectiveness of system functioning and links output information back to the inputs (Parillo, 1993). Feedback may be positive, negative, or neutral and is reintroduced into the system as input data in order to improve, adjust, modify, or make corrections as needed. For example, if an occupational health goal is thwarted because employees do not have appropriate personal protective equipment or cannot participate in occupational health programs (e.g., smoking cessation programs) on company time, the occupational health professional will need to reexamine and renegotiate approaches and strategies with management to achieve the desired goal or end point.

As another example of the system process (inputs→throughputs→outputs→feedback→inputs), an employee (*input*) diagnosed with high blood pressure visits the occupational health unit for blood pressure monitoring (*throughput*). The blood pressure is elevated, and the employee is referred (*throughput*) back to his primary health care provider for follow-up. The employee's medication is adjusted, and he returns to work with controlled blood pressure and fit for duty. Prevention of potential illness, such as a stroke, and injury may have occurred (*output*) as a result of the occupational and environmental health nurse's monitoring and referral intervention. This leads to information fedback into the system that monitoring for chronic disorders was effective (*feedback*).

CONCEPTUAL APPROACH TO OCCUPATIONAL HEALTH PROGRAMMING

The conceptual model shown in Figure 6-2 can serve as a guide for the application of the systems approach for assessing, analyzing, and developing occupational health and safety services and programs. The framework illustrates the interrelatedness of the system as a whole, its external environment, and the internal functioning of the

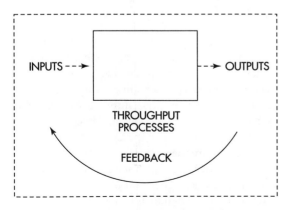

Figure 6-1 Systems framework environment.

system (through the flow of inputs, throughput processes and related interventions, and outputs) to achieve the goals or outcomes desired. The feedback mechanism represents a control function to improve the overall functioning of the system. As previously mentioned, all systems in systems theory are arranged in a hierarchical order; however, each subsystem, system, or suprasystem retains the functioning properties and elements of a system (i.e., contextual environment, system inputs, throughputs, outputs, and feedback). Thus, this model is an application of the systems approach to the occupational health unit viewed as the target

system, albeit a subsystem of the business or organization in which it functions.

ENVIRONMENTAL INFLUENCES

An examination of the model shows that the business and ultimately the occupational health unit are affected or influenced by external contextual factors, including population and health care trends, legislation/politics, the economy and economic forecasts, and technology and its advances. This relationship is depicted through environment-system interaction via the dotted interface line (see Figure 6-2). Examples of external contex-

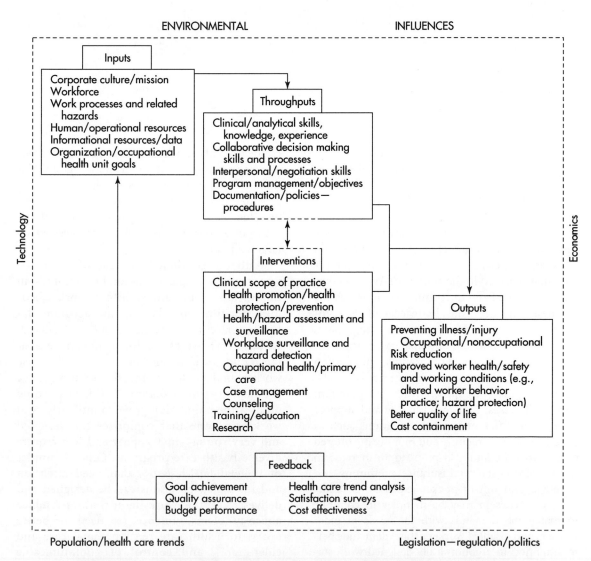

Figure 6-2   Conceptual framework for occupational health programs and services.

TABLE 6-1	Examples of External Environmental Influences		
POPULATION/HEALTH CARE TRENDS	LEGISLATION/REGULATION/ POLITICS	TECHNOLOGY	ECONOMY
Population demographics:	OSH Act	New/redesigned work processes	Increased health care costs
• Aging society	Hazard Communication Standard	New chemicals	Workers' compensation
• More women as workers	Americans With Disabilities Act	Computerization	Health insurance
• Ethnic diversity	Recordkeeping	Robotics/worker displacement	Cost containment
• Bipolarly aged society	Nurse Practice Acts	Communications	Managed care
• Increased chronic illness	Lobbying efforts by special interest groups	Distance education	Increased business costs
Bio/chemical terrorism	Political administration		
Rural/urban environments			
Community violence			

tual factors are shown in Table 6-1 and a description of each of these elements is provided here.

Population and Health and Health Care Trends

Population and health and health care trends are important factors affecting the business and occupational health unit because these indices are often reflected in the workforce. Workers typically are hired from the community in which the business is located; thus, knowledge of the community culture and population demographics can provide actual and anticipatory information about the workforce. For example, population data clearly indicate a continued increase in the aging of the population with concomitant chronic illnesses. This may indicate and support a need for different types of programs such as chronic disease screening and monitoring offered at the worksite and also point to an increase in health care costs via insurance premiums and coverage and out-of-pocket expenses. In addition, job redesign may be in order to continue to match job demands with the needs of older workers and disabled workers; this will include better attention to ergonomically designed work stations and work organization structures. Increased

ethnic diversity in the population and workforce will also require a better understanding of variations in ethnic culture; this understanding may provide more insight into how workers perceive or value health and/or how and under what circumstances health care delivery is received by targeted populations.

With the continued increase of women—who may be single heads of households—in the workforce, more flexibility in work schedules, flex-time, job sharing, and accommodations for child care must be considered. Evidence exists that employee concern regarding child care arrangements may increase worker anxiety, stress, and illness and reduce productivity (Mastroianni, 1992). Depending on how the population grows, a bipolarly aged workforce—one that comprises the very old and very young—may appear and will require diverse health care programs. Other examples of societal health issues that need attention and for which programs can be designed and delivered at the worksite include substance abuse problems, violence, the need for better access to health care (e.g., prenatal care and elder care), and control of communicable diseases.

Legislation/Regulation and Politics

The occupational and environmental health nurse must have a good understanding of another major group of contextual factors that include the laws, regulations, and quasi-regulations affecting industry and occupational health as well as the political influences affecting the processes of legislation and regulation. For example, over the past several decades several pieces of occupational health related legislation have been enacted; these include, among others, the Federal Coal Mine Safety and Health Act (1969), the Occupational Safety and Health Act (1970), the Noise Control Act (1972), the Toxic Substances Control Act (1976), the Hazard Communication Standard (1983), the Americans With Disabilities Act (1990), the Bloodborne Pathogens Standard (1991), and the Family and Medical Leave Act. Laws such as these and resultant regulations affect the workplace and workforce in terms of (1) mandated programs and requirements for occupational health and safety program initiatives and expansion, (2) program administration, (3) institution of preventive and control strategies to meet regulatory mandates and reduce worker exposures, and (4) acquisition of necessary resources to achieve occupational health requirements and goals. In addition, quasi-governmental agencies also affect industry entities. For example, the Joint Commission on the Accreditation of Health Care Organizations (JCAHO), while not regulatory, has the ability through its accreditation function to influence the standards and quality of care given by health care agencies. Understanding health care legislative reforms and changes in health care professional practice acts will have an important impact on the business community with regard to related health care costs and service delivery options.

The occupational and environmental health nurse is in a key position to help interpret the meaning of occupational health and safety and health care regulations with respect to appropriate and necessary health-related programs, strategies, and interventions and to help the company comply with regulatory requirements. The implementation of strategies to effect compliance with regulations may pose a significant economic burden on business and industry. Thus, health protection and health promotion programs must be cost-effectively designed to reduce work-related injuries and illnesses.

Political influences, such as special interest groups, can affect the passage of legislation; the occupational and environmental health nurse will want to recognize these influences and their impact and individually or collectively be involved in the political process to improve working conditions and worker and workforce health and safety. For example, the American Association of Occupational Health Nurses (AAOHN), through its governmental affairs program, monitors proposed legislation affecting occupational health and safety and provides testimony before congressional committees to influence passage, modification, or nonpassage of related legislative acts such as the Bloodborne Pathogens Standard or OSHA Reform Act. The impact of the current political administration will be significant. The occupational and environmental health nurse will want to keep abreast of these issues in order to effectively monitor and communicate the potential impact at the worksite.

Technology

Technological advances add to industries' capacity to develop and implement new or improved work processes, systems for more effective monitoring and analysis of work-related illness and injury trends, and enhanced computer applications for more efficient communications. New or redesigned work processes must be examined prior to implementation and continually monitored to determine the potential for work-related hazardous exposures. In addition, due to new or computerized manufacturing work processes, workers may be displaced, requiring job retraining and the acquisition of new skills, or workers may be terminated, with the loss not only of income but also of health insurance benefits, thus creating uncertainty and anxiety for workers (and families) and business.

Economics

Economic variables are of major contextual importance because they affect the overall health of the company in terms of profitability, growth, and expansion, which in turn affects the stability, morale, and productivity of a workforce. Thus, if the company is profitable, the size of the workforce will probably remain stable if not increase. However, with decreases in profits companies often downsize or resize to fit or balance the bottom line, and these corporate moves result in higher levels of unemployment and more uninsured individuals. In 1997 approximately $1.092 trillion, or 13.5% of the gross domestic product, was spent on health care costs (Levitt, 1998). Much of this cost was associated with increased health care costs related to medical technological advances and debilitating illnesses and was paid for by the employer through higher health care insurance premiums as well as escalating costs related to workers' compensation. As injury rates increase, workers' compensation insurance premiums also rise, adding to employer economic liabilities. In the context of economics the community employment rate and patterns are important measures to consider because these will affect the pool of potential workers at the company. This, complete with the work ethic present in potential employees, will affect the economic forecasts of the company. Employers must consider the value of implementing occupational health and safety programs, whether they are mandated regulatory programs or health promotion programs, and the potential savings derived despite their associated direct costs. However, occupational health professionals bear the responsibility for developing programs and services that are cost-effective. In addition, providing primary care services at the worksite can potentially decrease the utilization of costly external health care services and provide an effective cost containment strategy through more efficient resource use and decreased lost work time. Evidence exists to support the use of occupational and environmental health nurses and nurse practitioners at the worksite because they provide cost-effective services; thus, primary care services could be increased through utilization of these practitioners (Touger & Butts, 1989).

SYSTEM INPUTS

The inputs into the occupational health unit system are determined by the business or organization and include the corporate mission, philosophy, and culture; the workforce; the work, work processes, and related hazards; the available human and operational resources; the information resources; and the organizational and occupational health unit goals. System inputs interact together and with the environment and are ultimately transformed into system outputs (see Figure 6-2).

Corporate Mission, Philosophy, and Culture

The importance of understanding the corporate or company mission, philosophy, and culture cannot be overstated. The occupational and environmental health nurse will want to gather information about management's commitment to providing worksite health care programs, including occupational and nonoccupational health services. Management's commitment to occupational health is usually demonstrated through the establishment of and its participation on health and safety committees; resource allocation for occupational health and safety programs; inclusion of occupational health and employees in decision making processes regarding health and safety; promotion of health, wellness, and health risk reduction through company-sponsored health programs on company time; the incorporation of a concept of health that may extend beyond the workplace to include family participation in worksite health activities and industry-sponsored occupational health events, such as health fairs, or support for educational activities; and policy level placement of occupational health within the corporate structure.

Management's philosophy about work and health and their interrelationships as they affect workers' productivity, morale, and well-being will provide the underpinning for the success of the occupational health service. If management has a lukewarm attitude toward worker health, then occupational health services and programs are not likely to be viewed as a priority, except for meeting mandated programs. The occupational and environmental health nurse will want to influence management's perception about the value of occupational health and safety programs by demonstrating that these programs can be cost-effective, increase employee morale and productivity, and improve the company's image among the workforce and community.

The company culture is concerned with both management's and workers' attitudes, values, and beliefs about work and health. This may be witnessed in workers' participation in health and wellness programs, compliance with regulatory mandates, and overall observation of safe and healthful work practices. The occupational and environmental health nurse must understand the value of company culture because this can have a major impact on the success of any program. Organizational culture exerts considerable influence on types of changes made and behavior expressed. These points are described more fully in Chapters 9 and 13.

Workforce, Work, and Work-related Hazards

Workforce inputs must be examined so that the occupational and environmental health nurse can plan and implement effective occupational health and safety programs relative to the needs of the workers. The aggregate workforce should be viewed in terms of the size and distribution of the workforce, demographic characteristics (e.g., age, gender, ethnicity, and education), and health status indicators including lifestyle risk factors and morbidity and mortality trends and patterns. Workers perceptions about health, accident prevention, work and risk perception and acceptance, and related work practice behaviors also must be assessed. The health status and occupational history of workers also must be examined so that workers and jobs are appropriately matched. This is discussed in more detail in Chapter 10.

Workers are employed to produce a certain product or service. Depending on the type of work and related work processes, workers may potentially be exposed to various workplace hazards from biological, chemical, enviromechanical, physical, or psychosocial agents. For example, in the course of providing daily patient care nurses are at risk of biological agent exposure from potential exposure to blood or body fluids of patients. Farm workers may be at risk for neurological, hematological, or other adverse body system effects from chemical exposure to pesticides. Truck drivers may be at risk of back injury and cardiovascular stasis from prolonged sitting in awkward postures as well as injuries and deaths from motor vehicle accidents (highest cause of occupational fatalities). The occupational and environmental health nurse professional will need to have a thorough understanding of the industry's work processes, products and by-products, workers' job tasks and demands, and working conditions in order to recognize potential and actual hazards and design, implement, and monitor strategies to prevent potential hazard

exposure or alter existing hazardous conditions. This can be accomplished through a careful review of company information related to work processes, associated industry and governmental technical reports and health hazard evaluations, and direct observation from workplace walkthroughs. Depending on potential or actual exposures involved, the interaction of the worker with the work and its processes can clearly affect the health end points of the individual worker and the collective workforce. Hazard identification and evaluation are described more in-depth in Chapters 7 and 10.

Resources

Adequate human, operational, and capital resources are essential to an effective occupational health and safety program. With respect to human resources the best approach to comprehensive occupational health and safety programming is through a multidisciplinary effort. The core members of the occupational health and safety team include the occupational and environmental health nurse, occupational medicine physician, industrial hygienist, and safety specialist. Other team members may also include an ergonomist, toxicologist, and psychologist/employee assistance program (EAP) counselor. While the interdisciplinary approach to occupational health and safety management is the most effective, most businesses that employ occupational health and safety professionals primarily employ occupational and environmental health nurses. AAOHN surveys of its membership indicate that approximately 45% of the occupational and environmental health nurses employed tend to be the sole occupational and environmental health nurse at the worksite (AAOHN, 1999). Thus, the occupational and environmental health nurse is central to the management and coordination of occupational health unit activities. The occupational and environmental health nurse must have adequate and appropriate education, knowledge, and skills in the nursing, public health, occupational health, behavioral sciences and management concepts and principles; the nurse also must know about laws and regulations specific to occupational health. The knowledge and skills acquired are applied through the roles the nurse assumes in the occupational health setting, including direct care clinician, manager, educator, researcher, health promotion specialist, case manager, or consultant, all of which are described in great detail in Chapter 4.

As part of the core interdisciplinary team occupational medicine physicians may be employed full-time or part-time by the company to provide direct health care services or consultation in evaluating employee work-related illnesses and injuries requiring medical intervention. More often than not companies will have contractual relationships with community physicians or providers at health maintenance organizations to provide the services needed (Felton, 1990). The (collaborative) goal is a safe and rapid return of the ill or injured worker to work (McCunney, in press). Industrial hygienists help anticipate, recognize, evaluate, and control workplace hazards through walk-through observation of the workplace, measurement of workplace exposures, and recommendation and establishment of control strategies to prevent unnecessary exposures. Safety specialists conduct safety audits to identify hazardous and unsafe situations in the work environment, investigate accidents and work-related injuries, and institute worker training and education programs related to safety in the workplace. If the company does not employ these types of health care professionals, appropriate and specific services can be obtained from private consultants or through state health agencies.

The worker must be included as a member of the occupational health team if appropriate and realistic strategies for risk reduction and health improvement are to be developed and implemented. The team approach in assessing and evaluating work-related problems will lend itself to a broader perspective and interpretation of factors that affect worker health and also to a wider array of preventive and alternative control strategies.

Collaboration between professional disciplines and management is essential to effective, efficient programs and resource management. In addition to professional personnel, support personnel should be employed to handle the clerical and staff support tasks. This will ensure better use of occupational health professional skills and more efficient use of scarce resource dollars. Further information on occupational health and safety specialty areas can be found in this chapter and Chapter 7.

Operational resources include an adequate budget, facilities, equipment, and day-to-day operational supplies necessary to operate the occupational health and safety program. The occupational health unit budget should be developed based on established goals and objectives reflective of the needs for promoting and protecting worker health. The occupational and environmental health nurse manager must develop the budget or have input into the budget process because she or he is the person most familiar with the program unit goals and can most effectively manage the occupational health unit budget. In other words, the individual who controls the budget in essence controls the program.

Equipment needed in the occupational health unit can be expensive, so its purchase should be based on need and volume of use (i.e., occupational, nonoccupational, and health promotion activities). Extensive laboratory equipment is generally unnecessary where contractual laboratory services are more cost-effective and when the health care professional does not possess the skills necessary to conduct the test. As with any clinical setting up-to-date equipment should be provided. The occupational and environmental health nurse should develop and maintain an inventory of supplies and equipment necessary for the efficient and effective running of the occupational health services. An example of an inventory list of equipment/supplies can be found in Appendix 6-1.

Management should commit sufficient space for the occupational health unit. Facilities must be designed so that they meet the space needs of the staff and employee population while being comfortable and attractive. The size of the occupational health unit will vary and is often governed by space available. However, important factors in determining space allocation include the number of employees, work shifts, equipment used, storage needs, and scope and type of services to be provided. Guidotti et al. (1989) suggest that a more modern facility should provide a minimum of 1,500 square feet, with an additional 1.5 square feet, per employee above 200 employees.

Access to the occupational health unit is critical, and the unit should be located as central as possible to the majority of the workers. It should be barrier-free and equipped for handicapped individuals. The floor plan should be simple in design to facilitate the flow of work. Component areas include reception, record storage, diagnostic and treatment services, employee function areas (hygiene facilities, dressing rooms), counseling rooms, and conference space. Additional space for special program areas may be desirable depending on the types of services offered (e.g., physical therapy, fitness, library).

Information Resources

Information resources and data are needed to assist the occupational health professional in making decisions in occupational health programming. Examples of these resources include data on health, injury, and illness trends of the workforce; community health care service providers; health needs of the workforce for services and programs; health insurance and claims data; and costs of goods and services. Additional information resources include web-based technical resources, library/journal references, health and management-related materials, and computer linkages for data access and analysis and networking. Professional society and governmental resources provide numerous valuable tools, such as standards of care and code of ethics documents and health hazard evaluation reports produced by NIOSH.

Organizational/Occupational Health Goals

The last major system input is the establishment of occupational health unit goals. These goals must be congruent with the overall business or industry goals and should address such areas as high risk situations in terms of work-related illness/injury episodes and trends, worker needs, working conditions, and health promotion. The goals set the blueprint or direction, from which objectives will be derived for occupational health unit activities (throughput process), and the achievement of the throughput process will be measured as a system output. Although the goals for an occupational health program may vary depending on the type of industry and services provided, general goals include the following:

- Ensure a safe and healthful work environment;
- Protect employees from workplace hazards;
- Facilitate worker placement;
- Ensure adequate medical/health care and rehabilitation for the ill and injured worker;
- Promote optimal health of the worker/workforce;
- Build a corporate culture supportive of health.

SYSTEM THROUGHPUT PROCESSES AND INTERVENTIONS

System inputs interact and, as depicted in Figure 6-2, are transformed by utilizing a complex set of dynamic processes or throughputs to achieve the desired system output or outcome through organized, prioritized interventions. System throughput processes and interventions are variable and can be numerous, depending on the system and its needs. When considering the occupational health unit system inputs described, the following are examples of major throughput processes and interventions.

In the throughput process the occupational and environmental health nurse professional effectively utilizes knowledge, skills, and abilities to achieve the specified goals reflected in outputs. This includes (1) analyzing with other team members the interaction of system inputs; (2) setting achievable, programmatic objectives related to improved health and safety, such as developing an occupational health/medical surveillance program related to a specific OSHA standard, or developing a back injury prevention program within a specific time frame; (3) developing and implementing occupational health and safety policies and procedures; (4) identifying and prioritizing interventions related to scope of practice; (5) employing effective interpersonal skills to communicate to management and the workforce the value of and need for health programs and negotiating for additional or strategic resources; and (6) making collaborative decisions with the appropriate interdisciplinary team members, management, and workers regarding the development and implementation of effective strategies to improve worker health and safety, such as developing or using clinical guidelines or protocols for practice. This means that the occupational and environmental health nurse and other occupational health professionals must be adequately trained, skilled, and prepared and appropriately licensed and/or certified in order to identify and manage occupational health and safety problems, develop comprehensive and specific programs and services as required by law to meet worker needs, understand the business context for occupational health and safety programming, and continuously examine and monitor the effectiveness of decisions made. Both appropriate documentation, including recordkeeping and maintenance of administrative and legal reports, and utilization of computer-based record systems or programs for intervention are essential.

Interventions are tied to the throughput processes as products of the decision processes described earlier. Occupational and environmental health nurses practice within the legal framework of state nurse practice acts (see Chapter 15), the occupational and environmental health nursing scope of practice (Box 6-1 and see Chapter 3), the nursing process, the clinical nursing guidelines as appropriate (see Chapter 11), and the ethical parameters for practice derived from the AAOHN Code of Ethics (see Chapter 17). Interventions derived from the scope of practice are designed to meet the needs identified through throughput processes and lead to system outputs. Examples include health hazard assessments and surveillance; walk-throughs; health promotion, health protection and prevention programs, such as health appraisals, smoking cessation, wellness, hearing conservation, and health teaching and counseling regarding appropriate work practice and lifestyle risk factors; employee assistance programs; and delivery of occupational health and primary care and case management services for occupational and nonoccupational health services. Continuing training and education of the workforce and the occupational health professional is essential as a throughput process to improve and update knowledge, skills, and abilities related to the job. This training/education may include regulatory compliance training, disaster drills, or safety training or may be done through continuing education programs.

Research is also an important component in throughput processes; the occupational and environmental health nurse will need to read and implement, as appropriate, research findings relative to worker health and safety and also participate in the research process when feasible. For example, the nurse can identify researchable problems such as a cluster of repetitive motion problems reported by workers, participate in designing studies to address the problems, or test interventions to reduce the risk.

SYSTEM OUTPUTS

Through utilization of knowledge and skills in analysis, communication and negotiation techniques, decision making, interpersonal relationships, and collaboration, the occupational and environmental health nurse can improve her or his understanding of the interaction of the inputs, negotiate strategies, and design interventions that result in system outputs. These outputs reflect the product or service of the occupational health unit, a healthy worker and worker population and achievement of this desired end state. The major occupational health unit products or system outputs are related to the following factors:

1. Prevention of work-related illness and injury episodes
   - Decreased incidence and prevalence of work-related injuries, illnesses, and disabilities
   - Improved work practice controls and behaviors
   - Reduced premature morbidity and mortality related to hazardous exposure
   - Decreased workers' compensation claims
2. Improvement in the health and safety of the workforce and work environment
   - Improved population health and quality of life
   - Enhanced managerial commitment to a healthy, safe, supportive environment
   - Increased health promotion/health protection programs
   - Improved occupational health and safety risk reduction programs
   - Improved healthful working conditions and work environment
   - Increased compliance with health and safety strategies (mandated, recommended)
3. Cost-effective programming
   - Decreased health care costs (i.e., workers' compensation and health insurance premiums)
   - Decreased absenteeism and lost work time
   - Increased productivity

Box 6-1 **Scope of Practice in Occupational and Environmental Health Nursing**

- Worker/workplace assessment and surveillance
- Occupational health care and primary care
- Case management
- Health promotion/protection
- Counseling
- Management/administration
- Community orientation
- Research/trend analysis
- Legal/ethical monitoring

The occupational and environmental health nurse will want to determine if and to what extent outputs or outcomes have been achieved. This is best accomplished through ascertaining if occupational health services and programs were effective in meeting predetermined objectives, altering risk, improving health parameter measurements (e.g., morbidity and mortality trends), and reducing costs.

As previously described, in the process of transforming inputs into outputs objectives are determined in the throughput phase to meet occupational health and safety program goals. In the output phase the objectives should be measured for effective achievement. For example, if the occupational and environmental health nurse identified from system inputs that employees were potentially exposed to blood and were not using personal protection equipment or that complaints regarding repetitive motion disorders—later validated through examinations—had increased, objectives would be developed related to designing strategies to increase the use of protective equipment or to reduce the incidence of repetitively designed work, and these objectives would be measured as outputs.

SYSTEM FEEDBACK

The occupational health unit system is dependent on larger systems and influences—that is, the company and environment for its inputs and also for acceptance of its outputs (Gibson et al., 1985). The feedback or evaluation mechanism is designed so that the system can make adjustments that are more responsive to worker needs, organizational and occupational health goals, and environmental demands. Feedback is concerned with identifying and measuring goal/objective achievement or lack thereof, what needs to be altered or improved to correct deviations, or what successful endeavors need to be enhanced or promoted. For example, if musculoskeletal injury or pain complaints have increased, the nurse might be able to determine the cause as related to implementation of a new work process. Collaboration with industrial hygiene, safety, management, and workers to redesign or alter the process could be an effective strategy to eliminate the injury. In addition, if a hypertension screening program was implemented but was poorly attended, the nurse might find that the lack of participation was due to a problem with scheduling, which could be altered.

Measurement of illness/injury trend data over time can also provide information about the effectiveness of program strategies. For example, one can examine and analyze data collected from the OSHA log from one year to the next and use these data as a basis for comparison related to the effectiveness of interventions/programs instituted as a result of data analyzed. Development and measurement of objectives and analysis of epidemiologic trends are described in more detail in Chapters 13, 16, and 5 respectively.

Quality monitoring is an important aspect of the feedback process, which includes monitoring quality planning, control, and improvement functions. The outcome of this process is to determine if the results expected are achieved through quality health care at the most economical cost. The occupational and environmental health nurse will want to evaluate the effectiveness and benefits of outcomes achieved using cost-effectiveness and cost-benefit analyses. This approach can also be a mechanism used to demonstrate value.

In the feedback loop budget analysis should be performed to determine the budget's match with goals and objectives. This means examining expenditures as related to achievement of the objectives and determining budget deviations as overages or deficits in terms of allocated costs. This will also reflect the appropriateness of planning for programs and services.

Another important feedback mechanism with respect to the value of occupational health services and programs is the use of satisfaction surveys of workers and management (Rogers et al., 1993). Based on the satisfaction data obtained regarding how individuals feel about the delivery and quality of occupational health services, modifications or adjustments can be made to improve or enhance the program. Data from satisfaction surveys can be very powerful in supporting quality and cost findings and acknowledging the value of occupational health staff support in providing health care services.

Summary

The use of a conceptual approach to develop occupational health and safety programs and services provides a systematic method to examine and analyze the occupational health system within the context of the company and external environment. This will help to focus on system and environmental demands that are directed toward improving worker health and reducing work-related risks.

The occupational and environmental health nurse will want to thoroughly examine system inputs in order to determine what throughput skills (i.e., analysis, negotiation) need to be employed to achieve the outputs and outcomes desired. This approach will allow for a better understanding of how systems function and interact to achieve organizational and occupational unit goals.

References

American Association of Occupational Health Nurses. (1999). *Membership Statistics.* Atlanta, GA: Author.

Felton, J. S. (1990). *Occupational medical management.* Boston: Little, Brown & Company.

Gibson, J. L., Ivancevich, J. M., & Donnelly, J. H. (1985). *Organizations* (pp. 5-21). Plano, TX: Business Publications.

Griffith-Kenney, J. W., & Christensen, P. J. (1986). *Nursing process: Application of theories, frameworks, and models.* St. Louis, MO: Mosby.

Guidotti, T., Cowell, J., Jamieson, G., & Engleberg, A. L. (1989). *Occupational health services: A practical approach.* Chicago: American Medical Association.

Hall, J., & Weaver B. (1985). *Distributive nursing practice: A systems approach to community health.* Philadelphia: J. B. Lippincott.

Hazard, M. E. (1978). An overview of systems theory. *Nursing Clinics of Nursing America, 6*(3), 385-393.

Levit, K. C. (1998). National health expenditures in 1997: More slow growth. *Health Affairs, 17,* 99-110.

Mastroianni, K. (1992). Child day care arrangements and employee health. *AAOHN Journal, 40*(2), 78-83.

McCunney, R. (in press). *A practical approach to occupational and environmental medicine.* Boston: Little, Brown & Company.

Putt, A. (1978). *General systems theory applied to nursing.* Boston: Little, Brown & Company.

Rogers, B., Winslow, B., & Higgins, S. (1993). Employee satisfaction with occupational health services. *AAOHN Journal, 41*(2), 58-65.

Touger, G. N., & Butts, J. (1989). The workplace: An innovative and cost-effective practice site. *The Nurse Practitioner, 14*(1), 35-42.

von Bertalanffy, L. (1968). *General systems theory.* New York: George Brazillet.

6-1 Equipment and Supplies for an Occupational Health Unit

FURNISHINGS

Office

Desks
Chairs
Bookcases
Filing cabinets with locks
Storage cabinets with locks
Wall clocks
Word processor, typewriters, computer
Tables
Wastebaskets
In/Out baskets
Desk lamps
Bulletin boards
Calculators

Clinic

Stools, height appropriate to counter, with adjustable backs
Chart-holders, with priority and occupancy indicators
Stretcher, wheelchairs, beds
Sinks with surgical handles on faucets, towel racks
Examination tables
Chairs
Medication cabinet with locks
Pedal-operated wastebaskets with lid and liners
Health records filing cabinets
Instrument trays
Autoclave (optional)
Refrigerator
Oxygen unit

Major instruments

Wall-mounted otoscope/ophthalmoscope
Wall-mounted sphygmomanometer (blood pressure cuff)
Crash cart (cardiopulmonary resuscitation) must be fully equipped and provided with a seal to ensure that it is not opened and drugs and equipment are not used except in a true emergency
Scales

Electrocardiograph
Audiometer (optional)
Vision screening apparatus
Recording spirometry (optional)
Suction apparatus

Hand-held instruments

Irrigating syringe, suitable for removal of cerumen from ear
Assorted clamps
Dental mirror
Dynamometer (for measuring grip strength)
Flashlights
Laryngoscope (in crash cart)
Sphygmomanometer with varying cuffs (small, medium, large, [i.e., thigh])-band held
Magnifying lens
Percussion hammer
Scalpels
Surgical scissors
Ear specula
Nasal specula
Vaginal specula
Stethoscope
Tape measures
Thermometer
Tuning forks
Color vision chart (Ishihara plates)

SUPPLIES

Syringes
Needles
Gloves
Vacutainers and assorted blood-drawing apparatus
Tongue depressors
Cotton swabs
Gauze pads
Assorted dressings
Suture material and needles/suture removal materials
Specimen containers
Elastic bandages, in assorted sizes
Self-adhering gauze bandage rolls

Protective clothing
Large compresses
Butterfly closures (Steri-Strips)
Adhesive tape
Ace bandages
Portable emergency list
Stockinette bandage
Telfa pads of different sizes
Sling
Pressure bandages (2, 3, 4, and 6 inches in width)
Triangular bandages
Cold packs
Cervical collars
Surgical masks and hoods
Eye patches and pads
Cotton, in various forms
Inflatable splints
Various types of splints, such as wrist and leg
First aid boxes, first aid manual
First aid scissors, bandage scissors, straight scissors
First aid tweezers, splinter forceps, nail clippers
Basins of various sizes and capacities
Crutches
Instrument trays with covers
Heating pad set-up, hydroculator and pads
Finger cots

Antiseptics
Blankets
Examination gowns and paper sheets
Eye irrigating solutions
Facial tissue
Pillows with pillow cases
Safety pins
Sheets (including sterile burn sheet)
Towels (varying sizes)

MEDICATIONS COMMONLY USED IN AN OCCUPATIONAL HEALTH SERVICE

Acetylsalicylic acid 325 mg tablets (Aspirin)
Acetaminophen 325 mg tablets (Tylenol)
Actifed tablets
Chlorpheniramine maleate tablets (Chlor-Trimeton)
Dimenhydrinate tablets and suppositories (Dramamine)
Diphenhydramine hydrochloride 25 mg (Benadryl Caps); cream and injections 50 mg/ml
Epinephrine (Adrenalin)
Magnesia and alumina suspension (Maalox)
Kaopectate
Guaifenesin syrup 100 rag/5 ml (Robitussin)
Bacitracin 500 unit/g ointment (Baciguent)

7 Using Interdisciplinary Knowledge to Assess Work and the Work Environment

The Occupational Health and Safety Administration (OSHA) published "Guidelines on Workplace Safety and Health Program Management" (USDOL, 1989), which describes an effective program as one that looks beyond the specific requirements of the law in addressing general and specific workplace hazards. This supports the primary goal of a comprehensive occupational health program: to preserve, protect, and improve the health of the workforce. Doing so requires substantial knowledge in the occupational health sciences as well as an interdisciplinary approach to recognizing and understanding work-related risks and hazards so that effective occupational health and safety services can be delivered. Essential to the success of an effective program is a thorough assessment of the work and work environment to determine potential and actual work-related exposures and continuous monitoring to prevent and control workplace hazards. This complex process requires the knowledge and skills of many disciplines. Nursing's collaborative and interdependent relationship with occupational medicine and an understanding of the principles underlying the fields of safety, ergonomics, toxicology, and industrial hygiene are key to developing knowledge domains essential to occupational and environmental health nursing practice. This will further serve to foster increased collaboration among occupational health and safety professional disciplines to better understand the effects of work and workplace exposures on human health.

The occupational and environmental health nurse is often the only licensed health professional at the worksite and thus plays a critical role in worksite assessment. In order to relate any human response to a work-related exposure or within an occupational context, the occupational and environmental health nurse needs to be familiar with worker jobs and demands, steps in the work processes, and all aspects of the work environment. However, a team approach to worksite assessments and walk-throughs should be used whenever possible and may involve occupational health and safety professionals, workers, management, union representatives, and other health care professionals. This approach will add to the breadth and depth of the investigation, further the understanding of human consequences related to hazardous workplace exposures, and add input for remedies regarding hazard abatement. The ultimate goal is to ensure a safe and healthful work environment and thereby protect and promote the physical and mental well-being of the worker. With virtually thousands of new chemicals and work processes active in the occupational environment (Hall et al., 1997), all health care professionals must delineate new occupational hazards, detect existing problems, and develop and implement preventive strategies before human harm occurs. This requires the health care professional to identify high-risk occupations, work areas, materials, and processes; determine the effectiveness of existing health and safety programs and control measures; and recommend target areas for worksite and work process modification and/or training and education needs (Camp & Tanberg, 1985; Rogers, 1998). Guided by an interdisciplinary approach, a worksite assessment and a walk-through are essential to the identification of work-related hazards and will result in prevention and abatement strategies.

This chapter will focus on interdisciplinary fields of knowledge fundamental to occupational and environmental health nursing practice, which will enhance the nurse's knowledge of workplace hazards, mechanisms of exposures, and methods to control or minimize associated risks. The conduct of a worksite assessment and walk-through and essential components of hazard assessment and analysis will be discussed.

WORKPLACE HAZARDS

In order to begin a discussion of interdisciplinary fields of knowledge and risk assessment approaches, occupational health professionals must know what workplace exposure risks exist and how to recognize work-related hazards that contribute to a health risk environment. As a result of exposure to specific agents, the following workplace hazards can be potentiated:

1. *Biological/infectious hazards.* Infectious/biological agents, such as bacteria, viruses, fungi, or parasites, which may be transmitted to other individuals via contact with infected patients or contaminated body secretions/fluids
2. *Chemical hazards.* Varous forms of chemicals, including medications, solutions, gases, vapors, aerosols, and particulate matter, that are potentially toxic or irritating to the body system
3. *Enviromechanical hazards.* Factors encountered in the work environment that cause or potentiate accidents, injuries, strain, or discomfort (e.g., unsafe/inadequate equipment or lifting devices, slippery floors, work station deficiencies)
4. *Physical hazards.* Agents within the work environment, such as radiation, electricity, extreme temperatures, and noise, that can cause tissue trauma
5. *Psychosocial hazards.* Factors and situations that are encountered or associated with one's job or work environment and create or potentiate stress, emotional strain, and/or interpersonal problems

The occupational and environmental health nurse must have a good understanding of and accurately assess the potential for these workplace hazards and understand the role and skills of a variety of occupational health professionals in order to develop an effective and efficient risk reduction program.

OCCUPATIONAL MEDICINE

Since 1954 occupational medicine has been designated as a subspecialty of preventive medicine by the American Board of Preventive Medicine (McCunney, 1996). While some medical schools offer limited academic coursework in occupational medicine in the basic medicine curricula, postgraduate training in occupational medicine can be obtained through NIOSH Education and Research Centers and Training Project Grants located throughout the United States. These programs specialize in training aimed at preventing, treating, and controlling illnesses and injuries resulting from physical, chemical, and biological hazards in the workplace (McCunney, 1996). According to McCunney (2003), the number of specialists in the field of occupational medicine has increased nearly 200% during the last century, and the number of occupational medical residency programs has increased from only two or three in the early 1970s to about 40 U.S. medical centers offering training leading to Board certifications.

Felton (1990) defines occupational medicine as concerned with (1) the assessment, maintenance, restoration, and improvement of the health of the worker through the application of the principles of preventive medicine, emergency medical care, rehabilitation, and environmental medicine; (2) the promotion of productive and fulfilling interactions of workers with their work through the application of the principles of human behavior; and (3) the active appreciation of the social, economic, and administrative needs and responsibilities of both the worker and the work community. While occupational medicine is concerned with both the prevention and treatment of occupational disease and injury, the magnitude of occupational illness and injury is difficult to assess; this is particularly true for occupational illness. Each day in the United States an average of 9,000 workers sustain disabling injuries on the job, 16 workers die from a workplace injury, and 137 workers die from work-related diseases. However, the number of occupational diseases and injuries reported is much lower than estimated at 10 million work-related injuries and 430,000 new work-related illnesses occurring each year in the United States (US-DHHS, NIOSH, 1995). Although these statistics provide some idea of the scope and types of occupational health problems, they grossly underestimate the role of the workplace in causing new diseases and injuries and exacerbating existing ones. In addition, statistics do not represent the relative distribution of various work-related diseases. For example, because skin disorders are easy to recognize and relate to working conditions, their representation may overexaggerate their relative importance. The difficulty in obtaining accurate estimates of the frequency of work-related diseases is due to several factors, which include the following:

- Many problems do not come to the attention of health professionals and employers and therefore are not included in data collection systems.
- Recognition of disease as work-related is often difficult; the long period between initial exposure and onset of symptoms (or time of diagnosis) makes cause-effect relationships difficult to assess. Adding to this difficulty are the many occupational and nonoccupational hazards to which most workers are exposed.
- There may be a lack of knowledge about what is reportable as work-related (Figure 7-1).

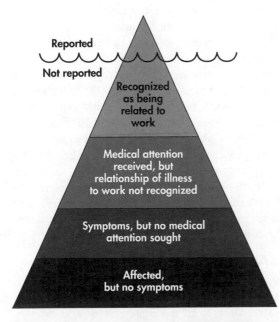

Figure 7-1 "The Iceberg" of occupational disease.

Industry has traditionally provided most employment in clinical occupational medicine. Physicians who work at the upper management level are more involved in questions of policy, whereas those at the plant level are more involved in clinical duties. Physicians also work for governmental agencies at federal and state levels. For example, physicians work with and assist in the functions of NIOSH and OSHA. Because NIOSH is primarily a research agency, its medical staff is devoted primarily to research which may take the form of health hazard evaluations or field investigations or involve basic scientific, surveillance, or epidemiologic investigations. Physicians at OSHA may be involved in setting standards, developing occupational health and safety regulations, and determining related policy.

A growing number of opportunities to practice occupational medicine can be found in clinical settings in the community. In some cases occupational medicine clinics exist as independent contractors that sell to client companies such services as preplacement and return to work evaluations, drug screening, and trauma care. Alternatively, some clinical occupational medicine units exist as parts of hospital staffs, usually within departments of medicine or family practice. Physicians may perform complex illness/injury management, evaluate patients for insurance companies (e.g., for disability impairment ratings), and participate in health/medical surveillance programs on a consultative basis (and subcontract with industrial hygiene and clinical laboratory facilities when appropriate).

Levy and Wegman (2000) state that physicians employed by companies have responsibilities in three general areas:

1. Prevention and early detection of occupational disease and injury
2. Diagnosis and treatment of occupational disease and injury (with emphasis on return of workers to their job)
3. Diagnosis and treatment of nonoccupational disease or injury in emerging situations or when community resources are unavailable

Clearly, some of these responsibilities represent overlapping or shared functions, particularly with nursing (and in some instances with other disciplines), within the parameters of state practice acts; thus, the need for close collaboration between occupational and environmental health nurses and occupational medicine physicians is imperative.

The occupational and environmental health nurse practicing in the clinical setting must be familiar with occupational diseases and injuries within the contexts of nursing practice and process and the exposures relevant to the workforce population served. For example, LaDou (1997) reports that workers in manufacturing have the largest number of occupational illnesses. Although these workers constitute only 20% of total employees, they account for 35% of occupational illnesses, with musculoskeletal disorders and skin rashes representing most cases. A major cause of occupational illnesses among production workers is exposure to toxic chemicals, such as solvents, acids, and those chemicals found in soaps, petroleum fractions, paints, plastics, and resins. Additional problems occur from exposure to dusts, gases, and metals. The occupational and environmental health nurse must be able to assess the problem and provide treatment or refer the injured or ill worker to the appropriate health care provider when necessary (or sometimes do both). The addition of reference sources in a variety of fields, such as textbooks in occupational medicine, safety, epidemiology, and toxicology, to the occupational health library will prove quite valuable.

A multidisciplinary approach to occupational health care is essential and requires occupational medicine physicians, nurses, safety specialists, industrial hygienists, and others whose knowledge is specific to the problem at hand to collaborate in recognizing, treating, and preventing occupational illness and injury. Felton (1990) points out that an effective occupational health service implies cooperative functioning of all members of the group charged with operation of a program in occupational health. There is much work to be done; promoting and protecting worker health and a philosophy of collaboration facilitates this effort.

SAFETY

Safety in the workplace is everyone's responsibility, and awareness of safety and health issues is key to accident prevention. An accident is an unanticipated, sudden event that results in an undesired outcome such as bodily injury, death, or property

damage (Keyserling, 2000). Work-related injuries can result from accidents such as a falling object crushing bones; however, many are caused by routine work activities such as repetitive trauma causing a musculoskeletal injury. Although the number of fatal occupational injuries has gradually declined in recent years, work-related illnesses and nonfatal injuries appear to be increasing. From data reported by the U.S. Department of Labor, Bureau of Labor Statistics (BLS) (2000) and the National Safety Council (1997) during 1997 alone, disabling injuries numbered 8 million, with more than 125 million lost work days. NIOSH estimates that at least 10 million injuries, about 3 million of which are severe, occur on the job each year. Every workday more than 10,000 people suffer injuries that result in lost work time. (Chapter 1 details specific data on work-related injuries and illnesses.) As work-related injuries continue to remain high, prevention of accidents and injuries at the worksite continues to be a major priority in occupational health. The American National Standards Institute (ANSI) classifies work injuries according to accident type (Table 7-1).

The principal responsibility of the safety professional is to design, implement, and evaluate strategies aimed at preventing and controlling workplace exposures that result in injuries and deaths and emphasize training and education of workers about job safety. According to Lack (1996), the key role in fulfilling this responsibility is that of program leader, not hazard controller, which is often the role many safety practitioners assume. Controlling hazards (i.e., unsafe conditions and unsafe work practices) is primarily the responsibility of employees and supervisors. They are closest to the hazards and have the greatest capability of recognizing and controlling them. There can never be enough safety and health professionals with enough authority present in the workplace to effectively control the myriad of hazardous exposures that can occur on any given workday. However, the safety and health professional should influence and assist managers, supervisors, and employees to successfully meet their responsibilities.

SAFETY PROGRAMS

An effective safety program requires a multidisciplinary effort. The emphasis and commitment on safety starts with top management and extends, by example, throughout the organization to man-

TABLE 7-1	Work Injuries According to Accident Type as Classified by the American National Standards Institute (ANSI)	
WORK INJURY TYPE		**EXAMPLES OF PREVENTIVE MEASURES**
Struck by: Incidents in which the worker is hit by a moving object or particle. Examples include falling or flying objects or moving equipment.		Side rails, nets, gratings, safety helmets, and steel-toed shoes.
Caught in, under, or between: Incidents involving an injury caused by crushing, squeezing, or pinching of a body part between a moving and stationary object or two moving objects. Examples include operations involving mechanical equipment such as power presses or calendars where tasks place workers' hands near moving parts.		Barrier guards and equipment enclosures, safety buttons, presence-sensing systems (electric eye), emerging stop buttons, and lockout switches.
Struck against: Incidents in which the worker collides with stationary objects. Examples include hitting head on low ceilings or body parts hitting equipment.		Improved work station and tool design and use of safety helmets or gloves.
Fall from elevation: Incidents in which the worker falls to a lower level and is injured on impact against an object on the ground. Examples include falls from ladders and other temporary work surfaces (scaffolds).		Guardrails and devices such as safety belts, harnesses, lanyards and lifelines.
Falls on same level: Incidents involving workers who lose their footing and fall to surfaces supporting them. Examples include loss of foot traction, walking on wet, oily surfaces or highly polished surfaces (usually from a non-skid surface), trips, and missteps.		Appropriate tread shoes, good housekeeping, maintenance, and lighting, and placement of warning or caution signs.
Motor vehicle accidents: (1) Incidents involving injury as a result of a vehicular crash due to changing environmental conditions (poor lighting, rain, ice) driver fatigue, or vehicle maintenance problems. (2) Incidents involving injury while person is operating a motor vehicle. Examples include internal accidents occurring at the worksite itself (e.g., while operating a forklift) and accidents external to the worksite on public roads.		Training techniques, driver selection processes, vehicle inspection and maintenance programs, seat belts, and daily limits on amount of driving.
Overexertion and repetitive trauma: Incidents involving worker injuries caused by excessive physical effort or highly repetitive patterns of localized muscle and joint usage resulting in back injuries, sprains, and strains. Examples include manual handling of materials, assembly line work, or jobs requiring awkward posture.		Ergonomically designed equipment, lifting devices, reductions in load weight, and job rotation.
Other causes of physical trauma: Incidents involving contact with electric current, temperature extremes, radiation, caustics, and toxic and noxious substances; tissue rubbing or abrading; bodily reaction; public transportation accident; other/unknown.		Appropriate measures to reduce the risk of injury (effective grounding of electrical equipment, insulation of all electric hand tools), safety equipment for body protection, (helmets), robots in extreme temperature situations, appropriate insulating materials, and covering of sharp objects with padding or handholds.

agers and other employees. The National Safety Council (1997) identifies the following five steps in planning systems for safety, health, and environmental management:

1. Work with senior management to shape and guide the organization's safety and health policy in order to build the commitment from top management; create a vision statement and define the safety, health, and environmental policy; make sure the policy is addressed in the business plan and aligned with the business strategy.
2. Identify and communicate the safety and health rules of everyone in the organization—spell out responsibilities; include accountabilities in each employee's job description and evaluate everyone, based on those accountabilities.
3. Analyze the work and the workplace continually to identify all existing and potential hazards—most analyses should be data driven, but some can be more imaginative (e.g., what-if accident scenarios); set priorities and focus on continuous improvement; write down the procedures for analysis and follow them.
4. Set goals and implement actions that will remove and prevent hazards; get everyone involved and use a continuous improvement process—the actions should include case management, workplace design, and improvement of accident investigation procedures; use data to measure and evaluate the results.
5. Train and coach managers, supervisors, and employees; provide thorough communication to create awareness; provide feedback to encourage learning and commend people for doing a good job.

Keyserling (2000) identifies the following basic policy/operational components that govern an effective safety program at the worksite:

1. A commitment to provide the greatest possible safety to all employees and ensure that all facilities and processes will be designed with this objective; similarly, purchasing policies that provide that all equipment, machines, and tools meet the highest safety standards
2. A requirement that all occupational injuries and accidents be reported and corrective action taken to ensure that similar incidents do not occur
3. Clear explanations to all employees of the safety and health hazards to which they are exposed and the establishment of training programs to inform employees of how to minimize their risk of being affected
4. Regularly scheduled systems safety analyses of all processes and work stations to identify potential safety hazards so that corrective actions can be taken before accidents occur
5. Disciplinary procedures for employees who engage in unsafe behavior and for supervisors who encourage or permit unsafe activities

While the chief executive officer is charged with the ultimate responsibility for the safety of all employees, this responsibility should be delegated and shared throughout the organization.

Larger companies may employ a full-time safety director to manage the safety program. Ideally, this person should be a Certified Safety Professional. The safety director works with all departments to ensure that related safety principles are being implemented and monitored on a daily basis. Typical responsibilities include developing and presenting safety training, inspecting facilities and operations for unsafe conditions and practices, conducting accident investigations, maintaining accident records and performing analyses to identify causal factors, and developing programs for hazard control. The safety director must work with the engineering and purchasing departments to ensure that equipment and facilities are designed and purchased in compliance with all applicable safety standards. The safety director also works closely with the occupational health staff to ensure that all injuries and illnesses are properly recorded and investigated.

Because of their direct contact with employees, line supervisors play a key role in the execution of safety programs. Line supervisors are responsible for ensuring that appropriate and safe equipment is available for employee use; that employees adhere to safety standards, regulations, and safe work practices; and that injuries are promptly reported and treated. Safety contests have been used to promote and encourage worksite safety practices; however, caution should be taken that these competitions do not undermine the safety effort through inaccurate or underreporting of injuries.

Occupational health personnel, including nurses and physicians, are integral to the safety program through identification of workplace hazards from observations and worker complaints, participation in company walk-throughs, and provision of primary treatment of injured employees. Health personnel must work closely with the line supervisors to help prevent repeated accidents and injuries by providing data related to the causes of workplace injuries and ensuring prompt injury reporting.

Employee participation in the safety program is essential to its success. Before starting a new assignment, a worker must be educated about specific hazards associated with the job. Training should include both hazard recognition and control techniques. If personal protective equipment is required to ensure safety, training must cover how to inspect, maintain, and wear such equipment. Training must emphasize the responsibility of each worker to maintain a safe workstation and comply with safe work practices. Part of this responsibility includes the necessity to report unsafe conditions to supervisors and employee safety representatives so that corrective action can be taken.

Each employee is an expert in his or her own job and must continue to be actively involved in inspection and systems safety analyses. This includes not only participation in safety education and training about specific job-related hazards but also involvement in the discussion and design of safer methods to perform the job and the evolution of prevention and control strategies.

Of particular importance in systems safety management is conducting a job safety analysis (JSA). The National Safety Council (1997) states that the JSA is a procedure used to review job methods and uncover hazards that (1) may have been overlooked in the layout of the facility or building and in the design of the machinery, equipment, tools, workstations, and processes; (2) may have developed after production started; or (3) resulted from changes in work procedures or personnel.

A JSA can be done through the following three basic steps (Figure 7-2):

1. Break the job down into successive steps or activities and observe how these actions are performed. Observe the employee performing the job and write down the basic steps. Videotaping the job may be helpful. To determine the basic job steps, ask "What step starts the job?" then, "What is the next basic step?" and so on. Completely describe each step and record any possible deviation from the regular procedure because this irregular activity may lead to an accident.

2. Identify the hazards and potential accidents. The purpose is to identify all hazards—both those produced by the environment and those connected with the job procedure. To do this, ask the following questions about each step:
   - Is there a potential for a slip or trip? Can the employee fall on the same level or to another?
   - Can strain be caused by pushing, pulling, lifting, bending, or twisting?
   - Is the environment hazardous to safety or health? For example, are there concentrations of toxic gas, vapor, mist, fume, dust, heat, or radiation?

   Close observation and knowledge of the particular job are required if the JSA is to be effective. The job observation should be repeated as often as necessary until all hazards and potential causes for accident or injury have been identified.

3. Develop safe job procedures to eliminate the hazards and prevent potential accidents; the principal solutions are as follows:
   - Find a new way to do the job.
   - Change the physical conditions that create the hazards.
   - Change the work procedure.
   - Reduce the activity frequency (particularly helpful in maintenance and materials handling).

SAFETY COMMITTEES

The establishment of a workplace safety (and health) committee is vital to transforming safety ideas into prevention and protection strategies in terms of policy, procedure, program development, and training and education about safety in the workplace. The safety committee can study and analyze safety and related health problems and recommend policies and programs for an improved safety program for the entire organization. The need for these policies and programs can be demonstrated from high or increased illness and injury rates, increased workers' compensation costs, or deficits that were noted from inspections for regulatory compliance and resulted in citations.

The safety committee should include the various levels of members of management, employees, occupational and environmental health nurse, physician, safety manager, other appropriate health care professionals, and union representatives, if applicable. A safety and health plan with specific goals and objectives should be established by the committee and with input from employees and all levels of management. The plan should be reviewed and updated annually and incorporated into the annual budget. Safety staff and health personnel generally know what should be done but often lack the support of line management needed to get it done. The safety committee can help to establish routine, effective lines of communication within all levels of the organization, from the ranking manager to the employee. This offers an excellent basis for training and informing personnel about safety and health procedures.

Boylston (1990) lists fundamental principles associated with safety and health management, including the following:

1. Safety and health maintenance is a line management function.
2. Safety and health maintenance is an inherent job responsibility.
3. Minimum acceptable safety and health standards must be established and maintained.
4. Safety responsibility and accountability must be achieved in the same manner as are responsibilities for production, quality, cost control, and personnel relations.

Boylston suggests that the safety and health committee be divided into the following eight task groups:

1. Safety activities
2. Rules and procedures
3. Inspections and audits

JOB SAFETY ANALYSIS	JOB TITLE (and number if applicable): Banding Pallets Page 1 of 2 JSA # 105	DATE: 00/00/00	[X] NEW [ ] REVISED
Instructions on Reverse Side	TITLE OF PERSON WHO DOES JOB: Bander	SUPERVISOR: James Smith	ANALYSIS BY: James Smith
Company/Organization: XYZ Company	PLANT/LOCATION: Chicago	DEPARTMENT: Packaging	REVIEWED BY: Sharon Martin
Required and/or Recommended Personal Protective Equipment: Gloves—Eye Protection—Long Sleeves—Safety Shoes		APPROVED BY: Joe Bottom	
Sequence of Basic Job Steps	Potential Hazards	Recommended Action or Procedure	
1. Position portable banding cart and place strapping guard on top of boxes.	1. Cart positioned too close to pallet (strike body and legs against cart or pallet, drop strapping gun on foot).	1. Leave ample space between cart and pallet to feed strapping—have firm grip on strapping gun.	
2. Withdraw strapping and bend end back about 3".	2. Sharp edges of strapping (cut hands, fingers, and arms). Sharp corners on pallet (strike feet against corners).	2. Wear gloves, eye protection, and long sleeves—keep firm grip on strapping—hold end between thumb and forefinger—watch where stepping.	
3. Walk around load while holding strapping with one hand.	3. Projecting sharp corners on pallet (strike feet on corners).	3. Assure a clear path between pallet and cart—pull smoothly—avoid jerking strapping.	
4. Pull and feed strap under pallet.	4. Splinters on pallet (punctures to hands and fingers). Sharp strap edges (cuts to hands, fingers, and arms).	4. Wear gloves—eye protection—long sleeves. Point strap in direction of bend—pull strap smoothly to avoid jerks	
5. Walk around load. Stoop down. Bend over, grab strap, pull up to machine, straighten out strap end.	5. Protruding corners of pallet, splinters (punctures to feet and ankles).	5. Assure a clear path—watch where walking— face direction in which walking.	
6. Insert, position, and tighten strap in gun.	6. Springy and sharp strapping (strike against with hands and fingers).	6. Keep firm grasp on strap and on gun—make sure clip is positioned properly.	

Figure 7-2 Sample of completed job safety analysis. *(From* Supervisors' Safety Manual *(9th ed.), by National Safety Council, 1997, Itasca, IL: Author.)*

4. Accident investigation
5. Education and training
6. Health and environment
7. Fire and emergency
8. Housekeeping

However, the division of tasks and groups may be dependent on the size of the company. Thus, in a smaller company task groups may be combined or composed of smaller numbers. Each task group must annually develop its goals and objectives, which then become part of the overall safety and health plan. The purpose and activities of each task area are briefly summarized below.

Safety activities involve overseeing the entire safety program to ensure program effectiveness in reducing illness and injury and include the following:

- Review annually safety program activities.
- Determine strategies to obtain employee input regarding program activities.

- Recommend special safety emphasis programs.
- Analyze workplace injuries to determine strategies for corrective actions.
- Publicize safety programs (e.g., on bulletin boards and in pamphlets, brochures).
- Disseminate safety information to employees.
- Coordinate safety awards/conferences/contests.

Rules and procedures communicate to all managers, supervisors, and employees safe ways to perform every job. Specific activities include the following:

- Recommend compliance procedures that can be followed.
- Audit the workplace for compliance with procedures and recommend corrective actions.
- Develop and review the safety manual and make it accessible in each department (Figure 7-3).
- Recommend necessary training and enforcement procedures.

SAFETY MANUAL CHECKLIST			Date:
			Page 1 of 3
Employer	**Facility**		**Unit**
Address			

General Information

Every employer should have a safety and health policies and procedures manual. A written manual is important to:

- Document company/governmental safety and health policies

- Train and educate employees as to safety and health policies

- Establish a safety and health management program that includes both management and hourly employees

- Enforce safety policies fairly and consistently

- Organize and address all safety and health issues

This manual should be developed with input from all levels of the organization. Every policy should be written and feasible, employees trained, and the policies enforced. A number of resources are available to obtain prepared policies that can be adapted to a worksite. Those resources include:

- Governmental Regulatory Agencies

- Industry Associations

- Safety and Industrial Hygiene Associations

- National Safety Council's *Accident Prevention Manual*

- OSHA, ANSI, NFPA, etc., Standards

Figure 7-3 Sample checklist form for safety and health manual. *(From* Managing Safety and Health Programs, *by R. Boylston, 1990, New York: Van Nostrand Reinhold.)*
Continued

SAFETY MANUAL CHECKLIST		Date:		
		Page 2 of 3		
Check When Complete	Subject	To Be Developed By	Dates	
			Target	Completed
	I. Safety and Health Program/Organization			
	A. Policy Statement			
	B. Central Safety Committee/Task Groups			
	1. Safety Activities Task Group			
	2. Rules and Procedures Task Group			
	3. Inspections and Audits Task Group			
	4. Fire and Emergency Task Group			
	5. Education and Training Task Group			
	6. Health and Environmental Task Group			
	7. Accident Investigation Task Group			
	8. Housekeeping Task Group			
	C. Plant Safety and Health Committee			
	II. Safety and Health Rules			
	A. General Plant Safety and Health Rules			
	B. Specific Division/Department Rules			
	III. Duties and Responsibilities			
	A. Chief Executive Officer, Ranking Official			
	B. Directors, Managers, and Supervisors			
	C. Employees			
	D. Plant Safety and Health Coordinator			
	E. Employee and Supervisory Performance Appraisals			
	F. Central Safety Committee and Task Group Responsibilities			
	IV. Safety and Health Training			
	A. Employee Selection and Placement			
	B. Safety Orientation and Training			
	C. Supervisory Safety Training			
	D. Employee Safety Meetings and Contacts			
	E. Special Safety and Health Training			
	1. Transfers			
	2. New Assignments			
	V. Accident/Incident Response			
	A. Accident Reporting			
	B. Accident Investigation			
	C. Injury and Illness Recordkeeping			
	D. Transportation of Injured/Ill Employees			
	E. Notification of Injured's Family			
	VI. Inspection and Audit Programs			
	A. Safety Audit and Inspection Procedure			
	B. Safety Inspection Checklists			
	C. Safety Audits of New or Modified Equipment and Facilities			
	D. Capital Project Insurance Review Procedure			
	E. Monitoring for Air Contaminants			
	F. Monitoring for Physical Health Hazards			
	VII. Effective Management Action			
	A. Corrective Action Procedures			
	B. Follow-up Assessments			
	C. Safety Work Orders			

Figure 7-3, cont'd   For legend see p.155.

SAFETY MANUAL CHECKLIST		Date:		
		Page 3 of 3		
Check When Complete	Subject	To Be Developed By	Dates	
			Target	Completed
	VIII. Safety Permits			
	A. Permit Systems			
	B. Confined Space Entry			
	C. Hot Work Permit			
	D. Electrical Hot Work Permit			
	E. Temporary Wiring Permit			
	IX. Electrical Safety			
	A. Hazardous Locations			
	B. Temporary Electrical Wiring			
	C. Electrical Safety for Employees			
	X. OSHA Inspections			
	XI. Contractor and Visitor Safety and Health			
	XII. Safety and Health Procedures			
	A. Emergency Action Plan			
	1. Fire and Explosions			
	2. Chemical Leaks and Spills			
	3. Meteorological Occurrences			
	4. Bomb Threats/Public Disorders			
	B. Hazard Communication Program			
	C. Locking and Tagging Procedure			
	D. Respiratory Protection Program			
	E. Job Safety and Health Analysis			
	F. Hearing Conservation Program			
	G. Medical Surveillance Program			
	H. Employee Exposure and Medical Records Policy			
	I. Confined Space Entry			
	J. Hot Work Procedures			
	K. Personal Protective Equipment			
	L. Barricade Procedures			
	M. Ladders, Scaffolds, Platforms, Manlifts			
	N. Office Safety			
	O. Walking and Working Surfaces			
	P. Manual Material Handling			
	Q. Machinery and Equipment			
	R. Compressed Gas Storage and Handling			
	S. Housekeeping			
	T. Railroad Safety			
	U. Forklifts, Industrial Trucks			
	V. Cranes and Hoists			
	W. Tools			
	X. Fall Protection			
	Y. Color Coding			
	Z. Excavating			
	AA. Traffic Rules			
	BB. Flammable and Combustible Liquids			
	CC. Open Flames and Sparks			
	DD. Fire Protection			
	EE. Compressed Air			
	FF. Process Hazards			
	GG. Fleet Safety and Vehicle Maintenance			
	HH. Asbestos Maintenance and Removal			

Figure 7-3, cont'd For legend see p.155.

Box 7-1 Minimum Safety Rules

1. All plant injuries must be reported immediately to supervision and medical staff.
2. Horseplay, scuffling, and fighting are prohibited.
3. Unauthorized operation or maintenance of equipment is prohibited.
4. Rings, bracelets, wristwatches, loose adornments, long hair (at or below shoulder), and loose clothing must not be worn within 3 feet of operating machinery or moving products.
5. All guards and safety devices must be in place before equipment is operated, except as provided in written approved procedures.
6. "Lock, tag, and try" procedures described in written company safety procedures must be followed by all employees to avoid injury while repairing, adjusting, or cleaning machinery or processes.
7. Roped off or barricaded areas may be entered only by permission of personnel working in the enclosed area or of the supervisor responsible for the work.
8. Safety spectacles must be worn as minimum eye protection for protection against flying objects, glare, and radiation, as specified by job safety procedures. Goggles are required for employees using air hoses to blow off equipment and for liquid splash protection.
9. Strike-anywhere matches, firearms, explosives, and ammunition are prohibited unless authorized.
10. Smoking is permitted only in designated areas. Cigarettes, cigars, and matches must be discarded only in ashtrays and specifically identified containers.
11. Posted speed limits for inplant and outside vehicles must be observed.
12. Intoxicants, narcotics, and persons under the influence of these are prohibited in the plant, except as authorized by medical staff.
13. Emergency exits, evacuation routes, and emergency equipment must not be obstructed.
14. Running in the plant is prohibited, except to prevent loss of life or serious injury.
15. All chemicals used in the plant must be approved through the Central Safety and Health Committee, and chemical containers must be identified.
16. All scissors, knives, razor blades, and sharp-pointed tools used by employees must be specifically approved by management for their intended use.

From *Managing Safety and Health Programs,* by R. Boylston, 1990, New York: Van Nostrand Reinhold.

- Review rules/procedures annually and update them with input from other groups.
- Review, evaluate, and recommend improvements in recordkeeping.
- Establish minimum safety rules (Box 7-1).

Inspection and audit involves identifying workplace hazards through systematic inspection and recommending corrective actions to correct defects and prevent occurrences (Figure 7-4). Specific activities include the following:

- Determine what is to be inspected and by whom.
- Develop an audit/inspection checklist and determine inspection frequency (i.e., periodic, special, continuous).
- Establish and participate in inspection procedures.
- Compile statistics on injury events.

- Highlight repeated injury events and problem areas and recommend control strategies.
- Ensure equipment maintenance.
- Monitor inspection outcomes for timely deficit correction.

Accident investigation involves determining cause for accident occurrence and formulating methods to prevent recurrence. Specific activities include the following:

- Investigate accident events promptly and document them.
- Review all accident reports to identify potential and actual causes and determine best control strategies.
- Discuss accident occurrence with employees and methods to reduce risk of recurrence.
- Observe work areas for contributing factors.

SAFETY AND HEALTH INSPECTION		Date:		Page 1 of 2
Organization		Location		Unit
Inspection Time—From To		Inspectors		

General—This safety and health inspection checklist is intended as a reminder for inspectors. It does not and cannot cover all safety and health items. Refer to specific standards, codes, and regulations for more details concerning safety and health inspection requirements.

No.	Item	Reference	Yes	No	Comments
	Rules and Procedures				
1.	Are rules and procedures known, understood, and followed?				
2.	Are assignments performed right—the safe way?				
	Housekeeping				
3.	Is the work area clean and orderly?				
4.	Are floors free from protruding nails, splinters, holes, and loose boards?				
5.	Are aisles and passageways kept clear of obstructions?				
6.	Are permanent aisles and passageways clearly marked?				
7.	Are covers or guardrails in place around open pits, tanks, and ditches?				
	Floor and Wall Openings				
8.	Are ladderways and door openings guarded by a railing?				
9.	Do skylights have screens or fixed railings to prevent someone from falling through?				
10.	Do temporary floor openings have standard railings or someone constantly on guard?				
11.	Are wall openings with a drop of more than 4 feet guarded by a standard railing?				
12.	Are open-sided floors, platforms, and runways with a drop of more than 4 feet guarded by a standard railing and toeboard?				
13.	Do all stairways with 4 or more risers have a handrail?				
14.	Are stairways strong enough? too steep? adequately illuminated? slip resistant?				
	Means of Exit				
15.	Are there enough exits to allow prompt escape?				
16.	Do employees have easy access to exits?				
17.	Are exits unlocked to allow egress?				
18.	Are exits clearly marked?				
19.	Are exits and exit routes equipped with emergency lighting?				
	Personal Protective Equipment				
20.	Is required equipment provided, maintained, and used?				
21.	Does equipment meet safety requirements? Is it reliable?				
	Employee Facilities				
22.	Are facilities kept clean and sanitary?				
23.	Are toilets kept clean and in good repair?				
24.	Are cafeteria facilities provided where toxic chemicals are used? Do employees use them?				
	Medical and First Aid				
25.	Is there a hospital, clinic, or infirmary nearby?				
26.	Are employees trained as first-aid practitioners present on each shift worked?				
27.	Are physician-approved first-aid supplies available?				
28.	Are first-aid supplies replenished as they are used?				

Figure 7-4 Sample checklist for safety and health inspection. *(From* Managing Safety and Health Programs, *by R. Boylston, 1990, New York: Van Nostrand Reinhold.)*

Continued

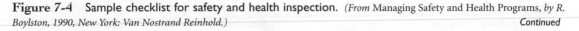

SAFETY AND HEALTH INSPECTION CHECK SHEET		No: Page 2 of 2			
No.	**Item**	**Reference**	**Yes**	**No**	**Comments**
	Fire Protection				
29.	Are fire extinguishers suitable for the type of fire most likely in that area?				
30.	Are enough extinguishers present to do the job?				
31.	Are extinguisher locations conspicuously marked?				
32.	Are extinguishers properly mounted and easily accessible?				
33.	Are all extinguishers fully charged and operable?				
34.	Are special-purpose extinguishers clearly marked?				
	Materials Handling and Storage				
35.	Is adequate clearance allowed in aisles where materials must be moved?				
36.	Are tiered materials stacked, interblocked, locked and limited in height to maintain stability?				
37.	Are storage areas kept free of tripping, fire, explosion, and pest hazards?				
38.	Is proper drainage provided?				
39.	Are signs warning of clearance limits posted?				
40.	Are powered industrial truck operators adequately trained?				
	Machine Guarding				
41.	Are point-of-operation guards in place and working on all operating equipment?				
42.	Are all belts and pulleys that are less than 7 feet from the floor (and within reach of workers) guarded?				
43.	Are spinning parts guarded?				
	Electrical				
44.	Are all machines properly grounded?				
45.	Are portable hand tools grounded or double insulated?				
46.	Are junction boxes closed?				
47.	Are extension cords out of the aisles (where they might be abused by heavy traffic)?				
48.	Are extension cords being used as permanent wiring? (It's a dangerous thing to do.)				

Figure 7-4, cont'd For legend see p. 159.

- Follow up to determine compliance with directives and abatement of hazard.
- Compile statistics for analysis.
- Maintain records.

Education and training involve helping employees recognize safety hazards and how to control them. Specific activities include the following:

- Manage and coordinate the safety education and training program related to, for example, new employees (Figure 7-5), regulations, work processes, and procedures, as well as employee transfers and national standards (e.g., ANSI).
- Establish a training schedule and assign administrative responsibilities.
- Maintain and store training records.

- Evaluate training effectiveness for content and instruction.

Health and environment involve coordinating all health and environmental activities in the organization and recommending measures for health promotion and protection, environmental protection, and hazard reduction or elimination. Specific activities include the following:

- Review safety program to ensure adequate health emphasis.
- Conduct on-site inspections with safety personnel to identify potential/actual exposures.
- Recommend control strategies to reduce health hazard exposures.

SUBJECT: NEW EMPLOYEE ORIENTATION AND TRAINING CHECKLIST

Name: _____ S.S.#: _____

Job Assignment: _____ Supervisor: _____

Employment Date: _____

1. By Personnel Department on the First Day of Employment
   - ☐ Management's safety and health philosophy
   - ☐ Management's, supervisor's, and employees' safety and health responsibilities
   - ☐ General plant safety and health rules
   - ☐ Hazard communication audiovisual presentation
   - ☐ Location and availability of the hazard communication program
   - ☐ Access to employee exposure and medical records

Completed by: _____ Date: _____

2. By New Employee's Immediate Supervisor
   A. First Day in Work Area   Date: _____
   - ☐ Introduction to operations where chemical and physical hazards are present—types of hazards encountered
   - ☐ Required work practices
   - ☐ Personal protective equipment
   - ☐ Emergency procedures
   - ☐ Detection of chemical hazards
   - ☐ Location and availability of Material Safety Data Sheets
   - ☐ Labeling systems

   B. One Week Follow-up   Date: _____
   - ☐ Review work practices and procedures with employee
   - ☐ Answer employee questions
   - ☐ Return complete checklist to Personnel Department for filing in employee personnel folder.

Completed by: _____ Date: _____

Employee's Signature: _____ Date: _____

Figure 7-5 New employee orientation and training checklist. *(From* Managing Safety and Health Programs, *by R. Boylston, 1990, New York: Van Nostrand Reinhold.)*

Fire and emergency include developing and implementing effective emergency management procedures to protect people, property, and environment. Specific activities include the following:

- Develop a written emergency plan and organize an emergency response program (e.g., safety, security, fire brigade), including damage control, follow-up, and operation resumption.
- Develop a proper training program.
- Conduct mock emergency preparedness situations.
- Disseminate to all employees the emergency plan (department contact person, report mechanisms, escape procedures, employee accountability, rescue/medical duties, training, evaluation).

- Evaluate new facilities, equipment, and work processes to identify potential emergency situations and controls.
- Evaluate procedures for emergency preparedness.

Housekeeping involves maintaining proper mechanisms for workplace cleanliness and orderliness to help enhance safety, productivity, and morale. Specific activities include the following:

- Observe workplace for safe and clean work surfaces.
- Ensure clutter-free stairways and corridors.
- Manage waste and spill refuse.
- Report noted deficits affecting worksite safety.

Within the context of a multidisciplinary effort the occupational and environmental health nurse has an important role contributing to the overall management of the safety program. The training and education of workers about safety issues, initiation of effective prevention strategies, and full participation on health and safety committees are part of the effort. The occupational and environmental health nurse will need to work with management to secure a commitment to an active safety program.

ERGONOMICS

Historical evidence exists in the early writings (1713) of Ramazzini (1940), in what we now refer to as ergonomic factors, regarding the effects of work on the worker.

The maladies that affect the clerks (aforesaid) arise from three causes: tint, constant sitting, secondly, the incessant movement of the hand and always in the same direction, thirdly, the strain on the mind from the effort not to disfigure the books by errors or cause loss to their employers when they add, subtract, or do other sums in arithmetics. (p. 254)

Ramazzini's perspective provides some insight into the long-standing problem of matching the worker to the job and work environment—rather than matching the job to the worker—within the context of effective, healthy, and safe human capabilities.

In today's work environment we continue to see the effects of repeated trauma from fast paced work and poorly designed workstation environments that result in work-related musculoskeletal disorders described as injuries and disorders of the soft tissue (muscles, tendons, ligaments, joints, and cartilage) and nervous system (NIOSH, 1997; USDOL, BLS, 2000). The Occupational Safety and Health Administration (USDOL, BLS, 2000) indicates that about 1.8 million workers report musculoskeletal disorders such as carpal tunnel syndrome, tendinitis, and back injuries each year with about 600,000 of those workers requiring work absence. OSHA estimates that another 1.8 million workers experience but do not report musculoskeletal diseases each year. In addition, the cost of musculoskeletal disorders is high:

- Musculoskeletal disorders account for 34% of all lost-workday injuries and illnesses.

- Musculoskeletal disorders account for $15 billion to $20 billion in workers' compensation costs and $1 of every $3 spent for workers' compensation. Total direct costs add up to as much as $50 billion annually.
- On average workers need 28 days to recover from carpal tunnel syndrome, longer than the time needed to recover from amputation or fractures.
- Workers with severe injuries can face permanent disabilities that prevent them from returning to their jobs or handling simple, everyday tasks.

Musculoskeletal disorders (Table 7-2) can cause a number of conditions including pain, numbness, tingling, stiff joints, difficulty moving, muscle loss, and sometimes paralysis. Resulting disorders include carpal tunnel syndrome, tendinitis, sciatica, herniated discs, and low back pain. Musculoskeletal disorders do not include injuries resulting from slips, trips, falls, or similar accidents. Work-related musculoskeletal disorders occur when the physical capabilities of the worker and physical requirements of the job are incongruent. Risk factors likely to cause musculoskeletal disorders include the following (NIOSH, 1997; USDHHS, NIOSH, 1996):

- *Awkward postures.* Body postures determine which joints and muscles are used in an activity and the amount of force or stresses that are generated or tolerated. For example, more stress is placed on the spinal discs when lifting, lowering, or handling objects with the back bent or twisted compared with when the back is straight. Manipulative or other tasks requiring repeated or sustained bending or twisting of the wrists, knees, hips, or shoulders also impose increased stresses on these joints. Activities requiring frequent or prolonged work over shoulder height can be particularly stressful. In addition, static postures, positions that a worker must hold for long periods of time, can restrict blood flow and damage muscles.
- *Forceful exertions.* Tasks that require forceful exertions, including lifting, pushing, and pulling, place higher loads of force on the muscles, tendons, ligaments, and joints. Increasing force means increasing body demands (e.g., greater muscle exertion along with other physiological changes necessary to sustain an increased effort). Prolonged or recurrent experiences of this type combined with inadequate time for rest

TABLE 7-2	Examples of Musculoskeletal Disorders			
BODY PARTS AFFECTED	**SYMPTOMS**	**POSSIBLE CAUSES**	**DISEASE NAME**	**WORKERS AFFECTED**
Thumbs	Pain at the base of the thumbs	Twisting and gripping	De Quervain's Disease	Butchers, house-keepers, packers, seam-stresses, cutters
Fingers	Difficulty moving finger; snapping and jerking movements	Repeatedly using the index fingers	Trigger Finger	Meatpackers, poultry workers, carpenters, electronic assemblers
Shoulders	Pain, stiffness	Working with the hands above the head	Rotator Cuff Tendinitis	Power press operators, welders, painters, assembly line workers
Hands, wrists	Pain, swelling	Repetitive or forceful hand and wrist motion	Tenosynovitis	Cake makers, poultry processers, meatpackers
Fingers, hands	Numbness, tingling; ashen skin; loss of feeling and control	Exposure to vibration	Raynaud's Syndrome (white finger)	Chain saw, pneumatic hammer, and gasoline-powered tool operators
Fingers, wrists	Tingling, numbness, severe pain; loss of strength, sensation in the thumbs, index, or middle or half of the ring finger	Repetitive and forceful manual tasks without time to recover	Carpal Tunnel Syndrome	Meat and poultry and garment workers, upholsters, assemblers, VDT operators, cashiers
Back	Low back pain, shooting pain or numbness in the upper legs	Whole body vibration	Back Disability	Truck and bus drivers, tractor and subway operators; warehouse workers; nurses aids; grocery cashiers; baggage handlers

or recovery can lead not only to feelings of fatigue but also to musculoskeletal problems.

* *Repetitive motions.* If motions are repeated frequently (e.g., every few seconds) and for prolonged periods such as an 8-hour shift, fatigue, irritation, muscle-tendon strain and nerve pressure can increase. Tendons and muscles can often recover from the effects of stretching or

forceful exertions if sufficient time is allotted between exertions. Awkward postures and forceful exertions increase the effects of repetitive motions from performing the same work activities.

* *Contact stresses.* Repeated or continuous contact with hard or sharp objects such as non-rounded desk edges or unpadded, narrow tool handles may create pressure over one area of the body

(e.g., the forearm or sides of the fingers) that can inhibit nerve function and blood flow.

- *Vibration.* Exposure to local vibration occurs when a specific part of the body comes in contact with a vibrating object, such as a power handtool. Exposure to whole-body vibration can occur while standing or sitting in vibrating environments or objects, such as when operating heavy-duty vehicles or large machinery or providing health care services aboard a helicopter.
- *Compression.* Grasping sharp edges, like tool handles, can concentrate force on small areas of the body, reduce blood flow and nerve transmission, and damage tendons and tendon sheaths.
- *Other conditions.* Workplace conditions that can influence the presence and magnitude of risk factors for musculoskeletal disorders can include cold temperatures, insufficient pauses and rest breaks for recovery, machine-paced work, and unfamiliar or unaccustomed work.
- In addition, nonoccupational risk factors including obesity, diabetes, arthritis, pregnancy, physical conditions, and stress can be contributory.

These risk factors, either alone or in combination, can subject workers' shoulders, arms, hands, wrists, backs, and legs to thousands of repetitive twisting, forceful, or flexing motions during a typical workday. To contribute to musculoskeletal disorders, however, these risk factors must be present for a sufficient duration, frequency, or magnitude. Box 7-2 shows occupations at high risk for musculoskeletal disorders. Data reflecting the burden of musculoskeletal disorders in pain, disability, and cost emphasize the need for finding effective solutions to

---

Box 7-2   **Top Ten Occupations for Musculoskeletal Disorders**

1. Nurses aides, orderlies, and attendants
2. Truck drivers
3. Laborers not involved in construction work
4. Assemblers
5. Janitors and cleaners
6. Registered nurses
7. Stock handlers and baggers
8. Construction laborers
9. Cashiers
10. Carpenters

From: U.S. Department of Labor, Bureau of Labor Statistics, 2000

---

manage musculoskeletal disorder hazards and problems in the workplace. One important solution is an ergonomically sufficient work environment.

The term *ergonomics* is derived from two Greek words, *ergos* meaning work and *nomos* meaning laws—thus, the laws of work. Ergonomics has been defined by several authors; however, Keyserling (2000) defines ergonomics as the study of humans at work in order to understand the interrelationships among people, their work environment (e.g., facilities, equipment, and tools), job demands, and work methods. The National Safety Council (1997) offers a simple but consistent definition: ergonomics is the science of designing the job and the workplace to fit the worker. The goal of ergonomics is to allow work to be done without undue stress. This encompasses the design of facilities (e.g., factories and offices), furniture, equipment, tools, and job demands and requires that they be compatible with human dimensions, capabilities, and expectations and also reduce stressors. All work, regardless of its nature, places both physical and mental stresses on the worker. Within the framework of these definitions the goal remains the same—to match job demands and requirements to the abilities and capabilities of the worker (Sluchak, 1992).

Keyserling and Armstrong (1992) state that ergonomics is a multidisciplinary science with the following four major areas of specialization:

1. *Human factors engineering* (sometimes called engineering psychology) is concerned with the information processing requirement of work. Major applications include designing displays (e.g., gauges, warning buzzers, signs, and instructions) and controls to enhance performance and minimize the likelihood of error.
2. *Anthropometry* is concerned with the measurement and statistical characterization of body size. Anthropometric data provide important information to the designers of clothing, furniture, machines, and tools.
3. *Occupational biomechanics* is concerned with the mechanical properties of human tissue, particularly the response of tissue to mechanical stress. A major focus of occupational biomechanics is the prevention of overexertion disorders of the low back and upper extremities.
4. *Work physiology* is concerned with the responses of the cardiovascular system, pulmonary system, and skeletal muscles to the

metabolic demands of work. This discipline is concerned with the prevention of whole body and localized fatigue.

Although ergonomics is concerned with matching work and job design to fit the capabilities of most people by adapting the product to fit the user, the design of the work environment should be flexible enough to consider the need for individual variation (Gauf, 1998; Sluchak, 1992). For example, two people with the same height and weight may have a different arm reach or strength, and accommodations for those differences should be available. In order to make these changes, anthropometric analysis—determining the relationship of the physical features of the human body (e.g., weight, size, range of motion) to the work and environment—may need to be taken into account.

Several studies cite numerous health problems, such as back injuries (Bigos, 1994; Silverstein & Kalat, 1998), carpal tunnel disorders (Gross et al., 1995; Osorio, 1993; Randolph, 2000; Stoy & Aspen, 1999), and neurologic problems (Mandel, 1987) as a result of ergonomic hazards. In addition, OSHA has written guidelines, *Ergonomics Program Management Guidelines for Meatpacking Plants,* to address growing concern regarding cumulative trauma disorders (CTDs) and other work-related musculoskeletal disorders in the meatpacking industry (USDOL, OSHA, 1991). However, these guidelines can be adapted for use in other settings. The OSHA ergonomic guidelines are intended to provide information to help employers determine if they have ergonomic-related problems in their workplaces, identify the nature and location of these problems, and implement measures to reduce or eliminate the problems. While the scope of these guidelines will not be fully described, the major elements will be reviewed. However, several authors provide an extensive discussion of the application of the guidelines (Hales & Bertsche, 1992; Ostendorf et al., 2000).

Critical to the development of any program is management's commitment and employee involvement. This is outlined by OSHA as follows:

1. Obtain management's commitment to reduce ergonomic hazards through active participation, policy development, resource allocation, and accountability for program implementation at all levels in the organization;

2. Develop a goal-directed written program for job safety, health, and ergonomics that is communicated to all employees;

3. Encourage employee involvement in the ergonomics program and decision making through mechanisms that bring their concerns to management and procedures that support the reporting, analysis, resolution and monitoring of ergonomic problems;

4. Develop mechanisms to evaluate program progress, including analysis of trends in illness/injury rates, employee surveys, and management's evaluation of job/worksite changes (USDOL, OSHA, 1991).

In keeping with OSHA's emphasis on management's commitment and employee involvement, successful program implementation is most often seen in the continuous improvement through gradual steps that focus on implementing employee education programs on ergonomics; customizing work areas with relatively inexpensive assistive devices or accommodations; increasing awareness so that new office or production designs incorporate ergonomic principles before a new facility is built or a process becomes operational; identifying health patterns or trends so that intervention strategies can be prioritized; and reporting to upper management the return on investment so that ergonomic strategies are viewed as cost-effective (Gauf, 1998; Hagberg et al., 1995; Travers, 1992).

The OSHA ergonomic guidelines (USDOL, OSHA, 1991) describe four major program elements including worksite analysis, hazard prevention and control, medical management, and training and education. Worksite analysis, which identifies existing hazards and conditions, operations that create hazards, and areas where hazards develop, should include the following:

1. An analysis of all illness and injury records will help find evidence of ergonomic deficiencies and trends related to specific departments, jobs, and titles.

2. Jobs, operations, processes, and work stations or methods that contribute to ergonomic musculoskeletal disorders must be identified. For example, risk factors for back disorders include bad body mechanics, such as continued bending over at the waist; continued lifting from below the knuckles or above the shoulders; twisting at the waist, especially while lifting; lifting or mov-

ing objects of excessive weight or asymmetric size; prolonged sitting, especially with poor posture; lack of adjustable chairs, footrests, body supports, and work surfaces at work stations; poor grips on handles; and slippery footing.

3. Initial and periodic job hazard analysis must be performed in order to detect situations that place workers at risk of musculoskeletal disorders. This would include an analysis of the work environment, work station, and manual materials lifting. A checklist example is shown in Figure 7-6. Use of a videotape analysis method is recommended, if feasible. In addition, task

analysis will help differentiate and target specific activities related to the task demand that may be risk factor contributors (Figure 7-7). Figure 7-8 shows a computer workstation checklist.

A general ergonomic workplace analysis can be facilitated through use of a workplace checklist specific for ergonomic concerns (Box 7-3). This will help provide for a systematic analysis approach and obtain objective, quantifiable data.

As described in these OSHA ergonomic guidelines, hazard prevention and control of musculoskeletal disorders risks are accommodated

---

Answer the following questions based on the primary job activities of workers in this facility.
Use the following responses to describe **how frequently** workers are exposed to the job conditions described below:
Never (worker is never exposed to condition)
Sometimes (worker is exposed to the condition less than 3 times daily)
Usually (worker is exposed to the condition 3 times or more daily)

	Never	Sometimes	Usually	If USUALLY, list jobs to which answer applies here
1. Do workers perform tasks that are externally paced?				
2. Are workers required to exert force with their hands (e.g., gripping, pulling, pinching)?				
3. Do workers use handtools or handle parts or objects?				
4. Do workers stand continuously for periods of more than 30 min?				
5. Do workers sit for periods of more than 30 min without the opportunity to stand or move around freely?				
6. Do workers use electronic input devices (e.g., keyboards, mice, joysticks, track balls) for continuous periods of more than 30 min?				
7. Do workers kneel (one or both knees)?				
8. Do workers perform activities with hands raised above shoulder height?				
9. Do workers perform activities while bending or twisting at the waist?				
10. Are workers exposed to vibration?				
11. Do workers lift or lower objects between floor and waist height or above shoulder height?				
12. Do workers lift or lower objects more than once per min for continuous periods of more than 15 min?				
13. Do workers lift, lower, or carry large objects or objects that cannot be held close to body?				
14. Do workers lift, lower, or carry objects weighing more than 50 lb?				

Figure 7-6 Job conditions hazard identification checklist. (*Data from* Elements of Ergonomics Program, *by U.S. Department of Health and Human Services National Institute for Occupational Safety and Health, 1996, Cincinnati, OH: Author.*)

primarily through effective design of the work station, tools, and jobs through engineering controls and administrative/work practice controls. Engineering techniques, where feasible, are the preferred method of control and can be accomplished by designing or modifying the work station, work methods, and tools to eliminate excessive exertion and awkward postures and to reduce repetitive motion. Engineering control strategies include the following:

- Changing the way materials, parts, and products can be transported—for example, using mechanical assist devices to relieve heavy load lifting and carrying tasks, or using handles or slotted hand holes in packages requiring manual handling
- Changing the process or product to reduce worker exposures to risk factors—for example, maintaining the fit of plastic molds to reduce the need for manual removal of flashing or us-

"No" responses indicate potential problem areas that should receive further investigation.		
1. Does the design of the primary task reduce or eliminate		
bending or twisting of the back or trunk?	☐ yes	☐ no
crouching?	☐ yes	☐ no
bending or twisting the wrist?	☐ yes	☐ no
extending the arms?	☐ yes	☐ no
raised elbows?	☐ yes	☐ no
static muscle loading?	☐ yes	☐ no
clothes wringing motions?	☐ yes	☐ no
finger pinch grip?	☐ yes	☐ no
2. Are mechanical devices used when necessary?	☐ yes	☐ no
3. Can the task be done with either hand?	☐ yes	☐ no
4. Can the task be done with two hands?	☐ yes	☐ no
5. Are pushing or pulling forces kept minimal?	☐ yes	☐ no
6. Are required forces judged acceptable by workers?	☐ yes	☐ no
7. Are the materials		
able to be held without slipping?	☐ yes	☐ no
easy to grasp?	☐ yes	☐ no
free from sharp edges and corners?	☐ yes	☐ no
8. Do containers have good handholds?	☐ yes	☐ no
9. Are jigs, fixtures, and vises used where needed?	☐ yes	☐ no
10. As needed, do gloves fit properly, and are they made of the proper fabric?	☐ yes	☐ no
11. Does the worker avoid contact with sharp edges when performing the tasks?	☐ yes	☐ no
12. When needed, are push buttons designed properly?	☐ yes	☐ no
13. Do the job tasks allow for ready use of personal equipment that may be required?	☐ yes	☐ no
14. Are high rates of repetitive motion avoided by		
job rotation?	☐ yes	☐ no
self-pacing?	☐ yes	☐ no
sufficient pauses?	☐ yes	☐ no
adjusting the job skill level of the worker?	☐ yes	☐ no
15. Is the employee trained in		
proper work practices?	☐ yes	☐ no
when and how to make adjustments?	☐ yes	☐ no
recognizing signs and symptoms of potential problems?	☐ yes	☐ no

Figure 7-7 Task analysis checklist. *(Data from* Elements of Ergonomics Programs, *by U.S. Department of Health and Human Services, National Institute for Occupational Safety and Health, 1996, Cincinnati, OH: Author.)*

"No" responses indicate potential problem areas that should receive further investigation.		
1. Does the workstation ensure proper worker posture, such as		
horizontal thighs?	☐ yes	☐ no
vertical lower legs?	☐ yes	☐ no
feet flat on floor or footrest?	☐ yes	☐ no
neutral wrists?	☐ yes	☐ no
2. Does the chair		
adjust easily?	☐ yes	☐ no
have a padded seat with a rounded front?	☐ yes	☐ no
have an adjustable backrest?	☐ yes	☐ no
provide lumbar support?	☐ yes	☐ no
have casters?	☐ yes	☐ no
3. Are the height and tilt of the work surface on which the keyboard is located adjustable?	☐ yes	☐ no
4. Is the keyboard detachable?	☐ yes	☐ no
5. Do keying actions require minimal force?	☐ yes	☐ no
6. Is there an adjustable document holder?	☐ yes	☐ no
7. Are arm rests provided where needed?	☐ yes	☐ no
8. Are glare reflections avoided?	☐ yes	☐ no
9. Does the monitor have brightness and contrast controls?	☐ yes	☐ no
10. Do the operators judge the distance between eyes and work to be satisfactory for their viewing needs?	☐ yes	☐ no
11. Is there sufficient space for knees and feet?	☐ yes	☐ no
12. Can the workstation be used for either right-handed or left-handed activity?	☐ yes	☐ no
13. Are adequate rest breaks provided for task demands?	☐ yes	☐ no
14. Are high stroke rates avoided by		
job rotation?	☐ yes	☐ no
self-pacing?	☐ yes	☐ no
adjusting the job skill level of the worker?	☐ yes	☐ no
15. Are employees trained in		
proper postures?	☐ yes	☐ no
proper work methods?	☐ yes	☐ no
when and how to adjust their workstations?	☐ yes	☐ no
how to seek assistance for their concerns?	☐ yes	☐ no

Figure 7-8 **Computer workstation checklist.** *(Data from* Elements of Ergonomics Programs, *by U.S. Department of Health and Human Services, National Institute for Occupational Safety and Health, 1996, Cincinnati, OH: Author.)*

ing easy-connect electrical terminals to reduce manual forces
- Modifying containers and parts presentation, such as height-adjustable material bins
- Changing workstation layout, which might include using height-adjustable workbenches or locating tools and materials within short reaching distances
- Changing tool designs—for example, pistol handle grips for knives to reduce wrist bending

postures required by straight-handle knives or squeeze-grip-actuated screwdrivers to replace finger-trigger-actuated screwdrivers
- Changing assembly access and sequence—for example, removing physical and visual obstructions when assembling components to reduce awkward postures or static exertions

Administrative controls are management-directed work practices and policies aimed to reduce

---

Box 7-3   General Ergonomic Risk Analysis Checklist

Put a check before each question if your answer is yes. A yes response indicates that an ergonomic risk factor may be present and requires further analysis.

MANUAL MATERIAL HANDLING

— Is there lifting of tools, loads, or parts?
— Is there lowering of tools, loads, or parts?
— Is there overhead reaching for tools, loads, or parts?
— Is there bending at the waist to handle tools, loads, or parts?
— Is there twisting at the waist to handle tools, loads, or parts?

PHYSICAL ENERGY DEMANDS

— Do tools and parts weigh more than 10 lb?
— Is reaching greater than 20 in?
— Is bending, stooping, or squatting a primary task activity?
— Is lifting or lowering loads a primary task activity?
— Is walking or carrying loads a primary task activity?
— Is stair or ladder climbing with loads a primary task activity?
— Is pushing or pulling loads a primary task activity?
— Is reaching overhead a primary task activity?
— Do any of the above tasks require five or more complete work cycles to be done within a minute?
— Do workers complain that rest breaks and fatigue allowances are insufficient?

OTHER MUSCULOSKELETAL DEMANDS

— Do manual jobs require frequent, repetitive motions?
— Do work postures require frequent bending of the neck, shoulder, elbow, wrist, or finger joints?
— For seated work, do reaches for tools and materials exceed 15 in from the worker's position?
— Is the worker unable to change his or her position often?
— Does the work involve forceful, quick, or sudden motions?
— Does the work involve shock or rapid buildup of forces?
— Is finger-pinch gripping used?

— Do job postures involve sustained muscle contraction of any limb?

COMPUTER WORKSTATION

— Do operators use computer workstations for more than 4 hours per day?
— Are there complaints of discomfort from those working at these stations?
— Is the chair or desk nonadjustable?
— Is the display monitor, keyboard, or document holder nonadjustable?
— Does lighting cause glare or make the monitor screen hard to read?
— Is the room temperature too hot or too cold?
— Is there irritating vibration or noise?

ENVIRONMENT

— Is the temperature too hot or too cold?
— Are the worker's hands exposed to temperatures less than 70° F?
— Is the workplace poorly lit?
— Is there glare?
— Is there excessive noise that is annoying, distracting, or producing hearing loss?
— Is there upper extremity or whole body vibration?
— Is air circulation too high or too low?

GENERAL WORKPLACE

— Are walkways uneven, slippery, or obstructed?
— Is housekeeping poor?
— Is there inadequate clearance or accessibility for performing tasks?
— Are stairs cluttered or lacking railings?
— Is proper footwear worn?

TOOLS

— Is the handle too small or too large?
— Does the handle shape cause the operator to bend the wrist in order to use the tool?
— Is the tool hard to access?
— Does the tool weigh more than 9 lb?
— Does the tool vibrate excessively?
— Does the tool cause excessive kickback to the operator?
— Does the tool become too hot or too cold?

GLOVES

— Do the gloves require the worker to use more force when performing job tasks?
— Do the gloves provide inadequate protection?

Modified from "Checklist for General Ergonomic Risk Analysis," University of Utah Research Foundation, http://ergoweb.com/; *Elements of Ergonomic Programs,* by U.S. Department of Health and Human Services, National Institute for Occupational Safety and Health, 1996, Cincinnati, OH: National Institute for Occupational Safety and Health.

Continued

Box 7-3 General Ergonomic Risk Analysis Checklist—cont'd

___ Do the gloves present a hazard of catch points on the tool or in the workplace?

ADMINISTRATION

___ Is there little worker control over the work process?

___ Is the task highly repetitive and monotonous?

___ Does the job involve critical tasks with high accountability and little or no tolerance for error?

___ Are work hours and breaks poorly organized?

Modified from "Checklist for General Ergonomic Risk Analysis," University of Utah Research Foundation, http://ergoweb.com/; *Elements of Ergonomic Programs,* by U.S. Department of Health and Human Services, National Institute for Occupational Safety and Health, 1996, Cincinnati, OH: National Institute for Occupational Safety and Health.

---

or prevent exposures to ergonomic risk factors. Although engineering controls are preferred, administrative controls can be helpful as temporary measures until engineering controls can be implemented or when engineering controls are not technically feasible. Since administrative controls do not eliminate hazards, management must assure that the practices and policies are followed. Common examples of administrative control strategies for reducing the risks of musculoskeletal disorders are as follows:

- Reducing shift length or curtailing the amount of overtime
- Rotating workers through several jobs with different physical demands to reduce the stress on limbs and body regions
- Scheduling more breaks to allow for rest and recovery
- Broadening or varying the job content to offset certain risk factors (e.g., repetitive motions, static, and awkward postures)
- Adjusting the work pace to relieve repetitive motion risks and give the worker more control of the work process
- Training in the recognition of risk factors for musculoskeletal disorders and instruction in work practices that can ease the task demands or burden
- Reducing the total number of repetitions per employee by such means as decreasing production rates and limiting overtime work
- Increasing the number of employees assigned to a task to alleviate severe conditions, especially in lifting heavy objects
- Using effective housekeeping programs to minimize slippery work surfaces and related hazards such as slips and falls.

Travers (1992) identifies several common ergonomic concerns and associated corrective measures in the office environment (Table 7-3).

An effective ergonomic health and medical program should encompass a multidisciplinary approach and include early identification, evaluation, treatment, follow-up, rehabilitation, and recording of signs and symptoms by health care providers knowledgeable in these areas and with respect to the company's operations, work practices, and light duty jobs. A survey of employees can be conducted to measure employee awareness of work-related disorders and report the location, frequency, and duration of discomfort (Figure 7-9). Body diagrams can be used to facilitate and clarify information gathering. A physician or occupational and environmental health nurse with appropriate ergonomics prevention/management training should oversee the program. The health/medical management program as identified by OSHA (USDOL, OSHA, 1991) should include the following:

- Injury and illness recordkeeping
- Early recognition and reporting
- Systematic evaluation and referral
- Conservative treatment
- Conservative return to work
- Systematic monitoring
- Adequate staffing and facilities

In an effective program health care providers should conduct periodic, systematic, workplace walk throughs to remain knowledgeable about operations and work practices, identify potential light duty jobs, and maintain close contact with employees. Health care providers also should be involved in identifying risk factors for muscu-

TABLE 7-3 Common Ergonomic Concerns and Corrective Measures*

PROBLEMS	RECOMMENDATIONS
Chair not adjusted; feet not flat on the floor; inadequate lumbar support	ENGINEERING CONTROLS 1. Adjust height and position of chair so that feet are flat on floor, arms are close to the body 2. Adequate lumbar support by using a rolled towel, pillow, cushion, or lumbar support 3. Footrest ADMINISTRATIVE CONTROLS 1. Employee education on adjusting chair and the importance of assuming varied postures throughout the course of any day
Keyboard too high, causing wrists and elbows to be in nonneutral positions	ENGINEERING CONTROLS 1. Lower keyboard by using desk drawer, articulating shelf, or lowering desk or table; or raise chair and use a footrest 2. Position keyboard and other input devices to avoid reaching motions ADMINISTRATIVE CONTROLS 1. Employee education on reasons for setting up areas to foster neutral body positions 2. Work practice changes so that no one position is assumed for long periods of time
Glare on terminal screen from overhead lighting or reflections from direct sunlight	ENGINEERING CONTROLS 1. Place screen perpendicular to the light source 2. Close blinds on windows or rearrange office setup to decrease glare from sunlight ADMINISTRATIVE CONTROLS 1. Regularly clean screen so vision is not hampered by smudge marks or an accumulation of dust 2. Have vision checked for viewing distance to screen; if needed, obtain glasses for specific viewing distance
Terminal screen too low	ENGINEERING CONTROLS 1. Raise terminal by using terminal stand, wooden box, or two-leveled stand
Contact with sharp edges	ENGINEERING CONTROLS 1. Pad edge of table or desk with foam robber, cushion, towel, or wrist support. ADMINISTRATIVE CONTROLS 1. Employee education on how to set up work area, symptoms, reasons for symptoms, and ways to avoid discomfort

From "Implementing Ergonomic Strategies in the Workplace: An Occupational Health Nursing Perspective," by P. H. Travers, *AAOHN Journal, 40,* 129-137. 1992. Reprinted by permission of the American Association of Occupational Health Nurses.
*These are examples of some of the solutions that can be implemented.

Symptoms Survey: Ergonomics Program

DATE ___ / ___ / ___

Plant	Dept #	Job #	Job Name

_____ years _____ months
Time on THIS job

Shift	Supervisor		Hours worked/week

Other jobs you have done in the last year (for more than 2 weeks)

Plant	Dept #	Job #	Job Name	_____ months _____ weeks Time on THIS job

Plant	Dept #	Job #	Job Name	_____ months _____ weeks Time on THIS job

(If more than 2 jobs, include those you worked on the most)

Have you had any pain or discomfort during the last year?
　　□ Yes　　　　　　□ No (if NO, stop here)

If YES, carefully shade in the area of the drawing which bothers you the MOST.

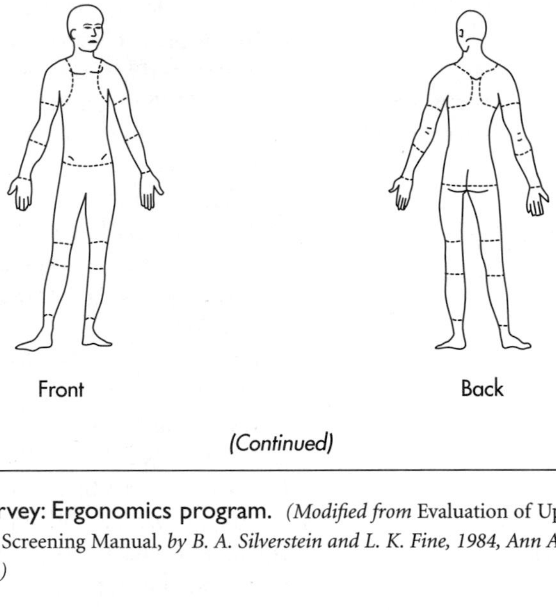

Front　　　　　　　　　　Back

(Continued)

Figure 7-9　Symptoms survey: Ergonomics program. *(Modified from* Evaluation of Upper Extremity and Low Back Cumulative Trauma Disorders: A Screening Manual, *by B. A. Silverstein and L. K. Fine, 1984, Ann Arbor, MI: University of Michigan, School of Public Health.)*　　　　　　Continued

loskeletal disorders in the workplace as part of the ergonomic team. The ergonomist or other qualified person should analyze the physical procedures used in the performance of each job, including lifting requirements, postures, hand grips, and frequency of repetitive motion. The ergonomist and health care providers should develop a list of jobs with the lowest ergonomic risk. For such jobs the ergonomic risk should be described. This information will assist health care providers in recommending assignments to limited duty or restricted duty jobs. The limited duty job should therefore not increase ergonomic stress on the same muscle-tendon groups. All

(Complete a separate page for each area that bothers you)

Check area: ☐ Neck ☐ Shoulder ☐ Elbow/Forearm ☐ Hand/Wrist ☐ Fingers
☐ Upper Back ☐ Low Back ☐ Thigh/Knee ☐ Low Leg ☐ Ankle/Foot

1. Please put a check by the word(s) that best describe your problem.
   ☐ Aching   ☐ Numbness (asleep)   ☐ Tingling
   ☐ Burning   ☐ Pain   ☐ Weakness
   ☐ Cramping   ☐ Swelling   ☐ Other
   ☐ Loss of Color   ☐ Stiffness

2. When did you first notice the problem? _____ (month) _____ (year)

3. How long does each episode last? (Mark an X along the line)

   _____/_____/_____/_____/_____
   1 hour   1 day   1 week   1 month   6 months

4. How many separate episodes have you had in the last year? _____

5. What do you think caused the problem? _____
   _____

6. Have you had this problem in the last 7 days?   ☐ Yes   ☐ No

---

7. How would you rate this problem? (Mark an X on the line)
   NOW

   _____
   None   Unbearable

   When it was the WORST

   _____
   None   Unbearable

---

8. Have you had medical treatment for this problem?   ☐ Yes   ☐ No
   8a. If NO, why not? _____
   8b. If YES, where did you receive treatment? _____
       1. Company Medical ☐   Times in past year _____
       2. Personal doctor ☐   Times in past year _____
       3. Other ☐   Times in past year _____

   8c. If YES, did the treatment help?   ☐ Yes   ☐ No

9. How much time have you lost in the last year because of this problem? _____ days

10. How many days in the last year were you on restricted or light duty because of this problem?
    _____ days

11. Please comment on what you think would improve your symptoms.
    _____
    _____
    _____
    _____

Figure 7-9, cont'd   For legend see opposite page.

new and transferred workers who are to be assigned to positions involving exposure of a particular body part to ergonomic stress should receive baseline health surveillance prior to assignment.

Employees should be encouraged to report symptoms so that adequate evaluation, treatment, and follow-up of the specific condition can be provided to prevent irreversible tissue damage and functional impairment.

In the work setting the health care professional must be knowledgeable and skilled to recognize symptoms and make appropriate decisions regarding the cause of the illness or injury and on-site treatment versus referral. The OSHA Ergonomics Guidelines Medical Management Section (USDOL, OSHA 1991) outlines specific management approaches and provides a useful algorithm for management of upper extremity cumulative trauma disorders.

Training and education is the final critical component of an ergonomics program for employees potentially exposed to musculoskeletal disorder risk. Training allows managers, supervisors, and employees to understand ergonomic solutions and hazards associated with a job or production process, ways to prevent and control these hazards, and their health/medical consequences. Employees with potential musculoskeletal disorder risk should be given formal instruction on the hazards associated with their jobs and related equipment. New employees and reassigned workers should receive an initial orientation and hands-on training prior to being placed in a full production job. On-the-job training should emphasize employee development and use of safe and efficient techniques.

Supervisors are responsible for ensuring that employees follow safe work practices and receive appropriate training to enable workers to follow

---

Box 7-4 General Workstation Design Principles

1. Make the workstation adjustable, enabling both large and small persons to fit comfortably and reach materials easily.
2. Locate all materials and tools in front of the worker to reduce twisting motions. Provide sufficient work space for the whole body to turn.
3. To avoid static loads, fixed work postures, and job requirements in which operators must frequently or for long periods, do the following:
   - Lean to the front or side;
   - Hold a limb in a bent or extended position;
   - Tilt the head forward more than 15 degrees; or
   - Support the body's weight with one leg.
4. Set the work surface above elbow height for tasks involving fine visual details and below elbow height for tasks requiring downward forces and heavy physical effort.
5. Provide adjustable, properly designed chairs with the following features:
   - Adjustable seat height
   - Adjustable up and down back rest, including a lumbar (lower back) support
   - Padding that will not compress more than an inch under the weight of a seated individual
   - Stability to floor at all times (5-leg base)
6. Allow the workers, at their discretion, to alternate between sitting and standing. Provide floor mats or padded surfaces for prolonged standing.
7. Support the limbs: provide elbow, wrist, arm, foot, and back rests as needed and feasible.
8. Use gravity to move materials.
9. Design the workstation so that arm movements are continuous and curved; avoid straight-line, jerking arm motions.
10. Design so arm movements pivot about the elbow rather than around the shoulder to avoid stress on shoulder, neck, and upper back.
11. Design the primary work area so that arm movements or extensions of more than 15 inches are minimized.
12. Provide dials and displays that are simple, logical, and easy to read, reach, and operate.
13. Eliminate or minimize the effects of undesirable environmental conditions such as excessive noise, heat, humidity, cold, and poor illumination.

Modified from design checklists developed by Dave Ridyard, CPE, CIH, CSP. Applied Ergonomics Technology, 270 Mather Road, Jenkintown, PA 19046-3129; *Elements of Ergonomics Programs,* by U.S. Department of Health and Human Services, National Institute for Occupational Safety and Health, 1996, Cincinnati, OH: National Institute for Occupational Safety and Health.

through. Supervisors, therefore, should undergo training comparable to that of the employees; supervisors should also receive additional training so they can recognize early signs and symptoms of musculoskeletal disorders, recognize and correct hazardous work practices, and reinforce the employer's ergonomic program, especially through the ergonomic training of employees as necessary. Resolution of ergonomic problems is best accomplished through a team problem solving approach. General workstation design principles are shown in Box 7-4. S. Rodgers (1992) provides several examples of approaches that address ergonomic problems by utilizing a team oriented framework (Box 7-5).

TOXICOLOGY

Toxicology is the study of the harmful effects of chemicals on biological systems, and a toxic agent is one capable of producing a harmful response in a biological system (Stine & Brown, 1996). Chemicals achieve their effect on biological systems through a series of events and reactions (Figure 7-10). This includes concentration of the agent in the environment, exposure to the host and entry into the body, and internal distribution in and effect on the target organ (Gibaldi & Perrier, 1982).

Industrial toxicology is the subdiscipline of toxicology primarily concerned with evaluating human

---

Box 7-5 **Examples of Approaches to Finding Ergonomic Solutions**

WORKPLACE DESIGN

1. Work height adjustments
   a. Adjust the work surface height.
      (1) Adjustable height surface.
      (2) Cut off or add blocks to work surface to change present height or use platform under supply bins.
   b. Adjust height of person relative to work surface.
      (1) Platforms
      (2) Chair adjustability
   c. Change the location of the operation to another part of the line where the height is more appropriate.
2. Reach improvements
   a. Make work height adjustments.
      (1) Adjust work surface.
      (2) Adjust position of person relative to work surface.
   b. Reduce forward reach requirements.
      (1) Work surface design changes (e.g., cut-outs)
      (2) Provision of reach extenders
3. Orientation of workplace and location of supplies
   a. Redesign line supply systems.
      (1) Conveyors
      (2) Location relative to line
   b. Provide for resupply of parts from existing storage.
      (1) Hoists
      (2) Roller conveyor sections
      (3) Hoppers

ENVIRONMENTAL DESIGN

1. Lighting
   a. Improve quality of lighting.
      (1) Task lighting
      (2) Type of lighting
      (3) Glare reduction
   b. Use specialized lighting for inspection.
      (1) Lighting angle adjustment
      (2) Special light sources (e.g., polarized light, projected stripes)
2. Temperature and humidity
   a. Modify ventilation systems.
      (1) Provide two-speed fans.
      (2) Alter duct or thermostat locations.
   b. Provide localized cooled or heated areas.
      (1) Break areas
      (2) Spot cooling or heating
   c. Vary workload requirements during hotter weather.
      (1) Alternate tasks for recovery from heat exposure.
      (2) Implement work practices to reduce heat illness.

EQUIPMENT DESIGN AND SELECTION

1. Tools
   a. Choose best tool for task.
      (1) Specialized tools—bend tool not wrist
      (2) Computer torque tools
      (3) Triggering versus push-to-start tools

Modified from "A Functional Job Analysis Technique, by S. Rodgers, 1992, *Occupational Medicine: State of the Art Reviews,* 7(4): 679-712.

Continued

Box 7-5 Examples of Approaches to Finding Ergonomic Solutions—cont'd

  b. Maintain tools.
    (1) Reduce vibration.
    (2) Keep torque capabilities.
2. Provide protective equipment.
  a. Vibration protection—Sorbothane/Viscolas
  b. Stall bars on tools
  c. Choice of gloves
  d. Choice of eye wear
3. Reduce complexity of information.
  a. Use understandable, action-oriented language.
  b. Provide troubleshooting aids.
  c. Use legible presentation.
    (1) Character size versus distance
    (2) Code use—shape, color, size, alphanumeric
    (3) Color contrast
    (4) Proper lighting
    (5) Reduce numbers of unnecessary quantitative displays

JOB DESIGN

1. Provide worker control.
  a. Reduce tight external pacing.
    (1) Incorporate in-process inventory or off-line areas in highly paced operations.
    (2) Provide easy access to parts, close to line.
    (3) Allow for some working ahead of or behind line speed.

    (4) Provide a "floater" to help reduce pressure on line workers.
  b. Provide training for new or transferred employees.
    (1) Provide some off-line training initially.
    (2) When job, equipment, or methods change, provide some time for learning during its implementation.
2. Reduce manual lifting demands.
  a. Find ways to slide the load rather than lift it.
    (1) Design to minimize handling.
    (2) Adjust heights to permit horizontal transfer at about 75-100 cm (30-40 in.) above the floor.
    (3) Use bail-beating tables or roller conveyor sections to move parts between locations.
  b. Use bulk transfer devices to handle parts.
    (1) Hoppers, super sacks
    (2) Lowerators
    (3) Hoists, magnets
3. Train workers to increase their work capacities.
  a. Provide on-the-job work-related fitness programs.
  b. Identify skills and strengths/endurances for jobs that are difficult to redesign. Determine what capabilities are needed and look for people with those capabilities.

Modified from "A Functional Job Analysis Technique, by S. Rodgers, 1992, *Occupational Medicine: State of the Art Reviews*, 7(4): 679-712.

health effects posed by chemical exposure in the workplace (Williams & Burson, 1985). Paracelsus (1493-1541) noted that "all substances are poisons; there is none which is not a poison. It is the dose only that distinguishes a poison and a remedy" (Ottoboni, 1991, p. 31). Thus, most all chemicals have the potential to create a toxic situation, wherein a toxic effect potentiates damage—measured in terms of a loss, reduction, or change in function—to an organism. However, effects that are considered adverse in one person may be desirable or therapeutic in another (Gochfeld, 1992b).

Everything in our physical world—the food we eat, the water we drink, the clothes we wear, the medicines we use, and all the materials of

daily living—are composed of chemicals. More than 6 million synthetic chemicals have been registered by the American Chemical Association, and the number of naturally occurring chemicals in the environment is unknown (Ottoboni, 1991). Workers are exposed to a variety of chemicals in the production of materials in the work environment, and the occupational and environmental health nurse may be the first person to assess the exposure. Thus, the occupational and environmental health nurses must have an understanding of general principles related to toxicological concepts. However, for a more in-depth discussion, the reader should consult a toxicology reference.

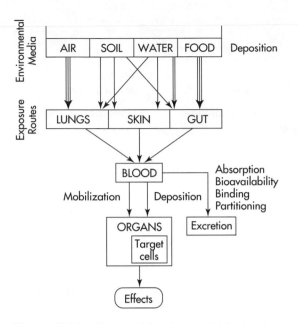

Figure 7-10 Chemical distribution: Multiplicative effect. *(From "Toxicology," by M. Gochfeld, in J. Last and R. Wallace [Eds.],* Maxcy-Rosenau-Last Public Health and Preventive Medicine *[13th ed., p. 316], 1992, Norwalk, CT: Appleton & Lange. Reproduced with permission of the McGraw-Hill Companies.)*

CHEMICAL CLASSIFICATIONS AND EFFECTS

Chemicals may be classified in several different ways. The American National Standards Institute has adopted the following definitions, which reflect the nature of the chemical's substance (Frumkin, 2000):

1. *Dusts.* Solid particles generated by handling, crushing, grinding, rapid impact, and detonation of organic or inorganic materials such as rocks, ore, metal, coal, wood, and grain. Dusts do not tend to flocculate except under electrostatic forces; they do not diffuse in air but settle under the influence of gravity.
2. *Fumes.* Solid particles generated by condensation from the gaseous state, generally after volatilization from molten metals, and often accompanied by a chemical reaction such as oxidation. Fumes flocculate and sometimes coalesce.
3. *Mists.* Suspended liquid droplets generated by condensation from the gaseous state to the liquid state or by breaking up a liquid into a dis-

persed state, such as by splashing, foaming, or atomizing.
4. *Vapors.* The gaseous form of substances that are normally in the solid or liquid state and can be changed to these states by either increasing the pressure or decreasing the temperature. Vapors diffuse.
5. *Gases.* Normally formless fluids that occupy the space of enclosure and can be changed to the liquid or solid state only by the combined effect of increased pressure and decreased temperature. Gases diffuse.

In addition, classification may be according to the duration of exposure, that is, acute or chronic toxicity, or by target site of action, either local or systemic (Table 7-4). Exposure to a high dose over a short time is an acute exposure, whereas chronic exposure usually involves continuous or periodic small doses over an extended period. With respect to endpoint health effect, the liver is of particular concern because many substances are directly transported to the liver for intermediary metabolism. The liver may detoxify harmful chemicals that are of themselves toxic or convert benign substances into a biologically harmful metabolite (Gochfeld, 1992b; Stine & Brown, 1996). The toxicity of a substance is its ability to damage an organ system, disrupt a biochemical process, such as hematopoietic mechanisms, or disturb an enzyme system.

Toxicity is not a direct estimate of hazard (Stine and Brown, 1996). For any substance the term *hazard* can be used to describe the actual risk of poisoning. Toxicity is only one variable in predicting how hazardous a substance will be during practical use. Another significant variable is the potential level of human exposure to the substance; this must be predicted based on factors such as the concentration and circumstances of use of the substance. Although the intrinsic toxicity of a substance cannot be altered because it is a basic property of that substance, reducing the practical risk of exposure can reduce the hazard of a toxic substance. A simple example is the invention of childproof packaging of nonprescription drugs, which reduces the hazard associated with some drugs by making access to the drug more difficult. In another example hazards posed by pesticide exposure to the pesticide applicator have been reduced by preparing the pesticide in dissolvable polymer bags containing premeasured quantities designed

TABLE

TABLE 7-4 Classification of Toxic Agents by Exposure and Effect		
CLASSIFICATION	**EXAMPLE: WELDING ON ZINC**	**EXAMPLE: CARBON TETRACHLORIDE**
Acute toxicity: Adverse toxic effects occurring from a short-term, usually single high-dose exposure to a toxic chemical, resulting in often severe symptoms developing rapidly. Effect is often reversible.	Symptoms of metal-fume fever	Depression of mental capacity
Chronic toxicity: Adverse toxic effects occurring from repeated or continuous exposure, usually low level, over a relatively long period of time. Effect is often irreversible.	Latent pneumoconiosis, pulmonary fibrosis	Liver or kidney damage
Local toxicity: Effect occurring at the site of application or exposure between the toxicant and biological system.	Burn	Irritation of eyes and throat
Systemic toxicity: Effect occurring within the body as a result of absorption and distribution of the toxicant via the bloodstream to susceptible organs that are the sites of action.	Gastrointestinal symptoms, musculoskeletal aches	Central nervous system depressant

to be dropped into the sprayer tank without being opened. This innovation greatly reduced the risk of exposure to formulated pesticide concentrates by eliminating measuring and mixing by the applicator. Toxic chemical exposure may range from minor, such as an irritation, to serious, such as liver or kidney damage or cancer, or to death from organ failure (Table 7-5).

Health effects from chemical exposure may be manifested as mutagenic, carcinogenic, or teratogenic and should be differentiated. A mutagen is a substance that interacts with genetic material and causes point mutations, chromosomal damage, or interference with cell development and division (Stine & Brown, 1996; Williams & Burson, 1985). Mutagen examples include antineoplastic agents and cigarette smoke. Alterations in the DNA affect the somatic, reproductive, or germ cells. Adverse effects on germ cells may be transmitted to offspring (Figure 7-11).

A carcinogen is a substance that, through the processes of initiation and promotion, is capable of causing cancer. Initiation is the process by which the genetic material of the cell is altered, predisposing it to cancer, and a process to which humans are exposed all their lives. The changes that constitute initiation may be reversed by repair mechanisms or may lie dormant, perhaps controlled by the immune system. This is followed by the stage of promotion, whereby initiated cells are stimulated or allowed to become cancerous (Armitage, 1985; Christani & Monson, 1997; Frumkin, 2000). Examples of substances known or suspected of being carcinogenic as reported by the National Toxicology Program (2000) in their annual report are shown in Box 7-6.

A teratogen is a substance that interferes with embryonic or fetal development and may cause major structural birth defects, slowed maturation, embryonic death, or even postnatal behavioral or learning dysfunction (McMartin et al., 1998; Stine & Brown, 1996). Teratogenesis will be discussed in more detail later.

TABLE 7-5 Selected Chemical Agents Related to Specific Target Organ Systems Effects

METAL	RENAL SYSTEM	NERVOUS SYSTEM	LIVER	GI TRACT	RESPIRATORY SYSTEM	HEMATOPOIETIC SYSTEM	BONE	ENDOCRINE SYSTEM	SKIN	CARDIOVASCULAR SYSTEM
Aluminum		+			+					
Arsenic		+	+	+	+	+		+	+	
Beryllium					+				+	
Bromide		+								
Cadmium	+	+	+	+	+		+		+	+
Chromium	+	+			+				+	
Cobalt		+		+	+			+	+	+
Copper				+		+				
Fluoride		+	+	+	+		+		+	
Iron		+		+	+	+		+		
Lead	+	+		+		+		+		
Manganese		+		+	+					
Mercury	+	+		+	+					
Nickel		+		+	+				+	
Selenium	+			+	+				+	
Silver				+	+				+	
Thallium	+	+	+	+	+	+	+			
Zinc				+			+			

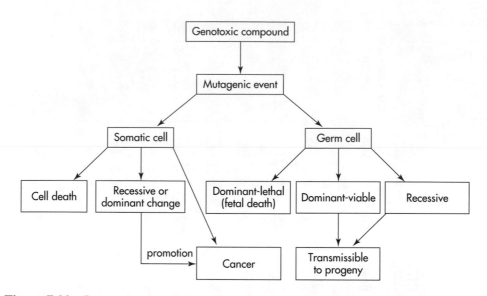

Figure 7-11 Potential consequences of a mutagenic event in somatic and germinal cells.
(From Industrial Toxicology, *by P. Williams and J. Burson, 1985, New York: Van Nostrand Reinhold.)*

Box 7-6 **Known or Reasonably Anticipated Carcinogens Listed in the Ninth Annual Report of the National Toxicology Program, 2000**

1. Substances or groups of substances and medical treatments that are known to be carcinogenic

Aflatoxins
4-Aminobiphenyl
2-Aminonaphthalene
Analgesic mixtures containing phenacetin
Arsenic and certain arsenic compounds
Asbestos
Azathioprine
Barium chromate
Benzene
Benzidine
bis(chloromethyl) ether and technical-grade chloromethyl methyl ether
1,3-Butadiene
1,4-Butanediol dimethylsulfonate (Myleran) (Busulfan)
Cadmium and cadmium compounds
Chlorambucil
1-(2-Chloroethyl)-3-(4-methylcyclohexyl)-1-nitrosourea (MeCCNU)
Chromium and certain chromium compounds
Coke oven emissions
Conjugated estrogens
Cyclophosphamide
Cyclosporin A
Diethylstilbestrol

Dyes that metabolize to benzidine
  Direct Black 38
  Direct Blue 6
Environmental tobacco smoke
Erionite
Ethylene Oxide
Melphalan
Methoxsalen with ultraviolet A therapy (PUVA)
Mustard gas
2-Naphthylamine
Radon
Silica, crystalline (respirable size)
  Quartz
Smokeless tobacco
Solar radiation and related forms
Soots, Tars, Mineral Oils
Strong inorganic acid mists containing sulfuric acid
Tamoxifin
Thiotepa
Thorium dioxide
Tobacco smoking
Tridymite
Vinyl chloride

Modified from *Ninth Annual Report on Carcinogens,* by U.S. Department of Health and Human Services, National Toxicology Program, 2000. Washington, DC: Author.

Continued

Box 7-6 **Known or Reasonably Anticipated Carcinogens Listed in the Ninth Annual Report of the National Toxicology Program, 2000—cont'd**

---

2. Substances or groups of substances and medical treatments that may reasonably be anticipated to be carcinogens

Acetaldehyde
2-Acetylaminofluorene
Acrylamide
Acrylonitrile
Adriamycin
2-Aminoanthraquinone
o-Aminoazotoluene
1-Amino-2-methylanthraquinone
Amitrole
o-Anisidine hydrochloride
Azacitidine
Benzotrichloride
Beryllium and certain beryllium compounds
bis(chloroethyl) nitrosourea
Bromodichloromethane
Butylated hydroxyanisole
Carbon tetrachloride
Ceramic fibers (respirable size)
Chlorendic acid
Chlorinated paraffins (C$_{12}$,60% chlorine)
1-(2-Chloroethyl)-3-cyclohexyl-
   1-nitrosourea (CCNU)
Chloroform
3-Chloro-2-methylpropene
4-Chloro-*o*-phenylenediamine
Chloroprene
p-Chloro-*o*-toluidine
p-Chloro-*o*-toluidine-hydrochloride
Chlorozotocin
C. I. basic red 9 monohydrochloride
Cisplatin
p-Cresidine
Cupferron
Dacarbazine
Danthron
DDT
2,4-Diaminoanisole sulfate
2,4-Diaminotoluene
1,2-Dibromo-3-chloropropane
1,2-Dibromoethane (EDB)
1,4-Dichlorobenzene
3,3'-Dichlorobenzidine and
   3,3'-dichlorobenzidine dihydrochloride
1,2-Dichloroethane
Dichloromethane (methylene chloride)
1,3-Dichloropropene (technical grade)
Diepoxybutane
Diesel exhaust particulates
Di(2-ethylhexyl)phthalate

Diethyl sulfate
Diglycidyl resorcinol ether
3,3'-Dimethoxybenzidine
4-Dimethylaminoazobenzene
3,3'-Dimethylbenzidine
Dimethylcarbamoyl chloride
1,1-Dimethylhydrazine
Dimethyl sulfate
Dimethylvinyl chloride
1,4-Dioxane
1,6 Dinitropyrene
1,8 Dinitropyrene
Disperse Blue 1
Epichlorohydrin
Estrogens (not conjugated): Estradiol-17β
Estrogens (not conjugated): Estrone
Estrogens (not conjugated): Ethinylestradiol
Estrogens (not conjugated): Mestranol
Ethyl acrylate
Ethylene thiourea
Ethyl methanesulfonate
Formaldehyde (gas)
Furan
Glasswool (respirable size)
Glycidol
Hexachlorobenzene
Hexachloroethane
Hexamethylphosphoramide
Hydrazine and hydrazine sulfate
Hydrazobenzene
Iron dextran complex
Isoprene
Kepone (chlordecone)
Lead acetate and lead phosphate
Lindane and other hexachlorocyclohexane
   isomers
2-Methylaziridine (propyleneimine)
4,4'-Methylenebis (2-chloroaniline) (MBOCA)
4-4'-Methylenebis (N,N-dimethyl)
   benzenamine
4,4'-Methylenedianiline
Methyl methanesulfonate
N-Methyl-*N*'-nitro-N-nitrosoguanidine
Metronidazole
Michler's ketone
Mirex
Nickel and certain nickel compounds
Nitrilotriacetic acid
o-Nitroanisole

Continued

Box 7-6 **Known or Reasonably Anticipated Carcinogens Listed in the Ninth Annual Report of the National Toxicology Program, 2000—cont'd**

6-Nitrochrysene	Dibenz[*a,j*]acridine
Nitrofen	Dibenz[*a,h*]anthracene
Nitrogen mustard hydrochloride	7H-Dibenzo[*c,g*]carbazole
2-Nitropropane	Dibenzo[*a,e*]pyrene
1-Nitropyrene	Dibenzo[*a,h*]pyrene
4-Nitropyrene	Dibenzo[*a,i*]pyrene
N-Nitrosodi-*n*-butylamine	Dibenzo[*a,l*]pyrene
N-Nitrosodiethanolamine	Indeno[1,2,3-*cd*]pyrene
N-Nitrosodiethylamine	5-Methylchrysene
N-Nitrosodimethylamine	Procarbazine hydrochloride
N-Nitrosodi-*n*-propylamine	Progesterone
N-Nitroso-*N*-ethylurea	1,3-Propane sultone
4-(*N*-Nitrosomethylamino)-1-(3-pryidyl)-	β-Propiolactone
1-butanone	Propylene oxide
N-Nitroso-*N*-methylurea	Propylthiouracil
N-Nitrosomethylvinylamine	Reserpine
N-Nitrosomorpholine	Saccharin
N-Nitrosonornicotine	Safrole
N-Nitrosopiperidine	Selenium sulfide
N-Nitrosopyrrolidine	Silica, Cristobalite
N-Nitrososarcosine	Streptozotocin
Norethisterone	Sulfallate
Ochratoxin A	2,3,7,8-Tetrachlorodibenzo-p-dioxin (TCDD)
4,4'-Oxydianiline	Tetrachloroethylene (perchloroethylene)
Oxymetholone	Tetraflouroethylene
Phenacetin	Tetranitromethane
Phenazopyridine hydrochloride	Thioacetamide
Phenolphthalein	Thiourea
Phenoxybenzamine hydrochloride	Toluene diisocyanate
Phenytoin	*o*-Toluidine and o-toluidine hydrochloride
Polybrominated biphenyls (PBBs)	Toxaphene
Polychlorinated biphenyls (PCBs)	Trichloroethylene
Polycyclic aromatic hydrocarbons, 15 listings	2,4,6-Trichlorophenol
Benz[*a*]anthracene	1,2,3 Trichloropropane
Benzo[*b*]fluoranthene	tris(1-aziridinyl)phosphine sulfide
Benzo[*j*]fluoranthene	tris(2,3-dibromopropyl) phosphate
Benzo[*k*]fluoranthene	Urethane
Benzo[*a*]pyrene	4-Vinyl-1-cyclohexene diepyoxide
Dibenz [*a, h*]acridine	

Modified from *Ninth Annual Report on Carcinogens*, by U.S. Department of Health and Human Services, National Toxicology Program, 2000. Washington, DC: Author.

The scheme of classification relative to how substances are used is essential for government regulation of such items as foods, drugs, cosmetics, pesticides, industrial chemicals, and medical devices. A substance that is claimed to be a food is governed by the food laws; the exact same substance, packaged and labeled as a drug, is governed by the drug laws, not the food laws. The laws that pertain to a substance depend on what use the manufacturer specifies for the product. For example, hydrochloric acid is regulated as a household product when it is present in cleaning compounds, as a drug when it is used to treat people with low gastric acidity, as a hazardous industrial chemical

TABLE 7-6 **Ranking System for Acute Chemical Toxicity**

TOXICITY RATING OR CLASS	PROBABLE ORAL LETHAL DOSE FOR AVERAGE ADULT	EXAMPLE OF SUBSTANCE
1. Practically nontoxic	>15 g/kg (more than 1 quart)	Sugar
2. Slightly toxic	5-15 g/kg (between 1 pint and 1 quart)	Salt
3. Moderately toxic	0.5-5 g/kg (between 1 ounce and 1 pint)	2,4-D (herbicide)
4. Very toxic	50-500 mg/kg (between 1 teaspoonful and 1 ounce)	Arsenic acid
5. Extremely toxic	5-50 mg/kg (between 7 drops and 1 teaspoonful)	Nicotine
6. Supertoxic	<5 mg/kg (a taste [<7 drops])	Botulism toxin

From *The Work Environment: Occupational Health Fundamentals,* by D. Hartsen, Chelsea, MI: Lewis. 1991.

when it is used in electroplating, and as a pesticide adjuvant when it is used to enhance the germicidal activity of chlorine in swimming pools. Hydrochloric acid is natural when produced by the stomach and synthetic when made in the laboratory (Ottoboni, 1991). Ottoboni lists the following harmful properties of chemicals:

- Explosiveness and reactivity
- Flammability and combustibility
- Radioactivity
- Corrosiveness
- Irritation
- Sensitization and photosensitization
- Toxicity

In addition, a poison is different from a toxin. A poison is a chemical that produces illness or death when taken in very small quantities (Ottoboni, 1991). A poison is defined legally as a chemical that has an LD_{50} of 50 milligrams (mg) or less of chemical per kilogram (kg) of body weight. An LD_{50}, also called median lethal dose, is the quantity of a chemical administered in one dose that is lethal for 50% of test animals within a 14-day period (Ottoboni, 1991). LD refers to the lethal dose, LC to the lethal concentration, and subscript 50 to the percentage of the animals for which the dose was lethal. LD_{50} is also used to express acute inhalation toxicity, which refers to the lethal concentration of an airborne contaminant. The smaller the LD_{50}, the greater the toxicity, and conversely, the larger the LD_{50}, the

less the toxicity. LD_{50}s and LC_{50}s are obviously unknown for humans for any chemical, because humans cannot be placed in these types of experimental conditions to test lethal doses. However, this concept is important because data from animal experiments are extrapolated to humans to estimate toxicity. For toxic effects one assumes that a person is at least as sensitive to the toxicity as the test species is and may be more susceptible. A relative ranking system of acute chemical toxicity is shown in Table 7-6.

DOSE-RESPONSE

Lioy (1990) describes an exposure-effect relationship on a continuum from point source emission to human contact exposure to potential dose to the body biologically effective/response dose to the target system early expression of disease health effect on endpoint. The degree to which a substance or chemical is harmful is determined by the dose of that chemical and the relationship of that dose to producing an adverse biological or health effect (Stine & Brown, 1996). This is in contrast to an effective dose (ED) in which the response is a desirable one. This concept of dose-response is the hallmark of toxicology and is critically important as the basis for determining the relative safety of a chemical compound in the living organism (Hansen, 1991). Most often the response is measured as the percentage of exposed animals that show a particular effect.

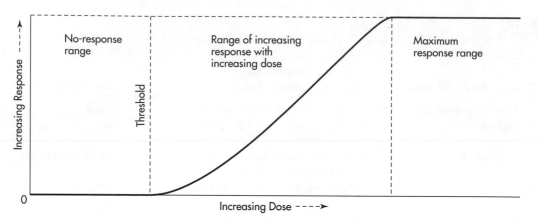

Figure 7-12 Dose-response curve.

Generally, higher levels of toxic exposure will invoke greater responses such as when higher concentrations of inhaled carbon monoxide produce higher carboxyhemoglobin levels (Becker, 1990). A dose-response graph (Figure 7-12) quantifies the relationship of the biological or health effect as a result of dose levels. The typical dose-response curve is demonstrated by the sigmoidal shape shown.

Important to the dose-response concept is the threshold dose or level at which no effect is observed. In the figure the lower end of the curve reflects the existence of a threshold dose (no effect noted) and is followed by a sharp rise in the curve, often displayed as a linear phase, where the increase in response is proportional to the dose increase. The upper end displays a flattening of the curve or ceiling level of maximal response that cannot be increased by greater doses. This level might correspond to the death of an individual. In the dose-response relationship it is necessary to know the endpoint of measurement, which may be, for example, the presence of a lesion (e.g., tumor), a biological, physiological, or behavioral alteration (response dose or effective dose), or death (lethal dose). Figure 7-13 shows a dose-response relationship between exposure to antineoplastic agents and urine mutagenicity in a population of exposed nurses (Rogers & Emmett 1987).

In addition to dose-response relationships, the concept of latency, the time between exposure and effect, is an important variable in interpreting presumed cause-effect relationships. If the latency period is very short (e.g., acute exposure to hydrogen sulfide), the effect is immediately measurable. In other situations, such as asbestos-induced mesothelioma, the latency period may be as long as 40 years (Selikoff & Lee, 1978). For diseases with long latency periods the exposure may not necessarily be associated with the outcome. Thus, the occupational and environmental health nurse must be familiar with and document exposures in order to investigate cause-effect relationships through epidemiologic studies.

ROUTES OF EXPOSURE

In the workplace chemicals enter the body primarily through inhalation, dermal absorption, and oral ingestion. Although chemicals can enter the body through other routes (e.g., injection), this is uncommon as a workplace exposure, except in the health care setting where needlestick injuries present a route of exposure (Rogers, 2000).

Inhalation is the major route of entry of the gases, vapors, mists and airborne particulate matter encountered in the workplace. Gases, vapors, and mists can cause damage to the respiratory tract; they also can pass through the lung to the bloodstream for distribution to other parts of the body, where they cause systemic poisoning. Highly soluble irritant gases, such as hydrogen fluoride, ammonia, and sulfuric acid, often produce an immediate irritation, while less soluble gases, such as nitrogen dioxide and phosgene, reach the alveoli and dissolve slowly, causing acute pneumonitis and pulmonary edema several hours later (Frumkin, 2000).

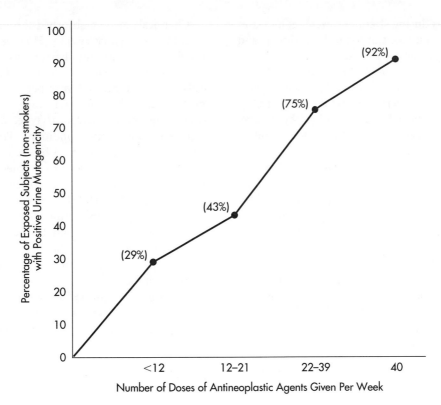

Figure 7-13 Percentage of positive urine mutagenicity results for exposed subjects (nonsmokers) by total number of doses of antineoplastic agents given. *(From Handling Antineoplastic Agents: Urine Mutagenicity in Nursing Personnel, by B. Rogers and E. Emmett, 1987, Image 19(3), 108-113.)*

Asphyxiants exert toxicity through interruption of oxygen to the tissues. Simple asphyxiants, such as carbon dioxide and nitrogen, cause hypoxia by displacing oxygen in the ambient air and can be a problem in confined spaces. Chemical asphyxiants block the delivery of oxygen at the cell site. Carbon monoxide, which is a product of incomplete combustion found in coke ovens and foundries, interferes with oxygen transport by binding to the hemoglobin to form carboxyhemoglobin. Cyanide and hydrogen sulfide are other examples of chemical asphyxiants (Becker, 1990; LaDou, 1997).

The delivery of gases, vapors, and mists to body tissues may be enhanced by rapid deep breathing, which occurs with strenuous exercise or a poorly designed or poorly fit respirator. In addition lipid-soluble subtances cross the alveolar membrane to the bloodstream and deposit themselves in fatty depots, thus allowing the blood to clear or free itself for another pick-up as it passes again through the lung. Examples of lipid-soluble substances include chloroform, carbon disulfide, and halogenated hydrocarbons (Williams & Burson, 1985).

Inhaled particles exert their adverse effects primarily through deposition in the lung tissue. The three basic regions of the lung are the nasopharyngeal region, tracheobronchial region, and alveolar region. The location and extent of deposition are influenced by the anatomy of the respiratory tract, particle size, and ventilation (Frumkin, 2000). For example, because the nasopharynx has sharp bends and nasal hairs, deposition may be enhanced, which may account, in part, for the increased incidence of nasal cancer in some groups occupationally exposed to dust-containing carcinogens, such as wood dusts, cork dusts, and fiberboard (Wills, 1982).

The effective anatomy of the respiratory tract changes significantly with a simple shift from nose breathing to mouth breathing, which occurs normally during physical exertion. This bypasses the more efficient filtration of larger particles by the nasopharynx and results in greater deposition in the tracheobronchial tree. Through such a transition workers performing physical labor may lose the benefit of a major natural defense mechanism (Frumkin, 2000). In addition, deep breathing, as during strenuous exercise, increases the amount of inhaled air to the distal airways and promotes alveolar deposition.

Particle deposition is also influenced by its shape and density. As indicated in a classic report by Brain and Valberg (1979), the efficiency of deposition of particles is determined by its size, shape, and density (Figure 7-14). Deposition of particles with an aerodynamic diameter of several micrometers (μm) is high, diminishes at about 1.0 μm and increases again below 0.5 μm. Those particles with an effective aerodynamic diameter between 0.5 and 5.0 mm (the respirable fraction) can be maintained in the alveoli and bronchioles, thus setting the stage for pneumoconiosis. Particle filtration in the upper airways and cilial action are important clearance mechanisms. Cilial action may be significantly compromised in smokers or in workers who have been continually exposed to some form of toxic material.

Chemicals may be absorbed through the skin into the circulatory system. However, the skin provides a significant barrier to absorption primarily because layers of epidermal and dermal cells in general are not very permeable to toxicants, although this will vary considerably depending on the chemical type, duration of exposure, and skin condition. Percutaneous absorption can be increased by damage or abrasion to the skin, increased skin wetness, or vascularization. Certain organic solvents, such as dimethyl sulfoxide (DMSO), also appear to act as delipidizing agents that reduce the barrier function of the stratum corneum, the outermost layer (Frumkin, 2000). Once a chemical penetrates the skin, it enters the bloodstream and is distributed throughout the body.

Ingestion is the third route of exposure for toxicants. While this route is generally not as significant in the workplace, chemicals can enter the

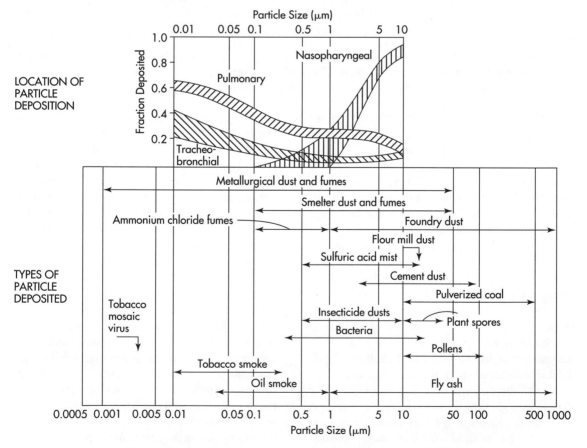

Figure 7-14 Respiratory deposition of inhaled particles influenced by particle shape and size.
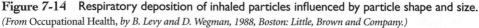
(From Occupational Health, *by B. Levy and D. Wegman, 1988, Boston: Little, Brown and Company.)*

body via contaminated food or water or inhaled particulates collected in the nasopharyngeal region and later swallowed (e.g., lead). Workers who mouth breath, chew gum or tobacco, or place contaminated fingers or materials in their mouths are also at risk for exposure through ingestion.

Gastric juices can help minimize toxicity through detoxification of the substances; thus, absorption into the bloodstream may be decreased. However, where substances are metabolized by the liver and the rate of passage is slowed, the length of time during which the compound is available for absorption is increased; such is the case with mercury or lead (Lewis, 1997).

FACTORS INFLUENCING TOXICITY

In addition to factors related to agent, dose, and route of exposure, several other factors influence toxicity. These include age, gender, ethnicity, nutrition, state of health, individual susceptibility, and previous or concurrent exposures.

Age

Although data are insufficient, evidence exists that infants and children are at greater risk of toxic insult from chemical exposure than are adults. Because infants have a less efficient biotransformation process than do adults and cells divide more rapidly in growing children than in adults, infants and children are more vulnerable to attack by chemical carcinogens than are adults (Loomis & Hayes, 1996; Ottoboni, 1991). Although not reported, the influence of the aging process on the metabolism of toxic materials should be considered. In addition, degenerative changes occurring in organ and immunologic systems may predispose older workers to harmful effects from toxic exposures. Further, the effects of age on healing processes may be an important consideration during the healing phase.

Gender

Gender differences related to toxic effects have been shown in numerous animal studies. However, in humans differences between the sexes relate primarily to their reproductive roles. While most current knowledge about reproductive toxicity comes from experimental animal studies, epidemiologic studies form the basis for occupational exposure associations in humans related to reproductive toxicity (Loomis, 1996; Olshan,

1993; Rogers & Emmett, 1987; Rowland et al., 1992; Schenker et al., 1995; Schnorr, 1993; Taskinen et al., 1994).

Reproductive toxicity

Prevention of reproductive system disorders is an important public health priority. The problems affect both men and women. In the United States approximately one in seven married couples is involuntarily infertile. Between 10% and 20% of pregnancies end in clinically recognized spontaneous abortion, and rates of very early periimplantation loss are even higher. Among newborns in the United States approximately 7% are of low birth weight (less than 2,500 g), and 3% have major congenital malformations (Paul & Frazier, 2000). The occupational health professional must have a good understanding of the reproductive processes in both the male and the female, a thorough knowledge of chemical exposures encountered in the workplace, and how or if these exposures may in any way compromise the reproductive system or outcome. The reproductive process is highly complex and dynamic. Damage by physical or chemical agents to the sperm, ovum, or the fertilized ovum may cause infertility, spontaneous abortion, or birth defects or may result in germ cell mutations that are passed on to future generations.

Because a variety of events occur at so many different times during the prenatal period, it stands to reason that the timing of exposure to a teratogen is critical in determining the potential effects. Exposure during the early stages (prior to implantation) is most likely to lead to embryonic death. Exposure during the late stages (in humans, the third trimester) is most likely to lead to growth retardation. It is during the middle stage, organogenesis, that exposure is most likely to lead to structural defects. Exposure to a teratogen during the critical period for a particular organ system may lead to malformations in that system. For example, exposure to the rubella virus during the first 8 weeks of pregnancy frequently produces defects of the visual and cardiovascular systems, the same exposure during weeks 8 to 10 leads to hearing impairment. Critical periods in humans may vary in length from as long as several weeks to as short as a day (Stine & Brown, 1996). When considering occupational exposures that may damage reproductive processes, the hazard to both men and women must be examined (Frazier & Hagl, 1998). For example, the risk of adverse pregnancy outcome after preconception exposure of men to toxic agents is an area of active research (Lahdetie, 1995; Nelson et al., 1996). A number of mechanisms have been postulated for these male-mediated effects, including germ cell mutagenesis. Increased rates of pregnancy loss have been reported among the wives of men exposed to lead, inorganic mercury, organic solvents, and other agents. Some studies suggest that certain paternal occupations pose an increased risk for congenital malformations and childhood cancers, but more research is needed. Tables 7-7 and 7-8 present examples of exposures and reproductive toxicity.

In utero development of the male reproductive system in the fetus begins about 7 weeks after

---

TABLE 7-7 Selected Occupational Agents with Suspected Effects on Pregnancy

Chemical Agent (Illustrative Exposures)	Reported Effects
Heavy metals	Neurobehavioral deficits in infants (with prenatal lead exposure, deficits reported at cord blood lead levels as low as 10-20 μg/dL)
Organic solvents (glycol ethers, toluene, xylene)	Spontaneous abortion; fetal loss rates increased in semiconductor workers exposed to EGEE/EGMEA; modestly increased risk of birth defects for mixed solvent exposure; toluene abuse (fetal solvent syndrome)
Antineoplastic agents (cisplatin, doxorubicin, fluorouracil, methotrexate)	Spontaneous abortion
Other pharmaceuticals (antivirals such as ribavirin; estrogenic or antiestrogenic compounds such as tamoxifen; immunosuppressive agents such as cyclosporine)	Spontaneous abortion; sperm effects in male animals and teratogenesis in female animals have been noted at high doses
Carcinogens and mutagens (ethidium bromide, aflatoxin B$_1$)	Human data limited; sperm effects noted in male animals, and teratogenesis and cancer in offspring of exposed female animals
Waste anesthetic gases (nitrous oxide [N$_2$O])	Spontaneous abortion
Sterilants and disinfectants (ethylene oxide, formaldehyde)	Spontaneous abortion
Polychlorinated biphenyls (PCBs) (chlorodiphenyls, chlorobiphenyls)	Congenital PCB syndrome at high doses; excreted efficiency into breast milk; low-level dietary exposure related to mild neonatal growth and neurobehavioral deficits in some studies
Pesticides (organochlorines such as lindane; organophosphates such as chlorpyrifos; N-methyl carbamates such as carbaryl; fungicides such as benomyl; herbicides such as 2,4-D)	Both male and female reproductive effects have been noted in animal studies for a number of pesticides; there are also some positive studies in workers; review data for each compound

From "Reproductive disorders," by M. Paul and L. Frazier, in B. Levy and D. Wegman (Eds.), *Occupational Health: Recognizing and Preventing Work-related Disease and Injury.* Philadelphia, Lippincott Williams & Wilkins. 2000.
EGEE/EGMEA, ethylene glycol monomethyl ether and its acetate.

TABLE 7-8   Adverse Reproductive Outcomes for Selected Chemicals Used in the Workplace

Chemical Agent	Infertility	Fecundity	Menstrual Disorders	Prematurity, Low Birth Weight	Spontaneous Abortion/Stillbirth	Birth Defects	Contaminated Breast Milk	Animal Studies
Anesthetic Agents	+				+			+
Anilene			+					
Antineoplastics					+/+	+		+
Arsenic					+			+
Benzene			+			+	+	+
Boron		M						+
Cadmium	+	M		+			+	+
Carbon Disulfide		M	+		+			+
Chloroprene	+	M	+		+			
Chromium								+
CO				+				
Copper							+	+
DDT							+	+
Dieldrin								+
Ethylene Dibromide	+	M						+
Ethylene Oxide					+			+
Formaldehyde			+	+				
Lead	+	M	+		+/+	+	+	+
Manganese	+	M						+
Mercury		F		+			+	+
Nickel							+	+
Selenium								+
Toluene		M	+	+				
Vinyl Chloride					+/+			+
Xylene								+

Data from *Occupational and Environmental Medicine,* by J. LaDou, Stamford, CT, Appleton & Lange, 1997; "Reproductive Disorders," by M. Paul and L. Frazier, in B. Levy and D. Wegman (Eds.), *Occupational Health: Recognizing and Preventing Work Related Disease and Injury,* Philadelphia: Lippincott Williams & Wilkins, 2000; *Principles of Toxicology,* by K. E. Stine and T. M. Brown, New York: Lewis. 1996.

+, Effect reported; M, male; F, female.

TABLE 7-9	Selected Occupational Agents With Suspected Effects on Male Reproductive Function	
ADVERSE EFFECTS	**EXAMPLES***
Decreased libido, hormonal alterations	Lead, mercury, manganese, carbon disulfide, estrogen agonists (e.g., polychlorinated biphenyls and organohalide pesticides); workers manufacturing oral contraceptives
Sperm toxicity	Lead, dibromochloropropane (DBCP), carbaryl, toluenediamine and dinitrotoluene, ethylene dibromide, plastic production (styrene and acetone), ethylene glycol monoethyl ether, welding, perchloroethylene, mercury, heat, military radar, Kepone, bromine, radiation (Chernobyl), carbon disulfide, 2,4-dichlorophenoxy acetic acid (2,4-D)
Spontaneous abortion in partner	Solvents, lead, mercury; workers in rubber and petroleum industries.
Altered sex ratio in offspring	Dibromochloropropane (DBCP)
Congenital malformations in offspring	Pesticides, chlorophenates, solvents; firefighters, painters, welders, auto mechanics, motor vehicle drivers, sawmill workers and workers in aircraft, electronics, forestry and logging industries
Neurobehavioral disorders in offspring	Alcohols, cyclophosphamide, ethylene dibromide, lead, opiates
Childhood cancer in offspring	Solvents, paints, pesticides, petroleum products; welders, auto mechanics, motor vehicle drivers, machinists and workers in aircraft and electronics industries

Modified from "Reproductive disorders," by M. Paul and L. Frazier, in B. Levy and D. Wegman, *Occupational Health: Recognizing and Preventing Work Related Disease and Injury,* Philadelphia: Lippincott Williams & Wilkins. 2000.
*Some human evidence, albeit limited, is available for all examples listed except those associated with neurobehavioral disorders in offspring; animal evidence is available for these paternal exposures.
*NIOSH has included these agents on its list of male reproductive hazards (www.cdc.gov/niosh/malrepro.html).

conception, with development of the male sex organs and testicular descent by 7 months gestation (Colie, 1993). During this process the phase of spermatogenesis in the male (stem germ cell to mature sperm) takes about 70 to 80 days, during which constant cell division makes the male reproductive system highly susceptible to chemical insult. Chemicals reach the testes by systemic blood distribution through inhalation, ingestion, or transpercutaneous absorption. Several male reproductive toxins have been occupationally identified (Table 7-9), including lead, selected halogenated pesticides, and possibly the organic solvents carbon disulfide (CS_2) and dinitrotoluene (Nelson, 1996; Levy et al., 1999).

The term *perinatal toxicology* designates the study of toxic responses to occupational and environmental agents when exposure occurs from the time of conception through the neonatal period

(Ottoboni, 1991). Exposures of the conceptus during specific periods of gestation elicit different responses. Fertilization of the ovum by the sperm occurs in the fallopian tube and is followed by implantation; the developing embryo is highly susceptible to both genetic abnormalities and toxic insults. Organogenesis occurs between days 17 and 56 (Paul & Frazier, 2000) and is followed by a slower development and maturation period, including neurological and sexual organ development. During this period of fetal development toxic exposures can result in neurologic, immunologic, developmental, and endocrine deficits and cancer in the offspring (Colt & Blair, 1998; Williams & Burson, 1985). Figure 7-15 depicts the stages of gestation and the biological responses associated with exposures to reproductive toxins during specific periods (Scialli, 1993; Williams & Burson, 1985).

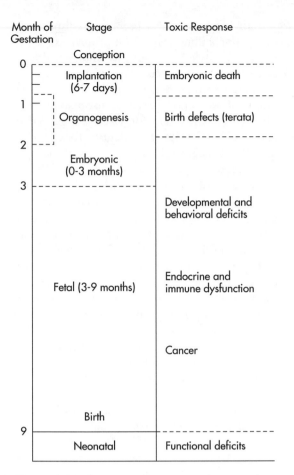

Figure 7-15 Stages of gestation and potential biological responses related to reproductive toxin exposure. *(From* Industrial Toxicology, *by P. Williams and J. Burson, 1985, New York: Van Nostrand Reinhold.)*

Teratogenesis is the process by which a physical or chemical foreign agent produces an abnormality in an organism developing in utero. Teratogens are agents that give rise to malformed or otherwise abnormal fetuses. Some chemicals and certain physical agents, such as natural and artificial radiation, can behave as teratogens. Chemical teratogens may or may not be mutagens, and chemical mutagens are not necessarily teratogens. X-rays may be both mutagens and teratogens. Chemical teratogen examples include antineoplastic agents, organic solvents, and polychlorinated biphenyls (PCBs). High doses of a teratogen may result in embryolethality (Gochfeld, 1992a).

During the critical period of embryonic development cells undergo differentiation and mobilization into tissue groups that differentiate further into major organs and cartilage (preskeleton). The critical stage of organ development for the human is the first 3 months (first trimester) of pregnancy. The kind of abnormality produced depends on what organ system is undergoing the most rapid development at the time of exposure to the teratogen. For example, exposure to high doses of vitamin A on the eighth day of gestation in rats results in skeletal malformations, whereas the same doses on the twelfth day result in cleft palate (Williams & Burson, 1985).

For reasons previously stated, the embryo is more susceptible to physical and chemical teratogens than is the mother. Overt toxicity and birth defects are not correlated, and, conversely, a number of chemicals producing toxic effects in the mother do not have adverse effects on the embryo. Maternal and placental metabolism of a chemical and the ability of a chemical to move from maternal blood across the placenta into the embryo's blood influence the amount and chemical form of an agent interacting with the rapidly dividing and differentiating cells. Teratogenic effects of a chemical occur within a relatively narrow range of concentration, between intermediate doses that kill the embryo and low doses that have no apparent effect (Ottoboni, 1991). Studies report reduced fertility among dental assistants exposed to nitrous oxide (Rowland, 1992) and spontaneous abortion in women exposed to glycol ethers while working in the semiconductor industry (Gray et al., 1995) and following exposure to organic solvents (McMartin et al., 1998; Khattak et al., 1999).

Mechanisms of teratogenesis are not well understood; however, changes in or inhibition of DNA and RNA, alteration in the structural formation of nucleic acids, or inhibition of enzymatic functions have been implicated. Spontaneous abortions have also been reported as a result of worker exposure to lead, copper, cadmium, anesthetic gases and antineoplastic agents (Paul & Frazier, 2000; Rogers & Emmett, 1987) (see Table 7-7). Chemicals can also produce fetal malformations by several nonteratogenic mechanisms, including preconception parent germ cell mutation and inadequate placental development with resultant disruption in the maternal-fetal nutrient flow and oxygen deficit (Paul & Frazier, 2000).

Prevention of reproductive disorders from workplace exposures should be a workplace priority, which the occupational and environmental health nurse can facilitate. The identification of potential hazardous conditions through worksite assessment with industrial hygiene and safety personnel and the evaluation of Material Safety Data Sheets will be important. To promote and protect reproductive health, programs for reproductive health surveillance can be instituted in the workplace. The components of the program will be influenced by the nature of the exposures and the workers affected. At the very minimum a reproductive health questionnaire (Figure 7-16) should be added to the occupational health history, in addition to periodic examinations and environmental and biological monitoring to detect exposures (Weeks et al., 1991). Counseling of workers for reproductive toxicity problems will be important because they may feel anxious and vulnerable. Perception of risk may be incorrect, and counseling may help sort through the facts. When exposures are of concern, occupational health professionals should work with employees, employers, and regulatory agencies to eliminate potential hazards by using engineering and administrative controls as well as personal protection equipment. Education of workers regarding potentially harmful exposures must be an integral component to any reproductive health program.

Nutrition

Nutritional status plays an important role in the ultimate toxic performance of chemicals. A good diet supplies the necessary metals for the biotransformation processes (i.e., those reactions that break down and transform substances into metabolites for excretion from the body) and prevents protein deficiencies that would reduce the ability of the body to supply key enzymes (Stine & Brown, 1996).

Health Status

Responses to a toxic exposure are influenced by physical and emotional health. For example, due to already compromised organ systems, individuals with preexisting liver, lung, or immunologic disease may be at greater risk of further injury from a toxic exposure. The integrity of the body system will have a major determination on a person's ability to withstand repeated toxic insults, particularly if previous exposures have occurred.

Individuals may also become predisposed to occupational illness as a result of toxic exposures through lifestyle habits such as smoking, alcohol abuse, or lack of exercise. For example, cigarette smoking has important interactive effects on the health of workers exposed to toxic substances. The National Institute for Occupational Safety and Health (NIOSH) has identified six mechanisms by which smoking interacts with occupational exposures. First, certain toxic agents in the workplace, such as carbon monoxide and cadmium, are also present in tobacco or smoke, thereby increasing these exposures. Second, workplace chemicals may be pyrolyzed into more harmful agents because the temperature of a burning cigarette reaches 1,600° F. Third, tobacco products serve as vectors by becoming contaminated with workplace agents like lead and pesticides, which may enter the body through inhalation, ingestion, or skin absorption. Fourth, there may be additive effects from smoking and exposure to other substances such as chlorine, cotton dust, and coal dust. Fifth, the effects may be synergistic between smoking and asbestos, gold, and rubber industry exposures. Sixth, smoking increases accident rates through loss of attention, preoccupation with the hand, irritation of the eyes, coughing, and fires. Smoking, of course, is associated with the development of lung cancer, increased mortality for workers exposed to asbestos, and increased risk of developing byssinosis in textile workers (Levy & Wegman, 2000). In addition, selected medication, such as Isoniazide, may pose an interactive effect when coupled with exposure to certain toxins, such as pesticides and cigarette smoke.

Individual Susceptibility

Individual susceptibility is an important variable in a response to chemical exposure (Ottoboni, 1991; Stine & Brown, 1996). For example, some individuals respond very differently to the same medications or may have different reactions when exposed to various odorous substances, such as perfumes. Other examples related to genetic predisposition include individuals who have red blood cells that are more fragile than usual due to a certain enzyme deficiency and thus are more susceptible to chemicals that cause hemolysis. People who have a genetic deficiency of a certain DNA repair process suffer from xeroderma

Occupational Health History
for
Reproductive Surveillance in the Workplace

Name _____ Date _____

Duration of Employment _____

Job Title _____

Description of Job Duties _____
_____
_____

Total Work Hours per Week _____ Shift Work? Yes _____ No _____

Do you work overtime? Yes _____ No _____

If yes, how many hours usually per week? _____

1. Physical Requirements of Job. Please indicate and describe if you engage in any of the work activities that are listed below and the approximate number of hours each week you do the activity.

   Bending _____   Sitting _____
   Climbing _____   Standing _____
   Lifting _____   Stooping _____
   Pulling _____   Twisting _____

2. Job Exposures. Please indicate if you have any of the following exposures and describe them by giving the amount and duration of the exposure.

   Chemicals (topical) _____   Psychological Stress _____
   _____   _____

   Dust, Fumes, Vapors _____   Radiation _____
   _____   _____

   Infectious Agents _____   Sharp Objects _____
   _____   _____

   Metals _____   Temperature Extremes _____
   _____   _____

   Noise _____   Vibration _____
   _____   _____

3. Do you use any of the following protective measures in the workplace?

   Apron/Coat _____   Gloves _____
   Ear Protection _____   Lifting Devices _____
   Eyewear _____   Respirator _____
   Face Mask _____   Ventilation _____

4. Do you have any exposures at home/community (e.g. lead paint)? _____
   _____

5. Do you have any hobby exposures? _____
   _____
   _____

6. Cigarette Smoke: Active (No. of packs per day)_____
                  Passive _____

7. Alcohol (quantity per day) _____

8. Please answer the following questions related to pregnancy and pregnancy outcomes in the past year.
   A. Have you and your spouse/partner had any problems with fertility or becoming pregnant? Yes _____ No _____
   B. Have you had any miscarriages? Yes _____ No _____
   C. Have you had a baby born to full term? Yes _____ No _____
   D. Have you had a premature or low birth weight baby (born weighing less than 5 lbs. or before the eighth month)?
      Yes _____ No _____

9. Have you had any child born with a birth defect? Yes _____ No _____

Figure 7-16 Occupational health history for reproductive surveillance in the workplace.

pigmentosum, a disease that renders them very susceptible to the carcinogenic effects of ultraviolet radiation on the skin. Albinos and fair-skinned people in general are more susceptible to the damaging effects of sunlight.

In addition, individuals may be hypersusceptible, which indicates an unusually high response to some dose of a substance. This may be a genetic predisposition to a toxic effect or a response that is uncharacteristic of the "average" person. Hypersensitivity is a form of hypersusceptibility that is characterized by an acquired, immunologically mediated sensitization to a substance and is usually manifested by respiratory or dermatologic responses in the workplace (Stine & Brown, 1996). For example, toluene diisocyanate (TDI), used in the manufacture of polyurethane, will evoke an asthmatic reaction in a small number of exposed workers even at permissible exposure levels (Christiani & Wegman, 2000). The complexity of the immune system allows for many possible mechanisms by which drugs and toxicants can produce immunosuppression. Benzene, for example, is generally cytotoxic to bone marrow and affects production of white cells, red cells, and platelets. Benzene's mechanism of action is not completely clear, but it appears that a metabolite of benzene and not benzene itself is responsible for the toxicity. Alkylating agents (which disrupt DNA replication and thus prevent cell division), antimetabolites (which inhibit the synthesis of nucleic acids, again interfering with DNA replication), and radiation exposure also produce general immunosuppression through effects on bone marrow (Stine & Brown, 1996).

Work History

A worker's prior occupational exposures may have a significant effect on her or his susceptibility to occupational disease from further occupational exposures. Many forms of occupational cancer are characterized by long latency periods—as long as 35 to 40 years—before the disease is clinically evident; the leading example of exposure resulting in cancer would be exposure to asbestos. Consequently, an individual with a history of previous toxic exposures may be considered by employers to be a high risk (Frumkin, 2000; Lilis, 1992).

A prior exposure to a carcinogen also may combine with a later exposure (even to a different agent) to produce an effect that neither exposure alone would have produced. For example, the incidence of leukemia among radiation-exposed survivors at Hiroshima and Nagasaki has been shown to increase with occupational exposure to benzene years after the radiation exposure (Upton, 2000).

In addition, exposure to different toxic substances at the same time is common in many industrial settings. The physiological effects of combined exposures may, in some instances, produce a synergistic effect that is greater than simply an additive effect of the single agents alone. For example, it is a well-established fact that smoking potentiates the carcinogenic effects of asbestos resulting in a lung cancer incidence 20 to 30 times greater than in nonsmokers (Selikoff & Lee, 1978).

A great deal remains to be learned about individual reactions to chemicals. Gathering and interpreting data and recognizing important cues indicative of a potential exposure can help reduce associated risks. The occupational and environmental health nurse must be vigilant for signs and symptoms triggered by seemingly innocuous exposures.

INDUSTRIAL HYGIENE

Because of the nature and complexity of hazards in the work environment, the occupational and environmental health nurse works closely with industrial hygienists who are familiar with workplace exposures and related health effects in order to develop an effective risk management program. According to Smith and Schneider (2000) industrial hygiene is the environmental science of anticipating, recognizing, evaluating, and controlling health hazards in the work environment with the objectives of protecting workers' health and well-being and safeguarding the community at large. Industrial hygiene encompasses the study of chronic and acute conditions emanating from hazards posed by physical agents, chemical agents, biological agents, and stress in the occupational environment and also concerns itself with the outdoor environment. For example, an industrial hygienist determines the composition and concentrations of all contaminants in a workplace where there have been complaints of eye, nose, and throat irritation and determines whether the contaminant exposures exceed the permissible exposure limits set by the Occupational Safety and Health Administration (OSHA) and other national limits. This definition is supported in the mission of the American Industrial Hygiene Association (AIHA) (Rose, 1997), which was initially formed in 1939 with the following four major goals:

1. The advancement and application of industrial hygiene and sanitation through the interchange and dissemination of technical knowledge on these subjects
2. The furthering of the study and control of industrial health hazards through determination and elimination of excessive exposures
3. The correlation of such activities as conducted by diverse individuals and agencies throughout industry and educational and governmental groups
4. The uniting of persons with these interests

However, occupational and environmental health nurses and other members of the occupational health and safety team play an integral role in identifying and managing workplace exposures and hazards. Further, depending on the size of the company and the scope and nature of the workplace hazards, an industrial hygienist may or may not be employed by the company. Thus, the occupational and environmental health nurse may play a larger role in the identification and management of workplace hazards and should be able to secure external industrial hygiene consultation. Therefore, the nurse must be familiar with all aspects of the work and work environment in order to accurately assess workplace hazards or provide data needed for effective consultation or do both.

The AIHA further specifies that the industrial hygienist works to accomplish the following:

1. Anticipate potential workplace hazards that might be prevented;
2. Recognize the environmental factors and stresses associated with work and work operations and understand their effect on people and their well-being;
3. Evaluate on the basis of experience and with the aid of quantitative measurement techniques the magnitude of these stresses in terms of the ability to impair people's health and well-being;
4. Prescribe methods to eliminate, control, or reduce such stresses when necessary to alleviate their effects.

The focus of hazard recognition is placed increasingly on the anticipation of occurrence of hazards early in the development of an industrial process in order to redesign or alter a process prior to implementation (Horstman, 1992). The importance of collaboration among professionals, including the occupational and environmental health nurse, safety specialist, physician, and management, in this process is essential to securing a safe and healthful work environment.

ANTICIPATION

Anticipation of hazards has become an important responsibility of the industrial hygienist. Anticipation refers to the application and mastery of knowledge that permits the industrial hygienist to foresee the potential for disease and injury (Smith & Schneider, 2000). The industrial hygienist should therefore be involved at an early stage in the planning of technology, process development, and workplace design. For example, an electronics company was developing a new process for making microcomputer chips. The process involved dissolving a photographic masking agent in toluene and then spraying the mask on a large surface covered with chips. The company's hygienist noted that this process would expose the workers to potentially high airborne levels of toluene and suggested they substitute xylene, which has a lower vapor pressure, and modify the process to use smaller amounts of solvent, which would reduce the amount of hazardous waste generated by the process.

An overview of the production process may be most easily obtained by describing the complete flow from raw material to final product. Production can be subdivided into its component processes. In this stepwise fashion the processes involving hazards can be recognized, worker exposures can be evaluated, and the exposures in nearby areas can be assessed (Smith & Schneider, 2000). The industrial hygienist should have sufficient experience, knowledge, and resources to anticipate potential hazards in the work environment.

HAZARD RECOGNITION

The process of hazard recognition and identification involves reviewing job classifications and determining potential hazards; reviewing background and toxicologic information on processes and associated hazards; visiting the relevant work unit to observe work processes, practices, and control measures; formulating plans to determine the exposure levels through ambient/environmental sampling; and examining worker complaints related to workplace exposures (Smith & Schneider, 2000). Use of a worksite walk-through checklist as described in a later section may aid in the recognition process.

Specific exposures can be identified in relation to various steps involved in the work processes. The goal is to discover potential illness-producing processes and operations, record the nature of the processes and operations, and determine approaches necessary to deal with them effectively and efficiently. Becoming familiar with the process requires the accumulation and comprehension of information from and about various aspects of the process's exposure conditions. These include a reasonable understanding of (1) the fundamental process being operated by workers whose exposures are being evaluated; (2) the physical facilities in which the process is housed or operated; (3) all chemical substances associated with the process, including raw materials, intermediates, by-products, and products; (4) the health hazards associated with all of the chemicals; (5) the nature of the jobs and job duties required of the workers in the plant; (6) controls in place to protect workers; (7) the health status of workers associated with the process; (8) results of past evaluations; and (9) any other hazards associated with the opera-

tion. Examples of some common work processes and related hazards are shown in Table 7-10.

It is important to determine if all hazardous chemicals are identified, catalogued in a list, and if the inventory is periodically updated. One of the major tools that can be utilized to aid in the initial identification of chemical hazardous materials is the Material Safety Data Sheet (MSDS). The MSDS is a document prepared by the manufacturer that describes the physical and chemical properties of products, their physical and health-related hazards, and precautions for safe handling and use. All facilities are required by law to have an MSDS for each hazardous chemical that is used in the facility (U.S. Department of Agriculture, 1987). While the MSDS may provide valuable information about the toxicities and health effects of material substances, it may also be out of date or incomplete (Smith & Schneider, 2000). Thus, other sources of information should also be utilized. MSDSs may appear in different formats; however, the OSHA Hazard Communication Standard (29CFR 1910-1200 [g]) requires that certain information be supplied (Box 7-7). Appendixes 7-1 and 7-2 are examples of MSDSs. Hazard recognition requires skill in assessing the work and work environment and investigating conditions that may contribute to health risks. This should be done using a multidisciplinary context. A full-scale worksite assessment and walk-through survey, described in detail later in this chapter, is a major component of the hazard recognition process.

TABLE 7-10   **Some Common Work Processes and Related Hazards**

WORK PROCESSES	COMMON HAZARD
Abrasive blasting	Silica and metal dust
Cosmetology	Chemical exposures
	Repetitive bending, standing
Farming	Pesticide exposure
	Heat exposure
	Heavy lifting
	Hazardous equipment
Grinding, polishing, and buffing	Inhalation of toxic dusts from metals and abrasives
Painting	Inhalation of solvents as mists, vapors, toxic substances
Meat wrapping	Lifting, standing, repetitive motion, fume exposure from wrap
Welding	Inhalation of metal fumes, toxic gases, materials

HAZARD EVALUATION

Evaluation of health hazards at the worksite follows hazard recognition. The evaluation of recognized or suspected hazards by the hygienist uses techniques based on the nature of the hazards, the emission sources, and the routes of environmental contact with the worker. For example, air sampling shows the concentrations of toxic particulates, gases, and vapors that workers may inhale; skin wipes measure the degree of skin contact with toxic materials that may penetrate the skin; and noise dosimeters record and electronically integrate workplace noise levels to determine daily exposure (Smith & Schneider, 2000). Biological samples (blood or urine), while part of the health/medical surveil-

lance program, can provide data when there are multiple routes of entry. Exposure measurements are intended to evaluate the dose delivered to the worker. Both acute and chronic exposures should be considered in the evaluation because they may be associated with different types of adverse health effects. In the evaluation process the following important questions should be considered:

1. *What are the potential or actual agents/exposures?* Determine what categories of agents or factors are present at the worksite and have the potential to cause an illness or injury (e.g., biological, chemical, enviromechanical, physical, psychosocial) that requires evaluation.
2. *Where and when does the exposure occur?* Determine the location of the exposure and the degree or magnitude of exposure associated with a particular work process, work area or department, work shift, or seasonal variation.
3. *Which workers are exposed and how does exposure occur?* Identify not only those workers involved with the work processes under investigation but also if other workers in close proximity may also be exposed. Determine all routes of exposure (e.g., ingestion, inhalation, skin contact) and levels of compliance with work practice and safety standards.
4. *What is the evidence of exposure?* Determine if there are obvious signs of hazards or exposures such as dusts, smoke, broken machinery, and slippery floors or if previous air sampling or other industrial hygiene surveys have been conducted and, if so, evaluate their findings. Evaluate if worker health complaints such as skin rash, cough, dyspnea, headaches, dizziness, anorexia, fatigue, eye irritation, or numbness/tingling of extremities are exposure-related and if the complaints resolve in the absence of exposure. Conduct biological and environmental sampling and analyze and interpret results in terms of existing health standards or known effects.
5. *What control measures are present, available, and effective?* Assess if engineering controls (e.g., ventilation systems) are appropriate, operable, and effective; if appropriate personal protective equipment is available and utilized; and if hygiene and appropriate work practice measures are observed.

Box 7-7 OSHA Required Information for Material Safety Data Sheets

- Identity of the material as listed on the label
- Chemical and common names of all ingredients that have been determined to be health hazards
- Physical and chemical characteristics of the hazardous chemical
- Physical hazards of the hazardous chemical (e.g., fire, explosion, inactivity)
- Health hazards of the hazardous chemical, including signs/symptoms of exposure, and health conditions generally recognized as being aggravated by the exposure
- Primary routes of entry
- OSHA permissible exposure limit, American Conference of Governmental Industrial Hygienists (ACGIH) threshold limit value, and any other applicable exposure limits
- Carcinogenic status (confirmed or potential) of the hazardous chemical
- Precautions for safe handling, including measures taken during equipment repair and procedures for clean-up of spills/leaks
- Applicable control measures (i.e., engineering, work practice, protective equipment)
- Emergency and first-aid procedures
- Date of preparation (or last change) of the MSDS
- Name, address, and telephone number of the chemical manufacturer, importer, employer, or other parties responsible for MSDS preparation and distribution

Hazard evaluation must take into account the changing nature of the work environment, such as operations, processes, materials, production schedules, routes of exposure, and control measures (DiNardi, 1997). Decisions as to whether a hazard exists are based on three sources of information (Smith & Schneider, 2000): (1) scientific literature and various exposure limit guides such as the threshold limit values (TLVs), which are a set of consensus standards about exposures established, revised, and published yearly by the American Conference of Governmental Industrial Hygienists (ACGIH); (2) legal requirements of OSHA and other federal, state, and local statutes and regulations; and (3) evaluative results of the exposed worker based on examinations by qualified licensed health care professionals. Consequently, the evaluation component should take into account information relative to hazard recognition (work and worksite assessment) and exposure data derived through sampling techniques to arrive at meaningful control strategies. A brief description of exposure indices and sampling techniques as evaluation tools follows.

THRESHOLD LIMIT

The concept of threshold limit is important in an exposure-effect relationship and implies a threshold limit of effect (and conversely no effect) wherein a certain level or dose of exposure will produce a measurable effect in a target organ system. Worker exposures should be held to the lowest minimum possible, but in some cases workers may be exposed to ambient levels greater than zero. Thus, threshold limit values (TLVs) are used in the workplace by industrial hygienists and others trained in the science as a guide to the maximum tolerable exposure limit (American Conference of Governmental Industrial Hygienists [ACGIH], 2000). The TLVs assume an 8-hour work day, 5 days per week. Exposing employees to amounts above the TLVs is believed to be potentially harmful (Kayafas, 1989; Verma & Verrall, 1985).

The TLVs are based on animal toxicity data and limited epidemiologic studies. Animal experiments have shortcomings in extrapolating data to the human workforce (Danse, 1991), because the dose, routes of exposure, and toxicokinetics may differ considerably in humans. In addition, they do not necessarily address the sensitive populations in the workforce, those with prior exposure

or preexisting disease, or exposures from other sources such as second jobs, hobbies, or home exposures. The American Conference of Governmental Industrial Hygienists (ACGIH) categorizes the TLVs in the following three ways:

1. *Threshold limit value-time weighted average (TLV-TWA).* The time-weighted average concentrations for a normal 8-hour workday and a 40-hour workweek, to which nearly all workers may be repeatedly exposed, day after day, without adverse effects

2. *Threshold limit value-short term exposure limit (TLV-STEL).* Provided that the daily TLV-TWA also is not exceeded, the concentration to which workers can be exposed continuously for a short period of time without suffering from (a) irritation, (b) chronic or irreversible tissue change, or (c) narcosis of sufficient degree to increase the likelihood of accidental injury, impair self-rescue, or materially reduce work efficiency

   A STEL (short term exposure limit) is defined as a 15-minute time-weighted average (TWA) exposure that should not be exceeded at any time during a workday even if the TWA is within the TLV. Exposures at the STEL should not be longer than 15 minutes and should not be repeated more than four times per day. There should be at least 60 minutes between successive exposures at the STEL. An averaging period other than 15 minutes may be recommended when this is warranted by observed biological effects.

3. *Threshold limit value-ceiling (TLV-C).* The concentration that should not be exceeded even instantaneously

The Occupational Safety and Health Administration has adopted permissible exposure limits (PELs) for chemical exposure, most of which are based directly on the TLV list of the ACGIH in effect in 1968. Since that time, the TLVs have been updated yearly, but most PELs have not changed (Silverstein, 1988). Thus, the TLVs may be more restrictive than PELs. The National Institute for Occupational Safety and Health (NIOSH) has published recommended exposure limits (RELs) that are TWA concentrations for up to a 10-hour workday during a 40-hour workweek. The occupational and environmental health nurse should be familiar with these terms and their meaning;

however, evaluation of results should be done by a health professional trained in industrial hygiene. A listing of the ACGIH-TLVs may be found in the *Threshold Limit Values and Biological Exposure Indices* (ACGIH, 2000). OSHA-PELs and NIOSH-RELs are found in the *NIOSH Pocket Guide to Chemical Hazards* (USDHHS, NIOSH, 1999).

SAMPLING METHODS AND TECHNIQUES

Quantifying exposures is usually done by the industrial hygienist through sampling methods and devices. Two basic types of samples are used to evaluate employees' exposures to gases and vapors: integrated and grab (Soule, 1991; Todd, 1997). *Integrated sampling* for gases and vapors involves the passage of a known volume of air through an absorbing medium to remove the desired contaminants from the air during a specified period of time. With this technique the contaminants of interest are collected and concentrated over a period of time to obtain the average exposure levels during the entire sampling period. *Grab sampling* techniques involve the direct collection of an air-contaminant mixture into a device such as a sampling bag, syringe, or evacuated flask over a short interval of a few seconds or minutes. Thus, grab samples represent the atmospheric concentrations at the sampling site at a given point in time.

Integrated sampling, covering the entire period of exposure, is required because airborne contaminant concentrations during a typical work shift vary with time and activity (Todd, 1997). Instantaneous measurements (grab samples) taken at any given period, therefore, do not reflect the average exposure of the worker for the entire shift and may not capture intermittent high or low exposures. Most integrated sampling is done to determine the 8-hour time-weighted average (TWA) exposure, and results are compared with the OSHA PELs, the threshold limit values (TLVs) of the American Conference of Governmental Industrial Hygienists (ACGIH), or other applicable limits or guidelines such as the NIOSH recommended exposure limits.

Most integrated sampling methods published by OSHA or NIOSH use active sampling techniques. *Active sampling* is defined as the collection of airborne contaminants by means of a forced movement of air by a sampling pump through an appropriate collection device, such as a sorbent tube, treated filter, or impinger containing a liquid medium.

Among the most important developments in air sampling technology in recent years is the development of passive sampling devices. *Passive sampling* is the collection of airborne gases and vapors at a rate controlled by a physical process such as diffusion through a static air layer or permeation through a membrane without the active movement of air through an air sampler. Many types of passive samplers are commercially available using either solid sorbents or liquid absorbers.

Grab samples are collected to measure gas and vapor concentrations at a point in time and are therefore used to evaluate peak exposures for comparison to ceiling limits. Grab samples can be used to identify unknown contaminants, to evaluate contaminant sources, or to measure contaminant levels from intermittent processes or other sources. Grab or instantaneous samples of air to be analyzed for its gaseous components are collected using rigid containers, such as syringes or partially evacuated flasks or cans, or nonrigid containers, such as sampling bags.

Direct-reading instruments (real-time monitors) are among the most important tools available to industrial hygienists for detecting and quantifying gases, vapors, and aerosols (Todd, 1997). These instruments permit real-time or near real-time measurements of contaminated concentrations in the field, thus eliminating the lag time encountered when samples are collected on media and analyzed by a laboratory. Using direct-reading instruments allows for air contaminants to be sampled and analyzed within the instrument itself in a relatively short time (seconds to minutes). Results are usually indicated on an analog or digital display, a graph, or by a color change that is compared with a calibrated scale. Real-time monitors generally can be used to obtain short-term or continuous measurements. Some monitors have data-logging capabilities that allow digital storage of data. While a data logger does not enhance the accuracy of a measurement, it frees the industrial hygienist from manually recording data and allows for a variety of statistical analyses.

Direct-reading instruments range in size from small personal monitors to hand-held monitors to complex stationary installations with multipoint monitoring capability. Field monitoring instruments are usually light-weight, portable, rugged, weather and temperature sensitive, and are simple to operate and maintain. However, there is no magic black box that can measure all contaminants in air; in addition, instruments used for gases and vapors cannot be used for aerosols and vice versa. Table 7-11 shows commonly used direct-reading instruments for gases and vapors.

Direct-reading instruments provide powerful on-the-spot information and are ideal for situations where the industrial hygienist wants immediate data that are temporally resolved into short time periods. Personal direct-reading instruments, which can be placed on lapels or pockets, can be used for personal exposure monitoring and are available for a limited number of chemicals, particularly for gases that have high acute toxicity, such as carbon monoxide and phosgene (Todd, 1997).

When skin contact is the route of exposure, as is the case with pesticide exposure, cloth patches or wipe sampling of the exposed skin area can be used to determine the amount of contamination. Wipe sampling is also used to evaluate surface contamination and identify contaminated areas when a toxic spill has occurred.

Evaluation of physical agents, such as noise, may be measured with sound level meters that give a source level decibel readout or noise dosimeters that involve placing a small microphone close to the worker's ear to record noise exposure. The latter approach is preferred because it gives a more accurate and specific measure of individual exposure.

After sampling techniques have been selected, a sampling strategy will need to be developed in order to determine exposure routes and variations and time-weighted exposures. Exposure measurements are then compared with existing standards and guides to determine if exposures meet acceptable levels. Interpretation of results is critical to the evaluation process and should be a collaborative effort between the industrial hygienist, the occupational and environmental health nurse, and the physician in order to relate the exposure to the health effect.

CONTROL MEASURES

Once the hazard has been identified and evaluated, control measures, which usually require the expertise of the industrial hygienist, will need to be instituted to correct the problem. Hazard reduction can

TABLE 7-11	Commonly Used Direct-Reading Instruments for Gases and Vapors
INSTRUMENT	**COMMON ANALYTES**
Combustible gas detectors	Combustible gases and vapors (nonspecific)
Colorimetric detectors	Various vapors including formaldehyde, hydrogen sulfide, sulfur dioxide, toluene diisocyanate (specific)
Electrochemical sensors	Carbon monoxide, nitric oxide, nitrogen dioxide, hydrogen sulfide, sulfur dioxide (specific)
Infrared gas analyzers	Organic and inorganic gases and vapors (specific)
Metal oxide sensors	Hydrogen sulfide, nitro, amine, alcohol, and halogenated hydrocarbons (specific)
Thermal conductivity sensors	Carbon monoxide, carbon dioxide, nitrogen, oxygen, methane, ethane, propane, and butane
Portable gas chromatographs	Organic and inorganic gases and vapors (specific)
Electron capture detector	Halogenated hydrocarbons, nitrous oxide, and compounds containing cyano or nitro groups
Flame ionization detectors	Organic compounds including aliphatic and aromatic hydrocarbons, ketones, alcohols, and halogenated hydrocarbons
Photoionization detectors	Most organic compounds, particularly aromatic compounds

From "Direct Reading Instrumental Methods for Gases, Vapors, and Aerosols," by L. A. Todd, in S. DiNardi (Ed.), *The Occupational Environment: Its Evaluation and Control,* Fairfax, VA: American Industrial Hygiene Association. 1997.

be achieved through a variety of individual methods or a combination of methods. Jones et al. (1990) recommend the following practices:

- When selecting control methods, consider the specific hazardous work, processes, and number of employees involved, work environment, available control alternatives, and all exposure and sampling data.
- Consider all possible routes of exposure when developing and implementing prevention programs.
- Eliminate hazards where possible; in some cases, substitute a less hazardous process or material to considerably reduce the potential for harm; ensure that any substituted environment, method, or chemical is safer than that originally used and as safe as science/technology is able to provide.
- When possible, reduce hazards by process redesign, preventive maintenance, or equipment modification.
- When a hazard cannot be eliminated, control at the source of generation (usually the most effective means of exposure reduction); evaluate appropriate engineering controls, such as local exhaust ventilation, to reduce airborne hazard potentials at or near the source of generation.
- Initiate special control procedures for energy sources, especially noise, radiation, lighting, heat, and vibration.
- Examine and modify employee work practices as necessary to decrease exposure and hazard potentials.
- Use personal protective devices as a last resort or as an additional control measure if the foregoing methods prove to be unsuccessful, inappropriate, infeasible, or inadequate.
- Train employees to understand hazard potentials and the importance of appropriate control methods.

The following basic risk reduction approaches to controlling occupational health hazards are listed in hierarchical order of effectiveness (DiNardi, 1997):

1. *Elimination/substitution.* Eliminating, changing, or substituting the process or materials used in the process so that toxic substances are not used. Substitution can be done only if a useful substitute is available. An example includes substituting safe artificial insulation fibers for asbestos.

2. *Isolation and containment.* Removing the hazard to a location away from the worker and enclosing the hazard by placing a barrier between the exposure source and the worker. Examples include an enclosure to reduce or alter a noise source and a puncture-resistant container for needles/sharps (Rogers & Goodno, 2000).

3. *Engineering controls.* Designing and installing systems to limit or prevent the release of toxic materials in the worker's environment. For example, a local exhaust ventilation is designed to capture contaminants and remove them from the workplace.

4. *Work practice controls.* Educating and training workers about and ensuring compliance with the proper use of control strategies and effective work practice procedures, which may help to minimize exposure risk. Good hygiene, safe handling of potentially contaminated devices, and good housekeeping are examples.

5. *Administrative controls.* Limiting potential or actual hazard exposure so that the amount of exposure is reduced to or below permissible levels. For example, job rotation is used to avoid excessive exposure of any one individual. Obviously, this approach has limited utility and should not be considered a substitute for adequate exposure control. Placing warning signs about hazardous materials, prohibiting access to restricted areas, and maintenance of equipment are other examples.

6. *Personal protection.* Providing adequate and appropriate protective devices and utilizing these devices to minimize exposure to hazardous materials. Examples include the use of protective clothing, gloves, head protection, ear plugs, goggles/glasses, safety shoes, and barrier creams appropriate to the situation. The effectiveness of personal protective equipment is dependent on many factors, such as worker understanding and compliance, proper fitting devices, and state-of-the-art equipment.

The process of identifying and controlling hazards in the workplace is essential in providing a safe and healthful work environment. This is fostered by a multi-disciplinary effort among workers, management, and key health professionals, including occupational and environmental health nurses, industrial hygienists, physicians, safety professionals, ergonomists, and others. The occupational and environmental health nurse must be familiar with basic concepts and principles related to industrial hygiene, including hazard recognition, evaluation, and control, and ensure active participation in managing workplace hazards.

WORKSITE ASSESSMENT

The previous sections of this chapter have provided a discussion of the core occupational health and safety science disciplines as related to the foundational knowledge domains important to occupational and environmental health nursing practice. Armed with this knowledge and using an interdisciplinary approach to workplace hazard identification, a comprehensive worksite assessment and walk-through can be conducted to assess work-related hazards that need control. This is the focus of the remainder of this chapter. Also provided in Appendix 7-3 is a Worksite Assessment Guide, which can be used in assessment and walk-through activities.

MANAGEMENT PHILOSOPHY AND COMMITMENT

The first element in a discussion of the worksite assessment is the philosophy and commitment of management to the overall company health and safety program. The occupational health program is preventive in nature and not simply a tool to reduce compensation costs or improve the company safety record. However, is this view consistent with the business mission? The occupational and environmental health nurse must understand the prevailing philosophy of corporate management with respect to health and safety programming because this philosophy will set the stage for services delivered.

Although the mission of business and industry encompasses a profit motive, ideally, management's philosophy will embody a commitment to worker health promotion and protection. This commitment is reflected in policies and programs for a healthful work environment, available resources to support program activities (including adequate levels and types of health care professionals), promotion of education and research to improve worker health and safety, and a mechanism for quality assurance; each of these should be specified in clear goals and measurable objectives. The support for establishment of a Health and Safety Committee should also be evident because this committee is critical in helping management ensure a safe and healthful environment (Silverstein & Mirer, 2000). The committee should review accidents and data related to health and safety issues at work and make recommendations for corrective action and policy. In addition, management must be willing to delegate authority and responsibility for program management to the appropriate health care professionals if the program is to be successful (Felton, 1990).

Management's commitment can be demonstrated by active involvement in the health and safety program and might take the form of participation in health and safety meetings and walk-through surveys, and appropriate allocation of capital equipment, materials, and human resources to provide quality services and control measures for hazard abatement and risk reduction. If management displays a lukewarm attitude toward a comprehensive occupational health program, the occupational and environmental health nurse will need to educate management as to the benefits of the program, such as a decrease in work-related illnesses, injuries, and associated health care costs and an increase in employee morale and productivity. In addition, obtaining background information on the industry may provide a historical context about the evolution of the organizational culture and a perspective on how health and safety has been viewed; the occupational and environmental health nurse may find this information helpful when negotiating for program expansion. Sometimes information may be difficult to obtain because management may be uncertain as to how the data will be used. A meeting with management can facilitate an understanding of the assessment process.

Management's commitment should extend to encouraging employee involvement in the program operation and participation in health and safety program decision making. Employees' input regarding their jobs can provide firsthand information about work procedures and associated hazards (Harris, 2000). In addition, employee involvement should be sought for worksite inspections and recommendations regarding work modification, hazard control measures, and development of training programs for job safety.

WORKFORCE CHARACTERISTICS

Information about the demographic characteristics of the workforce, such as the number and distribution of employees by age, sex, ethnicity, department, job title/responsibilities, and shift of work, is an essential component of the worksite assessment. Knowledge of these characteristics will help to determine if there are patterns or trends in illnesses and injuries that may be associated with selected personal variables, certain jobs or departments, or rotation of work schedules and areas (Rogers & Travers, 1991). For example, a workforce primarily consisting of women will present different problems compared with a workforce made up of mostly men (e.g., certain reproductive toxicities), as will older workers compared with younger workers.

Additional information about the worker and job may be obtained from the *Dictionary of Occupational Titles,* which provides standardized occupational information based on on-site job analyses in order to give definitions of approximately 20,000 jobs (USDOL, 1995). This information can be useful not only in enumerating and categorizing the types of jobs specific to a particular industry but also in furthering the understanding of job tasks and functions for job hazard analyses.

The *Dictionary of Occupational Titles* groups jobs into occupations based on similarities of job performance, thus defining the structure and content of all listed occupations. Each occupation is given a nine-digit code number, for example, 652.382-010. These digits specify a particular occupational category, division, and group within the category (first three digits); worker functions as related to data, people, and things (middle three digits); and the job title (last three digits). Thus, the example code number specifies a *Machine trades occupation* in a *Printing occupation* involving *Printing machine occupations* (652), with work functions of *compiling* data, *taking instructions helping* people, and *operating/controlling* things (382). The final three digits (010) specify a code applicable to only one occupational title, *Cloth printer.* Each designated job specifies the duties and tasks of the worker and the machine equipment and materials used by the worker. Thus, the *Dictionary of Occupational Titles* provides a unique code and description for each occupation within a designated industry. The reader is referred to this source for more specific information.

OCCUPATIONAL HEALTH PROGRAMS

Within the scope of the workplace assessment is a review of the types of programs and services offered to determine if they are appropriate and responsive to the health promotion and protection needs of the workers; mandatory compliance programs are also reviewed. Health promotion programs, such as those that promote exercise and good nutrition, may improve the overall health and fitness of workers, thus decreasing vulnerability to exposure and injury; health protection strategies, such as use of universal precautions and protective equipment, may significantly reduce exposure levels.

Mandated programs, such as hearing conservation against noise, eye protection against flying particulates and chemical exposures, and respiratory protection against airborne agents (e.g., lead, silica, asbestos, cotton, and solvent vapor), must be monitored for compliance. Observation of employee work practices or behaviors that may contribute to health damage should be assessed within the context of the overall health program. For example, if the occupational and environmental health nurse observes poor lifting techniques that may contribute to back injuries or unsafe handling of laboratory specimens, compliance directives as well as counseling and health education programs on appropriate lifting and handling techniques may be in order, in addition to compliance directives. Specific safety programs such as lock out/tag out or an integration of behavioral-based safety efforts should be assessed for effectiveness, acceptance, and risk reduction outcomes.

An examination of written reports, logs, sampling data, health and exposure records, and insurance data can aid the occupational and environmental health nurse to better target specific areas for observation, investigation, or follow-up (Cahall, 1984). This type of review prior to any walk-through survey may provide information on specific work-related illnesses and injuries prevalent at the worksite, help identify trends in occupational health and safety unit visits or exposures. This information can aid in determining problem departments or work processes that could be creating or contributing to illness/injury events.

WORK AND WORK PROCESSES

In the United States industries are categorized by specific type according to the *Standard Industrial*

Classification (SIC) system (U.S. Office of Management and Budget [USOMB], 1987). The SIC was developed for use in the classification of establishments by the type of activity in which they are engaged; for purposes of facilitating the collection, tabulation, presentation, and analysis of data relating to establishments; and for promoting uniformity and comparability in the presentation of statistical data collected by various agencies of the U.S. government, state agencies, trade associations, and private research organizations.

The SIC is intended to cover the entire field of economic activities: agriculture, forestry, fishing, hunting, and trapping; mining; construction; manufacturing; transportation, communications, electric, gas, and sanitation; wholesale trade; retail trade; finance, insurance, and real estate; personal, business professional, repair, recreation, and other services; and public administration. Each operating establishment is assigned an industry code based on its primary activity, which is determined by its principal product or group of products produced or distributed or by its services rendered. The structure of the classification makes it possible to tabulate, analyze, and publish establishment data on a division, and within that division, on a two-digit major group, a three-digit industry group, or a four-digit industry code basis, according to the level of industrial detail considered most appropriate.

The 10 major establishment divisions and 1 division identified as nonclassifiable establishments (A-K) are shown in Table 7-12. Within each division as a whole are major groups, each specified by two-digit numbers that further narrow or define the industry division. For example, division E, *Transportation, communications, electric, gas, and sanitation,* is identified by SIC numbers 40 through 49. These major groups are then subdivided into industry groups as specified by the addition of a third digit and then further subdivided according to the primary products of the industry, hence a fourth digit. In this classification scheme the SIC number 47 specifies the major group *Transportation services,* the SIC number 472 the industry group *Arrangement of passenger transportation,* and SIC number 4724 *Travel agencies.* The SIC is used to promote the comparability of established data relative to the U.S. economy. In addition, data can be categorized according to work-related illnesses and injuries;

TABLE 7-12	Major Industrial Divisions Within the Standard Industrial Classification Systems
DIVISION	**INDUSTRY DESCRIPTION**
A	Agriculture, forestry, and fishing
B	Mining
C	Construction
D	Manufacturing
E	Transportation, communications, electric, gas, and sanitation
F	Wholesale trade
G	Retail trade
H	Finance, insurance, and real estate
I	Services
J	Public administration
K	Nonclassifiable establishments

thus, a high estimation of hazard/risk can be determined through analysis of SIC codes.

In any work setting health care professionals need to have a certain degree of suspicion about the degree of risk in the work environment in order to identify potential or actual workplace hazards (Burgess, 1995; DiNardi, 1997). This can be accomplished in part through a prior review of the work processes, materials, and products. Resource books and technical publications are helpful in describing the manufacturing or work processes and providing information about health hazards, acute and chronic symptoms related to selected exposures, and adverse health outcomes. NIOSH criteria documents and a review of Material Safety Data Sheets (MSDS) will also provide useful information about the composition (i.e., physical and chemical properties) of materials used in the work processes.

Recognizing certain workplace hazards requires knowledge of the raw material used. A complete inventory of all chemicals, raw materials, intermediates, byproducts, and products produced or used in the manufacturing process or work setting must be obtained for appropriate reference during the evaluation. In developing an inventory there is a tendency to begin by focusing on the chemicals that are present in greatest quantity and pay less attention to those present in only small amounts.

Experience has shown that high volume materials present only in closed systems may be much less of a problem than small quantities used in the open (Conrad & Soule, 1997). Although hazards from raw materials may be predicted from animal toxicity data, many materials used in industry may not have been adequately evaluated for possible harmful effects. By-products, intermediates, and final products formed by the raw materials may be difficult to determine. New products are being introduced constantly; these require the use of new raw materials—or at least new combinations and applications of older substances—and new processes. Some estimates suggest that new substances are introduced in industry at the rate of 1 every 20 minutes and that nearly 70,000 such materials are in use today.

New uses for physical agents in industrial processes are increasing at a rapid rate as well; examples include the expanding use of lasers, microwaves, and other forms of nonionizing radiation. These, too, are potentially hazardous unless management institutes proper control measures and, therefore, should be included in any inventory of potential stresses.

Each step from raw materials to finished product must be evaluated. The processes must be understood well enough to determine where contaminants are released, who is exposed, and to what degree. This may be dependent on or affected by such variables as room air currents, work practices/patterns (e.g., shift work, overtime), temperature, and environmental hygiene factors.

It should be emphasized that the toxicity of a substance is not necessarily the most important factor in determining the extent of a health hazard associated with the use of that material. The nature of the process in which that material is used or generated, the possibility of reaction with other agents (biological, physical, or chemical), the extent and duration of exposure, and the degree of effective ventilation and other control measures all relate to the potential hazard associated with the use of that material. Consideration should also be given to the type and degree of toxic response the material may elicit in both the average and the hypersusceptible worker (Danse, 1991; Olishifski, 1983).

Knowledge of the work processes and materials will aid in preparation of and preplanning for the worksite survey and in the organization and efficiency in the conduct of the survey. A map or lay-out of the work environment usually will provide a good description of the general operations involved and work areas that are high risk. This information will help the occupational and environmental health nurse avoid missing critical areas and functions in the operations of the plant and pinpoint potentially dangerous or hazardous conditions, such as repetitive operations on assembly lines or exposure to chemical or physical agents associated with a specific process such as crushing, grinding, heating, and electrolysis (Camp & Tanberg, 1985; Olishifski, 1983).

A flow sheet that identifies each step of the work process from start to finish should be obtained and reviewed prior to the survey. The flow sheet should indicate the fate of raw materials from the time they enter to the time they leave the worksite; how they are used and transformed in the process; the various pieces of equipment involved; and by-products produced at any step in the process (Verma & Verrall, 1985). An example of a flow process for pulp and paper is shown in Figure 7-17.

Ultimately, exposure is related directly to the job activities performed by the worker. As part of the familiarization process one must learn all about the workers' job activities and the consequent potential for exposure. A logical starting point for this effort is the formal job description; however, in many situations a formal job description does not exist, and even when it does, it often lacks the needed detail. Even with a formal, well-defined job description in hand, it is wise to talk to the employee and the employee's supervisor.

In addition, an analysis of each job and its related hazards provides valuable information. The job hazard analysis or job safety analysis (described in a previous section, Safety) is a tool that provides a blueprint about how to do a critical job in a safe and productive manner, identifies actual or potential sources of occupational health problems/hazards, and specifies recommendations for prevention and control measures. A job hazard analysis is best completed by the occupational health team or occupational health and safety committee so that employees can be involved in the process. Direct observation of the worker(s) performing the job or videotaping of job activities, which allows for a careful step-by-step review of the tasks performed, is essential for an accurate analysis. An example of a job hazard analysis tool is shown in Table 7-13. Analysis of

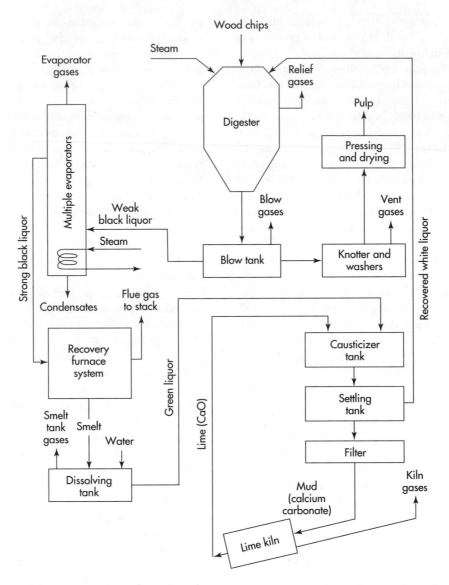

Figure 7-17   Flow process for pulp and paper operation. *(From* Recognition of Health Hazards in Industry *[2nd ed.], by W. A. Burgess, 1995, New York: John Wiley & Sons.)*

jobs performed at the worksite prior to the walk-through survey will assist in anticipating the physical and psychosocial demands placed on workers and detecting potential sources of injury and exposure.

Familiarization with control measures in use and their apparent effectiveness are necessary. Control measures mean the overall strategy for controlling potential hazards in the work environment as well as the specific components that make up that strategy. These include local exhaust and general ventilation, process isolation or enclosure, shielding

from heat, ionizing radiation, ultraviolet light or any other forms of radiant energy, protective clothing, and respiratory protective devices and other controls. A source of information often overlooked as part of the familiarization with a particular work environment is what is known about the workers from a general perspective of overall health status, including first aid treatments and other related information. However, employee written permission to review any health information is needed unless data can be supplied in aggregate form without identifiers.

TABLE 7-13   **Sample Job Hazard Analysis: Cleaning Inside Surface of Chemical Tank—Top Manhole Entry**

STEP	HAZARD	NEW PROCEDURE OR PROTECTION
1. Select and train operators.	Operator with respiratory or heart problem; other physical limitation Untrained operator— failure to perform task	Examination by industrial physician for suitability to work. Train operators. Dry run. (Reference: National Institute for Occupational Safety and Health (NIOSH) Doc. No. 80-406)

2. Determine what is in the tank, what process is going on in the tank, and what hazards this can pose.	Explosive gas
	Improper oxygen level
	Chemical exposure—
	Gas, dust, vapor:
	  irritant
	  toxic
	Liquid:
	  irritant
	  toxic
	  corrosive
	Solid:
	  irritant
	  corrosive
		Obtain work permit signed by safety, maintenance, and supervisors.
		Test air by qualified person.
		Ventilate to 19.5%-23.5% oxygen and less than 10% LEL of any flammable gas.
		Steaming inside of tank, flushing and draining, then ventilating, as previously described, may be required.
		Provide appropriate respiratory equipment—SCBA or air line respirator.
		• Provide protective clothing for head, eyes, body, and feet.
		• Provide parachute harness and lifeline.
		(Reference: OSHA standards 1910.106, 1926.100, 1926.21(b)(6); NIOSH Doc. No. 80-4061)
		• Tanks should be cleaned from outside, if possible.

3. Set up equipment.	Hoses, cord, equipment— tripping hazards Electrical-voltage too high, exposed conductors Motors not locked out and tagged	Arrange hoses, cords, lines, and equipment in orderly fashion, with room to maneuver safely. Use ground-fault circuit interrupter. Lockout and tag mixing motor, if present.
4. Install ladder in tank.	Ladder slipping	Secure to manhole top or rigid structure.
5. Prepare to enter tank.	Gas or liquid in tank	Empty tank through existing piping. Review emergency procedures. Open tank. Check of job site by industrial hygienist or safety professional. Install blanks in flanges in piping to tank. (Isolate tank.) Test atmosphere in tank by qualified person (long probe).

From U.S. Department of Labor, Occupational Safety and Health Administration, 1988.   *Continued*

TABLE 7-13	Sample Job Hazard Analysis: Cleaning Inside Surface of Chemical Tank—Top Manhole Entry—cont'd	
6. Place equipment at tank-entry position.	Trip or fall	Use mechanical-handling equipment. Provide guardrails around work positions at tank top.
7. Enter tank.	Ladder—tripping hazard Exposure to hazardous atmosphere	Provide personal protective equipment for conditions found. (Reference: NIOSH Doc. No. 80-406; OSHA CFR 1910.134) Provide outside helper to watch, instruct, and guide operator entering tank, with capability to lift operator from tank in emergency.
8. Clean tank.	Reaction of chemicals, causing mist or expulsion of air contaminant	Provide protective clothing and equipment for all operators and helpers. Provide lighting for tank (Class I, Div. I). Provide exhaust ventilation. Provide air supply to interior of tank. Frequent monitoring of air in tank. Replace operator or provide rest periods. Provide means of communication to get help, if needed. Provide two-man standby for any emergency.
9. Clean up.	Handling of equipment, causing injury	Dry run. Use material-handling equipment.

From U.S. Department of Labor, Occupational Safety and Health Administration, 1988.

WORKSITE WALK-THROUGH SURVEY

Walk-through surveys (Box 7-8) are conducted for many reasons and performed in the context of determining the breadth and depth of the assessment. The goals of walk-throughs are as follows

1. Identify and quantify potential and actual hazardous agents in the workplace and observe workers and their work practices;
2. Assess compliance status with respect to various occupational health standards;
3. Determine if the health and safety policies and programs have been successfully implemented;
4. Determine exposure in response to complaints;
5. Evaluate the effectiveness of engineering controls (Camp & Tanberg, 1985; DiNardi, 1997).

The walk-through may also help clarify a relationship between what may be presumed to be a nonoccupational complaint and a work-related exposure.

A general walk-through survey effort involves baseline and ongoing monitoring activities that are critical to an effective assessment of the complete operation at the worksite and related workplace hazards. In this survey regular and periodic exposure measurements of representative workers to selected agents are conducted, and the monitoring performed usually documents the average exposure condition of a population of workers being tracked over extended periods of time (DiNardi, 1997). In some instances unusual exposures occur that need to be assessed. These exposures include those that result from infrequent or nonroutine activities, cyclic or periodic

Box 7-8 Worksite Walk-Through Survey Checklist

1. Determine purpose of the survey
   - Comprehensive survey?
   - Evaluation of exposures of limited group of workers to specific agents?
   - Determination of compliance with specific recognized standards?
   - Evaluation of effectiveness of engineering controls?
   - Response to specific complaint?
2. Become familiar with worksite operations
   - Obtain and study process flow sheets and site layout.
   - Obtain a list of job classifications and the agents/environmental stresses to which workers are potentially exposed.
   - Compile an inventory of raw materials, intermediates, by-products, and products.
   - Review relevant toxicologic information.
   - Observe the activities associated with each job classification.
   - Review the status of workers' health.
   - Observe and review administrative and engineering control measures used.
   - Review reports of previous studies.
   - Determine the potential health hazards (e.g., chemical, physical) associated with worksite operations.
   - Review adequacy of labeling and warning.
3. Prepare for the walk-through
   Although each worksite has different operations, equipment, and physical layouts, certain items are quite common to many and deserve special mention. The following types of items should generally be considered when making an inspection:
   - Atmospheric conditions: dusts, gases, fumes, vapors, illumination
   - Pressurized equipment: boilers, pots, tanks, piping, hosing
   - Containers: all objects for storage of materials, such as scrap bins, disposal receptacles, barrels, carboys, gas cylinders, solvent cans
   - Hazardous supplies and materials: flammables, explosives, gases, acids, caustics, toxic chemicals
   - Buildings and structures: windows, doors, aisles, floors, stairs, roofs, walls
   - Electrical conductors and apparatus: wires, cables, switches, controls, transformers, lamps, batteries, fuses
   - Fire fighting equipment: extinguishers, hoses, hydrants, sprinkler systems, alarms
   - Machinery and parts: power equipment that processes, machines, or modifies materials (e.g., grinders, forging machines, power presses, drilling machines, shapers, cutters, lathes)
   - Material-handling equipment: conveyors, cranes, hoists, lifts
   - Hand tools: bars, sledges, wrenches, hammers, power tools
   - Structural openings: shafts, sumps, pits, floor openings, trenches
   - Transportation equipment: automobiles, trucks, railroad equipment, lift trucks
   - Personal protective clothing and equipment: goggles, gloves, aprons, leggings
4. Inspection
   - Determine which agents (e.g., chemical, physical) if any, are to be evaluated.
   - Arrange for appropriate personnel/professional to conduct measurements.
   - Obtain, as required, personal protective equipment (hard hat, safety glasses, goggles, hearing protection, respiratory protection, safety shoes, coveralls, gloves).
   - Sample each element referred.
   - Observe fire exits: clear marking, access, obstruction.
   - Inspect storage areas: clearance, obstruction, clutter, working signs, lifting.
   - Observe all machinery for guarding, tagging, lockout.
   - Observe all electrical equipment for proper grounding, loose wires, insulation.
   - Observe housekeeping procedures and outcomes: cleanliness, safety, clutter, labeling.

operations, or accidental or inadvertent releases or spills of substances. When investigating accidental exposures, past exposures should also be reviewed to determine if patterns of exposure or behavior are contributory. Here, workers and their work practices can also be observed to determine safe work task habits.

Compliance-related walk-throughs are done to determine the effects of mandated regulatory programs from agencies such as the Mine Safety and Health Administration (MSHA) and Occupational Safety and Health Administration (OSHA). For example, many OSHA standards define permissible exposure limits (PELs) that are not to be excluded. Noncompliance may suggest a possible weakness in the surveillance, evaluation, and control activities, or it could be that the apparent over-exposure is a rare, highly atypical event. In either case, evaluation and control strategies will need attention.

During the survey worksite operations and processes can be observed to determine problem areas, and newly added processes should be thoroughly examined in relation to worker task demand. A specific complaint survey is done to investigate a specific area of the work environment or particular operation based on worker complaints such as headaches, odors, skin irritations, or back problems, or complaints concerning a work process exposure or defect in the operations (Conrad & Soule, 1997). Employee complaints should always be evaluated not only because they may be real and warrant corrective action but also because they are believed to be real by the employee and therefore cause anxiety. The occupational health professional must be concerned not only with the physical facts but also with the social and psychological aspects of occupational health. When evaluating a health hazard based on a complaint, the employee should be directly talked to if at all possible. This will demonstrate that the complaint is being taken seriously and provide the opportunity to gather the facts directly from the person experiencing the effects. Whatever the outcome of the evaluation, the employee should be informed of the results. Finally, the occupational health team will want to conduct follow-up walk-throughs to validate that identified problems or hazards have been eliminated, policies regarding control strategies (e.g., use of hearing protection) have been implemented and adhered to, and safe work behaviors are in practice.

Once preparation and planning for the survey has been completed, the walk-through can be initiated and should start at the beginning of the production process where the raw products, materials, and supplies enter the worksite. Information about work processes obtained from the resource materials, flow diagrams, and inventory lists discussed previously will help identify potential problems. The occupational and environmental health nurse should become as familiar as possible with the total work process that is the focus of the survey. Walk-through surveys should be conducted with team members if at all possible, particularly the industrial hygienist and/or technical production personnel, especially when new processes are introduced or if a better understanding of existing processes and controls is needed.

An initial orientation to an industrial process should begin with an understanding of the general physical layout of the facilities (Conrad & Soule, 1997). The location of the particular building or buildings of interest in relation to other structures in the area, the general terrain surrounding the facilities, and the physical arrangement of the worksite itself must be assessed. Simple block flow diagrams with sufficient description of the individual activities making up the process are usually sufficient. With the aid of the floor plan, which can identify high risk areas, and the process flow sheet, a planned, systematic examination of the workplace, including area sampling, can be conducted to locate critical functions of the operation and potential sources of contaminants. Many potentially hazardous operations and sources of contaminants can be detected by visual observation. Dusty operations can be spotted easily, although this does not necessarily mean they are hazardous: dust particles that cannot be seen by the unaided eye are more hazardous than easily visible ones because they are more likely of respirable size. Potential for worker exposure—who and how many workers are exposed and the types of job categories involved—should be carefully noted.

An industry worksite checklist can be used to provide a more systematic method for and improved efficiency in data collection. However, a more specific guide may need to be developed for the worksite being surveyed. In addition, the occupational and environmental health nurse and/or team conducting the walk-through may need to look beyond the items identified in the checklist for conditions or processes that have changed since the last inspection. An experienced occupational health professional often can evaluate quite accurately and in some detail the magnitude of certain chemical and physical stresses associated with an operation without benefit of any instrumentation. In fact, the professional uses this qualitative evaluation every time a survey is made, whether it is intended to be the total effort of the work or a preliminary inspection prior to actual sampling and analysis of potential stresses. Qualitative evaluation can be applied by anyone familiar with an operation, from the worker to the professional investigator, to ascertain some of the potential problems associated with work activities.

An important aspect of the qualitative evaluation is an inspection of the control measures in use at a particular operation. In general, the control measures include such features as shielding from radiant or ultraviolet energy, local exhaust and general ventilation provision, respiratory protection devices, and other personal protective measures. General measures of the relative effectiveness of these controls are the presence or absence of accumulated dust on floors, ledges, and other work surfaces; the general condition of ventilation ductwork (e.g., holes, rust, damage); and the manner in which personal protective measures are accepted and used by workers.

Although the information obtained during a qualitative evaluation or walk-through inspection of a facility is important and always useful, only through quantitative measurements can actual levels of chemicals or physical agents be documented. The purpose of the quantitative evaluation is to develop information that will lead to decisions that will reduce or eliminate health risks to the workers. Sampling only produces data; data must be converted into information to be of value in the decision-making process.

The walk-through survey should be conducted at a time when the operation is in process in order to fully observe the processes, workers, and potential exposure points. Processes and job operations that are run only intermittently may present some of the greatest potential health hazards. Assessment of all shifts should be conducted. If work is done on the night shift or on weekends, a survey should also be made at these times to see if there are any differences in air contaminant concentrations at night as compared to regular daytime operations. Because the production rate may be significantly different on the night shift, conditions may be better or worse (Hansen, 1991; Jones et al., 1990).

Of particular concern during the walk-through survey are the work areas that have excessive exposures or poor work conditions such as excessive noise, excessive heat, inadequate ventilation, awkward operation positions, radiation exposure (ionizing and nonionizing), excessive air contaminants, and worker/machine interface. Exposure characteristics, exposure patterns, and working conditions, including the following, should be assessed:

- Types of agents in the work environment (biological, chemical, enviromechanical, physical, psychosocial)
- Potential hazards associated with each agent and unique work process, including work station design
- Types and numbers of workers exposed either directly or indirectly
- Concentration, frequency, occurrence (shift patterns), and location of exposure (microenvironmental and macroenvironmental)
- Routes of entry (inhalation, transdermal absorption, ingestion)
- Factors contributing to the exposure, such as performance of the job task, personal protective equipment, control mechanisms, individual susceptibility, and work practices
- Cleanliness of the work environment
- Equipment functioning and maintenance
- General environmental milieu
- Surveillance and monitoring activities

Sensory perception also provides valuable information for walk-through assessment purposes. For example, dusty operations can easily be seen; noise that exceeds the OSHA permissible exposure level (PELs) can be audibly detected; and vapors and gases exceeding the OSHA PELs are often odorous. Obvious exposures should provide direction for future exploration and investigation, including measurements of potential hazards with the aid of an industrial hygienist and/or safety specialist (Williams & Burson, 1985). Once a hazard has been identified, a more detailed analysis of the worksite, work processes, and practices can be conducted to determine the scope of the problem and potential strategies for abatement.

The walk-through assessment can aid in determining specific tasks or areas to inspect, and job observation can also be utilized to do the following:

- Improve job procedures and safe work behaviors;
- Determine compliance with safety rules and standards;

- Monitor work practices and use of personal protective equipment;
- Monitor effectiveness of training procedures and identify a need for retraining;
- Increase worker and management understanding of work-related hazards;
- Reinforce positive work behaviors (Rogers, 1990).

As mentioned previously, employee and management participation in the walk-through survey is especially important. Employee interest in identifying problems that need correction will be increased if their participation is not only requested but valued. This can be demonstrated by management's commitment to improving workplace health and safety. In addition, any changes or modifications recommended by the team or program manager should be implemented as soon as feasible. Otherwise, employees and the health care team may view this as an intellectual exercise only and without applied merit and sincere interest on the part of management. A system for monitoring and evaluating the effectiveness of the changes should also be implemented.

The frequency of worksite walk-through surveys should be determined by the nature of the work and major changes in procedures or materials; however, even a brief walk-through should be regularly conducted by the occupational and environmental health nurse. Worksite surveys serve to demonstrate to workers that health and safety at the worksite are important to management as well as the workers.

CONTROL, ABATEMENT, AND PROGRAM STRATEGIES

The use of control strategies should be considered in a hierarchical order of effectiveness. These were previously discussed in another section (Industrial Hygiene). Personal protective equipment is considered the least effective because it can only be effective if appropriate and reliable equipment is provided and if employees consistently use it (American Industrial Hygiene Association, [AIHA], 1997; Levy & Wegman, 2000). The following four important considerations deserve special attention when the decision has been made that a need exists for personal protective equipment:

1. Selection of the proper type of protective device
2. Employee fit with the equipment and instruction on its proper use

3. Enforcement of standards created
4. An effective system of equipment sanitation and maintenance

To ensure proper use of protective equipment, the occupational health professional must make sure that workers understand why protection is necessary so they will want to use it. In addition, special attention should be given to the ease and comfort with which this equipment can be used, so it will be used. Personal protective equipment can be misused or disused to varying degrees depending on a variety of program factors. Therefore, it behooves the occupational and environmental health nurse and other health professionals to constantly recognize that this approach to hazard control should always be secondary to a sincere effort to eliminate the exposure.

Once work-related problems/hazards are identified, steps can be taken for hazard abatement and risk reduction, including the institution of control measures, previously described in this chapter, the modification of existing health and safety programs or the development of new ones, and the improvement or implementation of worker and managerial training and education programs. Wherever possible, control strategies aimed at hazard elimination should be used.

Jensen and Sinkule (1988) state that the importance of education and training in occupational health is reflected in the disproportionately high injury rates among workers newly assigned to work tasks, with much of these rates related to inadequate knowledge of job hazards and safe work practices. Workers need training and education about general and specific hazards of the worksite and work processes, safety rules and procedures related to the particular work assignment, and prevention and control strategies, including work practice behaviors.

Supervisors and managers also have a responsibility to understand the work processes and related hazards and provide for health protection of the workforce through job training or retraining, formal health education sessions, and job hazard analyses. Occupational and environmental health nurses have the necessary skills to help develop and implement an effective occupational health and hazard control education program.

Once the walk-through survey is completed and all background data are collected and reviewed, results and recommendations should be described in a written report with a copy maintained in the occupational health unit. The report should have input from and discussion by all team members with recommendations for hazard abatement and improvement or modification of the occupational health and safety plan. A summary report should accompany the full report to management and should include costs and benefits associated with the recommendations.

Based on this comprehensive worksite assessment, the occupational and environmental health nurse should be in a better position to evaluate the occupational health and safety program and address the need for change that includes the following:

- Improvement of prevention and control strategies to reduce work-related hazards, ensure compliance-directed action, and validate worker exposure protection methods
- Development of new programs for health promotion, protection, and hazard control, such as disability management, prenatal care, disaster preparedness, substance abuse, and waste management
- Revision of policies and procedures for health and safety programming
- Procurement of additional resources for program management and expansion, including upgrading and maintenance
- Improvement and expansion of health and safety training and education programs
- Establishment of quality assurance and research programs to evaluate health program effectiveness and improve worker health

Summary

Effective assessment and management of workplace hazards and related health effects requires collaboration among several disciplines. The occupational and environmental health nurse is often the worksite's primary health care professional who is engaged in identifying work-related health hazards. The nurse must be familiar with key concepts and principles of related disciplinary knowledge that are foundations to the knowledge base in occupational health nursing. This will help to enhance skills and expertise in hazard recognition and control and risk reduction. Collaborative efforts to assess work-related hazards are essential in ultimately preventing unnecessary harm and

risk and protecting and promoting worker health and a safe and healthful work environment.

References

American Conference of Governmental Industrial Hygienists. (2000). *TLVs and BEIs.* Cincinnati, OH: Author.

American Industrial Hygiene Association. (1959). Definition, scope, function, and organization. *American Industrial Hygiene Association Journal, 20,* 428.

Armitage, P. (1985). Multistage models of carcinogenesis. *Environmental Health Perspectives, 63,* 195-201.

Becker, C. (1990). Gases. In J. LaDou (Ed.), *Occupational medicine* (pp. 432-442). Norwalk, CT: Appleton & Lange.

Bigos, S. (1994). *Acute low back problems in adults. Clinical Practice Guidelines # 14* (Agency for Health Care Policy and Research Publication No. 95-0642, pp. 1-160). Washington, DC: U.S. Department of Health and Human Services, Public Health Service, Agency for Health Care Policy and Research.

Boylston, R. (1990). *Managing safety and health programs.* New York: Van Nostrand Reinhold.

Brain, J. D., & Valberg, P. A. (1979). Aerosol deposition in the respiratory tract. *American Reviews of Respiratory Diseases, 120,* 1325-1373.

Burgess, W. A. (1995). *Recognition of health hazards in industry.* New York: John Wiley & Sons.

Cahall, J. (1984). Surveying the work environment to maintain the health of the worker. *AAOHN Update Series, 1*(23), 1-7.

Camp, J., & Tanberg, S. (1985). Assessment of the worksite: A guide for the occupational and environmental health nurse. *AAOHN Update Series, 2*(4), 2-7.

Christiani, D., & Wegman, D. (2000). Respiratory disorders. In B. Levy & D. Wegman (Eds.), *Occupational health* (4th ed., pp. 477-502). Boston: Little, Brown & Company.

Christiani, D. C., & Monson, R. R. (1997). Cancer in relation to occupational and environmental exposures [Special issue]. *Cancer Causes Control, 8*(3).

Colie, C.F. (1993). Male mediated teratogenesis. *Reproductive Toxicology, 7,* 3-9.

Colt, J. S., & Blair, A. (1998). Parental occupational exposure and risk of childhood cancer. *Environmental Health Perspectives, 106*(Suppl. 3), 909-925.

Conrad, R., & Soule, R. D. (1997). Principles of evaluating worker exposure. In S. DiNardi (Ed.), *The occupational environment—Its evaluation and control.* Fairfax, VA: American Industrial Hygiene Association.

Danse, I. (1991). *Common sense toxics in the workplace.* New York: Van Nostrand.

DiNardi, S. (Ed). (1997). *The occupational environment—Its evaluation and control.* Fairfax, VA: American Industrial Hygiene Association.

Felton, J. (1990). *Occupational medical management.* Boston: Little, Brown & Company.

Frazier, L. M., & Hagl, M. L. (1998). *Reproductive hazards of the workplace.* New York: John Wiley & Sons.

Frumkin, H. (2000). Toxins and their effects. In B. Levy & D. Wegman (Eds.), *Occupational health* (4th ed., pp. 309-334). Boston: Little, Brown & Company.

Gauf, M. (1998). *Ergonomics that work.* Horsham, PA: LRP.

Gibaldi, M., & Perrier, D. (1982). *Pharmakokinetics.* New York: Marcel Decker.

Gochfeld, M. (1992a). Environmental risk assessment. In J. Last & R. Wallace (Eds.), *Public health and preventive medicine* (13th ed., pp. 332-342). Norwalk, CT: Appleton & Lange.

Gochfeld, M. (1992b). Toxicology. In J. Last & R. Wallace (Eds.), *Public health and preventive medicine* (13th ed., pp. 315-324). Norwalk, CT: Appleton & Lange.

Gray, R. H., Corn, M., & Cohen, R. (1995). *The Johns Hopkins University retrospective and prospective studies of reproductive health among IBM employees in semiconductor manufacturing, May 1993.* Baltimore, MD: John Hopkins University Press.

Gross, A. S., Louis, D. S., Carr, K. A., & Weiss, S. A. (1995). Carpal tunnel syndrome: A clinicopathologic study. *Journal of Occupational Medicine, 37,* 437-441.

Hagberg, M., Silverstein, B., Wells, R. Smith, M. J., Hendrick, H. W., Carayon, P., & Rerusse, M. (1995). *Work related musculoskeletal disorders (WMSDs): A reference book for prevention.* Bristol, PA: Taylor & Francis.

Hales, T.R., & Bertsche, P. K. (1992). Managing of upper extremity cumulative trauma disorders. *AAOHN Journal, 40*(3) 118-128.

Hall, S. K., Chakaborty, J., & Ruch, R. (1997). *Chemical exposure and toxic responses.* New York: Lewis.

Hansen, D. (1991). *The work environment: Occupational health fundamentals.* Chelsea, MI: Lewis.

Harris, R. (Ed.). (2000). *Patty's industrial hygiene and toxicology: General principles* (Vol. 1). New York: John Wiley & Sons.

Horstman, S. (1992). Industrial hygiene. In J. Last & R. Wallace (Eds.), *Public health and preventive medicine* (13th ed., pp. 547-550). Norwalk, CT: Appleton & Lange.

Jensen, R., & Sinkule, E. (1988). Safety and education in the workplace. *Journal of Safety Research, 19,* 125-133.

Jones, S. E., Hosein H. R., Swain, G. R., & Yablonsky, S. F. (1990). *Occupational hygiene management guide.* Chelsea, MI: Lewis.

Kayafas, N. (1989). *Employee health and industrial hygiene.* Independence, MS: TIV Press.

Keyserling, W. M. (2000). Occupational safety: Preventing accidents and oven trauma. In B. Levy, & D. Wegman, (Eds.), *Occupational health* (4th ed., pp. 181-194). Boston: Little, Brown & Company.

Keyserling, W. M., & Armstrong, T. J. (1992). Ergonomics. In J. Last & R. Wallace (Eds.), *Public health and preventive medicine* (13th ed., pp. 533-546). Norwalk, CT: Appleton & Lange.

Khattak, S., K-Moghtader, G., McMartin, K., Barrera, M., Kennedy, D., & Koren, G. (1999). Pregnancy outcome following gestational exposure to organic solvents: A prospective controlled study. *Journal of the American Medical Association, 281,* 1106-1109.

Lack, R. W. (1996). *Essentials of safety and health management.* New York: Lewis.

LaDou, J. (1997). *Occupational and environmental medicine.* Stanford, CT: Appleton & Lange.

Lahdetie, J. (1995). Occupation- and exposure-related studies on human sperm. *Journal of Occupational and Environmental Medicine, 37,* 922-930.

Levy, B. & Wegman, D. (Eds.). (2000). *Occupational health: Recognizing and preventing work-related diseases.* Boston: Little, Brown & Company.

Levy, B. S., Levin, J. L., & Teitelbaum, D. T. (Eds.). (1999). Symposium: DBCP-induced sterility and reduced fertility among men in developing countries: A case study of the export of a known hazard. *Journal of Occupational and Environmental Health, 5,* 115-153.

Lewis, R. (1997). Metals. In J. Ladou (Ed.), *Occupational medicine* (pp. 297-326). Norwalk, CT: Appleton & Lange.

Lilis, R. (1992). Dims associated with exposure to chemical substances. In J. Last & R. Wallace (Eds.), *Public health and preventive medicine* (13th ed., pp. 403-432). Norwalk, CT: Appleton & Lange.

Lioy, P.J. (1990). Assessing total human exposure to contaminants. *Environmental Science Technology, 24*(7), 938-945.

Loomis, T. A., & Hayes, A. W. (1996). *Loomis' essentials of toxicology.* San Diego, CA: Academic Press.

Mandel, S. (1987). Neurologic syndrome from repetitive trauma at work. *Postgraduate Medicine, 82*(6), 87-92.

McCunney, R. (1996). *Occupational health services.* Chicago: American College of Occupational and Environmental Medicine.

McMartin, K. I., Chu, M., Kopecky, E., Einarson, T. R., & Koren, G. (1998). Pregnancy outcome following maternal organic solvent exposure: A meta-analysis of epidemic studies. *American Journal of Industrial Medicine, 34,* 288-292.

National Institute for Occupational Safety and Health. (1997). *Musculoskeletal disorders and workplace factors* (DHHS [NIOSH] Publication No. 97-141). Cincinnati, OH: Author.

National Safety Council. (1997). *Supervisors' safety manual* (9th ed.). Itasca, IL: Author.

Nelson, B. K., Moorman, W. J., & Schrader, S. M. (1996). Review of experimental male-mediated behavioral and neurochemical disorders. *Neurotoxicology Teratology, 18,* 611-616.

Olishifski, J. (1983). *Fundamentals of industrial hygiene.* Chicago: National Safety Council.

Olshan, A. F. (1993). Male-mediated developmental toxicity. *Annual Review Public Health, 14,* 159-181.

Osorio, A. (1993). Carpal tunnel syndrome among grocery store workers. In K. Steenland (Ed.), *Case studies in occupational epidemiology* (pp. 127-141). New York: Oxford University Press.

Ostendorf, J., Rogers, B., & Bertsche, P. (2000). Ergonomics: CTD management evaluation tool. *AAOHN Journal, 48*(1) 17-24.

Ottoboni, M. A. (1991). *The dose makes the poison.* New York: Van Nostrand Reinhold.

Paul, M., & Frazier, L. (2000). Reproductive disorders, In B. Levy & D. Wegman, *Occupational health: Recognizing and preventing work-related disease and injury* (pp. 589-603). Philadelphia: Lippincott Williams & Wilkins.

Ramazzini, B. (1940). Diseases of Workers (W. C. Wright, Trans.). Chicago: University of Chicago. (Original work published 1713)

Randolph, J. A. K. (2000). Carpal tunnel syndrome: Testing the sensitivity and validity of four "localized discomfort" instruments. *AAOHN Journal, 48*(8) 385-394.

Rodgers, S. (1992). A functional job analysis technique. *Occupational Medicine: State of the Art Reviews, 7*(4), 679-712.

Rogers, B. (1990). Occupational nursing practice, education and research: Challenges for the future. *AAOHN Journal, 38,* 581-585.

Rogers, B. (1998). Occupational health nursing expertise. *AAOHN Journal, 46*(10), 477-483.

Rogers, B., & Emmett, E. (1987). Handling antineoplastics agents: Urine mutagenicity in nursing personnel. *Image, 19*(3), 108-113.

Rogers, B., & Goodno, L. (2000). Evaluation of interventions to prevent needlestick injuries in health care occupations. *American Journal of Preventative Medicine, 18*(45) 90-98.

Rogers, B., & Travers, P. (1991). An overview of work-related hazards in nursing: Health & safety issues. *Heart & Lung, 20,* 486-497.

Roland, A. S., Baird, D. D., Weinberg, C. R., Shore, D. L., Shy, C. M., & Wilcox, A. J. (1992). Reduced fertility among women employed as dental assistants exposed to high levels of nitrous oxide. *New England Journal of Medicine, 327,* 993-997.

Rose, V. E. (1997). History and philosophy in industrial hygiene. In S. DiNardi, *The occupational environment—Its evaluation and control* (pp. 6-20). Fairfax, VA: American Industrial Hygiene Association.

Schenker, M. B., Gold, E. B., Beaumont, J. J., Eskenazi, B., Lasley, B. L., Hammond, S. K., McCurdy, S. A., Samuels, S. J., Saiki, C. L., & Swan, S. H. (1995). Association of spontaneous abortion and other reproductive effects with work in the semiconductor industry. *American Journal of Industrial Medicine, 28,* 639-659.

Schnorr, T. (1993). Video display terminals and adverse pregnancy outcomes. In K. Steenland (Ed.), *Case studies in occupational epidemiology* (pp. 7-20). New York: Oxford University Press.

Scialli, A. R. (Ed.). (1993). Pregnancy and the workplace. *Seminars in Perinatology, 17,* 1-57.

Selikoff, I. J., & Lee, D. H. (1978). *Asbestos and disease.* New York: Academic Press.

Silverstein, B., & Kalat, J. (1998). *Work-related disorders of the back and upper extremity in Washington State: 1989-1996* (Tech. Rep. No. 40-1-1997). Olympia, WA: Safety and Health Assessment and Research for Prevention (SHARP) Program, Washington State Department of Labor and Industries.

Silverstein, M., & Mirer, F. (2000). Labor unions and occupational health. In B. Levy & D. Wegman (Eds.), *Occupational health* (pp. 715-728). Boston: Little, Brown & Company.

Sluchak, T. J. (1992). Ergonomics: Origins, focus, and implementation considerations. *AAOHN Journal, 40*(3), 105-112.

Smith, T. J., & Schneider, T. (2000). Occupational hygiene. In B. Levy & D. Wegman, *Occupational health: Recognizing and preventing work-related disease and injury* (pp. 161-171). Philadelphia: Lippincott Williams & Wilkins.

Soule, R.D. (1991). Industrial hygiene sampling and analysis. In R. Harris (Ed.), *Patty's industrial hygiene and toxicology* (Vol. 1, pp. 73-135). New York: John Wiley & Sons.

Stine, K. E., & Brown, T. M. (1996). *Principles of toxicology.* New York: Lewis.

Stoy, D. W., & Aspen, J. (1999) Force and repetition management of hamboning: Relationship to musculoskeletal symptoms. *AAOHN Journal, 47*(6), 254-260.

Taskinen, H., Kyyronen, P., Hemminki, K., Hoikkala, M. Lajunen, K., & Lindbohm, M. L. (1994). Laboratory work and pregnancy outcome. *Journal of Occupational Medicine, 36,* 288-292.

Todd, L. A. (1997). Direct reading instrumental methods for gases, vapors, and aerosols. In S. DiNardi (Ed.), *The occupational environment—Its evaluation and control.* Fairfax, VA: American Industrial Hygiene Association.

Travers, P. H. (1992). Implementing ergonomic strategies in the workplace: An occupational health nursing perspective. *AAOHN Journal, 40,* 129-137.

Upton, A. (2000). Ionizing radiation. In B. Levy & D. Wegman (Eds.), *Occupational health* (4th ed., pp. 355-366). Boston: Little, Brown & Company.

U.S. Department of Agriculture. (1987). *Hazard communication: A program guide for federal agencies.* Washington, DC: U.S. Government Printing Office.

U.S. Department of Health and Human Services, National Institute for Occupational Safety and Health. (1995). *National occupational research agenda.* Cincinnati, OH: National Institute for Occupational Safety & Health.

U.S. Department of Health and Human Services, National Institute for Occupational Safety and Health. (1996). *Elements of ergonomic programs.* Cincinnati, OH: National Institute for Occupational Safety and Health.

U.S. Department of Health and Human Services, National Institute for Occupational Safety and Health. (1999). *Pocket guide to chemical hazards.*

(NIOSH Publication No. 90-117). Cincinnati, OH: Author.

U.S. Department of Labor. (1995). *Dictionary of occupational titles.* Washington, DC: U.S. Government Printing Office.

U.S. Department of Labor. (2000). *Ergonomics: The study of work.* Washington, DC: Occupational Safety and Health Administration.

U.S. Department of Labor, Bureau of Labor Statistics. News Release: *Lost-workingtime injuries and illnesses: Characteristics and resulting time away from work, 1998.* (2000). http://www.bls.gov.

U.S. Department of Labor, Occupational Safety and Health Administration. (1989). Guidelines on workplace safety and health program management: Issuance of voluntary guidelines. *Federal Register, 54,* 3904-3918.

U.S. Department of Labor, Occupational Safety and Health Administration. (1991). *Ergonomics program management guidelines for meatpacking plants* (Publication No. 3123). Washington, DC: Author.

U.S. Office of Management and Budget. (1987). *Standard industrial classification manual.* Springfield, VA: National Technical Information Service.

Verma, D., & Verrall, B. (1985). Principles of industrial hygiene. *AAOHN Update Series, 2*(26): 2-11.

Weeks, J., Levy, B., & Wagner, G. (1991). *Preventing occupational disease and injury.* Washington, DC: American Public Health Association.

Williams, P., & Burson, J. (1985). *Industrial toxicology.* New York: Van Nostrand Reinhold.

Wills, J. H. (1982). Nasal carcinoma in woodworkers: A review. *Journal of Occupational Medicine, 24,* 526-533.

7-1 An OSHA Material Safety Data Sheet

AN OSHA Material Safety Data Sheet

Material Safety Data Sheet
May be used to comply with
OSHA's Hazard Communication Standard,
29 CFR 1910.1200. Standard must be
consulted for specific requirements.

U.S. Department of Labor
Occupational Safety and Health Administration
(Non-Mandatory Form)
Form Approved
OMB No. 1218-0072

IDENTITY *(As Used on Label and List)*

Note: Blank spaces are not permitted. If any item is not applicable, or no information is available, the space must be marked to indicate that.

Section I

Manufacturer's Name	Emergency Telephone Number
Address *(Number, Street, City, State, and ZIP Code)*	Telephone Number for Information
	Date Prepared
	Signature of Preparer *(optional)*

Section II — Hazardous Ingredients/Identity Information

Hazardous Components (Specific Chemical Identity; Common Name(s))	OSHA PEL	ACGIH TLV	Other Limits Recommended	% (optional)

Section III — Physical/Chemical Characteristics

Boiling Point		Specific Gravity ($H_2O = 1$)	
Vapor Pressure (mm Hg)		Melting Point	
Vapor Density (AIR = 1)		Evaporation Rate (Butyl Acetate = 1)	

Solubility in Water

Appearance and Odor

Section IV — Fire and Explosion Hazard Data

Flash Point (Method Used)		Flammable Limits	LEL	UEL

Extinguishing Media

Special Fire Fighting Procedures

Unusual Fire and Explosion Hazards

Section V — Reactivity Data

Stability	Unstable		Conditions to Avoid
	Stable		

Incompatibility *(Materials to Avoid)*

Hazardous Decomposition or Byproducts

Hazardous Polymerization	May Occur		Conditions to Avoid
	Will Not Occur		

Section VI — Health Hazard Data

Route(s) of Entry:	Inhalation?	Skin?	Ingestion?

Health Hazards *(Acute and Chronic)*

Carcinogenicity:	NTP?	IARC Monographs?	OSHA Regulated?

Signs and Symptoms of Exposure

Medical Conditions
Generally Aggravated by Exposure

Emergency and First Aid Procedures

Section VII — Precautions for Safe Handling and Use

Steps to Be Taken in Case Material Is Released or Spilled

Waste Disposal Method

Precautions to Be Taken in Handling and Storing

Other Precautions

Section VIII — Control Measures

Respiratory Protection *(Specify Type)*

Ventilation	Local Exhaust		Special
	Mechanical *(General)*		Other

Protective Gloves	Eye Protection

Other Protective Clothing or Equipment

Work/Hygienic Practices

From *Material Safety Data Sheet*, by Occupational Safety and Health Administration, 1985, Washington DC: U.S. Department of Labor.

7-2 BOC Gases Material Safety Data Sheet

///// ///// ///// **BOC GASES**

MATERIAL SAFETY DATA SHEET

PRODUCT NAME: HYDROGEN SULFIDE

1. Chemical Product and Company Identification

BOC Gases
Division of,
The BOC Group, Inc.
575 Mountain Avenue
Murray Hill, NJ 07974

BOC Gases
Division of,
BOC Canada Limited
5975 Falbourne Street, Unit 2
Mississauga, Ontario L5R 3W6

TELEPHONE NUMBER: (908) 464-8100
24-HOUR EMERGENCY TELEPHONE
NUMBER: CHEMTREC (800) 424-9300

TELEPHONE NUMBER: (905) 501-1700
24-HOUR EMERGENCY TELEPHONE
NUMBER: (905) 501-0802
EMERGENCY RESPONSE PLAN NO: 2-0101

PRODUCT NAME: HYDROGEN SULFIDE
CHEMICAL NAME: Hydrogen Sulfide
COMMON NAMES/SYNONYMS: Dihydrogen Sulfide, Sulfur Hydride
TDG (Canada) CLASSIFICATION: 2.3 (2.1)
WHMIS CLASSIFICATION: A, B1, D1A, D2B

PREPARED BY: Loss Control (908) 464-8100/(905) 501-1700
PREPARATION DATE: 6/1/95
REVIEW DATES: 6/1/99

2. Composition, Information on Ingredients

EXPOSURE LIMITS[1]:

INGREDIENT	% VOLUME	PEL-OSHA[2]	TLV-ACGIH[3]	LD_{50} OR LC_{50} Route/Species
Hydrogen Sulfide FORMULA: H_2S CAS: 7783-06-4 RTECS #: MX1225000	>99.0	20 ppm Ceiling 50 ppm (10-min. max peak)	10 ppm TWA 15 ppm STEL	LC50: 712 ppm inhalation/rat (1 H)

[1]Refer to individual state of provincial regulations, as applicable, for limits which may be more stringent than those listed here.
[2]As stated in 29 CFR 1910, Subpart Z (revised July 1, 1993)
[3]As stated in the ACGIH 1998-1999 Threshold Limit Values for Chemical Substances and Physical Agents.

IDLH: 100 ppm

OSHA Regulatory Status: This material is classified as hazardous under OSHA regulations.

3. Hazards Identification

EMERGENCY OVERVIEW

Colorless, poison, highly flammable gas with rotten egg odor. Irritating to the eyes, mucous membranes and respiratory system. Can cause respiratory paralysis, sudden collapse, and death. Dangerous fire and explosion hazard. Avoid heat, sparks, and flames. Contents under pressure. Use and store below 125 °F.

ROUTE OF ENTRY:

Skin Contact	Skin Absorption	Eye Contact	Inhalation	Ingestion
Yes	No	Yes	Yes	No

Continued

HEALTH EFFECTS:

Exposure Limits Yes	Irritant Yes	Sensitization No
Teratogen No	Reproductive Hazard No	Mutagen No
Synergistic Effects None Reported		

Carcinogenicity: -- NTP: No   IARC: No   OSHA: No

EYE EFFECTS:
Low concentrations will generally cause irritation to the conjunctiva. Repeated exposure to low concentrations is reported to cause conjunctivitis, photophobia, tears, pain, and blurred vision.

SKIN EFFECTS:
May irritate the skin upon contact.

INGESTION EFFECTS:
Ingestion is unlikely. Hydrogen sulfide will irritate the mucous membranes causing a burning feeling with excess salivation likely. Irritation of the gastrointestinal tract may also occur.

INHALATION EFFECTS:
Lethal concentrations of hydrogen sulfide cause respiratory paralysis and breathing stops. Life threatening pulmonary edema is common following prolonged exposure to concentrations between 250 and 600 ppm. Edema has been reported following prolonged exposure at concentrations as low as 50 ppm.

Sense of smell becomes rapidly fatigued and cannot be used as warning of exposure.

MEDICAL CONDITIONS AGGRAVATED BY EXPOSURE:
May aggravate preexisting eye, skin, respiratory, and central nervous system (CNS) disorder.

NFPA HAZARD CODES		HMIS HAZARD CODES		RATINGS SYSTEM
Health:	4	Health:	2	0 = No Hazard
Flammability:	4	Flammability:	4	1 = Slight Hazard
Instability:	0	Reactivity:	0	2 = Moderate Hazard
				3 = Serious Hazard
				4 = Severe Hazard

4. First Aid Measures

EYES:
PERSONS WITH POTENTIAL EXPOSURE TO HYDROGEN SULFIDE SHOULD NOT WEAR CONTACT LENSES. Flush contaminated eyes with large amounts of water for at least 15 minutes. Part eyelids with fingers to ensure complete flushing. If irritation persists, seek medical attention immediately.

SKIN:
Flush affected area with water. If irritation persists, consult a physician.

INGESTION:
Not anticipated. Treat in a manner similar to inhalation exposure. Seek medical attention as soon as possible.

INHALATION:
PROMPT MEDICAL ATTENTION IS MANDATORY IN ALL CASES OF OVEREXPOSURE. RESCUE PERSONNEL SHOULD BE EQUIPPED WITH SELF-CONTAINED BREATHING APPARATUS AND SHOULD RECOGNIZE THE HAZARDS OF OVEREXPOSURE DUE TO OLFACTORY FATIGUE. An extreme fire hazard exists during rescue. Avoid use of rescue equipment which may contain ignition sources or cause static discharge. Victims should be assisted to an uncontaminated area and inhale fresh air. Quick removal from the contaminated area is most important. If breathing is difficult, administer oxygen. If breathing has stopped administer artificial resuscitation and supplemental oxygen or a mixture of 5% carbon dioxide in oxygen. Keep victim calm and warm. Further treatment should be symptomatic and supportive. Seek medical assistance immediately.

Note to physician: Acute hydrogen sulfide poisoning can be treated by induction of methemoglobinemia through parenteral injection of methemoglobin generating agents (i.e., sodium nitrile). This acts as an antidote by restoring the normal activity of the sulfide inhibited enzyme.

5. Fire Fighting Measures

Conditions of Flammability: Flammable		
Flash point: Not Available	Method: Not Applicable	Autoignition Temperature: 554°F (290°C)
LEL (%): 4.0		UEL (%): 44.0
Hazardous combustion products: Sulfur Compounds including sulfur dioxide		
Sensitivity to mechanical shock: None		
Sensitivity to static discharge: None		

FIRE AND EXPLOSION HAZARDS:
Hydrogen sulfide is heavier than air and may accumulate in low areas or travel along the ground to an ignition source and flash back. Product may explode or burn over a wide range of mixtures in air. Cylinder may rupture violently from pressure when involved in a fire situation.

EXTINGUISHING MEDIA:
Water, carbon dioxide, dry chemicals.

FIRE FIGHTING INSTRUCTIONS:
If possible, stop the flow of gas. Inerting the atmosphere to reduce oxygen levels may extinguish flame, allowing capping of leaking container. Do not attempt this unless specifically trained. Reduce the rate of flow and inject an inert gas, if possible, before completely stopping the flow to prevent flashback. Do not extinguish the fire until the supply is shut off as otherwise an explosive reignition may occur. If the fire is extinguished and the flow of gas continues, use increased ventilation to prevent build-up of explosive atmosphere.

Use water spray to cool surrounding containers. Be cautious of a Boiling Liquid Evaporating Vapor Explosion, BLEVE, if flame is impinging on surrounding containers. Direct 500 GPM water stream onto containers above liquid level with remote monitors. Limit the number of personnel in proximity of fire and evacuate surrounding areas in all directions.

Firefighters should wear respiratory protection (SCBA) and full turnout or Bunker gear. Continue to cool fire-exposed cylinders until well after flames are extinguished.

6. Accidental Release Measures

Immediately evacuate all personnel from affected area and extinguish all ignition sources. No smoking, sparks, flames, or flares in hazard area. Deny entry to unauthorized and unprotected personnel. Use appropriate protective equipment including respiratory protection. Stop or control the leak if it can be done without risk. Use water spray to knock down vapors and protect personnel. Dilute waters to nonflammable mixtures. Do not allow clean up waters to enter waterways and sewers. Consult a Hazmat specialist and the appropriate emergency telephone number in Section 1 or your closest BOC location. If leak is in user's equipment, be certain to purge piping with inert gas prior to attempting repairs.

7. Handling and Storage

Electrical Classification: Class I, Group C

Earth-ground and bond all lines and equipment associated with the Hydrogen Sulfide system. All equipment should be nonsparking or explosion proof.

Do not rely on the olfactory sense to detect the presence of hydrogen sulfide. Analytical devices and instrumentation are readily available for this purpose. Perform frequent analytical tests to be certain that the TWA is not exceeded. Many metals corrode rapidly with wet hydrogen sulfide. Anhydrous hydrogen sulfide can be handled in carbon steel, aluminum Inconel, Stellite and 304 and 316 stainless steels. Avoid hard steels which are highly stressed since they may be susceptible to hydrogen embrittlement from hydrogen sulfide. Multipoint air samplers with alarms for plant production units should be provided to constantly monitor the air in and around the units.

Use only in well-ventilated areas. Valve protection caps must remain in place unless container is secured with valve outlet piped to use point. Do not drag, slide, or roll cylinders. Use a suitable hand truck for cylinder movement. Use a pressure reducing regulator when connecting cylinder to lower pressure (<750 psig) piping or systems. Do not heat cylinder by any means to increase the discharge rate of product from the cylinder. Use a check valve or trap in the discharge line to prevent hazardous back flow into the system.

Continued

Protect cylinders from physical damage. Store in cool, dry, well-ventilated area away from heavily trafficked areas and emergency exits. Do not allow the temperature where cylinders are stored to exceed 125°F (52°C). Cylinders should be stored upright and firmly secured to prevent falling or being knocked over. Full and empty cylinders should be segregated. Use a "first in-first out" inventory system to prevent full cylinders being stored for excessive periods of time. Post "NO SMOKING OR OPEN FLAMES" signs in the storage area or use area. There should be no sources of ignition in the storage or use area.

Never carry a compressed gas cylinder or a container of a gas in cryogenic liquid form in an enclosed space such as a car trunk, van, or station wagon. A leak can result in a fire, explosion, asphyxiation, or a toxic exposure.

For additional storage recommendations, consult Compressed Gas Association Pamphlets P-1 and G-12.

8. Exposure Controls, Personal Protection

ENGINEERING CONTROLS:
Hood with forced ventilation. Use local exhaust to prevent accumulation above exposure limit.

EYE/FACE PROTECTION:
Gas tight chemical goggles or full-face piece respirator.

SKIN PROTECTION:
Protective gloves: Neoprene, butyl rubber, PVC, polyethylene.

RESPIRATORY PROTECTION:
Positive pressure air line with full-face mask and escape bottle or self-contained breathing apparatus should be available for emergency use.

OTHER/GENERAL PROTECTION:
Safety shoes, safety showers and an emergency eyewash station should be available. Personnel with potential exposure to hydrogen sulfide should work in pairs, wear a gas mask with an all purpose canister or light three minute unit with a self contained air supply for instantaneous use, and carry wet lead acetate paper on wrists or belt for detection of dangerous concentrations of hydrogen sulfide. (turns black in the presence of minute amounts of hydrogen sulfide)

9. Physical and Chemical Properties

PARAMETER	VALUE	UNITS
Physical state (gas, liquid, solid)	: Vapor	
Vapor pressure	: 267 (1840 kPa)	psia
Vapor density at STP (Air = 1)	: 1.21	
Evaporation point	: Not Available	
Boiling point	: −76	°F
	: −60	°C
Freezing point	: −117.8	°F
	: −82.2	°C
pH	: Not Available	
Specific gravity	: Not Available	
Oil/water partition coefficient	: Not Available	
Solubility (H_2O)	: Soluble	
Odor threshold	: Not Available	
Odor and appearance	: Colorless vapor with rotten egg odor.	

10. Stability and Reactivity

STABILITY:
Stable

INCOMPATIBLE MATERIALS:
Dangerously reactive when mixed with concentrated nitric acid or other strong oxidizing agents. Vapors will ignite spontaneously when mixed with vapors of chlorine, oxygen difluoride or nitrogen trifluoride.

HAZARDOUS DECOMPOSITION PRODUCTS:
Oxides of sulfur.

HAZARDOUS POLYMERIZATION:
Will not occur.

11. Toxicological Information

INHALATION:
Inhalation of 1000-3000 (dogs) was lethal. Respiration ceased after several breaths at 3000 ppm and death occurred within 15-20 minutes at concentrations of 1000 ppm.

SKIN AND EYE:
Concentrations of 50-500 ppm cause eye and respiratory irritation. Ocular toxicity has been reported at hydrogen sulfide concentrations ranging from 5-30 ppm.

CHRONIC:
Hydrogen sulfide is not considered a cumulative poison; however, headaches, fatigue, dizziness, irritability, and loss of libido have been reported following chronic exposure. It is unclear whether low level exposures, repeated unmeasured acute exposures, or preexisting neurological disease are responsible for the above symptoms.

12. Ecological Information

No data given.

13. Disposal Considerations

Do not attempt to dispose of residual waste or unused quantities. Return in the shipping container PROPERLY LABELED, WITH ANY VALVE OUTLET PLUGS OR CAPS SECURED AND VALVE PROTECTION CAP IN PLACE to BOC Gases or authorized distributor for proper disposal.

14. Transport Information

PARAMETER	United States DOT	Canada TDG
PROPER SHIPPING NAME:	Hydrogen Sulfide	Hydrogen Sulphide, liquefied
HAZARD CLASS:	2.3	2.3 (2.1)
IDENTIFICATION NUMBER:	UN 1053	UN 1053
SHIPPING LABEL:	POISON GAS, FLAMMABLE GAS	POISON GAS, FLAMMABLE GAS

Additional Marking Requirement: "Inhalation Hazard"
    If net weight of product ≥100 pounds, the container must be also marked with the letters "RQ".
Additional Shipping Paper Description Requirement: "Poison-Inhalation Hazard, Zone B"
    If net weight of product ≥100 pounds, the shipping papers must be also marked with the letters "RQ".

15. Regulatory Information

Hydrogen sulfide is listed under the accident prevention provision of section 112(r) of the Clean Air Act (CAA) with a threshold quantity (TQ) of 10,000 pounds.

SARA TITLE III NOTIFICATIONS AND INFORMATION:
Hydrogen sulfide is listed as an extremely hazardous substance (EHS) subject to state and local reporting under Section 304 of SARA Title III (EPCRA). The presence of hydrogen sulfide in quantities in excess of the threshold planning quantity (TPQ) of 500 pounds requires certain emergency planning activities to be conducted.

Releases of hydrogen sulfide in quantities equal to or greater than the reportable quantity (RQ) of 100 pounds are subject to reporting to the National Response Center under CERCLA, Section 304 SARA Title III.

SARA TITLE III—HAZARD CLASSES:
Acute Health Hazard
Fire Hazard
Sudden Release of Pressure Hazard

SARA TITLE III—SECTION 313 SUPPLIER NOTIFICATION:
This product contains the following toxic chemicals subject to the reporting requirements of section 313 of the Emergency Planning and Community Right-To-Know Act (EPCRA) of 1986 and of 40 CFR 372:

CAS NUMBER	INGREDIENT NAME	PERCENT BY VOLUME
7783-06-4	Hydrogen sulfide	>99.0

This information must be included on all MSDSs that are copied and distributed for this material.

Continued

16. Other Information

ACGIH	American Conference of Governmental Industrial Hygienists
DOT	Department of Transportation
IARC	International Agency for Research on Cancer
NTP	National Toxicology Program
OSHA	Occupational Safety and Health Administration
PEL	Permissible Exposure Limit
SARA	Superfund Amendments and Reauthorization Act
STEL	Short Term Exposure Limit
TDG	Transportation of Dangerous Goods
TLV	Threshold Limit Value
WHMIS	Workplace Hazardous Materials Information System

Compressed gas cylinders shall not be refilled without the express written permission of the owner. Shipment of a compressed gas cylinder that has not been filled by the owner or with his/her (written) consent is a violation of transportation regulations.

DISCLAIMER OF EXPRESSED AND IMPLIED WARRANTIES:
Although reasonable care has been taken in the preparation of this document, we extend no warranties and make no representations as to the accuracy or completeness of the information contained herein and assume no responsibility regarding the suitability of this information for the user's intended purposes or for the consequences of its use. Each individual should make a determination as to the suitability of the information for their particular purpose(s).

MSDS: G-94
Revised: 6/1/99

From BOC Gases, Division of BOC Group Inc., Murray Hill, NJ.

7-3 Worksite Assessment Guide

DATE_____

NAME OF INDUSTRY/WORKSITE _____

ADDRESS _____

TELEPHONE ( ) _____

Hours of Operation _____

Days of Operation _____

SIC Code _____

Parent Company _____

Name/Location of Corporate Office _____

_____

PERSON COMPLETING GUIDE _____

Describe the historical development of the company (including parent company and subsidaries).

_____

_____

_____

THE WORK

Identify the major products of the industry.

_____

_____

_____

_____

_____

_____

Describe each stage of the operational processes, raw materials used, and byproducts produced. Is there an inventory of chemicals in the processes? How is this managed?
How are materials stored?

_____

_____

_____

_____

_____

Continued

Do workers consider the work stimulating? (Describe) _____

_____

_____

_____

_____

Do workers take pride in the final product? _____

_____

_____

_____

_____

In general, what are the different types of jobs? _____

_____

_____

_____

_____

_____

THE WORK ENVIRONMENT

Describe the general conditions of the work environment including physical (temperature, lighting, noise, ventilation), and psychosocial (stress) characteristics, eating and hygiene facilities, and housekeeping.

_____

_____

_____

_____

_____

_____

_____

Describe the mechanism for disposal of waste products. Are there problems with pollution?

_____

_____

_____

_____

_____

Are safety signs posted and apparent when needed? _____

_____

_____

_____

_____

_____

Is the company unionized? If yes, please describe its influence and relationships. _____

_____

_____

_____

_____

_____

Describe the physical arrangements of the health unit (equipment, space, and physical location within the organization).

_____

_____

_____

_____

_____

_____

WORKER POPULATION

Total Number Employees   _____

Percent Men   _____

Percent Women   _____

Age Range   _____

Average Age   _____

Percent Nonproduction
Employees   _____

Percent Production
Employees   _____

Additional relevant comments about the characteristics of the workforce.

_____

_____

_____

_____

_____

Continued

Shift Work: Percent Employees First Shift   _____

                Percent Employees Second Shift   _____

                Percent Employees Third Shift   _____

Do workers rotate shifts? _____   If yes, what percentage of workers rotate shifts? _____

HUMAN RESOURCES/MANAGEMENT

	Number employed full-time	Number employed part-time (hours per week)	Contractual	Job descriptions available
Occupational Health Nurse	_____	_____	_____	_____
Nurse Practitioner	_____	_____	_____	_____
Licensed Practical Nurse	_____	_____	_____	_____
Physician	_____	_____	_____	_____
Industrial Hygienist	_____	_____	_____	_____
Safety Specialist	_____	_____	_____	_____
Clerical	_____	_____	_____	_____
Ergonomist	_____	_____	_____	_____
Other (specify)	_____	_____	_____	_____

Describe the corporate/company philosophy and commitment to the occupational/safety program.

_____

_____

_____

_____

_____

Are there written policies and procedures regarding operation of the health unit? If yes, describe how these were developed (i.e., decision making process).

_____

_____

_____

_____

_____

_____

_____

Describe narratively the management style and line and staff functions that operate with respect to the occupational health and safety program. Attach a diagram of the organizational structure.

_____

_____

_____

_____

_____

_____

Describe the focus, frequency, and outcomes of industrial hygiene and safety inspections and indicate occupational health nursing's involvement.

_____

_____

_____

_____

_____

_____

Describe the record system in the health unit (including logs, records, reports). What is the policy regarding confidentiality of health records and is this observed?

_____

_____

_____

_____

_____

_____

HEALTH/DISABILITY INSURANCE

What type of employee health insurance does the company have (e.g. third party, self-insured)?

_____

What are average annual company expenditures for health insurance claims?

$_____

Percentage Hospital Claims   _____

Percentage Ambulatory Care Claims   _____

Continued

What are the major categories of expenditures for these claims (specify illnesses, injuries, etc.)?

_____

_____

_____

_____

_____

What are the average annual company expenditures for worker's compensation claims?

$_____

What are the major categories of expenditure for worker's compensation claims (specify illnesses, injuries, etc.)?

_____

_____

_____

_____

_____

_____

OCCUPATIONAL HEALTH & SAFETY PROGRAMS

Give an overall description of the occupational health and safety program and health promotion/health protection activities. What are the major objectives for the health program? Describe monitoring/surveillance activities and disability and disaster preparedness programs.

_____

_____

_____

_____

_____

_____

_____

_____

_____

_____

_____

_____

_____

_____

_____

_____

_____

OCCUPATIONAL HEALTH & SAFETY SERVICES

HEALTH PROMOTION/PROTECTION PROGRAMS

Please indicate which of the following services are provided (check):

_____Breast cancer screening	_____Monitoring/surveillance of employees
_____Case management	_____Periodic exams by nurse
_____Cervical cancer screening	_____Periodic exams by physicians
_____Chest x-ray	_____Physical therapy
_____Cholesterol screening	_____Prenatal instruction
_____Colon cancer screening	_____Preplacement exams by nurse
_____Diabetes management	_____Preplacement exams by physician
_____Diabetes screening	_____Pulmonary function tests
_____Disability management	_____Reproductive health
_____Emergency care and follow-up	_____Respiratory protection program
_____Employee assistance program	_____Retirement planning
_____Exercise/fitness program	_____Return to work
_____First aid/CPR for employees	_____Smoking cessation program
_____General health counseling	_____Stress management program
_____General health education	_____Travel health
_____Glaucoma screening	_____Treatment of nonoccupational
_____Hazardous materials	illness/injury
management (hazard	_____Treatment of occupational illness/injury
communication)	_____Tuberculin testing
_____Healthy back program	_____Urine drug testing
_____Health risk appraisals	_____preplacement
_____Hearing protection program	_____for cause
_____Hepatitis screening	_____random
_____HIV screening	_____Vision protection program
_____HIV counseling	_____Weight reduction program
_____Home visiting	_____Other (specify)_____
_____Hypertension management	
_____Hypertension screening	
_____Immunizations	

When are group health education/promotion programs conducted?

_____ Percent on company time

_____ Percent on employee time

_____ Not offered

Comments: _____
_____
_____
_____
_____
_____
_____

Continued

Please indicate what, if any, mandated programs are in place and to what extent they are observed and enforced.

_____

_____

_____

_____

_____

_____

Do workers use appropriate personal protective equipment? (Describe.)

_____

_____

_____

_____

_____

_____

What other control measures are in place? (Describe.)

_____

_____

_____

_____

_____

Are OSHA regulations adhered to? (Describe.)

_____

_____

_____

_____

_____

_____

Is there a fire safety program; how often are fire drills and inspections conducted?

_____

_____

_____

_____

_____

_____

Estimate the number of visits made to the health unit by employees.

_____ Number of weekly visits   _____ Percent of visits handled by nursing staff

_____ Percent of visits for preventive screening   _____ Percent of visits handled by physician staff

_____ Percent of visits for illness/injury

What are the most common illnesses reported?

_____

_____

_____

_____

_____

_____

What are the most common injuries reported?

_____

_____

_____

_____

_____

_____

HEALTH/SAFETY HAZARD SURVEY

Describe potential/actual health hazards (i.e., biological, chemical, enviromechanical, physical, psychosocial, etc.) to which workers are exposed, the extent of the exposure and the mechanism(s) for hazards, abatement, and jobs that are high risk. Identify the nursing role in handling these hazards and your recommendations for improvement, if any. Use the back of this page or additional sheets if needed.

_____

_____

_____

_____

_____

Developed by Bonnie Rogers
Copyright © 1985
Last revision 1999
Do not reproduce without permission

Environmental Health

Human exposures to hazardous agents in the air, water, soil, and food, and to physical hazards in the environment are major contributors to illness, disability, and death worldwide. According to the World Health Organization (1997), "in its broadest sense, environmental health comprises those aspects of human health, disease, and injury that are determined or influenced by factors in the environment. This includes the study of both the direct pathological effects of various chemical, physical, and biological agents, as well as the effects on health of the broad physical and social environment, which includes housing, urban development, land-use and transportation, industry, and agriculture." Because the impact of the environment on human health is so great, protecting the environment has long been a mainstay of public health practice.

The public has only recently become aware of the environment's role in health. Publication of Rachel Carson's *Silent Spring* in the early 1960s, followed by the well-publicized poor health of residents of western New York's Love Canal, a significant toxic waste site, awakened public consciousness of environmental issues (Commissioned Corps of USPHS, 2000). However, there have been successes in environmental health. The sanitation movement of the 1800s resulted in enormous reductions in mortality due to infectious diseases and resulted in increases in life expectancy from 47 years in 1900 to almost 77 years in 1997. Since the mid-1970s stronger environmental laws in the United States have resulted in cleaner air, safer drinking water, and recovery of some water bodies that in 1970 were unsafe for fishing and swimming (Goldman, 2000) (Table 8-1).

ENVIRONMENTAL HEALTH HAZARDS

Environmental hazards are ubiquitous and complex. Since the mid-1970s, 80,000 chemicals have been produced in the United States (USEPA, 2000a), but many have never been in commerce. More than 15,000 high volume production (production of more than 10,000 pounds per year) artificial chemicals are in use, and hundreds more are introduced each year. More than half of them have never been tested for human toxicity (Landrigan et al., 1999). The capacity to produce new chemicals has exceeded the capacity to test them. In addition, the United States imports or produces at more than 1,000,000 pounds per year about 3,000 chemicals, with about 40% having no testing data related to basic toxicity and only 7% having a complete set of basic screening information (USEPA, 2000a).

Many acute and chronic health problems have their roots in the environment (Nadakavukaren, 2000) as a result of a battery of exposures such as lead poisoning, pesticides in food and water, air pollution, and toxic waste disposal. As summarized by Chalupka (2001a), the following environmental conditions affect human health:

- Approximately 113 million people live in areas of the United States designated as *non-attainment areas* by the EPA for one or more of the six commonly found air pollutants for which the federal government has established health based standards (USDHHS, 2000). A non-attainment area is any area that does not meet the national primary or secondary ambient air quality standard for the pollutant or contributes to ambient air quality in a nearby area that does not meet either of those air quality standards.

TABLE 8-1	Landmark Federal Environmental Legislation

YEAR	LEGISLATION
1948	Water Pollution and Control Act
1962	Health Service for Agricultural Migratory Workers Act
1969	National Environmental Policy Act
1969	Coal Mine Health and Safety Act
1970	Clean Air Act
1970	Poison Prevention Packaging Act
1970	Occupational Safety and Health Act
1970	Hazardous Materials Transportation Control
1970	Environmental Protection Agency
1971	Lead-Based Paint Poisoning Prevention Act
1972	Federal Water Pollution Control Act Amendments
1972	Noise Control Act
1976	Resource Conservation and Recovery Act
1976	Toxic Substances Control Act
1977	Clean Water Act
1980	Agency for Toxic Substances and Disease Registry
1980	Low Level Radiation Waste Policy Act
1980	Comprehensive Environmental Response, Compensation, and Liability Act (i.e., Superfund)
1996	Safe Drinking Water Act

- Approximately 17.3 million Americans have asthma, often triggered by or exacerbated by indoor and outdoor air pollution; this represents a 75% increase from 1980 to 1994 (IOM, 2000). Up to 26% of asthma cases are estimated to be work-related, with more than 250 agents contributing to the asthma occurrence (CDC, 1998a).
- As of November 1999, 41 states have issued 2,073 fish advisories for mercury, a potent bioaccumulative neurotoxin. These advisories inform the public that concentrations of mercury have been found in local fish at levels of public health concern necessitating limiting or avoiding consumption of certain fish. Ten states have issued statewide advisories for mercury in their freshwater lakes and rivers (USEPA, 2000b).

- 1,200 National Priorities List (NPL) sites are located in the United States. Also known as Superfund sites, these are hazardous waste sites posing a significant risk to human health (USDHHS, 2000). Approximately 3 million to 4 million children live within 1 mile of these sites (Agency for Toxic Substances and Disease Registry [ATSDR], 1999; Landrigan et al., 1999).

Environmental hazards may be encountered at home, work, or in the community via contaminated air, soil, water, and food. Routes of exposure include inhalation, such as of dust or fumes; ingestion, such as of pesticide residues on fruits and vegetables; and dermal absorption, such as through direct skin contact with caustic household cleansers. Environmental hazards may be artificial (e.g., pesticides, auto emissions) or natural (e.g., arsenical contamination of drinking water resulting from regional geologic formation). Whether or not toxic agents pose a threat to human health depends on the distribution of substances in the environment (Figure 8-1). For example, lead released from a smelter vaporizes into the air and can be inhaled. Movement of lead from the soil to surface or groundwater may result in human exposure through contaminated drinking water or crop irrigation use. Although lead found in soil is not absorbed by plant roots, it can contaminate food crops through resuspension in water and, when deposited on vegetation, ultimately exposes humans through the ingestion of contaminated leafy vegetables. Soil also can be directly ingested, particularly by children at play in areas of contamination (Blumenthal & Ruttenber, 1995). Particulate matter released into the air can settle on soil or plants to be ingested by humans or resuspended by motion (e.g., vehicular traffic or construction activities) and inhaled (Chalupka, 2001a). Table 8-2 identifies several examples of environmental health problems (Stevens & Hall, 2001).

In *Healthy People 2010* specific objectives related to environmental health (Box 8-1) are presented here and discussed, with specific outcomes to be achieved. Figure 8-2 (USDHHS, 2000) identifies sources of environmental hazards that will be briefly discussed.

OUTDOOR AIR QUALITY

With the onset of the Industrial Revolution air pollution became a major public health problem. In October 1948 in Donora, Pennsylvania, an air

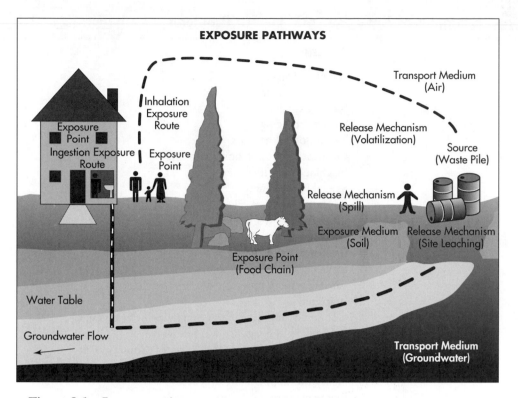

Figure 8-1 **Exposure pathways.** *(From* Public Health Assessment Guidance Manual, *by Agency for Toxic Substances and Disease Registry, 1993, Boca Raton, FL: Lewis.)*

pollution episode resulted in the deaths of 19 people in a community of 14,000 (Committee of the Environmental and Occupational Health Assembly of the American Thoracic Society, 1996). Causing premature death, cancer, and long-term damage to respiratory and cardiovascular systems, air pollution continues to be a widespread public health and environmental problem in the United States.

Air toxins reach the general population via direct assimilation into the pulmonary system and insidiously through bioaccumulation and subsequent ingestion of food, including fish and human milk, or through bioconcentration as toxins are deposited into the air from industrial processes or municipal waste incineration and redeposited on land or water (Nadakavukaren, 2000). So-called priority air pollutants are very important in causation and prevention of asthma and other chronic lung diseases. The six priority air pollutants regulated under the Clean Air Act are ozone, sulfur dioxide, respirable particulate matter, nitrogen dioxide, carbon monoxide, and lead. Priority air pollutants are regulated by the EPA strictly on a public health basis, with an adequate margin of

safety to protect the population and special attention given to protection of vulnerable populations. Air pollutants, especially those that are the product of uncontrolled coal combustion, are responsible for increased levels of morbidity and mortality in children (Bates, 1995).

Although some progress toward reducing unhealthy air emissions has been made, a substantial air pollution problem remains, with millions of tons of toxic air pollutants released into the air each year (USEPA, 1997b). Motor vehicles account for approximately one fourth of emissions that produce ozone and one third of nitrogen oxide emissions; particulate and sulfur dioxide emissions from motor vehicles represent approximately 20% and 4%, respectively. Some 76.6% of carbon monoxide emissions are produced each year by transportation sources (USEPA, 1997a).

Unhealthy air is expensive. The estimated annual health costs of human exposure to all outdoor air pollutants from all sources range from $40 billion to $50 billion, with an associated 50,000 premature deaths (American Lung Association, 1990).

TABLE 8-2   Examples of Environmental Health Problems

AREA	PROBLEMS
Living patterns	Drunk driving
	Second-hand smoke
	Noise exposure
	Urban crowding
	Technological hazards
Work	Occupational toxic poisoning
	Machine-operating hazards
	Sexual harassment
	Repetitive motion injuries
	Carcinogenic work sites
Atmospheric quality	Gaseous pollutants
	Greenhouse effect
	Destruction of the ozone layer
	Aerial spraying of herbicides and pesticides
	Acid rain
Water quality	Contamination of drinking supply by human waste
	Oil spills in the world's waterways
	Pesticide or herbicide infiltration of ground water
	Aquifer contamination by industrial pollutants
	Heavy metal poisoning of fish
Housing	Homelessness
	Rodent and insect infestation
	Poisoning from lead-based paint
	Sick building syndrome
	Unsafe neighborhoods
Food quality	Malnutrition
	Bacterial food poisoning
	Food adulteration
	Disrupted food chains by ecosystem destruction
	Carcinogenic chemical food additives
Waste control	Use of nonbiodegradable plastics
	Poorly designed solid waste dumps
	Inadequate sewage systems
	Transport and storage of hazardous waste
	Illegal industrial dumping
Radiation	Nuclear facility emissions
	Radioactive hazardous wastes
	Radon gas seepage in homes and schools
	Nuclear testing
	Excessive exposure to x-rays
Violence	Proliferation of handguns
	Increasing incidence of hate crimes
	Pervasive images of violence in the media
	High rates of homicide among young black males
	Violent acts against women and children

From "Environmental Health," by B. Stevens and J. Hall, in M. Nies and M. McEwen (Eds.) *Community Health Nursing*, Philadelphia: Saunders. 2001.

Box 8-1 *Healthy People 2010* – Environmental Health Objectives

OUTDOOR AIR QUALITY

8-1 Reduce the proportion of persons exposed to air that does not meet the U.S. Environmental Protection Agency's health-based standards for harmful air pollutants

8-2 Increase use of alternative modes of transportation to reduce motor vehicle emissions and improve the nation's air quality

8-3 Improve the nation's air quality by increasing the use of cleaner alternative fuels

8-4 Reduce air toxic emissions to decrease the risk of adverse health effects caused by airborne toxics

WATER QUALITY

8-5 Increase the proportion of persons served by community water systems who receive a supply of drinking water that meets the regulations of the Safe Drinking Water Act

8-6 Reduce waterborne disease outbreaks arising from water intended for drinking among persons served by community water systems

8-7 Reduce per capita domestic water withdrawals

8-8 (Developmental) Increase the proportion of assessed rivers, lakes, and estuaries that are safe for fishing and recreational purposes

8-9 (Developmental) Reduce the number of beach closings that result from the presence of harmful bacteria

8-10 (Developmental) Reduce the potential human exposure to persistent chemicals by decreasing fish contaminant levels

TOXICS AND WASTE

8-11 Eliminate elevated blood lead levels in children

8-12 Minimize the risks to human health and the environment posed by hazardous sites

8-13 Reduce pesticide exposures that result in visits to a health care facility

8-14 (Developmental) Reduce the amount of toxic pollutants released, disposed of, treated, or used for energy recovery

8-15 Increase recycling of municipal solid waste

HEALTHY HOMES AND HEALTHY COMMUNITIES

8-16 Reduce indoor allergen levels

8-17 (Developmental) Increase the number of office buildings that are managed using good indoor air quality practices

8-18 Increase the proportion of persons who live in homes tested for radon concentrations

8-19 Increase the number of new homes constructed to be radon resistant

8-20 (Developmental) Increase the proportion of the nation's primary and secondary schools that have official school policies ensuring the safety of students and staff from environmental hazards, such as chemicals in special classrooms, poor indoor air quality, asbestos, and exposure to pesticides

8-21 (Developmental) Ensure that state health departments establish training, plans, and protocols and conduct annual multi-institutional exercises to prepare for response to natural and technological disasters

8-22 Increase the proportion of persons living in pre-1950s housing that has been tested for the presence of lead-based paints

8-23 Reduce the proportion of occupied housing units that are substandard

INFRASTRUCTURE AND SURVEILLANCE

8-24 Reduce exposure to pesticides as measured by urine concentrations of metabolites

8-25 (Developmental) Reduce exposure of the population to pesticides, heavy metals, and other toxic chemicals, as measured by blood and urine concentrations of the substances or their metabolites

8-26 (Developmental) Improve the quality, utility, awareness, and use of existing information systems for environmental health

8-27 Increase or maintain the number of territories, tribes, and states, and the District of Columbia that monitor diseases or conditions that can be caused by exposure to environmental hazards

8-28 (Developmental) Increase the number of local health departments or agencies that use data from surveillance of environmental risk factors as part of their vector control programs

From *Healthy People 2010*, by U.S. Department of Health and Human Services, 2000, Washington, DC: Author.

Continued

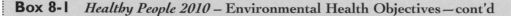

Box 8-1   *Healthy People 2010* – Environmental Health Objectives—cont'd

GLOBAL ENVIRONMENTAL HEALTH

8-29 Reduce the global burden of disease due to poor water quality, sanitation, and personal and domestic hygiene

8-30 Increase the proportion of the population in the United States-Mexico border region that have adequate drinking water and sanitation facilities

From *Healthy People 2010,* by U.S. Department of Health and Human Services, 2000, Washington, DC: Author.

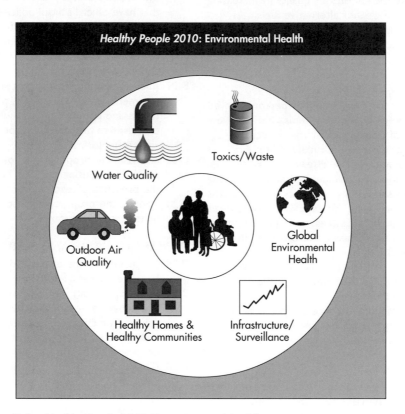

Figure 8-2   *Healthy People 2010:* Environmental health. *(From* Healthy People 2010, *by U.S. Department of Health and Human Services, 2000, Washington, DC: Author.)*

WATER QUALITY

Although 70% of the earth is covered by water, only 3% of that amount is fresh water, and two thirds of that amount is frozen in glaciers, leaving only approximately one half of 1% of the water on the earth available for human use (Chalupka, 2001b). The United States Great Lakes contain one fifth of the world's fresh water (Chlorine Chemistry Council, 2000).

Contamination of water can come from both point (e.g., industrial wastewater, municipal wastewater treatment discharge) and nonpoint (e.g., agricultural runoff, soil contamination) sources. Both point and nonpoint sources can contaminate surface waters directly and seep into underground aquifers to contaminate groundwater. Groundwater supplies serve half of the U.S. population. Mixed surface and groundwater supplies serve the other half (Etzel & Balk, 1999).

Biological and chemical contamination significantly reduce the value of surface waters (streams, lakes, and estuaries) for fishing, swimming, and other recreational activities. Synthetic organic chemicals contaminating surface and groundwater include industrial solvents, PCBs, pesticides, and DBPs. Originating from chemical manufacturing, petroleum refining, iron and steel production, wood pulp processing, textile manufacturing, and agriculture, these chemicals enter surface water through surface runoff, direct and indirect discharge, or volatilization and subsequent fallout during precipitation episodes. Groundwater can also be contaminated through downward percolation of chemicals after rains or poor waste disposal practices. In addition, chemicals such as tetrachloroethylene (TCE) can also enter drinking water supplies as leachate from polyvinyl chloride (PVC) water mains (USEPA, 1999). Showering, swimming, and other recreational water activities may result in exposure through inhalation, dermal absorption, and ingestion. When a pregnant woman ingests food or water in which pollutants have bioaccumulated, fetal exposure may occur. In addition, chronic exposure by the mother before the pregnancy may adversely affect the fetus. Polychlorinated biphenyls (PCBs) and heavy metals such as lead and mercury accumulate in the body and are not excreted easily (Etzel & Balk, 1999). During the summer of 1997, blooms of *Pfiesteria piscicida* were implicated as the likely cause of fish kills in North Carolina and Maryland. The development of intensive animal feeding operations has worsened the discharge of improperly or inadequately treated wastes, which presents an increased health threat in waters used either for recreation or for producing fish and shellfish (Minority Staff Report, 1997).

Waterborne infectious diseases have been estimated to kill as many as 900 Americans and sicken another 900,000 annually (American Society for Microbiology, 1999). The microbial contaminants of greatest concern in drinking water include bacteria, viruses, and protozoa that are usually of human or animal fecal origin (Craun, 1986). Recent bacterial drinking water disease outbreaks in the United States have been attributed to *Shigella sonnei, Giardia intestinalis,* and *Escherichia coli (E. coli)* serotype O157:H7 (CDC, 2000). *Pseudomonas* spp.,

E. coli O157:H7, *Shigella sonnei, Leptospira,* and *Legionella* infections have accounted for the majority of recreational water outbreaks. *Cryptosporidium parvum* and enteric protozoa are also a major cause of recreational water outbreaks (CDC, 2000). Clinical manifestations of cryptosporidiosis include profuse, watery diarrhea and cramping abdominal pain. Malaise, fever, anorexia, nausea, and vomiting occur less often. In children anorexia and vomiting may precede diarrhea. In immunologically healthy individuals symptoms fluctuate but usually resolve within 30 days. However, immunocompromised individuals may be unable to clear the parasite, and the disease may become prolonged and fulminant, chronic, or even contribute to death (Chin, 2000). Most outbreaks usually involve only a few individuals. However, in 1993 more than 403,000 people became sick during a single episode of waterborne cryptosporidiosis (CDC, 2000).

In the United States disinfection is usually done through chlorination. The advantage of chlorination is that it leaves a residual level in the water that prevents contamination downstream of the drinking water treatment plant. Providing drinking water free of disease-causing agents, whether biological or chemical, is the primary goal of all water supply systems.

TOXICS AND WASTE

Critical information on the levels of exposure to hazardous substances in the environment and their associated health effects often is lacking. As a result efficient health-outcome measures of progress in eliminating health hazards in the environment are unavailable. The identification of toxic substances and waste, whether hazardous, industrial, or municipal, that pose an environmental health risk represents a significant achievement in itself. Table 8-3 shows the priority list of the top 20 hazardous substances identified by ATSDR (ATSDR 1999).

Toxic and hazardous substances, including low-level radioactive wastes, deposited on land often are carried far from their sources by air, groundwater, and surface water runoff into streams, lakes, and rivers where they can accumulate in the sediments beneath the waters. Ultimate decisions about the cleanup and management of these sites must be made keeping public health concerns in mind.

The introduction and widespread use of pesticides in the American landscape continues in

TABLE

8-3   Agency for Toxic Substances and Disease Registry 1999 Priority List of Top 20 Hazardous Substances by Rank Order

HAZARDOUS AGENTS	SOURCES	EXPOSURE PATHWAYS	SYSTEMS AFFECTED
1. Arsenic	Manufacture of pigments, glass, pharmaceuticals, insecticides, fungicides, rodenticides; tanning	Ingestion, inhalation	Neuromuscular, skin, GI
2. Lead	Storage batteries; manufacture of paint, enamel, ink, glass, rubber, ceramics, chemicals	Ingestion, inhalation	Hematological, renal, neuromuscular, GI, CNS
3. Mercury	Electronics, paints, metal and textile production; chemical manufacturing; pharmaceutical production	Inhalation, percutaneous and GI absorption	Pulmonary, CNS, renal
4. Vinyl chloride	Production of polyvinyl chloride and other plastics; chlorinated compounds; used as a refrigerant	Inhalation, ingestion	Hepatic, neurologic, pulmonary
5. Benzene	Manufacture of organic chemicals, detergents, pesticides, solvents, paint removers	Inhalation, percutaneous absorption	CNS, hematopoietic
6. Polychlorinated biphenyls (PCBs)	Formerly used in electric equipment	Inhalation, ingestion	Skin, eyes, hepatic
7. Cadmium	Electroplating, solder	Inhalation	Pulmonary, renal
8. Benzo(a)pyrene	Emissions from refuse burning and autos; used as laboratory reagent; found on charcoal-grilled meats and in cigarette smoke	Inhalation, ingestion, and percutaneous absorption	Pulmonary, skin, eyes (BaP is a probable human carcinogen)
9. Polycyclic aromatic hydrocarbons (PAHs)	In coal tar, crude oil, creosote, roofing tar; also in manufacture of dyes, plastics, pesticides	Inhalation, ingestion, percutaneous absorption	Reproductive, skin
10. Benzo(b)fluoranthene	Cigarette smoke	Inhalation	Pulmonary
11. Chloroform	Aerosol propellants, fluorinated resins; produced during chlorination of water; used as a refrigerant	Inhalation, percutaneous absorption, ingestion	CNS, respiratory, mucous membranes, cardiac

From *Promoting Children's Health: Progress Report of the Child Health Workgroup Board of Scientific Counselors,* by Agency for Toxic Substances and Disease Registry, 1999, Atlanta, GA: Author.
CNS, central nervous system; *GI,* gastrointestinal; *CVS,* cardiovascular system.

TABLE 8-3

Agency for Toxic Substances and Disease Registry 1999 Priority List of Top 20 Hazardous Substances by Rank Order—cont'd

HAZARDOUS AGENTS	SOURCES	EXPOSURE PATHWAYS	SYSTEMS AFFECTED
12. DDT, p,p′ 1,1,1-trichloro-2,2-bis (p-chlorophenyl) ethane	Insecticide on agricultural crops; may be found on contaminated foods, meat, fish, poultry	Inhalation, ingestion, percutaneous absorption	CNS, hepatic
13. Arochlor 1260 (see PCBs)	Dielectric in capacitors and transformers; casting processes; heat exchange fluid; hydraulic fluid	Percutaneous, ingestion, inhalation	Hepatic, reproductive
14. Arochlor 1254 (see PCBs)	Dielectric in capacitors and transformers; casting processes; heat exchange fluid; hydraulic fluid	Percutaneous, ingestion, inhalation	Hepatic, reproductive
15. Trichloroethylene	Solvent in metal degreasing, dry cleaning, food extraction; manufacture of paint, adhesives, varnishes, inks	Inhalation, percutaneous absorption	CNS, skin, CVS
16. Chromium (+6)	Stainless and heat resistant steel and alloy steel; metal plating; chemical and pigment manufacturing; photography	Inhalation, ingestion	Pulmonary, renal
17. Dibenzo [a,h] anthracene	Major component of polynuclear aromatic hydrocarbons (AKA, PAHs); often bound to small particulate matter in urban air, industrial emissions, and cigarette smoke	Inhalation	Hepatic
18. Dieldrin	Insecticide on agricultural crops; may be found on contaminated foods, meat, fish, poultry	Inhalation, ingestion, percutaneous absorption	CNS
19. Hexachlorobutadiene	Manufacturing of rubber compounds, lubricants, heat transfer liquid, and hydraulic fluid; solvent	Inhalation, ingestion	Renal, hepatic

From *Promoting Children's Health: Progress Report of the Child Health Workgroup Board of Scientific Counselors,* by Agency for Toxic Substances and Disease Registry, 1999, Atlanta, GA: Author.
CNS, central nervous system; *GI,* gastrointestinal; *CVS,* cardiovascular system.

Continued

| TABLE 8-3 | Agency for Toxic Substances and Disease Registry 1999 Priority List of Top 20 Hazardous Substances by Rank Order—cont'd | | |

HAZARDOUS AGENTS	SOURCES	EXPOSURE PATHWAYS	SYSTEMS AFFECTED
20. DDE, p, p' 1,1-dichloro-2,2-bis (chlorophenyl) ethylene	Insecticide on agricultural crops; may be found on contaminated foods, meat, fish, poultry	Inhalation, ingestion, percutaneous absorption	CNS, hepatic

From *Promoting Children's Health: Progress Report of the Child Health Workgroup Board of Scientific Counselors,* by Agency for Toxic Substances and Disease Registry, 1999, Atlanta, GA: Author.
CNS, central nervous system; *GI,* gastrointestinal; *CVS,* cardiovascular system.

agricultural, commercial, recreational, and home settings. As a result these often very toxic substances pose a potential threat to people using them, especially if they are handled, mixed, or applied inappropriately or excessively. A pesticide is a chemical or biological agent used to control or kill a nonhuman organism considered by humans to be a pest—that is, inimical to human interest. Thus, the term *pesticide* encompasses insecticides, fungicides, herbicides, rodenticides, antimicrobial disinfectants, and biocides. Pesticides are applied extensively to food crops in nations around the world. More than 400 different pesticidal active ingredients, formulated into thousands of products, are registered for use on food in the United States. Pesticides are used at all stages of food production to protect against pests in the field and in shipping and storage (Goldman, 2000).

More than 620 chemicals are registered with the EPA as pesticides in the United States (Goldman, 1998), and when mixed with each other and inert ingredients, they produce more than 20,000 commercial pesticide products available in the marketplace (Goldman, 1998; Landrigan et al., 2000). Pesticides are widely used in homes, schools, and workplaces and have the potential to either benefit or harm human health. They may assist in the prevention of the spread of disease, improve crop yield, and be toxic to humans (Zahm & Ward, 1998).

As little as 1% of pesticides, with the exception of poison baits, reach targeted pests. The remaining 99% contaminate surfaces and air if sprayed indoors. If sprayed outdoors, the remaining 99%

fall on outdoor furniture and play areas and non-targeted organisms, plants, and animals (Etzel & Balk, 1999), and pesticides can contaminate drinking water as they enter groundwater, wells, and rivers. An estimated 50% of all the pesticides ingested in a lifetime are ingested in the first 5 years of life (ATSDR, 1999). Many pesticides are carcinogenic in animal bioassays, and some are known to be human carcinogens. Of the 51 pesticides evaluated by the National Cancer Institute and the U.S. National Toxicology Program, 24 demonstrated carcinogenicity in chronic bioassays. Many of these are still registered for use on food in the United States (Zahm & Ward, 1998).

Pesticides cause many health problems. The most important acute effects related to food contamination are cholinesterase inhibition (from high levels of organophosphates or carbamates) and developmental toxicity (due to exposure to teratogens during a sensitive period in utero). Important chronic health risks include developmental neurotoxicity, endocrine effects, and cancer. Because these effects may have a long latency period and occur after years of exposure, they may be difficult to attribute to exposure to residues in food. The EPA sets standards for allowable levels of pesticides on food. More research is needed to understand the long-term effects of chronic pesticide exposure. Epidemiologic studies have found associations between some childhood cancers, including leukemia, neuroblastoma, non-Hodgkin's lymphoma, Wilms' tumor, soft tissue sarcoma, and germ cell (testes), and pesticide exposure (Buckley et al., 2000; Kristensen et al., 1996; Leiss & Savitz, 1995; Meinert, 2000; Pagoda & Preston-Martin, 1997; Sharpe et al., 1995; Zahm & Ward, 1998).

Children are at increased risk for pesticide poisoning because of their smaller size and because pesticides may be stored improperly or applied to surfaces that are readily accessible to children. A substantial number of preschool children are exposed to or poisoned by pesticides each year. Based on calls to poison control centers, 125,000 such exposure-related cases were estimated for 1989. Based on a 1% statistical sample of the nation's emergency departments, 11,600 pesticide exposures occurred in 1985 in this age group. Of these cases 10% were admitted for hospitalization and 25% reported symptoms. Insecticides and rodenticides accounted for 87% of these cases, and ingestion had occurred in 76% of the cases. From 1977 to 1982 an estimated 900 childhood hospitalizations per year occurred due to pesticides (Blondell, 1997; Litovitz, 1997). The Toxic Exposure Surveillance System Poison Control Centers in the United States report more than 129,000 pesticide poisonings each year, with approximately 20% of individuals requiring treatment in emergency rooms (USDHHS, 2000). Workers should be aware of the risks of bringing pesticides home from the workplace for use at home and reusing chemical containers or contaminated equipment from the workplace.

HEALTHY HOMES AND COMMUNITIES

To provide a healthy environment within the nation's communities, potential risks in the places people spend the most time—their homes, schools, and offices/worksites—must be considered. These risks include indoor air pollution; inadequate heating, cooling, and sanitation; structural problems; electrical and fire hazards; lead-based paint; and hazardous household substances, such as cleaning products and pesticides. More than 6 million housing units across the country meet the Federal Government's definition of substandard housing (Bureau of Census, 1997).

In 1996 the American Association of Poison Control Centers reported more than 2 million poison exposures from 67 participating poison control centers. The site of exposure was a residence in 91% of cases (Litovitz et al., 1997). Occupational studies have proven to be import-

ant in assessing health risks from some exposures, such as radon. Studies of underground miners of uranium and other ores demonstrated that radon decay products could damage cells and cause lung cancer. The EPA used the quantitative dose-response relationship between radon levels and cancer to estimate that approximately 15,000 lung cancers every year are attributable to indoor radon. For other risks direct study of the general population has been important (National Academy of Sciences, [NAS], 1999).

Indoor environments may contain several airborne pollutants, including biological materials, vapors, gases, and particulate matter. Common sources of air pollution in the home include environmental tobacco smoke, wood and gas stoves, radon, and construction materials and home furnishings that release organic vapors and gas. Animal dander, mold spores, bacteria, and the fecal material of house dust mites and other insects are among the biological agents and allergens in the home. Natural and mechanical ventilation may even bring particulate matter from the outdoors (IOM, 2000; Moeller, 1997; O'Reilly et al., 1998).

Environmental tobacco smoke is one of the most common hazardous pollutants found indoors and is associated with a number of risks. Children with higher levels of exposure to environmental tobacco smoke show decreased growth, increased incidence of ear infections, increased incidence and severity of respiratory infections, and exacerbation of asthma. In addition, they are much more likely to become smokers and to begin smoking earlier than other children. Epidemiologic studies have shown that nonsmoking adults who are married to smokers have a higher incidence of lung cancer as well. Environmental tobacco smoke is not just a problem in the home but also in other indoor spaces, such as vehicles (USDHHS, 1986). A home environmental assessment guide is shown in Box 8-2.

INFRASTRUCTURE AND SURVEILLANCE

Preventing health problems caused by environmental hazards requires having enough personnel and resources to investigate and monitor environmental exposures. This means developing effective programs in environmental health hazard reduction; advocating laws, regulations, and public policy to prevent and control environmental health

---

Box 8-2 Home Environmental Assessment

GENERAL OBSERVATIONS

Examine areas in the immediate vicinity of the home to answer the following:

- Are water hazards present?
- Are automobile, farm, or other large equipment left in hazardous condition or in places where children could gain access?
- Are garbage/waste storage containers adequate?
- Are garages, sheds, or other outbuildings safe?
- Are chemical storage areas securely locked and adequately maintained?
- Where are pets or livestock kept; are they safe?
- Are there areas where rodents could live around home or outbuildings?
- What is the general age and condition of home (e.g., presence of peeling paint, metal edges from siding)?

Consider whether any of the aforementioned items constitute a health threat to any family members or to the community in general.

FAMILY MEMBERS

- Does anyone in the family have asthma, allergies, chronic bronchitis, burning eyes, coughing, or sneezing that happens most often while at home?
- Does anyone smoke inside the home?

HOUSING/HOUSEHOLD

- Is furniture made of particle board?
- Is there new carpet in the home?
- Are there leaks, drips, or standing water in or around the home?
- Are there hazardous household products?
- Are hazardous household products stored and disposed of properly?

- Are hazardous household products accessible to children?
- Are labels read for hazard and protection actions?
- Are space heaters that burn kerosene, propane, or natural gas, or a wood stove or fireplace used in a closed room without fresh air?
- How often are furnace, flues, and chimneys inspected and cleaned?
- Are there pets inside the house?
- Is the home tested for radon gas?
- Does the home's air ever smell musty, damp, smoky, or like chemicals?
- Does water come from a public water supply, such as the city water company or from a private water supply, such as a well or a spring?

EXTERNAL CONDITIONS

- Does the home have loose or torn screens or broken windows or gaps or holes in the building that let in pests?
- How is garbage, trash managed?
- Are airborne pesticides, like flea bombs or roach sprays, used inside the home?
- Are flea collars, sprays, or powder used on pets?
- Are pesticide labels read?
- Are children or pets in the room when pesticides are used?
- Are fruits and vegetables washed thoroughly before eating?
- Are pesticides stored in different containers from the ones in which they came?
- Are pesticides stored where children can reach them or near food?
- How are empty pesticide containers disposed of, and are they placed where children can reach them?

---

hazards; and educating the public about environmental health hazards. Efforts need to be developed and coordinated to ensure adequate resources are available to accomplish these tasks.

GLOBAL ENVIRONMENTAL HEALTH

Increased international travel and improvements in telecommunications and computer technology are making the world a smaller place. The term

global community has real significance because shared resources—air, water, and soil—draw people together. Actions in every country affect the environment and influence events around the world. For example, in 1996 the United States exported more than $2.5 billion worth of pesticides (SRI International, 1998). Exported pesticides that are not registered or pesticides that are restricted for use in the United States are often used by developing countries. Their use not only endangers populations in those countries but also can contaminate food being exported from those countries to the United States. Sensitive populations, such as children, pregnant women, and the elderly, may be at increased risk from these environmental exposures.

TRENDS

During the 1990s progress in improving environmental health was mixed. The decline in childhood lead poisoning in the United States represents a public health success. In 1984 between 2 million and 3 million children age 6 months to 5 years had blood lead levels (BLLs) greater that 15 μg/dL, and almost a quarter of a million had BLLs above 25 μg/dL, a level which can damage vital organs and the brain (ATSDR, 1989). By the early 1990s fewer than 900,000 children had BLLs above 10 μg/dL, the current standard for identifying children at risk. This dramatic reduction is the result of research to identify persons at risk, professional and public education campaigns, broad-based screening measures to find those at risk, and effective community efforts to clean up problem areas, namely substandard housing units (CDC, 1997; USDHHS, 2000).

Since the mid-1980s asthma rates in the United States have risen to the level of an epidemic (Last, 1998). Asthma and other respiratory conditions often are triggered or worsened by airborne substances, such as tobacco smoke, ozone, and other particles or chemicals. Based on existing data, an estimated 17.3 million people had asthma in 1998, including more than 5 million children age 18 years and under (CDC, 1998a). Between 1980 and 1993 the overall death rate for asthma increased 52%, from 12.8 to 19.5 per million population; for people age 18 years and under, the death rate increased 67%, from 1.8 to 3.0 per million population. The direct economic and health care costs of asthma and other respiratory conditions can be large. In 1990 the estimated total cost of asthma was $6.2 billion; the total cost was projected to rise to $14.5 billion by the year 2000. The indirect costs of asthma, measured in reduced quality of life and lost productivity, include the estimated 10 million school days that children miss each year. Lost productivity from missed work days of parents caring for children with asthma is estimated to be $1 billion, not including the cost of lost productivity from adults with asthma who miss work (Weiss et al., 1992).

Urban sprawl has become an increasingly important concern in the United States for several reasons: increased outdoor air pollution in major urban areas, reduced quality of life due to the loss of free time and the stress of increased commuting time, and less green space in major metropolitan areas. Between 1983 and 1995 the average annual vehicle miles traveled increased 80% (Summary of Travel Trends, 1999). These conditions lead to negative health conditions, such as asthma and injuries from road rage due to traffic-related stress. In addition, sprawl diminishes the amount of land available for prime recreational and agricultural uses and can bring two land uses together that do not coexist well. Examples include when new residential development in an area that was previously agricultural exposes new residents to sounds, smells, and substances, such as pesticides, that can pose a possible hazard to their health, or when urban sprawl and development reduces or eliminates land used for nature's wildlife creating road accidents from animals forced onto highways and roads.

To be successful, programs to improve environmental health must be based on scientific evidence. The complex relationship between human health and the acute and long-term effects of environmental exposures must be studied so prevention measures can be developed. Surveillance systems to track exposures to toxic substances, such as commonly used pesticides and heavy metals, must be developed and maintained. To the extent possible, these systems should use biomonitoring data, which provide measurements of toxic substances in the human body. A mechanism is needed for tracking the export of pesticides restricted or not registered for use in the United States.

Toxic air pollutants are those pollutants known or suspected to cause cancer or other serious health effects, such as reproductive effects or birth defects, or cause adverse environmental effects (USDHHS, 2000). The degree to which a toxic air pollutant affects a person's health depends on many factors, including the quantity of pollutant to which the person is exposed, the duration and frequency of exposures, the toxicity of the chemical, and the person's state of health and susceptibility. Examples of toxic air pollutants include benzene, which is found in gasoline; perchloroethylene, which is emitted from some dry cleaning facilities; and methylene chloride, which is used as a solvent and paint stripper by a number of industries. Examples of other air toxics include dioxin, asbestos, toluene, and metals such as cadmium, mercury, chromium, and lead compounds.

The USEPA (2000b) reported that about 40% of the nation's surface waters (streams, lakes, and estuaries) are too polluted for fishing, swimming, or other uses designated by states and tribes. Water quality in lakes, streams, and estuaries affects both their recreational and food production use. States and tribes have water-quality management programs that address recreational use and fish and shellfish harvesting. The USEPA establishes water-quality objectives for these bodies of water and monitors progress toward these goals. Discharging inadequately treated or inappropriate quantities of human, industrial, or agriculture wastes reduces the ability of water to provide conditions that support the growth and harvesting of fish and shellfish for human consumption. Such discharging also prevents water's use as a recreational resource.

Indoor allergens, such as those from house dust mites, cockroaches, mold, rodents, and pets, can worsen symptoms of respiratory conditions, such as asthma and allergies. These allergies are an important public health issue because most people spend the majority of their time indoors, both at home and at work. Fortunately, effective methods to reduce exposure to some of these allergens exist (e.g., placement of impermeable covers on mattresses and pillows reduces dust mite allergen exposures in beds).

NURSING AND ENVIRONMENTAL HEALTH

As described in Chapter 2, nursing's efforts in environmental health has its underpinnings with the work began by Florence Nightingale, the founder of modern nursing, who advocated and emphasized the importance of the following five environmental health dimensions:

1. Pure fresh air
2. Pure fresh water
3. Efficient, sanitary drainage
4. Cleanliness and hygiene
5. Direct light (Nightingale, 1859)

In the following passage from *Notes on Nursing; What It Is And What It Is Not*, Nightingale (1859), stresses the importance of these five environmental dimensions and relates how deficiencies in or neglect of these contexts will ultimately result in disease, illness, lack of comfort, and death:

In watching disease, both in private houses and in public hospitals, the thing which strikes the experienced observer most forcibly is this, that the symptoms or the sufferings generally considered to be inevitable and incident to the disease are very often not symptoms of the disease at all, but of something quite different— of the want of fresh air, or of light, or of warmth, or of quiet, or of cleanliness, or of punctuality and care in the administration of diet, of each or of all of these. And this quite as much in private as in hospital nursing.

The very first canon of nursing, the first and the last thing upon which a nurse's attention must be fixed, the first essential to the patient, without which all the rest you can do for him is as nothing, with which I had almost said you may leave all the rest alone, is this: TO KEEP THE AIR HE BREATHES AS PURE AS THE EXTERNAL AIR, WITHOUT CHILLING HIM. Yet what is so little attended to? Even where it is thought of at all, the most extraordinary misconceptions reign about it. Even in admitting air into the patient's room or ward, few people ever think, where that air comes from. It may come from a corridor into which other wards are ventilated, from a hall, always unaired, always full of fumes of gas, dinner, of various kinds of mustiness; from an underground kitchen, sink, washhouse, water-closet, or even, as I myself have had sorrowful experience, from open sewers loaded with filth; and with this the patient's room or ward is aired, as it is called—poisoned, it should rather be said. (p. 8)

Registered nurses occupy a unique position among health care providers. In both rural and urban settings nurses are often the initial, and sometimes the only, point of contact for people seeking medical care. Estimated at 2.2 million, nurses are also the largest group of professional health care providers in the United States (IOM,

1995). In occupational health practice nurses outnumber physicians by six to one. The close interaction of nurses with patients and the on-site aspects of nursing care provide tremendous opportunities for nurses to detect previously unrecognized health problems, including those related to environmental exposures, and to initiate appropriate interventions. Finally, a good fit exists between environmental health concerns, the historical development of the nursing profession, and core nursing values. On a daily basis regardless of specialty or practice site, nurses meet people who are at risk or ill because of hazards in the environment, such as contaminated food or drinking water, toxic waste, occupational exposures to harmful substances and conditions, lead and radon in the home, and health-threatening conditions related to poverty. The health benefits to patients from nurses' education and involvement in addressing environmental health concerns are potentially enormous (IOM, 1995).

With environmental influences on health so widespread and so consequential, an understanding of environmental health is important in all areas of nursing practice, including assessment, diagnosis, planning, intervention, and evaluation. This is already recognized to a large extent in community and public health nursing and in occupational and environmental health nursing. For example, occupational and environmental health nurses routinely take environmental influences and concerns into account when assessing a patient's health status. The same approach needs to be used more widely in other areas of nursing practice (Nyman et al., 2001).

Nurses caring for economically disadvantaged patients should be aware that vulnerable populations often face an increased risk of exposure to hazardous environmental pollutants (IOM, 1995). For example, low income and minority populations are more likely to (1) live near or work in heavily polluting industries, hazardous waste dump sites, and incinerators (2) live in substandard houses with friable asbestos and deteriorating lead paint and have yards with contaminated soil, and (3) be exposed to toxic chemicals through diets that include seafood or fish taken from local waters designated unfit for swimming and fishing (ATSDR, 1992). Thus, the environmental burden weighs heavily upon minorities and the economically disadvantaged because they

are exposed to a disproportionate number and intensity of environmental pollutants in food, air, water, homes, and workplaces. Inequalities of this kind have generated sharp controversies, often cast in terms of environmental justice, about legislative and regulatory measures that can be used to decrease the burden of pollution on disadvantaged communities.

Accurately quantifying the burden of morbidity and mortality related to environmental exposures is impossible for several reasons: poor compliance with reporting requirements for occupational illness, long latency periods between initial exposure and resulting disease, inability of health care providers to recognize environmental causes of diseases, and absence of national reporting systems for environmentally related illnesses. The extent of the problem is further obscured by the multifactorial causes of many environmentally related diseases (e.g., lung cancer caused by exposure to asbestos is more likely to occur among people who smoke tobacco) (IOM, 1995).

The workplace is an important setting to consider when studying environmentally related illness; environmental hazards and exposures can be substantial in occupational settings. At present workplace injuries and fatalities are the most well-documented indices of adverse effects of the environment on health (NIOSH, 2000).

Individuals vary widely in their susceptibility to adverse health effects following exposure to toxic substances. Personal characteristics such as age, gender, weight, genetic composition, nutritional status, physiologic status (including pregnancy), preexisting disease states, behavioral and lifestyle factors, and concomitant or past exposures may all affect human responses to environmental conditions. The manner in which these characteristics may enhance or decrease susceptibility to environmental hazards is in some cases fairly obvious, while in others it is less obvious. For example, adverse reproductive capacity varies by gender and exposure (Table 8-4). The unique vulnerabilities of individuals at two extremes of the life cycle, that is young children and the aged, are similar in many ways due either to the immaturity or normal decline in functioning of major physiologic processes.

Elderly populations have progressively decreasing function of major system processes, resulting in impaired host defenses, impaired immune system

TABLE 8-4

Environmental and Occupational Exposures Associated With Adverse Reproductive Capacity

	FEMALES			MALES	
AGENT	**OUTCOMES**	**STRENGTH OF ASSOCIATION***	**AGENT**	**OUTCOMES**	**STRENGTH OF ASSOCIATION***
Anesthetic gases†	Reduced fertility, spontaneous abortion	1.3	Boron	Decreased sperm count	1.0
Arsenic	Spontaneous abortion, low birth weight	1.0	Benzene	None	NA†
Benzo(a)pyrene	None	NA‡	Benzo(a)pyrene	None	NA
Cadmium	None	NA	Cadmium	Reduced fertility	1.0
Carbon disulfide	Menstrual disorders, spontaneous abortion	1.0	Carbon disulfide	Decreased sperm count, decreased sperm motility	2.3
Carbon monoxide	Low birth weight, fetal death (high doses)	1.0	Carbon monoxide	None	NA
Chlordecone	None	NA	Carbon tetrachloride	None	NA
Chloroform	None	NA	Carbaryl	Abnormal sperm morphology	1.0
Chloroprene	None	NA	Chlordecone	Decreased sperm count, decreased sperm motility	2.0
Ethylene glycol ethers	Spontaneous abortion	1.0	Chloroprene	Decreased sperm motility, abnormal morphology, decreased libido	2.0
Ethylene oxide	Spontaneous abortion	1.0	Dibromochloropropane (DBCP)	Decreased sperm count, azoospermia, hormonal changes	2.0
Formamides	None	NA	Dimethyl dichlorovinyl phosphate (DDVP)	None	NA
Inorganic mercury‡	Menstrual disorders, spontaneous abortion	1.0	Epichlorohydrin	None	NA
Lead‡	Spontaneous abortion, prematurity, neurologic dysfunction in child	2.0	Estrogens	Decreased sperm count	2.0

Agent	Female reproductive effect	Strength of evidence*
Organic mercury	CNS malformation, cerebral palsy	2.0
Physical stress	Prematurity	2.0
Polybrominated biphenyls (PBBs)	None	NA
Polychlorinated biphenyls (PCBs)	Neonatal PCB syndrome (low birth weight, hyperpigmentation, eye abnormalities)	2.0
Radiation, ionizing	Menstrual disorders, CNS defects, skeletal and eye anomalies, mental retardation, childhood cancer	2.0
Selenium	Spontaneous abortion	3.0
Tellurium	None	NA
2,4-Dichlorophen-oxyacetic acid (2,4-D)	Skeletal defects	4.0
2,4,5-Trichlorophen-oxyacetic acid	Skeletal defects	4.0
Video display terminals	Spontaneous abortion	4.0
Vinyl chloride‡	CNS defects	1.0
Xylene	Menstrual disorders, fetal loss	1.0

Agent	Male reproductive effect	Strength of evidence*
Ethylene oxide	None	NA
Ethylene dibromide (EDB)	Abnormal sperm motility	1.0
Ethylene glycol ethers	Decreased sperm count	1.0
Heat	Decreased sperm count	2.0
Lead	Decreased sperm count	2.0
Manganese	Decreased libido, impotence	1.0
Polybrominated biphenyls (PBBs)	None	NA
Polychlorinated biphenyls (PCBs)	None	NA
Radiation, ionizing	Decreased sperm count	2.0

Data from *Occupational and Environmental Medicine*, by J. LaDou, 2000, Stamford, CT: Appleton & Lange; *Occupational Health* by B. Levy, and D. Wegman, 2000. Boston: Little, Brown, & Company; *Promoting Children's Health: Progress Report of the Child Health Workgroup Board of Scientific Counselors*, by Agency for Toxic Substances and Disease Registry, 1999, Atlanta, GA: Author; *Public Health Assessment Guidance Manual*, by Agency for Toxic Substances and Disease Registry, 1993, Boca Raton, FL: Lewis.

*1, limited positive data; 2, strong positive data; 3, limited negative data; 4, strong negative data.

† Not applicable because no adverse outcomes were observed.

‡ Agents that may have male mediated effects. Source ATSDR (1993).

Note: Major studies of the reproductive health effects of exposure to dioxin are currently in progress.

function, and changes in their ability to detoxify chemicals (Tarcher, 1992).

Changes in the stratum corneum of the skin can increase the percutaneous absorption of chemicals. Structural and functional changes that occur in the lung with advanced age, including loss of elasticity and impaired ciliary action, can result in more rapid absorption and decreased clearance of foreign substances in the lung. A decline in the metabolic clearance of certain drugs that require oxidative mechanisms for biotransformation has been noted in aged populations that may also result in a decreased ability to detoxify environmental toxins. Declines in blood flow to both liver and kidney, in part due to declining cardiac output estimated at 1% annually after age 30, may result in a decreased ability to detoxify and eliminate toxic substances from the body among aged populations. Immune system function is also impaired with aging, including a reduction in cell-mediated immunity. Body composition changes occur with aging, with a marked increase in adipose tissue mass and decline in lean body mass . . . As a result of changes in body composition, water soluble drugs and chemicals have a smaller volume of distribution and greater serum levels, while lipid-soluble substances have an increased volume of distribution. This spectrum of physiologic changes in the aged may increase or decrease both their susceptibility to, and the magnitude of, adverse health outcomes associated with exposure to environmental hazards.

Children . . . have a higher basal metabolic rate than adults, which affects the absorption and metabolism of toxicants. Children also have a different breathing zone than adults; they are closer to the floor, where dust, dirt, and toxic heavy metals such as lead are deposited. The rapid growth and differentiation of cells in young children leaves them more susceptible to genetic alterations associated with many chemical exposures (Reigart & Roberts, 1999). An increased rate of cell proliferation can indirectly lead to carcinogenesis by increasing the likelihood that spontaneous mutation will occur or by decreasing the time available to repair DNA damage (NRC, 1993). Moreover, the normal hand-to-mouth activity of toddlers increases the likelihood of exposure through in-

gestion of toxic substances. Because some toxicants are retained in "biologic sanctuaries" (e.g., lead in bone and polycyclic aromatic hydrocarbons in fat), they can cause low-dose chronic exposure for a much longer period of time than would be experienced by exposed adults (CEHN, 1999). (IOM, 1995, pp. 33-34)

GENERAL ENVIRONMENTAL HEALTH COMPETENCIES IN NURSING

The environment is one of the primary determinants of the health status of individuals and populations. There is increased awareness of the need for the preservation of environmental resources in addition to concern about the adverse effects of the degradation of home, community, and global environments on human health. Increasingly, occupational and environmental health nurses will need to have the basic competencies in environmental health.

In its report *Nursing, Health, and the Environment* the Institute of Medicine provides several recommendations related to environmental health and nursing in nursing practice, education, and research (Box 8-3) and also outlines four general competencies relevant to nursing practice (Box 8-4). To discuss each of these in great detail is impossible in one chapter; however, each competency area is briefly addressed.

BASIC KNOWLEDGE

Nurses must have basic knowledge about environmental health integrated into practice. For individuals to be harmed by environmental contamination, several factors must be in place, including an exposure source, environmental media for transport and release mechanism, route of exposure, dose concentration, and receptor population. To reduce or eliminate health hazards, the exposure pathway must be interrupted through control and prevention strategies. For example, waste products can be disposed of through incineration or, if disposed of in water, must be adequately treated to ensure that the dosage in water is not great enough to cause harm or that the waste product can be altered to a less toxic form (Cary & Mood, 2000). Whatever intervention mechanism is used, an interdisciplinary approach will be vital. If environmental health

---

Box 8-3   **Summary Listing of Institute of Medicine Recommendations for Environmental Health and Nursing**

NURSING PRACTICE

Recommendation 3.1: Environmental health should be reemphasized in the scope of responsibilities for nursing practice.

Recommendation 3.2: Resources to support environmental health content in nursing practice should be identified and made available.

Recommendation 3.3: Nurses should participate as members and leaders in interdisciplinary teams that address environmental health problems.

Recommendation 3.4: Communication should extend beyond counseling individual patients and families to facilitating the exchange of information on environmental hazards and community responses.

Recommendation 3.5: The concept of advocacy in nursing should be expanded to include advocacy on behalf of groups and communities, in addition to advocacy on behalf of individual patients and their families.

Recommendation 3.6: Conduct research regarding the ethical implications of occupational and environmental health hazards and incorporate findings into curricula and practice.

NURSING EDUCATION

Recommendation 4.1: Environmental health concepts should be incorporated into all levels of nursing education.

Recommendation 4.2: Environmental health content should be included in nursing licensure and certification examinations.

Recommendation 4.3: Expertise in various environmental health disciplines should be included in the education of nurses.

Recommendation 4.4: Environmental health content should be an integral part of lifelong learning and continuing education for nurses.

Recommendation 4.5: Professional associations, public agencies, and private organizations should provide more resources and educational opportunities to enhance environmental health in nursing practice.

NURSING RESEARCH

Recommendation 5.1: Multidisciplinary and interdisciplinary research endeavors should be developed and implemented to build the knowledge base for nursing practice in environmental health.

Recommendation 5.2: The number of nurse researchers should be increased to prepare to build the knowledge base in environmental health as it relates to the practice of nursing.

Recommendation 5.3: Research priorities for nursing in environmental health should be established and used by funding agencies for resource allocation decisions and to give direction to nurse researchers.

Recommendation 5.4: Current efforts to disseminate research findings to nurses, other health care providers, and the public should be strengthened and expanded.

From *Nursing, Health, and the Environment,* by Institute of Medicine, 1995, Washington, DC: National Academy Press.

---

concerns are to be included in practice in meaningful ways, nurses will need to function as members of professional teams. For effective teamwork all health professionals—nurses, physicians, and allied health personnel—need to place a greater emphasis on skills required for interprofessional collaboration, such as negotiation, critical thinking, and mutual problem solving. In addition, there must be opportunities for interdisciplinary interaction throughout professional education and clinical practice, and existing barriers to interdisciplinary practice must be removed.

ASSESSMENT AND REFERRAL

The second general environmental health competency is assessment and referral. The human response to environmental conditions varies with personal characteristics, including age, weight, gender, nutritional status, physiological status, preexisting disease states, concomitant or previous exposures, and even behavioral and lifestyle factors; these will need to be assessed. Assessment includes several elements such as individual health assessments, community assessments, and environmental health site assessments. In conducting these

Box 8-4 General Environmental
Health Competencies for Nurses

BASIC KNOWLEDGE AND CONCEPTS

All nurses should understand the scientific principles and underpinnings of the relationship between individuals or populations and the environment (including the work environment). This understanding includes the basic mechanisms and pathways of exposure to environmental health hazards, basic prevention and control strategies, the interdisciplinary nature of effective interventions, and the role of research.

ASSESSMENT AND REFERRAL

All nurses should be able to successfully complete an environmental health history, recognize potential environmental hazards and sentinel illnesses, and make appropriate referrals for conditions with probable environmental etiologies. An essential component of this is the ability to access and provide information to patients and communities and to locate referral sources.

ADVOCACY, ETHICS, AND RISK COMMUNICATION

All nurses should be able to demonstrate knowledge of the role of advocacy (case and class), ethics, and risk communication in patient care and community intervention with respect to the potential adverse effects of the environment on health.

LEGISLATION AND REGULATION

All nurses should understand the policy framework and major pieces of legislation and regulations related to environmental health.

From *Nursing, Health, and the Environment,* by Institute of Medicine, 1995, Washington, DC: National Academy Press.

assessments, an environmental exposure history must be taken. Environmental health components of history taking can be integrated into the routine assessment of patients by including questions about prior exposure to chemical, physical, or biological hazards and about temporal relationships between the onset of symptoms and activities performed before or during the occurrence of symptoms. During an assessment the nurse should be alert to patterns of comorbidity among patients, family members, workers, and communities, which may indicate environmental causes (Rogers, 1994). Nurses also conduct assessments during visits to

patients in their homes and places of work, gaining first hand information about environmental factors that may adversely affect health. In addition, the nurse will want to gather as much information as possible about exposure sources and related health effects. Box 8-5 presents detailed information related to occupational and environmental exposure assessment; Appendix 8-1 presents an excerpt for conducting an exposure history as part of *Case Studies in Environmental Medicine* developed by ATSDR (ATSDR, 1992, 2000).

Many federal, state, and local agencies can supply vast amounts of information about specific exposures. For example, the Agency for Toxic Substances and Disease Registry (ATSDR) was created by Superfund legislation in 1980 as a part of the U.S. Department of Health and Human Services. ATSDR's mission is to prevent or mitigate adverse human health effects and diminished quality of life resulting from exposure to hazardous substances in the environment. In order to carry out its mission and serve the needs of the people, ATSDR conducts activities in public health assessments, health investigations, exposure and disease registry, emergency response, toxicological profiles, health education, and applied research (ATSDR, 1992). Table 8-5 identifies resource information areas within ATSDR. The National Institute of Environmental Health Sciences is the principal federal agency for biomedical research on the effects of chemical, physical, and biological agents on human health and well-being. Research results form the basis for environmental programs for environmentally related diseases and policy and legislative action.

States also provide valuable environmental health information. For example, states may have separate priority sites and listings that are handled by state environmental agencies. These sites do not receive federal attention or funding but may be a priority within the state. Regardless, state environmental agencies often have valuable information about environmental contamination in their communities, including environmental monitoring data, health advisories, previous studies, and other data bases. State health agencies may have useful epidemiologic information, including disease registries and other statistics. Many states also have environmental epidemiologists who can be instrumental in identifying and analyzing an environmental contamination of potential health concern.

Box 8-5 Detailed Interview for Occupational and Environmental Exposures

ADULT PATIENT
OCCUPATIONAL EXPOSURE

- What is your occupation? (if unemployed, go to next section)
- How long have you been doing this job?
- Describe your work and hazards you are exposed to (e.g., pesticides, solvents or other chemicals, dust, fumes, metals, fibers, radiation, biological agents, noise, heat, cold, vibration).
- Under what circumstances do you use protective equipment (e.g., work clothes, safety glasses, respirator, gloves, hearing protection)?
- Do you smoke or eat at the worksite?
- List previous jobs in chronological order, include full-time and part-time, temporary, second jobs, summer jobs, and military experience. (Because this question can take a long time to answer, one option is to ask the patient to fill out a form with this question on it prior to the formal history taking by the clinician. Another option is to take a shorter history by asking the patient to list only the prior jobs that involved the agents of interest. For example, one could ask for all current and past jobs involving pesticide exposure.)

ENVIRONMENTAL EXPOSURE HISTORY

- Are pesticides (e.g., bug or weed killers, flea and tick sprays, collars, powders, shampoos) used in your home or garden or on your pet?
- Do you or any household member have a hobby with exposure to any hazardous materials (e.g., pesticides, paints, ceramics, solvents, metals, glues)?
- Ask the following if pesticides are used:
  - Is a licensed pesticide applicator involved?
  - Are children allowed to play in areas recently treated with pesticides?
  - Where are the pesticides stored?
  - Is food handled properly (e.g., washing of raw fruits and vegetables)?
- Did you ever live near a facility which could have contaminated the surrounding area (e.g., mine, plant, smelter, dump site)?
- Have you ever changed your residence because of a health problem?
- Does your drinking water come from a private well, city water supply, or grocery store?
- Do you work on your car?

- Which of the following do you have in your home: air conditioner, air purifier, central heating (gas or oil), gas stove, electric stove, fireplace, wood stove, or humidifier?
- Have you recently acquired new furniture or carpet or remodeled your home?
- Have you weatherized your home recently?
- Approximately what year was your home built?

SYMPTOMS AND MEDICAL CONDITIONS (if employed)

- Does the timing of your symptoms have any relationship to your work hours?
- Has anyone else at work suffered the same or similar problems?
- Does the timing of your symptoms have any relationship to environmental activities listed above?
- Has any other household member or nearby neighbor suffered similar health problems?

NONOCCUPATIONAL EXPOSURES POTENTIALLY RELATED TO ILLNESS OR INJURY

- Do you use tobacco? If yes, in what forms (cigarettes, pipe, cigar, chewing tobacco)? Approximately how much tobacco do you smoke or use per day? At what age did you start using tobacco? Are there other tobacco smokers in the home?
- Do you drink alcohol? How much per day or week? At what age did you start?
- What medications or drugs are you taking? (Include prescription and nonprescription uses.)
- Has anyone in the family worked with hazardous materials that they might have brought home (e.g., pesticides, asbestos, lead)? (If yes, inquire about household members potentially exposed.)

PEDIATRIC PATIENT (QUESTIONS ASKED OF OR ABOUT PARENT OR GUARDIAN)
OCCUPATIONAL EXPOSURE

- What is your occupation and that of other household members? (If no employed individuals, go to next section.)
- Describe your work and hazards you are exposed to (e.g., pesticides, solvents or other chemicals, dusts, fumes, metals, fibers, radiation, biological agents, noise, heat, cold, vibration).

Modified from "Environmental and Occupational History," by A. M. Orsorio, in J. Rout Reigard and J. R. Roberts (Eds.), *Recognition and Management of Pesticide Poisonings* (5th ed., 735-R-98-003), 1999, Washington, DC: Environmental Protection Agency.

Continued

Box 8-5   Detailed Interview for Occupational and Environmental Exposures—cont'd

ENVIRONMENTAL EXPOSURE HISTORY

- Are pesticides (e.g., bug or weed killers, flea and tick sprays, collars, powders, shampoos) used in the patient's home or garden or on the patient's pet?
- Does the patient or any household member have a hobby with exposure to any hazardous materials (e.g., pesticides, paints, ceramics, solvents, metals, glues)?
- Ask the following if pesticides are used:
  - Is a licensed pesticide applicator involved?
  - Are children allowed to play in areas recently treated with pesticides?
  - Where are the pesticides stored?
  - Is food handled properly (e.g., washing of raw fruits and vegetables)?
- Has the patient ever lived near a facility which could have contaminated the surrounding area (e.g., mine, plant, smelter, dump site)?
- Has the patient ever changed residence because of a health problem?
- Does the patient's drinking water come from a private well, city water supply, or grocery store?
- Which of the following are in the patient's home: air conditioner, air purifier, central heating (gas or oil), gas stove, electric stove, fireplace, wood stove, or humidifier?

- Has new furniture or carpet recently been acquired or remodeling been done recently in the patient's home?
- Has the home been weatherized recently?
- Approximately what year was your home built?

SYMPTOMS AND MEDICAL CONDITIONS

- Does the timing of symptoms have any relationship to environmental activities listed above?
- Has any other household member or nearby neighbor suffered similar health problems?

NONOCCUPATIONAL EXPOSURES POTENTIALLY RELATED TO ILLNESS OR INJURY

- Are there tobacco users in the patient's home? If yes, in what forms (cigarettes, cigar, chewing tobacco)?
- What mediations or drugs is the patient taking? (Include prescription and nonprescription uses)
- Has anyone in the family worked with hazardous materials that they might have brought to the patient's home (e.g., pesticides, asbestos, lead)? (If yes, inquire about household members potentially exposed.)

Modified from "Environmental and Occupational History," by A. M. Orsorio, in J. Rout Reigard and J. R. Roberts (Eds.), *Recognition and Management of Pesticide Poisonings* (5th ed., 735-R-98-003), 1999, Washington, DC: Environmental Protection Agency.

Additional environmental and health information is often available at the local level as well. Local health department sanitarians or other environmental professionals can provide valuable information on community contamination, toxic waste problems, and local ordinances. An example of a case study investigated by a local health department is shown in Box 8-6 (ATSDR, 1991). Birth, death, or other vital records may show trends in health outcomes, which may help assess environmental health at the community level.

Referral is an important skill for the occupational and environmental health nurse because it relies on the nurse's judgment that an intervention other than or in addition to nursing is needed. Referral resources may be individual or community-level directed. Thus, the nurse will need to have an inventory of occupational and environmental medical practitioners whom a patient with signs and symptoms of an environmental exposure could see for medical intervention. Additional resources, such as federal, state, and local agencies that can provide expertise in dealing with environmental problems, will be critical. This may include local health departments and environmental protection agencies; emergency centers and poison control centers; agricultural extension services; occupational and environmental health experts

TABLE 8-5	ATSDR* Information Resources	
RESOURCE NAME	**PHONE NUMBER**	**DESCRIPTION OF RESOURCE**
ATSDR* *Case Studies in Environmental Medicine*	ATSDR Division of Health Education: (404) 498-0101	Self-instruction publications designed to increase the primary care provider's knowledge of hazardous substances in the environment and aid in the evaluation of potentially exposed patients (*Case Studies* available for over 30 hazardous substances)
ATSDR *Public Health Statements*	ATSDR Division of Toxicology: (404) 498-0160	Document describing a substance's relevant toxicological properties in a nontechnical, question and answer format (*Public Health Statements* available for 80 hazardous substances)
ATSDR *Toxicological Profiles*	ATSDR Division of Toxicology: (404) 498-0160	Document providing information on the health effects of a substance by route of exposure, levels of a substance in the human body and in the environment that are associated with health effects, chemical and physical information, and regulations and advisories for the substance (*Toxicological Profiles* available for over 100 hazardous substances)
ATSDR Emergency Response Line	ATSDR Division of Health Assessment and Consultation: (404) 498-0007	Assistance on health issues pertaining to the release or threat of release of hazardous materials; assistance provided to federal, state, and local agencies, first responders, hospitals, private industry, and the general public
ATSDR Division of Health Assessment and Consultation Community Involvement Liaison	ATSDR Division of Health Assessment and Consultation: (404) 498-0007	Information on ATSDR's public health assessment and consultation process

*Agency for Toxic Substances and Disease Registry web address: http://www.atsdr.cdc.gov/

in schools of medicine, nursing, and public health; and professional and voluntary agencies with environmental health information and guidance resources. Appendix 8-2 provides a list of poison control centers and agency and Appendix 8-3 a list of organizational environmental health resources. However, many resources are available through the Internet and can be located through common search engines.

ADVOCACY, ETHICS, AND RISK COMMUNICATION

Interventions in environmental health problems often require nurses and other health care professionals to assume the roles of advocate, activist, and policy planner on behalf of an individual patient or population of patients (IOM, 1995) and use skills based in advocacy, ethics, and risk communication, skills that constitute the third general competency. Patient advocacy, or bringing

Box 8-6 Illustrative Case Study

A female infant born weighing 7 pounds, 9 ounces, appeared healthy during her first month at home. However, she became ill at 3 weeks of age and developed diarrhea and vomiting after feeding. At 6 weeks of age she was hospitalized for treatment of vomiting, failure to thrive, and dehydration. She weighed 6 pounds, 10 ounces, and had no other signs of infection. The infant was rehydrated and returned to her home the following day. After 6 days at home, she was readmitted with recurrence of symptoms and a diagnosis of failure to thrive. Her blood hemoglobin level was normal; however, her methemoglobin level was 21.4 % (normal level, 0%-3%). She was diagnosed with methemoglobinemia and treated with oral fluids and oxygen, and within 24 hours her methemoglobin level dropped to 11.1 %. The family began using bottled water to dilute the formula, and symptoms did not recur. The family's home was situated on a river bank near 100 acres of corn and alfalfa. Water was supplied by a shallow 28-foot standpoint well. Water samples collected from the well during the infant's hospitalization were analyzed and found to contain excess levels of nitrates, and water samples from the kitchen faucet were found to contain excess levels of copper. On the basis of these analyses, the health department recommended that the family use bottled water for drinking and food preparation.

a patient's concerns to the attention of the physician within the health care setting, is familiar to most, if not all, nurses. However, advocacy that goes beyond the confines of the health care system is a new kind of activity for many nurses who may feel ill-equipped for translating research and practice issues into health policy terms. Appendix 8-4 provides a position statement by the International Council of Nurses that speaks to these issues.

The nurse advocate provides information on technical matters as well as on the decision process and may speak on behalf of the community in policy discussions about environmental health. The nurse can be a welcomed partner in facilitating the public input process, which may be the activity and interaction that is most uncomfortable for environmental scientists. The public generally has known and had experience with nurses as empathetic listeners and professionals with the community's interests at heart. Having a nurse as a facilitator of the dialogue allows people to relax a little, knowing they will be heard. Increased civility and respectful attention can lead to better outcomes in public dialogue. The skillful nurse advocate and facilitator can be instrumental in shifting the organizational culture of regulatory agencies and regulated industries to view public participation as valued rather than required and in promoting dialogues in which new and useful information leads to better decisions (Cary & Mood, 2000).

Occupational and environmental health nurses are obligated to practice using an ethical framework to provide competent and safe practice and protect clients from health hazards. This practice is vital in the area of environmental health. Nurses may find themselves in situations where they wish to advocate for clients or communities who are at risk for adverse environmental exposures. All individuals have the right to know about actual or potential health exposures in order to make informed decisions about the protection of their health and that of their families and future offspring. For example, if a toxic spill occurs in a community or workers are exposed to chemical toxicants, the health professional has an ethical obligation to inform all parties of the potential consequences of the exposure. In some situations community leaders and company executives assume a paternalistic posture because they believe that they know what is best in terms of information disclosure. This attitude may place certain populations at greater risk due to both lack of access to health care and potential harm from continued exposure. Those living closest to a spill, those spending the most time near toxic substances during cleanup, and particularly sensitive populations, such as children and pregnant women living in the area near a chemical spill, may be at greater risk for adverse health effects than others in the community and should have full access to information about substances to which they have been potentially exposed. Nurses must be knowledgeable about potential hazards and may need to act autonomously in supplying the required information to community members on the basis of professional, ethical responsibilities—whether they are explicit or implicit in nature (IOM, 1995).

In communicating risk, nurses can educate individuals, families, workers, and communities about the possible adverse effects of exposure to environmental hazards and how to reduce or eliminate such exposures. This type of education is commonly referred to by public agencies and environmental health specialists as hazard or risk communication. Nurses can further develop this role by providing information to create environmentally safe homes, schools, day care settings, workplaces, and communities. Nurses can encourage citizens to live in an environmentally safe manner by limiting unnecessary exposure to chemicals or by carrying out routine duties in a manner that minimizes injury. Nurses can act as educators by speaking at community gatherings and becoming involved in community-level activities related to the environment and human health. They can also participate in risk or hazard communication activities for public health agencies.

The original focus of risk communication was on developing and delivering a message from an expert or agency to the public in order to help the public better understand a situation and its implications for their health and well-being. This definition is widening to incorporate a two-way dialogue between regulators or managers and the public. The interactive process of exchanging information on technical hazards and the human response, both physiological and emotional, calls for professionals who can listen, interpret, clarify, and reframe questions and information in emotionally charged and sometimes hostile situations. The basic patient education role of nurses, limited to individuals and families, will need to be expanded to include entire communities and the general public if nurses are to fill an essential niche in environmental health.

To the extent possible, the occupational and environmental health nurse should identify individuals and groups at potentially increased risk so appropriate primary and secondary prevention measures can be instituted. Examples of these preventive activities might include workplace smoking cessation programs in areas of high radon activity or community education programs to teach about safe use of pesticides and household chemicals in households with children. The ability to assess the target audience, develop a meaningful and understandable message, choose a method or media for conveying the message,

and conduct community-level conflict resolution are skills needed by nurses (IOM, 1995).

LEGISLATION AND REGULATION

The fourth and final environmental health competency is the necessity to understand laws and regulations relevant to environmental health at federal, state, and local levels. Numerous laws and regulations spring up annually, and nurses need to have an understanding of how these laws affect individuals, business, communities, and professional practice. Environmental health laws are complex and may overlap each other; thus, the nurse will need to understand how the pieces fit together and how they affect people's lives and health. A working knowledge of environmental laws and regulations is essential if the nurse is to provide or facilitate community access to accurate information, guide communities through public participation and decision making processes, inform communities of their rights, and recognize policy gaps for attention and advocacy (Cary & Mood, 2000).

INTEGRATION OF ROLES

The basic competencies in environmental health for nurses (as recommended by the Institute of Medicine) provide occupational and environmental health nurses the opportunity to integrate skill sets into effective interventions at primary, secondary, and tertiary prevention levels. At the primary prevention level the occupational and environmental health nurse can help educate workers about potential environmental health hazards and pollutants and methods to reduce exposure in the workplace and community. Primary prevention can also include risk assessment, policy development at the worksite, and political activism in the community to reduce and control environmental health hazards, such as toxic waste disposal.

At the secondary prevention level the nurse can conduct or arrange for baseline and periodic screenings to monitor for early adverse health effects. Referral to appropriate health care providers and agencies will be needed in order to provide focused interventions to individuals needing treatment and to control and eliminate environmental exposures. Risk communication will be an important strategy.

Tertiary prevention occurs after exposure and its resultant effects and is designed to further minimize adverse sequelae. Rehabilitative interventions for individuals with lung or neurological diseases will be important to restoring the individual to optimal health. Working as a case manager with agencies, organizations, and health care professionals to coordinate needed services can provide the individual with reassurance, continuity of service, and focused counseling.

Summary

Occupational and environmental health nurses must have knowledge and competencies in environmental health because many environmental hazards originate in the workplace and extend into the community and because workers are also a part of a larger community environment. Occupational and environmental health nurses with expertise in the identification of hazardous chemical and physical exposures, as well as preventive strategies, are critical resources to their colleagues in the larger community and the global environment (Lipscomb, 1994; Rogers & Cox, 1998). Working in collaborative relationships with other disciplines can help best ensure a safe environment in which to live, work, and play.

References

Agency for Toxic Substances and Disease Registry. (1991). Nitrate/nitrite toxicity. In Agency for Toxic Substances and Disease Registry (Ed.), *Case studies in environmental medicine* (Vol. 16, pp. 1-24). Atlanta, GA: Author.

Agency for Toxic Substances and Disease Registry. (1992). *Clues to unraveling the association between illness and environmental exposure.* Atlanta, GA: Author.

Agency for Toxic Substances and Disease Registry. (1993). *Public health assessment guidance manual.* Boca Raton, FL: Lewis.

Agency for Toxic Substances and Disease Registry. (1998). *The nature and extent of childhood lead poisoning in children in the United States: A report to Congress.* Washington, DC: U.S. Department of Health and Human Services.

Agency for Toxic Substances and Disease Registry. (1999). *Promoting children's health: Progress report of the Child Health Workgroup Board of Scientific Counselors.* Atlanta, GA: Author.

Agency for Toxic Substances and Disease Registry. (2000). *Case studies in environmental medicine: Taking an exposure history.* Atlanta, GA: Author.

American Lung Association. (1990). *Health costs of air pollution.* New York: Author.

American Society for Microbiology. (1999). *Microbial pollutants in our nation's water: Environmental and public health issues.* http://www.asmusa.org/pasrc/pdfs/waterreport.pdf.

Bates, D. V. (1995). The effects of air pollution on children. *Environmental Health Perspectives, 103,* 49-53.

Blondell, J. (1997). Epidemiology of pesticide poisonings in the United States, with special reference to occupational cases. *Occupational Medicine, 12,* 209-220.

Blumenthal, D. S., & Ruttenber, J. A. (1995). *Introduction to environmental health* (2nd ed.). New York: Springer.

Buckley, J. D., Meadows, A. T., Kadin, M. E., LeBeau, M. M., Siegel, S., & Robison, L. L. (2000). Pesticide exposures in children with non-Hodgkin lymphoma. *Cancer, 89,* 2315-2321.

Bureau of the Census. (1997). *American housing survey for the United States in 1995* (Current housing reports H150/95RV). Washington, DC: U.S. Government Printing Office.

Cary, A., & Mood, L. (2000). Environmental health. In M. Stanhope & J. Lancaster (Eds.), *Community and public health nursing* (pp. 157-176) St. Louis, MO: Mosby.

Centers for Disease Control and Prevention. (1997). *Screening young children for lead poisoning: Guidance for state and local public health officials.* Atlanta, GA: Author.

Centers for Disease Control and Prevention. (1998a). Forecasted state-specific estimates of self-reported asthma prevalence—United States, 1998. *Morbidity and Mortality Weekly Report, 47,* 1022-1025.

Centers for Disease Control and Prevention. (1998b). Surveillance of work-related asthma in selected U.S. states using surveillance guidelines for State Health Departments—California, Massachusetts, Michigan, and New Jersey, 1993-1995. *Morbidity and Mortality Weekly Report, 48*(SS-3), 1-20.

Centers for Disease Control and Prevention. (2000). Surveillance for waterborne-disease outbreaks—United States, 1997-1998. *Morbidity and Mortality Weekly Report, 49*(SS-4), 1-35.

Chalupka, S. M. (2001a). Essentials of environmental health: Enhancing your nursing practice (Part I). *AAOHN Journal, 49,* 137-153.

Chalupka, S. M. (2001b). Essentials of environmental health: Enhancing your nursing practice (Part II). *AAOHN Journal, 49*(4), 194-212.

Children's Environmental Health Network. (1999). *Training manual on pediatric environmental health: Putting it into practice.* San Francisco: Children's Environmental Health Network/Public Health Institute.

Chin, J. (Ed.). (2000). *Control of communicable diseases manual* (17th ed.). Washington, DC: American Public Health Administration.

Chlorine Chemistry Council. (2000). Global water crisis. *Drinking Water & Health, 7*(1), 7.

Commissioned Corps of the United States Public Health Service, U.S. Department of Health and Human Services, 2000, June, http://www.os.gov/phs/corps/direct1.html#history.

Committee of the Environmental and Occupational Health Assembly of the American Thoracic Society. (1996). Health effects of outdoor air pollution: State of the art, Parts 1 and 2. *American Journal Respiratory Critical Care Medicine, 153,* 3-50, 477-498.

Craun, G. F. (1986). In G. F. Craun (Ed.), *Waterborne disease outbreaks in the United States* (pp. 52-74) Boca Raton, FL: CRC Press.

Etzel, R. A., & Balk, S. J. (1999). *Handbook of pediatric environmental health.* Elk Grove Village, IL: American Academy of Pediatrics.

Goldman, L. R. (1998). Linking research and policy to ensure children's environmental health. *Environmental Health Perspectives, 106*(Suppl. 3), 857-860.

Goldman, L. R. (2000). *Environmental health and its relationship to occupational health: Recognizing and preventing work-related disease.* (4th ed., pp.51-96). Philadelphia: Lippincott, Williams & Wilkins.

Institute of Medicine. (1995). *Nursing, health, and the environment.* Washington, DC: National Academy Press.

Institute of Medicine. (2000). *Clearing the air.* Washington, DC: National Academy Press.

Kristensen, P., Andersen, A., Irgens, L. M., Bye, A. S., & Sundheim, L. (1996). Cancer in offspring of parents engaged in agricultural activities in Norway: Incidence and risk factors in the farm environment. *International Journal of Cancer, 65*(1), 39-50.

Landrigan, P. J., Claudio, L., & McConnell, R. (2000). Pesticides. In M. Lippman (Ed.), *Environmental toxicants* (pp. 725-739). New York: Wiley-Interscience.

Landrigan, P. J., Suk, W. A., & Amler, R. W. (1999). Chemical wastes, children's health, and the Superfund Basic Research Program. *Environmental Health Perspectives, 107*(6), 423-427.

Last, J. M. (Ed.). (1998). *A dictionary of epidemiology.* Cambridge, England: Cambridge University Press.

Leiss, J. K., & Savitz, D. A. (1995). Home pesticide use and childhood cancer: A case control study. *American Journal of Public Health, 85*(2), 249-252.

Lipscomb, J. (1994). Environmental health: Assuming a leadership role. *AAOHN Journal, 42*(7), 314-315.

Litovitz, T. L., Smilkstein, M., Feldberg, L., Klein-Schwartz, W. Berlin, R., & Morgan, J. L. (1997). 1996 annual report of the American Association of Poison Control Centers: Toxic exposure surveillance system. *American Journal of Emergency Medicine 15,* 447-500.

Meinert, R., Schuz, J., Kaletsch, U., Kaatsch, P., & Michelis, J. (2000). Leukemia and non-Hodgkin's lymphoma in childhood exposure to pesticide: Results of a register-based control study in Germany. *American Journal of Epidemiology, 15,* 639-650.

Minority Staff Report for Senator Tom Harkin, (D-IA), Ranking Member United States Senate Committee on Agriculture, Nutrition, & Forestry. (1997). *Animal waste pollution in America: An emerging national problem: Environmental risks of livestock and poultry production.*

Moeller, D. W. (1997). *Environmental health.* Cambridge, MA: Harvard University Press.

Nadakavukaren, A. (2000). *Our global environment: A health perspective.* Prospect Heights, IL: Waveland Press.

National Academy of Sciences. (1999). *Health effects of exposure to radon: BEIR VI.* Washington, DC: Author.

National Institute for Occupational Safety and Health. (2000). *Worker health safety chartbook, 2000.* Washington, DC: Author.

National Research Council. (1993). *Measuring lead exposure in infants, children and other sensitive populations.* Washington, DC: National Academy Press.

Nightingale, F. (1859). *Notes on nursing: What it is and what it is not.* London: Harrison.

Nyman, C., Butterfield, P., & Shaffler, J. (2001). Environmental health. In K. Lundy & S. Jaynes (Eds.), *Community health nursing.* Boston: Jones and Bartlett.

O'Reilly, J., Hagan, P., Gots, R., & Hedge, A. (1998). *Keeping buildings healthy: How to monitor and prevent indoor environmental problems.* New York: Wiley-Interscience.

Pagoda, J. M., & Preston-Martin, S. (1997). Household pesticides and risk of pediatric brain tumors. *Environmental Health Perspectives, 105*(11), 1214-1220.

Reigart, J., & Roberts, J. (1999). *Recognition and management of pesticide poisonings.* Washington, DC: U.S. Environmental Protection Agency.

Rogers, B. (1994). Linkages in environmental and occupational health: Assessing, detecting, and containing exposure sources. *AAOHN Journal, 42*(7), 336-343.

Rogers, B., & Cox, A. R. (1998). Expanding horizons: Integrating environmental health in occupational health nursing. *AAOHN Journal, 46*(1), 9-13.

Sharpe, C. R., Franco, E. L., de Camargo, B., Lopes, L. F., Barreto, J. H., Johnson, R. R., & Mauad, M. A. (1995). Parental exposures and risk of Wilm's tumor in Brazil. *American Journal of Epidemiology, 141*(3), 210-217.

SRI International. (1998). Chemical Economics Handbook. http://www.ceh.sric.sri.com/Public/Reports/

Stevens, B., & Hall, J. (2001). Environmental health. In M. Nies & M. McEwen (Eds.), *Community health nursing.* Philadelphia: Saunders.

Summary of Travel Trends. (1999). *1995 nationwide personal transportation survey.* Oak Ridge, TN: Oak Ridge National Library.

Tarcher, A. B. (1992). *Principles and practice of environmental medicine.* New York: Plenum.

U.S. Department of Health and Human Services. (1986). *The health consequences of involuntary smoking: A report of the Surgeon General.* Washington, DC: Author.

U.S. Department of Health and Human Services. (2000). *Healthy people 2010.* Washington, DC: Author.

U.S. Environmental Protection Agency. (1997a). *National air quality and trends report.* Washington, DC: Author.

U.S. Environmental Protection Agency. (1997b). *National toxics inventory.* Washington, DC: Author.

U.S. Environmental Protection Agency. (1999). *Safe drinking water is in our hands: Existing standards and future priorities* (EPA815-F-99-004). Washington, DC: Author.

U.S. Environmental Protection Agency. (2000a). *Chemical hazard data availability study* (last revision 10-25-00). www.epa.gov/opptintr/chemtest/ hazchem.index.

U.S. Environmental Protection Agency. (2000b). *National listing of fish and wildlife advisories: Summary of 1999 data* (EPA-823-F-00-20). Washington, DC: Author.

Weiss, K. B., Gergen, P. J., & Hodgson, T. A. (1992). An economic evaluation of asthma in the United States. *New England Journal of Medicine 326,* 862-866.

World Health Organization. (1997). *Indicators for policy and decision making in environmental health.* Geneva, Switzerland: Author.

Zahm, S. H., & Ward, M. H. (1998). Pesticides and childhood cancer. *Environmental Health Perspectives, 106*(Suppl. 3), 893-908.

8-1 Taking an Exposure History*

ENVIRONMENTAL ALERT

- *Because many environmental diseases either manifest as common medical problems or have nonspecific symptoms, an exposure history is vital for correct diagnosis.*
- *The primary care clinician can play an important role in detecting, treating, and preventing disease due to toxic exposure by taking a thorough exposure history.*

USING THE EXPOSURE HISTORY FORM

A work and exposure history has three components: exposure survey, work history, and environmental history. The main aspects of an exposure history (summarized in the outline that follows) will be elicited through the administration of the exposure history form included. Although a positive response to any question on the form indicates the need for further inquiry, a negative response to all questions does not necessarily rule out a toxic exposure or significant previous exposure.

All patients should complete exposure history forms, although the form need not be evaluated extensively in every clinical situation. As in all data gathering activities, sound clinical judgment must be exercised.

COMPONENTS OF AN EXPOSURE HISTORY

Part 1. Exposure Survey
A. Exposures
   1. Current and past exposure to metals, dust, fibers, fumes, chemicals, biologic hazards, radiation, noise, vibration
   2. Typical work day (job tasks, location, materials, agents used)
   3. Changes in routine or processes
   4. Other employees or household members similarly affected
B. Health and safety practices at worksite
   1. Ventilation
   2. Medical and industrial hygiene surveillance
   3. Employment exams
   4. Personal protective equipment (e.g., respirators, gloves, coveralls)
   5. Lockout devices, alarms, training, drills
   6. Personal habits (Smoke? Eat in work area? Wash hands in solvents?)

Part 2. Work History
A. Description of all prior jobs including short-term, seasonal, and part-time employment and military service.
B. Description of present job(s)

Part 3. Environmental History
A. Present and prior home locations
B. Current and past exposures to home cleaning agents, pesticides, and hazardous wastes/spills
C. Jobs of household members
D. Home insulating, heating and cooling system
E. Water supply
F. Recent renovation/remodeling
G. Air pollution (indoor and outdoor)
H. Hobbies (painting, sculpting, welding, woodworking, piloting, autos, firearms, stained glass, ceramics, gardening)

---

*Note: This shortened document has been excerpted from *Case Studies in Environmental Medicine*'s "Taking an Exposure History," published by the Agency for Toxic Substances and Disease Registry (1992). The full document, which includes case studies and questions, can be obtained from ATSDR.

EXPOSURE HISTORY FORM

Part 1. Exposure Survey   Name:_____ Date:_____
Please circle the appropriate answer.   Birthdate:_____ Sex: M   F

1. Are you currently exposed to any of the
    following:

    Metals?   *no*   *yes*   Loud noise, vibration, extreme heat or cold?
                                                                              no   *yes*

    Dust or fibers?   *no*   *yes*   Biological agents?   *no*   *yes*
    Chemicals?   *no*   *yes*   2. Have you been exposed to any of above in the
                                                   past?   *no*   *yes*
    Fumes?   *no*   *yes*   3. Do any household members have
                                                   contact with metals, dust, fibers,
                                                   chemicals, fumes, radiation, or
    Radiation?   *no*   *yes*   biological agents?   *no*   *yes*

If you answered *yes* to any of the items above, describe your exposure in detail—how you were exposed
and to what you were exposed. If you need more space, please use a separate sheet of paper.

---

4. Do you know the names of the metals, dusts, fibers, chemicals, | If *yes*, list the
    fumes, or radiation that you are/were exposed to?   *no*   *yes* | materials and
                                                                               | agents
5. Do you get the material on your skin or clothing?   *no*   *yes* | below.

6. Are your work clothes laundered at home?   *no*   *yes*

7. Do you shower at work?   *no*   *yes*

8. Can you smell the chemical(s) or material(s)
    you are working with?   *no*   *yes*

---

9. Do you use protective equipment such as gloves, | If *yes*, list the
    masks, respirator, or hearing protectors?   *no*   *yes* | protective
                                                                               | equipment
10. Have you been advised to use protective equipment?   *no*   *yes* | used.

11. Have you been instructed in the use of protective
    equipment?   *no*   *yes*

12. Do you wash your hands with solvents?   *no*   *yes*

13. Do you smoke at the workplace?   *no*   *yes*

14. Do you eat at the workplace?   *no*   *yes*

EXPOSURE HISTORY FORM

15. Do you know of any coworkers experiencing similar or unusual symptoms?   *no*   *yes*

16. Are family members experiencing similar or unusual symptoms?   *no*   *yes*

17. Has there been a change in the health or behavior of family pets?   *no*   *yes*

18. Do your symptoms seem to be aggravated by a specific activity?   *no*   *yes*

19. Do your symptoms get either worse or better at work?   *no*   *yes*

    At home?   *no*   *yes*

    On weekends?   *no*   *yes*

    On vacation?   *no*   *yes*

20. Has anything about your job changed in recent months (such as duties, procedures, overtime?)   *no*   *yes*

If you answered *yes* to any of these questions, please explain.

Continued

Part 2. Work History
Occupational Profile
The following questions refer to your current or most recent job:

Name:_____ Date:_____
Birthdate:_____ Sex: M   F

Job title:_____

Type of industry:_____

Name of employer:_____

Date job began:_____

Are you still working in this job?
     yes   no

*If no, when did this job end?*_____

Describe this job:
_____
_____
_____
_____
_____
_____
_____
_____
_____
_____
_____
_____
_____
_____
_____
_____

Fill in the table below listing all jobs you have worked, including short-term, seasonal, and part-time employment, and military service. Begin with your most recent job. Use additional paper if necessary.

Dates of Employment	Job Title and Description of Work	Exposures*	Protective Equipment

*List the chemicals, dusts, fibers, fumes, radiation, biological agents (e.g., molds, viruses) and physical agents (e.g., extreme heat, cold, vibration, noise) that you were exposed to at this job.

Have you ever worked at a job or hobby in which you came in contact with any of the following by breathing, touching, or ingesting (swallowing)? If yes, please check the box beside the name.

☐ Acids	☐ Cadmium	☐ Ethylene dibromide	☐ Mercury	☐ Phosgene	☐ TDI or MDI
☐ Alcohols (industrial)	☐ Carbon tetrachloride	☐ Ethylene dichloride	☐ Methylene chloride	☐ Radiation	☐ Trichloroethylene
☐ Alkalies	☐ Chlorinated naphthalenes	☐ Fiberglass	☐ Nickel	☐ Rock dust	☐ Vinyl chloride
☐ Ammonia	☐ Chloroform	☐ Halothane	☐ PBBs	☐ Silica powder	☐ Welding fumes
☐ Arsenic	☐ Chloroprene	☐ Isocyanates	☐ PCBs	☐ Solvents	☐ X-rays
☐ Asbestos	☐ Chromates	☐ Ketones	☐ Perchloro-ethylene	☐ Styrene	☐ Others (specify)
☐ Benzene	☐ Coal dust	☐ Lead	☐ Pesticides	☐ Talc	
☐ Beryllium	☐ Dichloro-benzene	☐ Manganese	☐ Phenol	☐ Toluene	

Developed by ATSDR in Cooperation with NIOSH, 1992.

1. Have you ever been off work for more than one day because of an illness related to work?   *no*   *yes*
2. Have you ever been advised to change jobs or work assignments because of health problems or injuries?   *no*   *yes*
3. Has your work routine changed lately?   *no*   *yes*
4. Is there poor ventilation in your workplace?   *no*   *yes*

Part 3. Environmental History   *Please circle the appropriate answer.*
1. Do you live next to or near an industrial plant, commercial business, dump site, or nonresidential property?   *no*   *yes*
2. Which of the following do you have in your home?
   Please circle those that apply.
   Air conditioner   Air purifier   Central heating (gas or oil?)
   Gas stove   Electric stove   Fireplace
   Wood stove   Humidifier
3. Have you recently acquired new furniture or carpet or refinished furniture or remodeled your home?   *no*   *yes*
4. Have you weatherized your home lately?   *no*   *yes*
5. Are pesticides or herbicides (bug or weed killers; flea and tick sprays, collars, powders, or shampoos) used in your home or garden or on pets?   *no*   *yes*
6. Do you (or any household member) have a hobby or craft?   *no*   *yes*
7. Do you work on your car?   *no*   *yes*
8. Have you ever changed your residence because of a health problem?   *no*   *yes*
9. Does your drinking water come from a private well, city water supply, or grocery store?
   Please circle correct answer.   *no*   *yes*
10. Approximately what year was your home built? _____

If you answered *yes* to any of the questions, please explain.

APPENDIX 8-2 Poison Control Centers

ALABAMA
Alabama Poison Center
2503 Phoenix Dr.
Tuscaloosa, AL 35405
Emergency Phone: (800) 222-1222

Regional Poison Control Center
Children's Hospital
1600 7th Ave. S.
Birmingham, AL 35233
Emergency Phone: (800) 222-1222

ALASKA
Anchorage Poison Control Center
3200 Providence Dr.
P.O. Box 196604
Anchorage, AK 99519-6604
Emergency Phone: (800) 222-1222

ARIZONA
Arizona Poison and Drug Information Center
Arizona Health Sciences Center
1501 N. Campbell Ave., Room 1156
Tucson, AZ 85724
Emergency Phone: (800) 222-1222

Samaritan Regional Poison Center
Good Samaritan Regional Medical Center
1111 East McDowell—Ancillary 1
Phoenix, AZ 85006
Emergency Phone: (800) 222-1222

ARKANSAS
Arkansas Poison and Drug Information Center
College of Pharmacy
University of Arkansas for Medical Sciences
4301 W. Markham, Mail Slot 522
Little Rock, AR 72205
Emergency Phone: (800) 222-1222
TTY/TDD: (800) 641-3805

CALIFORNIA
California Poison Control System—
    Fresno/Madera Division
Valley Children's Hospital
9300 Valley Children's Pl., MB 15
Madera, CA 93638-8762
Emergency Phone: (800) 876-4766 (Cal. only)
TTY/TDD: (800) 972-3323

California Poison Control System—Sacramento
    Division
UC Davis Medical Center
2315 Stockton Blvd.
Sacramento, CA 95817
Emergency Phone: (800) 876-4766 (Cal. only)
TTY/TDD: (800) 972-3323

California Poison Control System—San Diego
    Division
University of California, San Diego, Medical
    Center
200 West Arbor Dr.
San Diego, CA 92103-8925
Emergency Phone: (800) 876-4766 (Cal. only)
TTY/TDD: (800) 972-3323

California Poison Control System—
    San Francisco Division
1001 Potrero Ave., Room 1E86
UCSF Box 1369
San Francisco, CA 94143-1369
Emergency Phone: (800) 876-4766 (Cal. only)
TTY/TDD: (800) 972-3323

COLORADO
Rocky Mountain Poison and Drug Center
1010 Yosemite Circle
Building 752
Denver, CO 80230-6800
Emergency Phone: (800) 222-1222

CONNECTICUT
Connecticut Poison Control Center
University of Connecticut Health Center
263 Farmington Ave.
Farmington, CT 06030-5365
Emergency Phone: (800) 222-1222
TTY/TDD: (866) 218-5372 (toll free)

DELAWARE
Poison Control Center
3535 Market St., Suite 985
Philadelphia, PA 19104-3309
Emergency Phone: (800) 222-1222
TTY/TDD: (215) 590-8789

DISTRICT OF COLUMBIA
National Capital Poison Center
3201 New Mexico Ave., NW
Suite 310
Washington, DC 20016
Emergency Phone: (800) 222-1222
TTY/TDD: (202) 362-8563 (TTY)

FLORIDA
Florida Poison Information Center—Jacksonville
655 West 8th St.
Jacksonville, FL 32209
Emergency Phone: (800) 222-1222
TTY/TDD: (800) 282-3171 (Fla. only)

Florida Poison Information Center—Miami
University of Miami, Department of Pediatrics
Jackson Memorial Medical Center
P.O. Box 016960 (R-131)
Miami, FL 33101
Emergency Phone: (800) 222-1222

Florida Poison Information Center—Tampa
Tampa General Hospital
P.O. Box 1289
Tampa, FL 33601
Emergency Phone: (800) 222-1222

GEORGIA
Georgia Poison Center
Hughes Spalding Children's Hospital
Grady Health System
80 Butler St., SE
P.O. Box 26066
Atlanta, GA 30335-3801
Emergency Phone: (800) 222-1222
TTY/TDD: (404) 616-9287 (TDD)

HAWAII
Hawaii Poison Center
1319 Punahou St.
Honolulu, HI 96826
Emergency Phone: (800) 222-1222

IDAHO
Rocky Mountain Poison and Drug Center
1010 Yosemite Circle
Building 752
Denver, CO 80230-6800
Emergency Phone: (800) 222-1222

ILLINOIS
Illinois Poison Center
222 S. Riverside Plaza, Suite 1900
Chicago, IL 60606
Emergency Phone: (800) 222-1222
TTY/TDD: (312) 906-6185

INDIANA
Indiana Poison Center
Methodist Hospital
Clarian Health Partners
I-65 at 21st St.
Indianapolis, IN 46206-1367
Emergency Phone: (800) 222-1222
TTY/TDD: (317) 962-2336 (TTY)

IOWA
Iowa Statewide Poison Control Center
St. Luke's Regional Medical Center
2720 Stone Park Blvd.
Sioux City, IA 51104
Emergency Phone: (800) 222-1222

KANSAS
Mid-America Poison Control Center
University of Kansas Medical Center
3901 Rainbow Blvd., Room B-400
Kansas City, KS 66160-7231
Emergency Phone: (800) 222-1222
TTY/TDD: (913) 588-6639 (TDD)

KENTUCKY
Kentucky Regional Poison Center
Medical Towers South, Suite 572
234 E. Gray St.
Louisville, KY 40202
Emergency Phone: (800) 222-1222

LOUISIANA
Louisiana Drug and Poison Information Center
University of Louisiana at Monroe
College of Pharmacy, Sugar Hall
Monroe, LA 71209-6430
Emergency Phone: (800) 222-1222

MAINE
Maine Poison Center
Maine Medical Center
22 Bramhall Street
Portland, ME 04102
Emergency Phone: (800) 222-1222
TTY/TDD: (877) 299-4447 (Me. only); (207)
   871-2879

MARYLAND
Maryland Poison Center
University of Maryland at Baltimore
School of Pharmacy
20 N. Pine St., PH 772
Baltimore, MD 21201
Emergency Phone: (800) 222-1222
TTY/TDD: (410) 706-1858 (TDD)

National Capital Poison Center
3201 New Mexico Ave., NW
Suite 310
Washington, DC 20016
Emergency Phone: (800) 222-1222
TTY/TDD: (202) 362-8563 (TTY)

MASSACHUSETTS
Regional Center for Poison Control and
    Prevention Serving Massachusetts and
    Rhode Island
300 Longwood Ave.
Boston, MA 02115
Emergency Phone: (800) 222-1222
TTY/TDD: (888) 244-5313

MICHIGAN
Children's Hospital of Michigan
Regional Poison Control Center
4160 John R. Harper Professional Office Building
Suite 616
Detroit, MI 48201
Emergency Phone: (800) 222-1222
TTY/TDD: (800) 356-3232 (TDD)

DeVos Children's Hospital
Regional Poison Center
1840 Wealthy SE
Grand Rapids, MI 49506-2968
Emergency Phone: (800) 222-1222
TTY/TDD: (800) 356-3232 (TTY)

MINNESOTA
Hennepin Regional Poison Center
Hennepin County Medical Center
701 Park Ave.
Minneapolis, MN 55415
Emergency Phone: (800) 222-1222
TTY/TDD: (612) 904-4691 (TTY)

MISSISSIPPI
Mississippi Regional Poison
    Control Center
University of Mississippi
    Medical Center
2500 N. State St.
Jackson, MS 39216
Emergency Phone: (800) 222-1222

MISSOURI
Cardinal Glennon Children's Hospital
Regional Poison Center
1465 S. Grand Blvd.
St. Louis, MO 63104
Emergency Phone: (800) 222-1222

MONTANA
Rocky Mountain Poison and Drug Center
1010 Yosemite Circle, Building 752
Denver, CO 80230-6800
Emergency Phone: (800) 222-1222

NEBRASKA
The Poison Center
Children's Hospital
8200 Dodge St.
Omaha, NE 68114
Emergency Phone: (800) 222-1222

NEVADA
Oregon Poison Center
Oregon Health Sciences University
3181 SW Sam Jackson Park Rd., CB550
Portland, OR 97201
Emergency Phone: (800) 222-1222

Rocky Mountain Poison and Drug Center
1010 Yosemite Circle, Building 752
Denver, CO 80230-6800
Emergency Phone: (800) 222-1222

NEW HAMPSHIRE
New Hampshire Poison Information Center
Dartmouth-Hitchcock Medical Center
One Medical Center Dr.
Lebanon, NH 03756
Emergency Phone: (800) 222-1222

NEW JERSEY
New Jersey Poison Information and
    Education System
201 Lyons Ave.
Newark, NJ 07112
Emergency Phone: (800) 222-1222
TTY/TDD: (973) 926-8008

NEW MEXICO
New Mexico Poison and Drug
    Information Center
Health Science Center Library, Room 130
University of New Mexico
Albuquerque, NM 87131-1076
Emergency Phone: (800) 222-1222

NEW YORK
Central New York Poison Center
750 E. Adams St.
Syracuse, NY 13210
Emergency Phone: (800) 222-1222

Finger Lakes Regional Poison and Drug
    Information Center
University of Rochester Medical Center
601 Elmwood Ave., P.O. Box 321
Rochester, NY 14642
Emergency Phone: (800) 222-1222
TTY/TDD: (716) 273-3854 (TTY)

Hudson Valley Regional Poison Center
Phelps Memorial Hospital Center
701 North Broadway
Sleepy Hollow, NY 10591
Emergency Phone: (800) 222-1222

Long Island Regional Poison and Drug
    Information Center
Winthrop University Hospital
259 1st St.
Mineola, NY 11501
Emergency Phone: (800) 222-1222
TTY/TDD: (516) 924-8811 (TDD Suffolk);
(516) 747-3323 (TDD Nassau)

New York City Poison Control Center
NYC Department of Labs
455 1st Ave., Room 123, Box 81
New York, NY 10016
Emergency Phone: (800) 222-1222
TTY/TDD: (212) 689-9014 (TDD)

Western New York Regional Poison
    Control Center
Children's Hospital of Buffalo
219 Bryant St.
Buffalo, NY 14222
Emergency Phone: (800) 222-1222

NORTH CAROLINA
Carolinas Poison Center
Carolinas Medical Center
5000 Airport Center Pkwy., Suite B
Charlotte, NC 28208
Emergency Phone: (800) 222-1222

NORTH DAKOTA
North Dakota Poison Information Center
Meritcare Medical Center
720 4th St. N.
Fargo, ND 58122
Emergency Phone: (800) 222-1222

OHIO
Central Ohio Poison Center
700 Children's Drive, Room L032
Columbus, OH 43205
Emergency Phone: (800) 222-1222
TTY/TDD: (614) 228-2272 (TTY)

Cincinnati Drug and Poison Information Center
Regional Poison Control System
3333 Burnet Ave.
Vernon Place—3rd Floor
Cincinnati, OH 45229
Emergency Phone: (800) 222-1222

Greater Cleveland Poison Control Center
11100 Euclid Ave.
Cleveland, OH 44106-6010
Emergency Phone: (800) 222-1222

OKLAHOMA
Oklahoma Poison Control Center
Children's Hospital of Oklahoma
940 NE 13th St.
Oklahoma City, OK 73104
Emergency Phone: (800) 222-1222
TTY/TDD: (405) 271-1122

OREGON
Oregon Poison Center
Oregon Health Sciences University
3181 SW Sam Jackson Park Rd., CB550
Portland, OR 97201
Emergency Phone: (800) 222-1222

PENNSYLVANIA
Central Pennsylvania Poison Center
Pennsylvania State University
Milton S. Hershey Medical Center
500 University Dr.
MC H043, PO Box 850
Hershey, PA 17033-0850
Emergency Phone: (800) 222-1222
TTY/TDD: (717) 531-8335 (TTY)

Pittsburgh Poison Center
Children's Hospital of Pittsburgh
3705 5th Ave.
Pittsburgh, PA 15213
Emergency Phone: (800) 222-1222

Poison Control Center
3535 Market St., Suite 985
Philadelphia, PA 19104-3309
Emergency Phone: (800) 222-1222
TTY/TDD: (215) 590-8789

PUERTO RICO
San Jorge Children's Hospital Poison Center
Calle San Jorge #252
Santurce, Puerto Rico 00912
Emergency Phone: (787) 726-5674

RHODE ISLAND
Regional Center for Poison Control and
  Prevention Serving Massachusetts and
  Rhode Island
300 Longwood Ave.
Boston, MA 02115
Emergency Phone: (800) 222-1222
TTY/TDD: (888) 244-5313

SOUTH CAROLINA
Palmetto Poison Center
College of Pharmacy
University of South Carolina
Columbia, SC 29208
Emergency Phone: (800) 222-1222

SOUTH DAKOTA
Hennepin Regional Poison Center
Hennepin County Medical Center
701 Park Ave.
Minneapolis, MN 55415
Emergency Phone: (800) 222-1222
TTY/TDD: (612) 904-4691 (TTY)

TENNESSEE
Middle Tennessee Poison Center
501 Oxford House
1161 21st Ave. S.
Nashville, TN 37232-4632
Emergency Phone: (800) 222-1222
TTY/TDD: (615) 936-2047 (TDD)

Southern Poison Center
University of Tennessee
875 Monroe Ave., Suite 104
Memphis, TN 38163
Emergency Phone: (800) 288-9999 (Tenn. only);
  (901) 528-6048

TEXAS
Central Texas Poison Center
Scott and White Memorial Hospital
2401 S. 31st St.
Temple, TX 76508
Emergency Phone: (800) POISON-1(Tex. only);
  (254) 724-7401

North Texas Poison Center
Texas Poison Center Network
Parkland Health & Hospital System
5201 Harry Hines Blvd.
P.O. Box 35926
Dallas, TX 75235
Emergency Phone: (800) 764-7661
  (Tex. only)

South Texas Poison Center
University of Texas Health Science Center—
  San Antonio
Department of Surgery, Mail Code 7849
7703 Floyd Curl Dr.
San Antonio, TX 78229-3900
Emergency Phone: (800) 764-7661 (Tex. only)
TTY/TDD: (800) 764-7661 (Tex. only)

Southeast Texas Poison Center
The University of Texas Medical Branch
301 University Blvd.
3.112 Trauma Building
Galveston, TX 77555-1175
Emergency Phone: (800) 764-7661 (Tex. only);
  (409) 765-1420
TTY/TDD: (800) 764-7661 (Tex. only)

Texas Panhandle Poison Center
1501 S. Coulter
Amarillo, TX 79106
Emergency Phone: (800) 764-7661 (Tex. only)

West Texas Regional Poison Center
Thomason Hospital
4815 Alameda Ave.
El Paso, TX 79905
Emergency Phone: (800) 764-7661 (Tex. only)

UTAH
Utah Poison Control Center
410 Chipeta Way, Suite 230
Salt Lake City, UT 84108
Emergency Phone: (800) 222-1222

VERMONT
Vermont Poison Center
Fletcher Allen Health Care
111 Colchester Ave.
Burlington, VT 05401
Emergency Phone: (800) 222-1222

VIRGINIA
Blue Ridge Poison Center
University of Virginia Health System
P.O. Box 800774
Charlottesville, VA 22908-0774
Emergency Phone: (800) 222-1222

National Capital Poison Center
3201 New Mexico Ave., NW
Suite 310
Washington, DC 20016
Emergency Phone: (800) 222-1222
TTY/TDD: (202) 362-8563 (TTY)

Virginia Poison Center
Medical College of Virginia Hospitals
Virginia Commonwealth University
P.O. Box 980522
Richmond, VA 23298-0522
Emergency Phone: (800) 222-1222

WASHINGTON
Washington Poison Center
155 NE 100th St., Suite 400
Seattle, WA 98125-8012
Emergency Phone: (800) 222-1222
TTY/TDD: (206) 517-2394; (800) 572-0638
  (WA only)

WEST VIRGINIA
West Virginia Poison Center
3110 MacCorkle Ave, SE
Charleston, WV 25304
Emergency Phone: (800) 222-1222

WISCONSIN
Children's Hospital of Wisconsin Poison Center
P.O. Box 1997, Mail Station 677A
Milwaukee, WI 53201-1997
Emergency Phone: (800) 222-1222
TTY/TDD: (414) 266-2542

University of Wisconsin Hospital and Clinics
Poison Control Center
600 Highland Ave., F6/133
Madison, WI 53792
Emergency Phone: (800) 222-1222

WYOMING
The Poison Center
Children's Hospital
8200 Dodge St.
Omaha, NE 68114
Emergency Phone: (800) 222-1222

OTHER
American Society for the Prevention of Cruelty
  to Animals
Animal Poison Control Center
1717 South Philo Rd., Suite 36
Urbana, IL 61802
Emergency Phone: (888) 426-4435

8-3 A Sampling of Agency and Organization Resources Relevant to Environmental Health

AGENCY FOR TOXIC SUBSTANCES AND DISEASE REGISTRY—ATLANTA, GEORGIA

The mission of the Agency for Toxic Substances and Disease Registry (ATSDR) is to prevent or mitigate adverse human health effects and diminished quality of life resulting from exposure to hazardous substances in the environment. ATSDR's Division of Health Education is mandated to assemble, develop, and distribute to the states, medical colleges, physicians, and other health professionals educational materials on medical surveillance, screening, and methods of diagnosis and treatment of injury or disease related to exposure to hazardous substances. ATSDR also provides training and education for primary care physicians to diagnose and treat illness caused by hazardous substances and supports curriculum development and applied research in the area of environmental health.

AMERICAN ACADEMY OF NURSE PRACTITIONERS—AUSTIN, TEXAS

The American Academy of Nurse Practitioners (AANP) was established to promote high standards of health care delivered by nurse practitioners. The AANP acts as a forum to enhance the identity and continuity of nurse practitioners while also addressing national and state legislative issues that affect its members.

AMERICAN ASSOCIATION OF OCCUPATIONAL HEALTH NURSES—ATLANTA, GEORGIA

The American Association of Occupational Health Nurses (AAOHN) is an organization of registered professional nurses employed by business and industrial firms; nurse educators, con-

sultants, and researchers; and others interested in occupational and environmental health nursing. The AAOHN provides continuing education and supports initiatives relevant to occupational and environmental health.

AMERICAN ASSOCIATION OF POISON CONTROL CENTERS—WASHINGTON, DC

The American Association of Poison Control Centers (AAPCC) aids in the procurement of information on the ingredients and potential acute toxicity of substances that may cause accidental poisonings and the proper management of such poisonings. The AAPCC has established standards for the poison information and control centers, which offer immediate information through hotlines around the country. The AAPCC also conducts educational programs and prepares visual aids on prevention of accidental poisonings, maintains a national poisoning database, and operates a nationwide speakers' bureau.

AMERICAN CANCER SOCIETY—ATLANTA, GEORGIA

The American Cancer Society (ACS) comprises volunteers who support education and research in cancer prevention, diagnosis, detection, and treatment. ACS provides special services to cancer patients while also establishing educational programs for health professionals and communities.

AMERICAN COLLEGE OF OCCUPATIONAL AND ENVIRONMENTAL MEDICINE—ARLINGTON HEIGHTS, ILLINOIS

The American College of Occupational and Environmental Medicine (ACOEM) is an association of approximately 6,500 physicians attempting to educate members and other physicians, employers, organizations, and the public about occupational and environmental health. The ACOEM has developed a continuing education course entitled *Core Curriculum in Environmental Medicine* in order to enhance physicians' critical thinking on environmental issues, improve their problem solving skills, and help them make more effective decisions about environmental concerns.

AMERICAN INDUSTRIAL HYGIENE ASSOCIATION—FAIRFAX, VIRGINIA

The goal of the American Industrial Hygiene Association (AIHA) is to promote the highest quality of occupational and environmental health and safety within the workplace and the community through advocacy. The association fosters active collaboration for the protection of worker rights, community health, and safe environment. Ethical practice of industrial hygiene is achieved through the anticipation, recognition, evaluation, and control of hazards arising from the workplace. A sound scientific basis for action, good business, and good occupational and environmental health and safety are closely linked.

AMERICAN LUNG ASSOCIATION—NEW YORK, NEW YORK

The American Lung Association (ALA) is a federation of state and local associations of physicians, nurses, and laymen interested in the prevention and control of lung disease. The ALA works with other organizations in planning and conducting programs in community services, research, and public, professional, and patient education. The ALA also makes recommendations regarding medical care of respiratory disease, occupational health, hazards of smoking, and air conservation.

AMERICAN NURSES ASSOCIATION— WASHINGTON, DC

The American Nurses Association (ANA) comprises registered nurses. The ANA seeks to promote the nursing profession through its sponsorship of the American Nurses Foundation (for research), American Academy of Nursing, Center for Ethics and Human Rights, International Nursing Center, Ethnic/Racial Minority Fellowship Programs, and the American Nurses Credentialing Center. The ANA supports efforts in occupational health and safety.

AMERICAN PUBLIC HEALTH ASSOCIATION—WASHINGTON, DC

The American Public Health Association (APHA) was founded in 1872 as a professional organization of physicians, nurses, educators, academicians, environmentalists, epidemiologists, new professionals, social workers, health administrators, optometrists, podiatrists, pharmacists, dentists, nutritionists, health planners, other community and mental health specialists, and any interested consumer. The APHA seeks to protect and promote personal, mental, and environmental health through the promulgation of health standards, establishment of uniform practices and procedures, development of etiology of communicable diseases, research in public health, and exploration of medical care programs and their relationships to public health.

ASSOCIATION OF OCCUPATIONAL AND ENVIRONMENTAL CLINICS— WASHINGTON, DC

The Association of Occupational and Environmental Clinics (AOEC) is dedicated to higher standards of patient-centered, multidisciplinary care emphasizing prevention and total health through information sharing, quality service, and collaborative research. As a national network of clinical facilities, the clinics vary greatly in orientation, physical facilities, and staff capabilities. However, every clinic does offer an on-site staff physician with either board certification or demonstrated expertise in occupational medicine. Clinics must also have industrial hygienists and other professionals with expertise in occupational and/or environmental health, such as nurses, social workers, and health educators, either on staff or available through a prearranged referral network. The AOEC supports nursing initiatives in occupational and environmental health.

ASSOCIATION OF TEACHERS OF PREVENTATIVE MEDICINE— WASHINGTON, DC

The Association of Teachers of Preventative Medicine (ATPM) is a national organization for medical educators, practitioners, and students committed to advancing the teaching of all aspects of preventive medicine. The scope of knowledge and competence distinctive to preventive medicine includes biostatistics, epidemiology, administration, environmental and occupational health, the application of social and behavioral factors in health and disease, and primary, secondary, and tertiary prevention measures within clinical medicine. The ATPM was founded in 1942 with three basic objectives: (1) advancing medical education; (2) developing instruction, scientific skills and knowledge in preventive medicine; and (3) exchanging experience and ideas among its members.

ASSOCIATION OF UNIVERSITY ENVIRONMENTAL HEALTH/SCIENCES CENTERS—NEW YORK, NEW YORK

The Association of University Environmental Health/Sciences Centers (AUEHSC) provides a forum for all of the university-based environmental health science centers supported by the National Institute of Environmental Health Sciences. The AUEHSC enables members to exchange information, work in collaboration on projects, and promote cooperation among centers.

CENTERS FOR DISEASE CONTROL AND PREVENTION—ATLANTA, GEORGIA

The Centers for Disease Control and Prevention (CDC) is charged with protecting the public health of the nation by providing leadership and direction in the prevention and control of diseases and other preventable conditions and responding to public health emergencies.

CENTER FOR SAFETY IN THE ARTS— NEW YORK, NEW YORK

The Center for Safety in the Arts (CSA) seeks to gather and disseminate information about health hazards encountered by artists, craftsmen, teachers, children, and others working with art materials. The CSA provides on-site assessments of the health and safety features of facilities used by artists, craftsmen, and students; responds to inquiries concerning art-related health hazards; and conducts consultation programs.

CHILDREN'S ENVIRONMENTAL HEALTH NETWORK—WASHINGTON, DC

The Children's Environmental Health Network (CEHN) is a national multidisciplinary project whose mission is to promote a healthy environment and protect the fetus and the child from environmental health hazards. The CEHN has worked on the national level since 1992 and has focused on the areas of research, policy, and education. The CEHN's goals are to promote the development of sound public health and child-focused national policy; stimulate prevention-oriented research; educate health professionals, policy makers and community members in preventive strategies; and elevate public awareness of environmental hazards to children.

COMMITTEES ON OCCUPATIONAL SAFETY AND HEALTH—NATIONWIDE

The Committees on Occupational Safety and Health (COSH) are nonprofit coalitions of local unions and individual workers, physicians, lawyers, and other health safety activists dedicated to the right of each worker to a safe and healthy job. Committees throughout the states provide health and safety training, technical assistance, consultations and on-site evaluations, and contract language assistance.

CONSUMER PRODUCT SAFETY COMMISSION—BETHESDA, MARYLAND

The Consumer Product Safety Commission (CPSC) provides information on health and safety effects related to consumer products. CPSC has direct jurisdiction over chronic and chemical hazards in consumer products; assists consumers in evaluating the comparative safety of consumer products; develops uniform safety standards for consumer products and minimizes conflicting state and local regulations; and promotes research and investigation into the causes and prevention of product-related deaths, illnesses, and injuries.

DEPARTMENT OF ENERGY— WASHINGTON, DC

The Department of Energy (DOE) provides the framework for a comprehensive and balanced national energy plan through the coordination and administration of the energy functions of the federal government. The DOE is responsible for the long-term, high risk research and development of energy technology; the marketing of federal power; energy conservation; the nuclear weapons program; the energy regulations programs; and a central energy data collection and analysis program.

The DOE's Office of Environment, Safety, and Health provides independent oversight of departmental execution of environmental, occupational safety and health, and nuclear/nonnuclear safety and security laws, regulations, and policies; ensures that departmental programs are in compliance with environmental, health, and nuclear/nonnuclear safety protection plans, regulations, and procedures; provides an independent overview and assessment of DOE-controlled activities to ensure that safety programs receive management review; and carries out legal functions of the nuclear safety civil penalty and criminal referral activities mandated by the Price-Anderson Amendments Act.

ENVIRONMENTAL PROTECTION AGENCY—WASHINGTON, DC

The Environmental Protection Agency (EPA) was established in 1970 in order to permit coordinated and effective governmental action on behalf of the environment. The EPA endeavors to abate and control pollution systematically by proper integration of a variety of research, monitoring, standard setting, and enforcement activities. As a complement to its other activities, the agency coordinates and supports research and antipollution activities by state and local governments, private and public groups, individuals, and educational institutions. The EPA also reinforces efforts among other federal agencies with respect to the impact of their operations on the environment, and it is specifically charged with publishing its recommendations concerning a proposal when it is unsatisfactory from the standpoint of public health or welfare or environmental quality. The EPA is designed to serve as the public's advocate for a livable environment.

FOOD AND DRUG ADMINISTRATION— WASHINGTON, DC

The Food and Drug Administration (FDA) inspects manufacturing plants and warehouses and collects and analyzes samples of foods, drugs, cosmetics, and therapeutic devices for adulteration and misbranding. Responsibilities also extend to sanitary preparation and handling of foods, waste disposal on interstate carriers, and enforcement of the Radiation Control Act as related to consumer products. Epidemiological and other investigations are conducted to determine causative factors or possible health hazards involved in adverse reactions or hazardous materials accidents. Investigators are located in resident posts in major cities throughout the country.

INTERNATIONAL COMMISSION ON OCCUPATIONAL HEALTH

The International Commission on Occupational Health (ICOH) was founded in 1906 to study new facts in the field of occupational health, draw the attention of all responsible to the results of study and investigation in occupational health, and organize meetings on national and international problems in this field. The ICOH has established several scientific committees, including the Scientific Committee on Occupational Health Nursing, that focus on specific occupational health problems and issues.

INTERNATIONAL LABOUR ORGANIZATION—GENEVA, SWITZERLAND

The International Labour Organization (ILO) exists to promote and realize standards, fundamental principles, and rights of people at work. To do this, the ILO assists members states as well as employers' and workers' organizations in ratifying ILO Conventions and implementing international labor standards. Since 1994 the ILO has been working to modernize and strengthen its labor standards system

MOTHERRISK PROGRAM—TORONTO, ONTARIO, CANADA

The Motherrisk program counsels callers about the safety of an exposure to drugs, chemicals, or radiation during pregnancy or breastfeeding. A team of physicians and information specialists gives advice on whether medications, x-rays, or chemicals in the work environment will harm the developing fetus or breast-fed baby.

NATIONAL ASSOCIATION OF SCHOOL NURSES—SCARBOROUGH, MAINE

The National Association of School Nurses (NASN) is made up of school nurses throughout the country who conduct comprehensive school health programs in public and private schools. The objectives of the NASN are to provide national leadership in the promotion of health services for schoolchildren, promote school health interests to the nursing and health community and the public, and monitor legislation pertaining to school nursing. The NASN also provides continuing education programs at the national level and assistance to states for program implementation. The NASN also certifies school nurses through its National Board for Certification of School Nurses. Besides establishing several workshops and grants for studying the female body, children, drug abuse, and skin care, the NASN bestows the annual School Nurse of the Year Award and Lillian Wald Research Award.

NATIONAL CANCER INSTITUTE— BETHESDA, MARYLAND

The National Cancer Institute (NCI) conducts and funds research on the causes, diagnosis, treatment, prevention, control, and biology of cancer and the rehabilitation of people with cancer. NCI also funds projects for innovative and effective approaches to preventing and controlling cancer, establishes multidisciplinary cancer care and clinical research activities in community hospitals, and supports cancer research training, clinical training, continuing education, and career development.

NATIONAL CENTER FOR ENVIRONMENTAL HEALTH— ATLANTA, GEORGIA

The mission of the National Center for Environmental Health (NCEH) is to promote health and quality of life by preventing or controlling disease, injury, and disability related to the interactions between people and their environment outside the workplace. To achieve these goals, NCEH directs programs both to prevent the adverse health effects of exposure to toxic substances and to combat the societal and environmental factors that increase the likelihood of exposure and disease. NCEH also works to prevent injuries and diseases resulting from natural or technological disasters and to prevent birth defects and developmental disabilities resulting from nutritional deficiencies or exposure to environmental toxins in utero or during early childhood.

NATIONAL ENVIRONMENTAL HEALTH ASSOCIATION—DENVER, COLORADO

The National Environmental Health Association (NEHA) is a professional society of people engaged in environmental health and protection for governmental agencies, public health and environmental protection agencies, industry, colleges, and universities. NEHA also conducts national professional registration programs and offers continuing education opportunities for interested professionals.

THE NATIONAL ENVIRONMENTAL EDUCATION AND TRAINING FOUNDATION—WASHINGTON, DC

The National Environmental Education and Training Foundation (NEETF) was chartered by Congress in 1990. NEETF is a private nonprofit organization that plays a unique role in the environmental education and training field. NEETF develops and supports environmental learning programs to meet social goals, such as improved health, better education, and "greener," more profitable business. In particular, NEETF addresses the needs of disadvantaged communities requiring cleaner local environments. NEETF makes challenge grants to innovative programs and in recognition of outstanding achievement in the field.

NATIONAL INSTITUTE FOR OCCUPATIONAL SAFETY AND HEALTH—WASHINGTON, DC

The National Institute for Occupational Safety and Health (NIOSH) was established by the Occupational Safety and Health Act of 1970 to conduct research on occupational diseases and injuries, respond to requests for assistance by investigating problems of health and safety in the workplace, recommend standards to the Occupational Safety and Health Administration (OSHA) and the Mine Safety and Health Administration (MSHA), and train professionals in occupational safety and health.

NATIONAL INSTITUTE OF ENVIRONMENTAL HEALTH SCIENCES—RESEARCH TRIANGLE PARK, NORTH CAROLINA

The National Institute of Environmental Health Sciences (NIEHS) is the principal federal agency for biomedical research on the effects of chemical, physical, and biological environmental agents on human health and well-being. The NIEHS supports research and training focused on the identification, assessment, and mechanism of action of potentially harmful agents in the environment. Research results form the basis for preventive programs for environmentally related diseases and for action by regulatory agencies.

The NIEHS currently sponsors several programs available to the medical school community, individual researchers, and other organizations or centers interested in studying the effects of the environment on health and how to better educate medical school students, employees, and the general public about environmental health risks and hazards.

NATIONAL INSTITUTES OF HEALTH— BETHESDA, MARYLAND

The National Institutes of Health (NIH) is the principal biomedical research agency of the federal government. Its mission is to pursue knowledge to improve human health. To accomplish this goal, NIH seeks to expand fundamental knowledge about the nature and behavior of living systems, apply that knowledge to extend the health of human lives, and reduce the burdens resulting from disease and disability. In the quest of its mission NIH supports biomedical and behavioral research around the world, trains promising young researchers, and promotes the acquisition and distribution of medical knowledge. Research activities conducted by NIH will determine much of the quality of health care for the future and reinforce the quality of health care currently available.

NATIONAL STUDENT NURSES' ASSOCIATION—NEW YORK, NEW YORK

The National Student Nurses' Association (NSNA) comprises students currently enrolled in state-approved nursing schools for the preparation of becoming registered nurses. NSNA seeks to aid in the development of the individual nursing student and urges students, as future health professionals, to be aware of and to contribute to improving the health care of all people. NSNA also encourages programs and activities in state groups concerning nursing, health, and the community.

NUCLEAR REGULATORY COMMISSION—WASHINGTON, DC

The Nuclear Regulatory Commission (NRC) licenses and regulates civilian use of nuclear energy to protect health and safety and the environment. This is achieved by licensing persons and companies to build and operate nuclear reactors and other facilities and to own and use nuclear materials. The NRC makes rules and sets standards for these types of licenses. It also carefully inspects the activities of the licensed persons and companies to ensure that they do not violate the NRC safety rules.

OCCUPATIONAL SAFETY AND HEALTH ADMINISTRATION— WASHINGTON, DC

The Occupational Safety and Health Administration (OSHA) was created within the Department of Labor under the Occupational Safety and Health Act of 1970 to enforce national occupational health and safety standards. OSHA encourages employers and employees to reduce workplace hazards, implements new or improved safety and health programs, provides training and research in occupational safety and health, requires a reporting and recording system to monitor job-related illnesses and injuries, develops mandatory job safety and health standards and enforces them effectively, and provides for the development, analysis, evaluation, and approval of state occupational safety and health programs.

PESTICIDE EDUCATION CENTER—SAN FRANCISCO, CALIFORNIA

Founded in 1933 to educate the public about the hazards and health effects of pesticides, the Pesticide Education Center (PEC) works with community groups, workers, individuals, and others harmed by or concerned about risks to their health from exposure to pesticides used in agriculture, home and garden, and other environmental and industrial uses. Its goal is to provide critical information about pesticides so that the public can make informed decisions and choices. The PEC provides information, curricular materials, and help with seminars and workshops on a nationwide basis.

SIGMA THETA TAU INTERNATIONAL— INDIANAPOLIS, INDIANA

Sigma Theta Tau International (STTI) was founded in 1922 as an honorary society for nurses. STTI provides members with the opportunity to access information through its libraries, references, and databases and also recognizes excellence in the field of nursing with grants for research. STTI seeks to promote the profession of nursing as leaders, advocates, and pertinent players in the care of the individual and the community's health.

SOCIETY FOR OCCUPATIONAL AND ENVIRONMENTAL HEALTH— McLEAN, VIRGINIA

The Society for Occupational and Environmental Health (SOEH) includes scientists, academicians, and industry and labor representatives who seek to improve the quality of both working and living places by operating as a neutral forum for conferences involving all aspects of occupational and environmental health. SOEH's activities include studying specific categories of hazards as well as developing methods for assessment of health effects and diseases associated with particular jobs.

TERATOGEN EXPOSURE REGISTRY AND SURVEILLANCE—BOSTON, MASSACHUSETTS

The Teratogen Exposure Registry and Surveillance (TERAS) is a network of geneticists and pathologists studying human embryos and fetuses exposed to teratogens. TERAS maintains information networks for consultation and evaluations.

8-4 Position Statement From the International Council of Nurses: The Nurse's Role in Safeguarding the Human Environment

The preservation and improvement of the human environment has become increasingly important for man's survival and well-being. The vastness and urgency of the task place on every individual and every professional group the responsibility to participate in the efforts to safeguard man's environment, to conserve the world's resources, to study how their use affects man, and how adverse effects can be avoided.

THE NURSE'S ROLE IS TO:

Help detect ill effects of the environment on the health of man, and vice-versa. The nurse should:

- Apply observational skills for the detection of ill effects of environment on the individual;
- Observe individuals in all settings for effects of pollutants in order to advise on protective and/or curative measures;
- Record and analyze observations made of ill effects on environment and/or pollutants on individuals;
- Be informed and report observations of the ecological consequences of pollutants and their adverse effects on the human being.

Be informed and apply knowledge in daily work with individuals, families, and/or community groups as to the data available on potential health hazards and ways to prevent and/or reduce them. The nurse should be informed about:

- The studies and identification of the environmental problems at local, national, and international level
- Their effects on man
- The standards for the protection of the human organism, especially from pollutants

- Ways to prevent and/or reduce health hazards

Be informed and teach preventive measures about health hazards due to environmental factors as well as about conservation of environmental resources to the individual, families, and/or community groups. The nurse can:

- Request and attend continuing education programs about the study of the environment and the application of this knowledge in daily life and work;
- Provide health education for both the general public and health personnel in order to create awareness of environmental issues and to involve the public with environmental management and control;
- Apply knowledge in areas where nursing intervention may prevent or reduce health hazards;
- Report on steps taken to control the significant environmental problems of the area.

Work with health authorities in pointing out health care aspects and health hazards in existing human settlements and in the planning of new settlements. Nurses can:

- Participate in exchange of information and experience about similar environmental problems with authorities in other areas;
- Cooperate with health authorities in the preparation of programs to enable national and local authorities to influence their own environments;
- Participate in the promotion of legislation to improve health care and reduce/prevent health

hazards, and encourage the enforcement of such legislation where/when appropriate;

- Participate in national/local predisaster planning and cooperate in international programs in case of disasters in other countries.

Assist communities in their action on environmental health problems. The nurse can assist communities in programs to:

- Reduce harmful pollutants (chemical, biological, or physical, e.g., noise) in air, soil, water, and food by industries or other human efforts;
- Improve nutrition;
- Encourage family planning;
- Assess environmental factors in work situations and pursue activities for the elimination or reduction of hazards;
- Educate the general public and all levels of nursing personnel in environmental and other health hazards, especially those related to unacceptable levels of contamination.

Participate in research providing data for early warning and prevention of deleterious effects of the various environmental agents to which man is increasingly exposed and research conducive to discovering ways and means of improving living and working conditions. The nurse, as principal investigator or in collaboration with other nurses or related professions, can carry out epidemiological and experimental research designed to provide data for:

- Early warning for prevention of health hazards
- Improving living and working conditions
- Monitoring the environmental levels of pollutants
- Measuring the impact of nursing intervention on environmental hazards

*From "Position Statement," by International Council of Nurses, in *The Nurse's Role in Safeguarding the Human Environment,* 1986, Geneva, Switzerland: Author.

ORGANIZATIONAL CULTURE

An organization is a group or a collection of groups interacting to achieve a common goal. Groups interact and articulate together in such a way that the behavior of one member or group influences the behavior of another. Every organization has cultural norms and values that hold the organization together, and the work of groups is to share common goals and values to facilitate goal achievement. According to Peters and Waterman (1982) in their highly influential book *In Search of Excellence,* companies with effective organizational systems have one thing in common: a shared understanding of the company's value system and reasons for existence (i.e., mission and strategies). How this is translated to the work environment is influenced by and affected through the organizational culture.

Organizational culture has been defined as the learned values, assumptions, and behaviors that knit an organizational community together (Kraut, 1996; McNeil & Garcia, 1991; Schein, 1985; Turnipseed, 1990) and is often viewed as the unwritten, feeling part of the organization (Daft, 1992). Organizational culture preserves and unifies the social structure through a system of norms, expectations, and assumptions about the way individuals feel or behave within a group. For example, if a healthy workforce and a healthful workplace are considered important and valued as goals within the organization, then these goals must be reflected in the actual infrastructure and physical and emotional environment of the company, and programs must be implemented and organizational behaviors modeled to support, promote, and protect worker health (e.g., hazard exposure control, nutrition awareness, stress man-

agement). Culture conceived of as shared key values and beliefs fulfills several important functions. First, it conveys a sense of identity for organization members. Second, it facilitates the generation of commitment to something larger than self. Third, it enhances social system stability, and fourth, it serves as a sense-making device that guides and shapes behavior (Richard, 1992; Smircich, 1983). Several beliefs have been linked that characterize "excellent" organizations (Plessinger, 1993):

- A clear, shared vision connects the corporate vision with day-to-day decisions and work.
- The leadership consistently communicates and reinforces the vision and values.
- Involved employees are a valued asset, not a cost. They assume responsibility for work, control their work environment, and are accountable for the outcomes.
- Employees maintain an external focus (e.g., customer, supplier, general public, community).
- Management understands what competencies are required to accomplish strategic objectives and where competence adds value.
- The organization is structured so that employees can respond quickly and positively to a changing environment.
- Good measures reinforce shared values.
- All members—top to bottom, managers and nonmanagers alike—are in alignment with overall goals and strategies.

In addition, the strength of a culture is associated with member stability. Over time the collective success of an organization's responses leads to greater member or worker stability, which in turn reinforces the development of automatic responses and assumptions about how to respond to situations. This leads to an ever stronger culture. However, this ongoing reinforcement can present a paradox in that the strength of an organization's culture can also block the organization's ability to adapt to a changing environment (Kraut, 1996).

In addition to the dominant culture in organizations there are subcultures and countercultures. Subcultures have the same elements as the dominant culture, including shared ideologies that may support or deviate from the dominant culture. Similar personal characteristics such as age, education, ethnicity, occupational training, and social class facilitate cultural groupings. Countercultures oppose the dominant culture and are often formed by rebellious innovators, chronically discontented employees, or through mergers and acquisitions (Trice & Beyer, 1993). Goodstein et al. (1992) term some members in the organization as heretics—that is, those who challenge the basic assumptions and beliefs of the system and the established order. Members who violate organizational norms are initially pressured to conform. If pressure does not produce the desired conformity, then severe sanctions may be imposed. However, it should be pointed out that large-scale cultural change requires heretical challenges that can precipitate the emergence of a new cultural order.

Organizational culture has often been thought of as the "soft" side of business and therefore much more difficult to measure than the "hard" quantitative areas like product output, expenditures, structures, and cost-benefit ratios. However, corporate leaders are recognizing that organizational culture is basic and foundational to the overall success and profitability of the company and requires attention, nurturing, and understanding.

Harrison and Stokes (1990) describe a typology of organizational cultures that involves four generic types: the power culture, the role culture, the achievement culture, and the support culture

---

Box 9-1 Typology of Organizational Cultures

1. *Power Culture.* This culture is based on an assumption that an inequality of resources such as money, privileges, security, and overall quality of life is natural. Hierarchical structure of the organization is accepted. Strong leaders are needed to manage these inequalities and provide balance to the system. These leaders are firm but fair in power cultures that work well. Poorly managed power cultures are ruled by fear, with power abused by the leaders and their followers for personal gain. Playing politics, manipulation, and infighting is common. Power cultures are best suited for start-up organizations in need of direction; however, as the organization expands, delegation and functional systems are needed for efficiency and continued growth.

2. *Role Culture.* The basis of this culture is that work is best accomplished through rules and procedures. Roles are identified and clearly delineate each person's responsibilities and rewards. The system is managed through task delegation rather than arbitrary (power) control from the top. Role cultures provide stability, justice, and efficiency. Bureaucracies are typical role-oriented cultures that are generally efficient because work is routine and can be managed by rules, regulations, and procedures. However, bureaucracies tend to be rigid and inflexible, thwarting creativity and innovation, which can hamper organizational growth and dynamism.

3. *Achievement Culture.* Within the organizational context this culture supports the notion that people want to make significant contributions to work and society and derive satisfaction from a job well-done and meaningful interactions with others in the work environment. The role of management in this culture is to support workers in achieving the organizational mission and to empower workers to achieve both organizational and professional goals. Sustaining a high level of energy and enthusiasm and dealing with a lack of attention to organizational structures and systems may be difficult.

4. *Support Culture.* This culture's primary motivation is to develop mutual trust and support between the organization and the individual. The valuing and nurturing of the human being is critical in this type of organization, with harmony, warmth, and caring deeply valued and confrontation avoided. This support culture meets important human needs often ignored in organizations; however, commitment to goal/task achievement may be compromised.

(Box 9-1). This model does not presume to categorize organizations by type but rather to assess the degree to which each of these four cultures are represented in an organization. While models will never fit any organization exactly, they are useful in understanding the focus and parameters of cultural norms. Organizations can also be described in terms of (1) anthropology (family, big daddy, prodigal son), (2) mechanism (assembly line, factory, well-oiled machine), (3) television (sitcom, soap opera), (4) military (battles, battle zone, captain, enemies, troops), (5) sports (quarterback, stars, teams), and (6) zoo (chicken, sly fox) (Decker & Sullivan, 1992; Huber, 1996; Swansburg & Swansburg, 1999; Trice & Beyer, 1993; Wilkens, 1989).

Organizational culture exerts a powerful influence on the types of decisions that are made, the kinds of information that are shared, when and in what manner information is disseminated, who is considered powerful, and what employee behaviors are deemed acceptable. The challenge for successful managers is to understand the organizational culture well enough to be able to tailor their behavior and strategies to comply with existing norms and values (del Bueno & Freund, 1986). How successful the occupational and environmental health nurse is will depend in part on successful interrelationships and interactions both vertically and horizontally within the organization and with external groups and constituents and on recognition and understanding of the dynamics of the organizational culture.

Most nurses work in traditional health care settings, such as hospitals, nursing homes, and public health agencies where health care is the primary service. In contrast, the occupational and environmental health nurse practices primarily in a business setting, where the provision of health care is not the primary product, rather a support service to the primary mission (McNeil & Garcia, 1991). Occupational health services and programs are aimed at ensuring a healthy workforce and a safe and healthful work environment in order to reduce or eliminate work-related illnesses and injuries and promote worker health and productivity. From this perspective it is important to recognize the value and relationship of the occupational health unit to the other organizational units. Understanding how the occupational health unit is perceived and fits into the total organization can help the occupational and environmental

health nurse determine the value and effectiveness of occupational health contributions.

CULTURE ASSESSMENT IN THE ORGANIZATION

Within the context of organizational culture it is important to examine organizational politics and related structures such as formal structure and formal and informal communication patterns, leadership styles/behaviors, work environment, projected/perceived image, status symbols, rituals and stories, and evidence of strategic planning (Beyers, 1984; Dieneman, 1989; Hein & Nicholson, 1986; McNeil & Garcia, 1991; Swansburg & Swansburg, 1999). A brief discussion of each of these factors follows. In addition, the concept of power is important because power sources clearly exert a major impact on the organization; these will be discussed in more detail. A detailed checklist for organizational assessment can be found in Appendix 9-1.

Assessment of organizational politics is a critical element and can reveal much information about power relationships, decision making roles and alliances, and who influences resource allocation. A certain amount of politics is inevitable in every organization, and the occupational and environmental health nurse must be able to recognize the power/politics game and players and develop political skills and savvy while maintaining integrity. del Bueno and Freund (1986) identify several strategies for dealing with organizational politics (Box 9-2).

While acquisition of resources may realistically be tied to political tactics and strategies, the organization's values and beliefs must be assessed with respect to political harnessing. Politicizing can breed contempt and distrust, or an employee can quickly become politically vulnerable or expendable or a scapegoat. The manager must be astutely aware of political interrelationships and agendas and use caution and assertiveness as appropriate and necessary.

Assessment of the organization's formal structure is an obvious and key element that can help the occupational and environmental health nurse understand the design, management, and visionary force supporting the organization, the decision making authority centers, and the occupational health unit's fits within the formal and

Box 9-2   Strategies for Dealing with Organizational Politics

- Establish alliances with superiors and peers but choose your friends and confidants carefully.
- Use all possible channels of communication, including formal, informal, and the grapevine.
- Know when to be fair to subordinates but recognize aggressive and manipulative individuals who may want to take over.
- Know how decisions are made, including the influence of powerful people and their biases (not necessarily based on ideas of merit).
- Be courteous, because this is a very powerful tool that increases others' self-esteem.
- Maintain a flexible/adaptable position and do not be uncompromising except on positions or issues that are morally or ethically essential.
- Use passive resistance or delay action when you are under pressure from demands that you cannot openly challenge.
- Project an image of status and power because too much modesty may be perceived as or mistaken for lack of power.

Modified from *Power and Politics in Nursing Administration: A Casebook,* by D. del Bueno and C. Freund, 1986, Owings Mills, MD: National Health.

policy making structure. Examples of key formal structure assessment elements include the mission/philosophy statements and organizational goals, the organizational chart, the key policy and procedure documents, and the job descriptions.

Assessment of both formal and informal communication structures and patterns is critical to understanding how information is disseminated, received, and interpreted. In all organizations the potential for communication breakdown and distortion always exists, and information may be directed without clarity. How vertical (upward and downward) information flows between managers and workers establishes the limits, accessibility, and flexibility with respect to organizational communications. Horizontal communication between workers reflects a degree of teamwork within and across groups. How individuals communicate with each other irrespective of the type of communication is a measure of the level of personal and professional respect encouraged and

supported within the organization. Examples of key formal communication assessment elements include memos, performance appraisal techniques and documents, one-to-one discussions, and meeting structures and frequency.

Informal communication structures are equally important because these represent the grapevine exchange of information, and these key data references determine how information is received, filtered, and interpreted. Informal communication channels can be skillfully manipulated through such strategies as withholding or leaking information to achieve hidden agendas. How workers and managers use the informal structure to pass along and collect information is important to assess. Examples of informal communication assessment elements include observations of social relationships on and off the job between and among coworkers and managers, who avoids whom, who criticizes and supports ideas, and who speaks out.

Leadership styles and behaviors ebb from the historical context of the organization. The organization itself is steeped in history and tradition and is characterized by certain modes of leadership behaviors that are often considered culturally institutionalized. As described previously, the organization has a style and value system with which the leaders articulate, and leaders are often selected to match this style and behavior unless a change in organizational philosophy and behavior is desired. Leaders help shape the culture by identifying and projecting a vision, demonstrating a philosophy, modeling values, setting policies, creating systems, and supporting a reward system. Thus, the occupational and environmental health nurse must recognize and understand organizational leadership behaviors and their impact on workers' behaviors and performance. Examples of leadership assessment elements include visioning; types of leadership styles (autocratic, democratic, situational, transformational); perception of uses of leadership styles (task vs. relationship oriented); intimidation, empowerment, or stabilizing tactics; role modeling behaviors (e.g., facilitating organizational norms/culture); treatment of employees personally and with regard to personal problems; and the value leaders place on worker health and safety as demonstrated by active program support.

Assessment of the work environment is particularly important because this can greatly affect the physical and mental well-being of the workplace inhabitants. The physical condition and hygiene of the environment may be perceived, to some extent, as reflecting how management feels about the workplace and the workers and how the employees feel about the workplace and themselves. Employee satisfaction with this aspect of the organizational culture is important to consider because it affects the productivity and cohesiveness of the organization (Blancett, 1992). Issues related to workplace safety and working conditions, work productivity, and stress production/management are important to assess. Examples of worksite environmental assessment elements include design and structure of existing buildings, adequacy of equipment and supplies, health and safety hazard identification, eating and comfort facilities, and location and adequacy of the occupational health unit.

Assessment of the image the organization portrays or strives to portray is important in determining how the organization desires to be perceived by the external community. In addition, the relationship of the organization to the external community is vital to assess because the organization is affected by the population characteristics of the community (e.g., age of residents, ethnic makeup, and values). Examples of key image assessment elements include slogans or phrases describing the organization, public relations activities, employee dress codes, organizational health consciousness (e.g., smoking, exercise), publications, and involvement in community activities.

Assessment of status symbols can provide information about who has power, who is considered successful, and the degree of corporate elitism. Examples of key status symbol assessment elements include the allocation and location of parking spaces; the size, appearance and location of office space; and the ability to determine one's working hours.

While the organizational culture is being assessed, rituals and stories must be considered. Rituals are time-honored customs that enable individuals to understand social relationships, reduce uncertainty and anxiety, and exert control (e.g., committee meetings that are routinely held without reason and/or productivity) (del Bueno & Freund, 1986). Examples of organizational rituals include holiday parties, company picnics, and participation in sports events.

Stories help describe conflicts, events, and relationships; reinforce the history of decision making; and facilitate the cultural linkages. Stories inform new employees about the organization, affirm important values and norms, and reveal what is unique about the organization's function in society (Conner & Lake, 1994). As stated by del Bueno and Freund:

> *It is not sufficient to have knowledge of the formal structure, the written rules and policies. These only represent the surface or the conscious life of the organization. Penetration beneath the surface level is necessary to understand the true reality of the organization, which consists of both the overt and the covert or the conscious and the unconscious. Linkage among values, beliefs, and actions are often explained by the organization's rituals, myths, and stories. A diverse sample of these and other indicators are necessary to form a true picture of an organization's culture.* (p. 20)

An important part of the organizational culture experience is the existence and viability of a strategic vision, because this implies a future-oriented organization. Strategic planning allows for an integration of a shared vision and shared values regarding the organization's future direction and should take into consideration any deliberate or planned changes needed if cultural ruts or barriers thwart process and long-range improvements. Strategic vision and planning must examine the core organization culture and fit with the organization's mission, goals and objectives, and relationship to its environment. Several questions to consider when assessing the organization's strategic status are shown in Box 9-3.

Box 9-3 Assessing Strategic Status

- Where is the enterprise currently?
- Where does the organization wish to be in the future?
- What steps are needed to achieve the desirable state?
- What is the environmental context?
- How do the internal strengths and weaknesses relate to the external opportunities and threats?

Changes in the external environment make it critical for organizations to develop a strategic vision, because this helps to define the organization for the future and shape services and ventures. Critical factors to consider and predict are information technology, regulations, and competitors. The strategic planning process does more than plan for the future; it helps an organization create its future.

If organizational change is needed, cultural groups will need to be identified. This will involve examining the norms and behaviors of the organizational members and asking what needs to be changed. This may include norms related to the following (Conner & Lake, 1994):

- *Task/task support.* Helping others, sharing information, and being concerned about efficiency
- *Task innovation.* Being creative, taking risks, and performing new activities
- *Social relationships.* Mixing business with nonbusiness activities and socializing with co-workers
- *Personal freedom.* Using self-expression, being autonomous in work decisions, and exercising judgment

Worker groups then identify the norms appropriate for the organization's success and implement and monitor culture changes. This will require management to support, facilitate, and enforce the changes, team building to support the organization's effort in the culture change, and strategic direction to set in motion goals, tasks, people, and resources to operationalize the culture change.

A concept closely related to organizational culture is that of the social climate of the environment or organization. Moos (1994) has examined the "personality" of a work setting or organization that affects the work environment, work outcomes, and job satisfaction, and has developed a Work Environment Scale (WES) that comprises subscales to measure the social environment of the work setting. The subscales assess three major dimensions: Relationships, Personal Growth, and System Maintenance and Change. The Relationship dimensions are measured by the Involvement, Peer Cohesion, and Supervisor Support subscales; the Personal Growth dimensions are measured by the Autonomy, Task Orientation, and Work Pressure subscales; and the System Maintenance and Change dimensions are measured by the Clarity, Control, Innovation, and Physical Comfort subscales. The WES can also be used to compare employee and manager perceptions and actual and preferred work environments, enhance organizational development, and identify interventions to foster job satisfaction and productivity, including evaluating organizational dynamics, planning for organizational change, encouraging teamwork and cohesiveness, facilitating organizational management, and planning for physical environmental change (Flarey, 1991). The complete instrument, which can be used to assess the work environment, can be obtained from Consulting Psychologists Press.

POWER CONCEPTS AND RELATIONSHIPS

The organizational culture gives rise to various forms of power and influence in the company and supports or negates actions taken by its employees. Power and influence are interrelated concepts. In organizations power can be derived from several sources (Box 9-4) (French & Raven, 1959; Hersey & Blanchard, 1996; Tomey, 2000; Yukl, 1989). Power generally refers to the capacity or ability of an individual or group to influence, modify, or control the behavior of another individual or group in such a way that desired results are achieved (Shortell, 1993). Power is derived from where individuals stand in the division of labor and the communications system of the organization. One's place in these structures fosters power from the ties one has to other influential people in the organization, the formal authority system of the organization, the ability to deal with important uncertainties or contingencies that face the organization, and the control over resources. Jurisdiction over resources is an important source of power within the structural framework, but only to the extent that one actually controls the resource and its use. Further, resources that serve as a basis of power must be critical for the organization; that is, the resource must be essential to the functioning of the organization, in short supply or concentrated in terms of the number of people who possess it, and nonsubstitutional (Shortell, 1993).

Box 9-4   Sources of Power

Legitimate Power is based on the position held by the leader. Normally, the higher the position, the higher the legitimate power tends to be. Leaders high in legitimate power induce compliance or influence others because others in the organization feel these leaders have the right, by virtue of position in the organization, to expect that suggestions will be followed.

Reward Power is based on the leader's ability to provide rewards for other people who believe that compliance will lead to positive incentives such as increased pay, promotion, or recognition.

Coercive/Punitive Power is based on fear. A leader high in coercive power is seen as inducing compliance because failure to comply will lead to punishment, such as undesirable work assignments, reprimands, or dismissal.

Information Power is based on the leader's possession of or access to information that is perceived as valuable by others. This power base influences others because they need this information or want to be in on things.

Expert Power is based on the leader's possession of expertise, skill, and knowledge, which through respect influences others and leads to compliance with the leader's wishes. A leader high in expert power is seen as possessing the expertise to facilitate the work behavior of others.

Referent Power is based on the leader's personal traits. A leader high in referent power is generally liked and admired by others because of personality, which allows for personal influence.

Connection Power is based on the leader's connections with influential or important persons inside or outside the organization. A leader high in connection power induces compliance from others because they aim at gaining the favor or avoiding the disfavor of the powerful connection.

Influence is considered the effect one party has on another. Even though simply stated, the process of influence may take different forms and result in different outcomes. For example, when one party (agent) is attempting to get another party (target) to accept an idea, proposal, or decision, the result may include a commitment to the decision or request with an enthusiasm to implement the decision; compliance with the decision but apathy or minimal effort toward decision implementation; or resistance to the proposal or decision through active opposition to implementation, such as making excuses, trying to influence withdrawal of the request, sabotaging the implementation plan, and refusing to carry out the request (Yukl, 1989).

POSITIONAL POWER

Formal authority or legitimate power is based on the leadership position held in the organization and the associated rights and responsibilities inherent in that position. The manager has the right to influence and make requests such as certain work assignments, and workers have an obligation to comply. Tied to formal authority is the manager's authority to make decisions regarding allocation of resources. The higher one's authority position in the organization, the more control she or he has over resources.

Power related to reward and punishment is based on the perceived credibility of the manager to effect the reward or punishment as promised. The capacity to provide compensation, promotions, more responsibility, or status symbols, such as larger office space or reserved parking, are examples of reward power. The organization also uses formal authority in the form of punishment or coercive power to influence workers, although this method of power is not very effective and is used infrequently (Katz & Kahn, 1978). Examples of coercive or punishment power include undesired assignments, withheld pay increases, and termination (Tomey, 2000). Punitive power, such as job dismissal for arbitrary reasons, is usually prohibited; however, in situations where workers do not perform their duties or thwart the organizational goals, some form of disciplinary or punitive action may be expected. A leader with substantive reward and punishment power is more likely to obtain worker compliance with requests and demands even when no explicit promises or threats have been made. However, workers are more likely to acknowledge being influenced by referent or expert power than to admit to succumbing to change based on compensation or fear of reprisal (Yukl, 1989).

One's access to and control over the distribution of vital information to others is an important source of power. Control of information downward can involve selective interpretation and filtering and may also involve distortion of information in an attempt to dictate a certain course of action. In addition, withholding information from workers may also serve to increase worker dependence on the leader or manager for decision making and, in effect, decrease worker autonomy.

PERSONAL POWER

Types of personal power, which are viewed as facilitating the work, include expert and referent power. Expert power is based on one's possession of expertise, knowledge, and skills in problem solving and task performance. Perceived expertise can be as influential as actual expertise; however, in the long term actual expertise will need to be demonstrated, and certainly expertise must be maintained. Specialized knowledge and skills will remain sources of power as long as dependence on the person who possesses these characteristics continues. Knowledge of the organization's history, rules, regulations, and work strategies helps in acquiring and retaining knowledge power over those without the knowledge to meet their responsibilities (Loveridge & Cummings, 1996).

Referent power is based on one's personal traits wherein the leader is liked and admired by others and symbolizes what others desire. This type of power is often dependent upon feelings of friendship and loyalty, and often the worker identifies with a likable leader, perceiving some of the same qualities in herself or himself. Referent power is an important source of upward, horizontal, and downward power in organizations; that is, praise, flattery, and loyalty given sincerely can be very influential at all levels (Kaplan, 1984; Tomey, 2000).

INTERPERSONAL POWER

The power of politics is pervasive in organizations and includes such strategies as co-optation, connection, and coalitions. Co-optation is a form of political action wherein the objective is to overcome the opposing party by encouraging the group or a member of the group to become a part of the project, committee, or function responsible for the decision making. The result then usually favors the proposed action through individual or group attitude change and ownership, and thus the member and/or group are co-opted to carry out the decision (Goodstein, 1992).

Connection power refers to the leader's connection to or relationship with other influential individuals who have the capacity to reward or disfavor, either internal or external to the organization. The leader is thus viewed as powerful by association, and workers, peers, or colleagues may feel they can gain by association with the leader.

Coalitions and alliances represent a political force that acts together to get what it wants either in supporting or opposing a particular change or program (Stevenson et al., 1985). In a coalition two or more groups (e.g., departments) unite, generally to achieve a common goal, such as better or increased human and physical resources. The literature attaches considerable significance to the importance of finding others with common interests and building long-term relationships with them. Such coalitions differ from ad hoc arrangements insofar as they imply future as well as present commitment. Alliances and coalitions are developed through several different mechanisms, including helping people to obtain positions of power through appointments and promotions and doing favors for those whose support is needed (Pfeffer, 1992). Another common example is the use of collective bargaining strategies to acquire more benefits, such as increased compensation or improved working conditions.

In organizations the use of power varies greatly, depending on individual relationships (i.e., upward, downward, lateral) and the cultural and situational context. Effective leaders are likely to use a mix of power tactics to effect change. Over time leaders gain and lose power in organizations, depending on such factors as loyalty, competence, and success. Political processes and other types of power are used to protect and increase one's power in organizations; how these processes are used and the consequences of any action must be recognized and understood.

Conflict in organizations exists, and potential or probable reasons for the conflict between individuals or groups are often attributable to power struggles related to philosophical differences, competing values, and competition for scarce resources. In working with people and organizations, the occupational and environmental health nurse manager can utilize skills and tactics to help prevent or resolve power struggles and conflicts as previously described by recognizing the context of the organizational culture.

Summary

Organizational culture is an important force in determining the direction, support, and influence of the health of the work environment. While health care managers and administrators spend a lot of time attending to management and delivery of workplace health services, they must carefully assess organizational culture and other variables such as formal and informal structures and power relationships in order to effectively understand decision making tactics and strategies used to effect change and productivity in organizations.

References

Beyers, M. (1984). Getting on top of organizational change. *Journal of Nursing Administration, 14,* 32-37.

Blancett, S. (1992). Satisfaction: It's more than effectiveness and efficiency. *Journal of Nursing Administration, 22,* 5.

Conner, P. E., & Lake, L. K. (1994). *Managing organizational change.* Westport, CT: Praeger.

Daft, R. L. (1992). *Organization theory and design.* St. Paul, MN: West.

Decker, P. J., & Sullivan, E. J. (1992). *Nursing administration.* Norwalk, CT: Appleton & Lange.

del Bueno, D., & Freund, C. (1986). *Power and politics in nursing administration: A casebook.* Owings Mills, MD: National Health.

Dieneman, J. (1989). Theoretical perspectives in organization science for nursing administration. In B. Henry, C. Arndt, M. Divincetti, & A. Marriner-Tomey (Eds.), *Dimensions of nursing administration.* Boston: Blackwell Scientific.

Flarey, D. (1991). The social climate: A tool for organizational change and development. *Journal of Nursing Administration, 21,* 37-44.

French, J., & Raven, B. (1959). The bases of social power. In D. Canwright (Ed.), *Studies of social power.* Ann Arbor, MI: Institute for Social Research.

Goodstein, L. D., Nolan, T. M., & Pfeiffer, J. W. (1992). *Applied strategic planning.* San Diego, CA: Pfeiffer & Company.

Harrison, R., & Stokes, H. (1990). *Diagnosing organizational culture.* Mountain View, CA: Harrison.

Hein, E., & Nicholson, J. (1986). Assessing organizational structure. In E. Hein & J. Nicholson (Eds.) *Contemporary leadership behavior: Selected readings* (pp. 353-362). Boston: Little, Brown & Company.

Hersey, P., & Blanchard, K. (1996). *Management of organizational behavior.* Englewood Cliffs, NJ: Prentice Hall.

Huber, D. (1996). *Leadership and nursing care management.* Philadelphia: W. B. Saunders.

Kaplan, R. E. (1984). Trade routes: The manager's network of relationships. *Organizational dynamics, Spring,* 37-52.

Katz, D., & Kahn, R. L. (1978). *The social psychology of organizations.* New York: John Wiley.

Kraut, A. I. (1996). *Organizational surveys: Tools for assessment and change.* San Francisco: Jossey-Bass.

Loveridge, C. E., & Cummings, S. H. (1996). *Nursing management in the new paradigm.* Gaithersburg, MD: Aspen.

McNeil, V., & Garcia, M. A. (1991). Enhancing program management through cultural organizational assessment. *AAOHN Update Series, 4*(6), 1-8. Skillman, NJ: Continuing Professional Education Center.

Moos, R. (1994). *Work environment scale manual* (4th ed.). Palo Alto, CA: Consulting Psychologists Press.

Peters, T. S., & Waterman, R. H. (1982). *In search of excellence: Lessons from America's best-run companies.* New York: Harper and Row.

Pfeffer, J. (1992). *Managing with power: Politics and influence in organizations.* Boston: Harvard Business School Press.

Plessinger, P. (1993). Organizational change: Pushing the right levers. *The Planning Forum Network, 6,* 5.

Richard, L. (1992). *Organization theory and design* (4th ed.). St. Paul: West.

Schein, E. (1985). *Organizational culture and leadership.* San Francisco: Jossey-Bass.

Shortell, S. M. (1993). *Health Care Management: Organizational Design and Behavior.* Albany, NY: Delmar.

Smircich, L. (1983). Concepts of culture and organizational analysis. *Administrative Science Quarterly, 28,* 339-358.

Stevenson, W., Pearce, J., & Porter, L. (1985). The concept of coalitions in organization and theory and research. *Academy of Management Review, 10,* 256-268.

Swansburg, R. C., & Swansburg, R. J. (1999). *Introductory Management and Leadership for Nurses: An Interactive Text.* Boston: Jones & Bartlett.

Tomey, A. M. (2000). *Guide to nursing management and leadership.* St. Louis: Mosby.

Trice, H. M., & Beyer, I. M. (1993). *The futures of work organizations.* Englewood Cliffs, NJ: Prentice Hall.

Turnipseed, D. (1990). Evaluation of health care work environments via a social climate scale: Re-suits of a field study. *Hospital Health Services Administration, 35,* 245-262.

Wilkins, A. L. (1989). *Developing corporate character.* San Francisco: Jossey-Bass.

Yuki, L. (1989). *Leadership in organizations.* Englewood Cliffs, NJ: Prentice Hall.

9-1 An Organizational Culture Checklist

What beliefs and norms organize and influence rules, policies, and behavior in your organization? What is the desired image? What is explicit and what is implicit? The following checklist is neither all-inclusive nor universally applicable. It may be helpful, however, for learning about and understanding your organization's culture and subcultures.

IMAGE

- How does the organization wish to be perceived? What word, slogans, or phrases are used in describing the organization? Examples: friendly, caring, innovative, safe, up-and-coming, biggest, oldest, dependable.
- Is money obviously being spent on creating this image with respect to decor, landscaping, equipment, signage, public relation activities, annual reports, or community activities?
- How does the public get access to the organization? Through a lobby, parking garage, clinic, or reception area? How comfortable, attractive, and secure is this access?
- How are visitors treated? Does the treatment depend on socioeconomic status?
- Is community involvement expected of employees? If so, does it depend on position or status in the organization?

DEPORTMENT

- Is there a dress code? How strictly is it enforced? Is it different for men and women? Do people dress formally/informally? Does this depend on status in the hierarchy?
- Is facial hair tolerated on men? Is hair length or style an issue? How much makeup and jewelry can women wear?
- Is touching acceptable or desirable? Only between same-sex employees or between opposite sexes? How much, if any, affection is acceptable?
- What kind of relationships are acceptable off the job between different sexes, at different job or position levels?

- Can people "let themselves go" at parties or social events?
- Is social drinking or smoking acceptable on the job?
- Are there off-limits places for employees?
- Does it matter whom you hang around with or does it depend on your position?
- Are there social stratifications? If so, what is the basis of this stratification: title, department, personal relationship?
- Is swearing or use of four-letter words acceptable? Can employees tell off-color or ethnic jokes? Is political correctness the norm?
- Do employees use first names or last names with each other? Does it depend on job position or gender? Does it depend on the setting (e.g., social gatherings versus work)?
- Are sexist behaviors tolerated? Does it depend on title or status?

STATUS SYMBOLS AND REWARD SYSTEMS

- Are there any acknowledged symbols of status such as space, titles, or special privileges?
- On what basis are promotions given: performance, longevity, loyalty? Are upper-level positions given to outsiders or only to those who have "earned their stripes"?
- Are there restricted areas or areas that are off-limits except for special groups, such as meeting rooms or lounge spaces?
- Do only specific individuals or positions warrant reserved parking or personal bathrooms or closets?
- What are the elitist committees, societies, projects, or events?
- Do certain people receive special perquisites such as a company car, country club membership, or professional association dues? Who are those individuals?
- What badges or physical indicators such as beepers, personal desktop computers, different uniforms, or clipboards set people apart as being special?

- Who gets sent to the fun cities for conventions and meetings?
- Do titles truly reflect status and authority in the organization?

ENVIRONMENT AND AMBIANCE

- Are there lounges or places for employees to relax? Where are they located? How attractive and comfortable are they?
- Are eating and drinking allowed in the work area?
- Are there public eating areas? Who has access? What is the appearance and ambiance?
- Can employees have plants, photographs, posters, or other individual touches in their work areas or offices?
- Is there a company color scheme? If so, is it subdued, bright, sterile?
- Is music provided or acceptable in work areas or offices?
- What are the norms in regard to starting time, quitting time, and "goof-off" time?
- Who eats with whom? Are there separate eating areas for special groups?
- How is office furniture arranged? Is open seating at tables or in a circle encouraged?

COMMUNICATION

- Is the norm for important communication verbal or written?
- Are written communications formal or informal? Is the preferred style narrative or memo? Is language to the point or circuitous?
- Is jargon acceptable or desirable? in the organization? with clients or outsiders?
- Are minutes of meetings kept? Are they circulated? If so, to whom? What kind of reports are important and what kind are filed in the wastebasket?
- Is rumor the usual method of information distribution?
- Are there bulletin boards, company newsletters, or house organs? How important or meaningful are these means of communication? What is their purpose: recognition, information, or both?
- Does important information flow from the top down or from the bottom up? Can the chain of command be circumvented without punishment?

- Where does important communication take place: in meetings, in the hall, at social functions, away from the place of business, in the men's room?

MEETINGS

- Are there unwritten rules about who speaks first and last at meetings?
- What meetings can you skip without being punished or is missing anything important?
- Is it permissible to come late or leave early, or does it depend on whose meeting it is?
- Where are people seated? Are there territorial rights? Are there established arrangements based on status or hierarchy?
- Is discussion allowed? Is the agenda predetermined and no adjustments permissible?
- Are refreshments provided? Who pours or serves the refreshments? Does everyone help himself?
- Are time limits strictly enforced?

RITES, RITUALS, AND CEREMONIES

- Are there established rituals that must be attended, such as Monday morning executive breakfast meetings, Friday afternoon drinks or beer bashes, Christmas parties, the annual picnic?
- Is orientation to the organization special? Who greets new employees? Is orientation different for different position levels?
- What does the organization do to recognize length of service? birth of employees' children? retirement? marriage? death in employees' families?
- Are there sports teams? How important is membership or participation?
- Are there rules or assumptions about how long you have to be employed before you are considered an insider?

SACRED COWS

(A sacred cow is a person, place, thing, or belief that cannot be discussed, attacked, or ignored. Sacred cows are revered and protected. Denial of the existence of sacred cows or failure to give fealty to them is fraught with risk.)

- Are there heroes, living or dead, in the organization who are revered and honored? How did these individuals get to be heroes?

- Are there any myths about the organization that must be perpetuated, such as, "We have a mission to the poor and needy"?
- Are there any subjects or ideas that are taboo, such as unionization or merit systems?
- Are there rules or policies that are sacrosanct and cannot be changed even if outdated, ineffective, or illogical?
- Are there relationships between departments, individuals, or groups that cannot be threatened, challenged, or questioned, such as between physicians and nurses or between lay members and professional or religious members of the board?
- If there is a difference between what we do and what we say, is it acceptable to acknowledge this inconsistency or is it taboo to suggest that such a situation even exists?
- Can employees speak freely to the media or are all public relations and statements carefully controlled?

SUBCULTURES

- Are there any? If so, what purpose do they serve? Is the purpose deliberate?
- If there are subcultures, are they subversive or covert? Are they tolerated or pointed to with pride as our unique group, department, or unit?

From *Power and Politics in Nursing Administration: A Casebook,* by D. del Bueno and C. Freund, 1986, Owings Mills, MD: National Health.

10 Workers as Clients: Health Assessment and Surveillance

Assessment, surveillance, management, and promotion of worker health is central to occupational and environmental health nursing professional practice. The development and conduct of worker health assessment, surveillance, and monitoring programs may be a joint effort among several health care disciplines; however, in most occupational health settings the occupational and environmental health nurse assumes major responsibility for the implementation and management of these programs. Depending on the knowledge, skills, and experience level of the occupational and environmental health nurse and/or specific conditions being evaluated, some functions, such as physical assessment/examination, may be performed by or shared collaboratively with other health care professionals. Written guidelines should be available to detail the processes and procedures necessary to carry out programs specific to each occupational health setting and to delineate roles and functions within the context of legal scope of practice and skill mix needed (e.g., nurse, physician, industrial hygienist).

A health assessment, monitoring, and surveillance program for workers is multidimensional and should provide for the following:

- Assessment of the worker by noting the demands of the job with the compatibility of the worker without risk to the worker or coworkers
- Collection and recording of baseline health status data for future comparative purposes, particularly in the event of disability, illness, or injury
- Documentation of preexisting or concurrent illnesses and injuries to be included in the worker health status data profile
- Proper placement of prospective workers in jobs that will match worker capabilities

- Promotion of continued safe and healthful employment for employees within the context of the work and working environments
- Detection of infectious or communicable diseases and referral for appropriate health care management
- Detection of nonoccupationally related acute and chronic conditions for appropriate management, referral, and/or monitoring
- Determination of any evidence of impaired health as a result of harmful work-related exposures and working conditions, and recommendations for corrective actions, worker removal, and/or job placement
- Adherence to compliance with government-mandated regulations
- Maintenance, improvement, or rehabilitation of employee health

Several benefits have been associated with the assessment and surveillance of worker health. These include the early recognition and prevention of work-related illness and injury, decreased absenteeism as a result of hiring workers who can safely perform the job, and identification of health status and lifestyle risk factors, which may be reduced through early medical referral, preventive strategies, and health counseling techniques, such as smoking cessation program efforts (Levy & Wegman, 2000; Matte et al., 1990; Meservy et al., 1997).

Depending on work-related exposures and health hazards, government-mandated surveillance activities, and company philosophy related to health, several types of health protection programs may be performed at the worksite. The most common types include worker placement assessments and periodic health surveillance and monitoring activities. Various definitions for

---

Box 10-1 Common Workplace
Assessments

Preplacement assessment is conducted in order to match the demands of the job with the employee's capabilities by evaluating existing health conditions with respect to potential aggravation by job duties and to provide baseline data for future comparisons.

Return to work assessment is conducted to evaluate any change in the employee's health status that might require a change in the work duties and to assure proper work placement to prevent further illness and injury.

Job transfer assessment is conducted to match the employee's capabilities with proposed new job when there has been a change in the employee's health status or in the work conditions that place the employee at health risk.

Periodic health monitoring is conducted, at intervals, to detect any previously unrecognized health problems or undiagnosed health effects and to determine if work-related health effects have occurred.

Health surveillance is conducted to target specific high-risk groups for specific adverse health effects tied to a particular occupational exposure.

---

these types of assessments, have been provided (Box 10-1) (Brown, 1981; Burkeen & Cooper, 1985; Felton, 1990; Freeman, 1983; Guidotti et al., 1989; McCunney, 2002). Special health assessments, such as fitness for duty or retirement assessments, may also be conducted.

WORKER PLACEMENT ASSESSMENT

Worker placement assessments are conducted to ensure that employees can perform a job without hazard to themselves or their coworkers. There are various reasons for performing worker placement assessments; however, the most common reasons include preplacement assessment, return to work evaluation, and job transfer assignment.

PREPLACEMENT ASSESSMENT

After an offer of employment is made, the preplacement assessment is conducted. It is designed to recommend placement of prospective workers into their positions of hire in accordance with their physical and emotional capacities and the physical, psychosocial, and environmental demands of the job (Cassidy, 1993; Felton, 1990; Hayes, 1993; Levy & Wegman, 2000). The assessment is also conducted to identify previously undiagnosed health problems, any health-related condition that may be aggravated by or compromise job duties, and potential situations that may affect the health and safety of coworkers. The critical determinants in the decision making processes are the individual's health, a thorough understanding of the job duties, and the work environment (McCunney, 2002). Preplacement assessments provide baseline data against which future evaluative data can be measured, and these assessments may also be part of certain legally mandated Occupational Safety and Health Administration (OSHA) standards' requirements (e.g., asbestos, benzene, lead).

In order to complete an accurate health assessment, occupational history and physical assessment, the occupational health professional must be given (by the employer) current information about the worker's job, such as a job description, job demand checklist or job task, and safety analysis, which might include a video observation. The analysis provides a definition of the work, how it is to be performed, the duration and frequency of the tasks, any specific activities to be conducted, such as repetitive movements and lifting or operation of equipment, the potential for exposure to hazardous agents, and recommendations for abatement. This analysis will help focus data collection relative to specific target body systems that may be affected by job demands. A job safety analysis form can be found in Chapter 7.

When the preplacement assessment is being conducted, subjective and objective data are incorporated to arrive at a diagnosis and plan of care to facilitate worker placement and health (Jarvis, 1996). Subjective data include information obtained from a comprehensive personal and family health history, a detailed occupational health history, and a general review of systems. The occupational and environmental health nurse should be thoroughly familiar with these assessment components. Various formats for obtaining pertinent historical and health status information are available and can be modified or tailored in terms of understanding and terminology to guide the data collection process and meet the needs of prospective employees completing the forms. A thorough personal history can help the health care provider determine if a health condition exists that creates incompatibility with the job (e.g., a job requiring heavy lifting and preexisting back injury); it also provides an opportunity to do health teaching and counseling (Burkeen & Cooper, 1985). An example of a comprehensive health history is shown in Box 10-2.

The occupational health history (Figure 10-1) is designed to help the occupational health care provider discover preexisting conditions that may be exacerbated by workplace exposures and conditions, determine relevance of previous work experiences that may affect health, identify asymptomatic employees with existing illnesses, and identify potentially synergetic risk factors (Ginetti & Greig, 1981; Goldman & Peters, 1981; LaDou, 2000; Papp & Miller, 2000; Rosenstock & Cullen, 1994). The occupational and environmental health nurse/examiner must understand the prospective employee's job title, duties, tasks, related demands, potential work-related hazards, and any physical and/or emotional capacities required in order to conduct an accurate assessment (Felton, 1990).

The occupational history has five key parts: a description of all the employee's pertinent jobs, both past and present; a review of exposures related to health; information on the timing of symptoms in relation to work; data on similar problems among coworkers; and information on nonwork factors, such as smoking habits and hobbies that may cause or contribute to disease or injury (Levy & Wegman, 2000). The history should include descriptions of all jobs held by the employee and in some cases information on summer and part-time jobs held while attending school. Job titles alone are not sufficient because the same job title may mean entirely different job responsibilities in two different companies. For example, a clerical position in a bank will have different exposures than the same title position in a hospital or laboratory setting. The occupational history can add to the description of the actual work performed with associated exposures and hazards. For the current job it may be useful to have the employee describe a typical work shift from start to finish and simulate the performance of work tasks by demonstrating actual work performed. Observational visits may be scheduled to see the work performed and are always informative. Routine as well as unusual and overtime tasks, such as cleaning out tanks or cleaning up spills, should also be noted, because they may be the most hazardous assignments.

The employee should be questioned carefully about working conditions and past or present biological, chemical, physical, and psychological exposures. Open-ended questions, such as, What have you worked with?, are asked initially and then are followed by more specific questions, such as, Have you ever been exposed to lead? It is often worthwhile to rephrase important questions and ask them at two points in the interview, because employees sometimes recall, upon repeat questioning, exposures that they initially overlooked. It is also important to inquire about unusual accidents or incidents that may be related to the problem (such as hazardous spills) or about introduction of new substances or changed processes at work (Levy & Wegman, 2000). Qualification of exposure in terms of exposure duration, skin contact, hand washing, and use of personal protective equipment will also be important assessment parameters.

Information on the relatedness of exposure to symptoms is often vital in determining whether a given disease or syndrome is work-related. The following questions are often useful: Do the symptoms begin shortly after the start of the workday? Do they disappear shortly after leaving work? Are they present during weekends or vacation periods? (Levy & Wegman, 2000). Latent periods will vary for certain exposures that produce diseases; thus, the occupational and environmental health professional will need to understand these important conditions. For example, certain irritants with low water-solubility produce severe pulmonary damage and even fatal pulmonary edema with onset about 12 to 18 hours after work ceases, whereas symptoms of byssinosis are characteristically worse on returning to work on Monday morning.

Knowledge of other workers at the same workplace or in similar jobs elsewhere who have the same symptoms or illness may be the most important clue to recognizing work-related disease and must be queried. Both acute and long-term consequences (e.g., cancer) should be discussed, if known. Nonwork exposures and activities should be discussed as a synergistic relationship between occupational and nonoccupational factors in disease causation. Questions about cigarette smok-

Box 10-2 Comprehensive Health History

Identifying data should include date of history and demographic information such as date of birth, sex, race/ethnicity, marital status, education, and occupation.

Major concerns should include detailed description of pertinent health problems or concerns, especially the onset and manifestation of the problem and treatment, if any, received.

Health history should include general state of health; all previous childhood and adult illnesses/injuries, immunizations; mental illness; hospitalizations and operations; allergies; current medications; and living patterns including diet, sleep, exercise, and use of coffee, alcohol, other drugs, and tobacco.

Family history should include age and health status of each immediate family member and (where relevant) causes of death as well as occurrence of relevant health conditions within the family such as arthritis, blood disorders, cardiovascular disease (i.e., stroke), diabetes, headaches, hypertension, kidney dysfunction, mental illness, or tuberculosis.

Psychosocial history should include an outline or description of important, relevant information about the employee such as recreation and leisure activities, lifestyle, and social support system.

Occupational history (see Figure 10-1).

Review of systems should include the following:

General	Usual weight or recent change, weakness, fatigue, fever
Skin	Rashes, itching, irritation, injury, color change, changes in hair or nails
Head	Headaches, head injury
Eyes	Pain, redness, itching, excessive tearing, discharge, vision blurred/impaired, cataracts, glaucoma, glasses, last eye examination
Ears	Pain, infection, discharge, tinnitus, vertigo, earaches, hearing loss, hearing aid
Nose/sinuses	Stuffiness, hay fever, epistaxis, sinus trouble
Mouth/throat	Condition of teeth and gums, frequent sore throats, hoarseness
Neck	Pain, swollen nodes, goiter, limited range of motion
Respiratory	Cough, sputum (color, quality), dyspnea, wheezing, asthma, pneumonia, tuberculosis, bronchitis, emphysema, smoking history, allergies
Cardiovascular	Coronary heart disease, hypertension, murmurs, dyspnea, orthopnea, edema, varicosities, thrombophlebitis, past electrocardiogram
Breasts	Pain, nipple discharge, dimpling, lumps, mastectomy
Gastrointestinal	Difficulty swallowing, change in appetite, pain, nausea, vomiting, diarrhea, constipation, change in bowel habits, rectal bleeding, hemorrhoids, jaundice, liver/hepatitis, gallstone
Urinary genito-reproductive	Frequency of urination, dysuria, hermaturia, nocturia, infections, incontinence
Male	Discharge from or sores on penis, history of sexually transmitted diseases, testicular pain/masses, sexual/reproductive difficulties, hernias
Female	Menstrual history/dysfunction, menopausal symptoms, post-menopausal bleeding, discharge, itching, history of sexually transmitted diseases, last Pap smear, obstetrical history, birth control methods, sexual/reproductive difficulties
Musculoskeletal	Back or neck pain, stiffness, injury, or abnormality; stiff, painful (arthritic), locking, dislocated, trick, or weak joints; flat feet; bone fracture, deformity, infection, or disease; amputations; difficulty working in certain body positions; bursitis
Neurologic	Fainting, blackouts, dizziness, loss of balance or poor coordination, seizures, paralysis, local weakness, numb places or situations
Mental status	Nervousness, depression, mood changes, anxiety, tension
Endocrine	Thyroid trouble, diabetes, heat or cold intolerance, excessive sweating, thirst, hunger, urination
Hematologic	Anemia, bleeding tendencies, past transfusions

Date: _____
What Is Your Current Job?
Job Title: _____
How Long At This Job? _____ (Years, Months)
Please Describe The Work You Do:

Exposures
In your current job have you had regular exposure to any of the following substances? Please circle them.

Chemicals or gases:	ammonia	formaldehyde	hydrogen sulfide	cyanide	insecticides
	sulfur dioxide	fluorides	nitrogen oxides	other:	
Fumes or dusts:	asbestos	talc	fiberglass	cotton dust	silica
	graphite	sawdust	plastics	vehicle exhaust	other:
Metals:	lead	mercury	nickel	cadmium	beryllium
	chromium	arsenic	aluminum	other:	
Solvents:	benzene	carbon disulfide	carbon tetrachloride	methyl chloroform	
	naphtha	toluene	trichloroethylene	xylene	other:
Infectious agents:	hepatitis B		HIV	other virus/bacteria	
	cytomegalovirus		tubercle bacillus (tuberculosis)		

Physical agents:

noise   radiation   vibrations
heat   cold   repetitive motion

Is protective equipment required/used in your job? Yes ___ No ___ If yes, please specify (circle all that apply)
gloves   goggles   face shield   hearing protection
respirator   apron/cover clothes   other:

Past Employment
Starting with the job before your current job and working back in time, provide the information requested below.
Please list all of the jobs you have held, including military occupations.
Job title:

Dates: From _____ To _____
Description of Work
Exposures (see list above)
Frequency of Exposures (daily, weekly)
Protective Equipment used (specify)
Any Illnesses or Injuries Experienced (describe)
Were any coworkers ill or injured from similar exposures? Yes ___ No ___
Do you have any hobbies? Yes ___ No ___ If yes, please describe.
Are chemical exposures involved? Yes ___ No ___If yes, please list.
Do you have any pets at home? Yes ___ No ___
Do you smoke? Yes ___ No ___ If yes, how long?
Does anyone in your household smoke? Yes ___ No ___
Do you have any health problems that you feel are associated with your work? Yes ___ No ___
Have you or a family member lived near any other industrial facilities, waste dump sites, etc. where hazardous substances may have been brought home? Yes ___ No ___
Any other types of exposures/concerns?

Figure 10-1   Occupational health history.

Continued

Company

Is there an occupational health program?

Does the company give physical examinations?

What is the industrial hygiene policy?

Are you informed of the results of examinations or of workroom air samplings?

Is there a safety program?

Job

What exactly were you doing when you became ill?

Were you working your regular shift?

What material do you work with?

If it is liquid, does it give off vapor (fumes) that can be breathed?

Does it ever spill on your skin?

Does it ever soak your clothing?

Has there ever been a spill at your work station?

If you used protective devices, are these maintained by the company?

Do you exchange your respirator when it gets dirty or when you smell the chemical through the mask?

Does the company ever hold information meetings to tell you about the material you work with?

Is any chemical being used near you by other employees?

Do you become ill during the week at work and then get better over the weekend?

Do you get sick when you return to work?

    After a weekend off?

    After your vacation?

Has any new substance been introduced that you work with?

Has the brand of any material been changed?

Has the equipment ever broken down?

Has anything interrupted the usual work process?

Have you ever changed jobs because of your health?

Has there ever been an OSHA inspection of your workplace?

    If so, what was found and what action was taken?

Is there an exhaust ventilation system used at your work station?

Does anyone ever take air samples where you work?

Have any of your fellow workers been ill in the same way you are? When?

Do you like your job?

Figure 10-1, cont'd   Occupational health history.

ing or exposure, hobbies (e.g., woodworking, gardening), or other nonwork factors, such as living near a toxic waste site or contaminated sources of water, are important to note. In addition, exposures external to the workplace (e.g., home use pesticides) can also be noted and assessed for relevance and interaction properties.

As part of the history taking, information should be collected through a complete review of systems in order to further explicate data needed for a complete health assessment. If previous health records need to be obtained, they should be requested with the prospective employee's written permission. A synthesis of data obtained from the personal and occupational histories and the review of systems can help (1) facilitate accurate diagnoses, (2) prevent occupational disease and aggravation of underlying medical conditions by workplace factors, (3) identify potential workplace hazards, (4) detect new associations between exposure and disease, and (5) establish the basis for compensation of work-related disease (Kemerer & Raniere, 1990; Rosenstock & Cullen, 1994).

As part of the health assessment, objective data are obtained through a physical examination systematically conducted to examine each organ system and through appropriate laboratory tests (McCunney, 2002). The examination must be performed by a practitioner who is skilled in physical assessment and has knowledge of the job demands and related exposures in question. The extent of the examination and tests should be determined by the details of the specific job, and emphasis should be placed on functional status capacity, particularly if warranted by the job demands. In other words, not every body system needs to be examined unless indicated by the job requirements and working conditions. For example, workers who drive heavy equipment or large trucks will generally require a fairly detailed physical examination and extensive laboratory and special clinical testing (i.e., audiogram, complete blood count [CBC], blood chemistry, electrocardiogram (ECG), urinalysis, vision/depth perception), whereas workers who perform office functions may require musculoskeletal, audiometric, visual, and manual dexterity assessments. Workers in jobs where silica or asbestos may be present will require special emphasis on pulmonary functioning, including spirometric evaluation and chest x-ray examination (Guidotti et al., 1989).

Laboratory and clinical measurements are often done during the preplacement assessment to establish baseline data that can be used for future comparisons, to comply with mandated regulations, and to detect early adverse health status indications (e.g., high blood pressure) in order to prevent detrimental health end points. As with the physical examination only laboratory tests necessary for an accurate assessment of the worker's ability to perform her or his job should be performed. This generally includes a complete blood count, urinalysis, and blood chemistry. Other clinical measurements such as spirometric and audiometric testing should be performed as appropriate to the job demands. These measurements require special practitioner knowledge and skills, and certification in these areas may be required. Chest roentgenograms and special blood testing (e.g., lead levels, carboxyhemoglobin levels) may also be part of the assessment package when tied to certain job exposures and conditions. In addition, tuberculin skin testing may be considered part of the overall preplacement assessment. Whatever the situation, the employee should be informed of the examination findings and referred for necessary follow-up of any abnormal findings. The preplacement assessment does not constitute a substitute for a complete health assessment by a personal health care provider but is directed at defining the applicant's abilities to perform the job and detecting conditions that prevent the employee from performing the work safely.

Appropriate recommendations as to the prospective employee's job compatibility requires professional judgment, reflecting an evaluation of all parts interacting as a whole (i.e., job demands, health history, and health status). An employee may be judged able to work in a specific job without restriction or may need reasonable modifications. An attempt to make these accommodations should be made, and the occupational and environmental health nurse has a key role in suggesting alternative modifications. In addition to substantial knowledge about the job duties and tasks, this requires that good communication skills be used with the supervisor, employee, and occupational health professionals.

Refusal to hire based on a health and physical examination should be based on an applicant's inability to perform the job safely. A prospective employee cannot be refused hire if the assessment reveals a chronic disease that may increase health insurance costs or if the prospective employee is disabled but can do the job with reasonable accommodation (Pimentel et al., 1992). The occupational and environmental health nurse should make certain that appropriate health information is fully documented and records are stored, maintained, and adequately secured.

Personal health information should be kept confidential, and data obtained from the assessment should not be given to the employer because this information is not needed for the worker placement decision. A recommendation as to applicant's suitability for the position, with requirements for work modification if appropriate, is all that is needed. In some situations the applicant has a right within the parameters of state laws to refuse the physical examination or parts of the examination, and this right must be observed. The occupational and environmental health nurse needs to be cognizant of these laws and document appropriately. In all instances the occupational health professional must act ethically and protect the individual's right to confidentiality of medical and health information and reveal only outcome information pertinent to the hiring decision. The occupational and health history can be used as a guide to obtaining a detailed interval history in conducting health assessments and to gathering data about significant health events that may have occurred since the last evaluation. Changes in lifestyle risk factors (e.g., weight, alcohol or drug consumption, nutrition and exercise, illness occurrence, or pregnancy) and changes in work conditions (e.g., shiftwork, number of work hours, increased work stress, or introduction of new work processes) are important to assess. Physical assessment procedures and laboratory tests should be thorough and complement the interval history with respect to new findings and potentially hazardous work exposures identified.

RETURN TO WORK ASSESSMENT AND JOB TRANSFER ASSESSMENT

Return to work assessments and examinations are part of the occupational health program of some companies and are performed to evaluate a worker after a severe illness, injury, or extended absence from work. This assessment is similar to the preplacement assessment, with a focus on whether there has been a change in the employee's health status that would potentiate risk to the

worker or to coworkers. The employee health problem can be such to require limited duty or work restrictions as determined and recommended by the occupational health professional. On occasion a worker may be unable to return to her or his usual job but may be able to perform less demanding work until fully recovered (Pimentel, 1995; Weeks et al., 1991). Depending on the company philosophy and policies, this approach is a useful option in returning the ill/injured employee to work as soon as possible, which may be in the form of modified, transitional, or limited duty.

Modified or transitional duty generally refers to some adaptation of the employee's original job. Limited duty, defined as a job appropriate to the injured worker's skills, interests, and capabilities, is a new job designed for an individual who cannot return to her or his original work area and is created for either a temporary (specified time period, such as a few weeks or months) or permanent placement (Pimentel et al., 1992; Randolph & Dalton, 1989).

Work hardening, used to facilitate or ease workers back into the workplace, is a progressive, individualized physical conditioning and training program in which the worker simulates work tasks. The intent is to gradually increase all physical and psychological requirements or aspects of the job so that the person will return to the usual job or achieve a level of productivity that is acceptable at the worksite.

To make appropriate recommendations about return to work, the health care provider must know the physical demands of the job that the worker is expected to perform. This knowledge also will allow the occupational and environmental health nurse to coordinate temporary alternative work or modified duty assignments for injured workers returning to work. Matching the work abilities and restrictions of the employee to the physical demands of the job is essential in keeping the employee in the position without increased risk of reinjury (Peters, 1990).

Rapid, safe return to work is an important factor in successful rehabilitation. Research has shown that the longer employees are off the job, the less likely it is that they will return at all. Kelsey and White (1980) have reported that the likelihood of return to work after 6 months of lost work days is only 50%. This drops to 25% after 1 year, and almost to 0% after 2 years off the job.

Return to work in a part-time position or in a modified duty program can be important in halting the deconditioning and psychological behavior patterns that hamper successful return to work.

When serious occupational injury or inadequate treatment results in chronic or debilitating physical problems and delayed recovery, both physical and psychological barriers must be addressed if the worker is to be successfully returned to previous job demand. Rehabilitative services, referrals, and case management services may be part of the return to work program and can help the employee with a less stressful return to work and the employer with less work time lost.

Job transfer assessments are conducted when the health status of the employee or the working conditions change, placing the worker at-risk of work-related illness or injury. A job transfer assessment is similar to the preplacement assessment in that its purpose is to determine the worker's fit with the proposed new job. Thus, the assessment should be conducted to match the job with the employee while ensuring health protection.

The occupational and environmental health nurse will find previously collected baseline data helpful for comparative purposes with respect to job placement parameters and recommendations. In addition, the recording and documentation of work-related illnesses and injuries must be sufficient so it may be used for determination of disability management or worker's compensation claims.

Regardless of the type of worker placement assessment performed, the goal is an appropriate match between the worker and the job demands. To complete a worker placement evaluation, the nurse must understand the working conditions and type of work duties performed. Much of this information can be obtained from the job description and job analysis specifications. Talking with employees who occupy the position and with supervisory staff will also help to clarify the details and demands of the job.

SCREENING, SURVEILLANCE, AND MONITORING

Periodic health assessments are conducted at intervals during the employment period to determine the worker's continued compatibility with the job assignment, to determine if adverse health effects have occurred that may be attributable to the work or working conditions, and to put in place specific programs to prevent serious health consequences from occurring. Periodic health assessments, performed for employees as fundamental strategies to optimize employee health, incorporate specific health interventions that include health screening, health/medical surveillance, and biological monitoring as key components of an effective early detection strategy. (Meservy et al., 1997; Miller, 1986; Ordin, 1992; U.S. Preventive Services Task Force, 1996). Although these terms are often used interchangeably, distinct differences in purpose exist, and each will be discussed.

According to OHSA (1999), screening is, in essence, only one component of a comprehensive health/medical surveillance program and can contribute significantly to the success of worksite health and safety programs. Screening is a method for detecting disease or body dysfunction before an individual would normally seek medical care. Screening tests are usually administered to individuals who do not have any symptoms but may be at high risk for certain adverse health outcomes. Detection examinations, tests, or procedures used in screening are generally not diagnostic but, rather, sort out those individuals presumptively positive for the screened attribute requiring further diagnostic confirmation (Smith & Schneider, 2000). The fundamental purpose of screening is early diagnosis and treatment of the individual and thus has a clinical focus (OSHA, 1999).

Surveillance is the analysis of health information to identify problems that may be occurring in the workplace and require targeted prevention; thus surveillance serves as a feedback loop to the employer. Surveillance may be based on a single case or sentinel event but more typically uses screening results from the group of employees being evaluated to detect abnormal trends in health status. Surveillance can also be conducted on a single employee over time. Review of group results helps to identify potential problem areas and the effectiveness of existing worksite preventive strategies. The fundamental purpose of surveillance is to detect and eliminate the underlying causes (i.e., hazards/exposures) of any discovered trends and thus has a prevention focus (OSHA, 1999).

Biological monitoring usually refers to the detection or measurement (or both) of agents or their metabolites in body fluids, expired air, and/or tissues as a means of evaluating exposure. Genetic monitoring, the measurement of changes in chromosomes or deoxyribonucleic acid (DNA) due to exposure to substances such as carcinogens, is a form of biological monitoring (Ashford, 1990). Genetic monitoring reflects "biological effective dose," and other forms of biological monitoring measure "internal dose."

To contrast health/medical surveillance and biological monitoring, surveillance activities are designed to identify adverse health effects, and biological monitoring reflects body burden or organ "target site" burden of the agent of interest. Biological monitoring studies do not solely and directly reflect adverse health effects (Hayes, 1993). Guidotti et al. (1989) defines monitoring as a strategy for observing the overall health experience of the individual or group without regard to any particular outcome, whereas surveillance is defined as the strategy used to determine the experience of a group of workers when the risk of a particular disease (outcome) is known to be increased in a particular industry.

SCREENING

To be of use in health surveillance, a screening test must be able to detect an exposure-related abnormality as early as possible, so that early diagnosis can be made and treatment or intervention instituted as appropriate. Matte et al. (1990) state that for a health effect to be screenable, a test must be available that can detect the toxic health effect before it would normally cause a worker to present for medical attention (i.e., during the preclinical phase), and at a time when intervention (reduction of exposure and/or medical treatment) is more beneficial than for advanced disease. Generally, the preclinical phase of an effect must be of sufficient duration (at least weeks or months) to be detected by a screening test given feasible intervals. Screening is of little help in preventing acute, severe health effects, such as cyanide poisoning, since the preclinical phase is too brief to be detected. Some acute but intermittent health effects, such as from solvent intoxication, may be amenable to screening by questionnaire, because workers may recall symptomatic episodes during screening examinations weeks or months after they occur. This information may be useful because such episodes may precede the development of chronic central nervous system toxicity (Matte et al., 1990).

For a test to be appropriate for screening, it must have sufficiently high sensitivity and specificity in order to correctly identify individuals with adverse health effects of exposure. Sensitivity is defined as the probability of the test to correctly identify persons with the problem or disease being investigated (true positives), and specificity is defined as the probability of the test to correctly identify persons without the problem or disease being investigated (true negatives). Given a certain amount of test imprecision and human biological variation, a useful screening test should reliably reproduce consistent results upon repeat testing. Important, practical principles should be considered when screening tests are selected and surveillance programs are developed for groups of people. These principles include the following:

- The condition and/or disease sought is an important health problem producing serious morbidity or mortality.
- Timing of the screening test should be targeted to the specific risks consistent with the exposure or occupation.
- Targeted conditions or diseases have a detectable asymptomatic preclinical phase that is reasonably common among the population to be screened, with treatment more effective if implemented at this point.
- Specific risks that are targeted for surveillance or monitoring should be consistent with the exposure or the occupation and should be reassessed periodically to ensure consistency with evolving knowledge.
- There should be reasonably effective treatment options for patients with identified conditions or diseases, such as medical removal from the exposure and medical therapies.
- Resources and facilities for diagnosis and treatment should be available.
- Test(s) and program(s) should be inexpensive, simple to administer, and acceptable to both participants and providers and require minimum employee work time.
- Tests are not associated with serious complications and are reasonably painless.
- Tests are accurate and reliable, with test outcomes that are highly sensitive and specific to the disease or condition in question.
- Professional personnel trained in administering and interpreting surveillance and monitoring procedures are available. (Note that training in occupational health frequently is a prerequisite to accurate interpretation of tests designed to monitor occupational diseases.)

- Test interpretation should be compared to established normal values in the targeted community—the workforce.
- The surveillance and monitoring program should be linked with a plan of care.
- Surveillance and monitoring programs should be ongoing, with the frequency of screening dependant on the incidence of the disease, the length of the preclinical but detectable phase, the level and frequency of exposure, and the worker turnover rate.
- The cost of case finding, including diagnosis and treatment, should be analyzed as compared with alternative methods and in conjunction with overall health care needs and resources for this population.
- Data should be used to protect other workers similarly exposed (Ashford, 1990; Halperin et al., 1986; Hayes, 1993).

HEALTH/MEDICAL SURVEILLANCE

Surveillance as defined by the Centers for Disease Control and Prevention (CDC) and the Council of State and Territorial Epidemiologists (CSTE) is an ongoing systematic collection, analysis, and interpretation of health data essential to the planning, implementation, and evaluation of public health practice and dissemination of information. The final link in the surveillance chain is the application of these data to prevention and control.

Public health surveillance, of which occupational surveillance is a subset, is focused on populations. Although the overriding goals of health/medical surveillance and public health surveillance—that is, prevention—are the same the specific goals are different (Levy & Wegman, 2000). The five goals of public health surveillance as it is applied to occupational disease include the following:

1. To identify illnesses, injuries, and hazards that represent new opportunities for prevention. New opportunities can arise from new problems, such as might occur from the introduction of a new hazardous machine, the belated identification of a long-standing but ignored problem, or the recurrence of a problem previously controlled.
2. To determine the magnitude and distribution of the problem in the workforce. Information on

magnitude and distribution is useful for planning intervention programs; although no hazard is acceptable, the more common and severe problems deserve more immediate attention.
3. To track trends in the magnitude of the problem as a rudimentary method of assessing the effectiveness (or ineffectiveness) of prevention efforts. Epidemics can be tracked on their rise or their decline.
4. To identify and target categories of occupations, industries, and specific worksites that require attention in the form of consultation, educational efforts, or inspection for compliance with established regulation.
5. To publicly disseminate information so that wise personal and societal decisions can be made.

Rernpel (1990) and Levy & Wegman (2000) offered definitions of occupational surveillance in the workplace that follow closely that of the CDC and CSTE but expand the definition specific to the worksite. Surveillance programs are targeted to specific high-risk groups defined by workplace assignment and exposure history. Thus, occupational surveillance is defined as the systematic and ongoing analysis, collection, and evaluation of employee health data to identify specific instances of illness or health trends suggesting an adverse effect of workplace exposures and the dissemination of information coupled with actions to reduce hazardous workplace exposures. A synthesis of these definitions makes it explicit that surveillance and prevention go hand in hand.

Health/medical surveillance programs in occupational health are conducted when workers are potentially exposed to health hazards. The nature and scope of occupational health/medical surveillance activities and the timing interval of the evaluation are determined by specific standards set forth by a legislative authority, such as OSHA, or in criteria documents developed by the National Institute for Occupational Safety and Health (NIOSH). At-risk employees are scheduled for evaluations at regular intervals, usually once a year, and the health history and physical examination are similar to that of the periodic health assessment with emphasis on the specific exposure being evaluated.

Surveillance activities are directed at watching over individuals and groups of workers at high risk for specific adverse health outcomes related to a particular occupational exposure. Surveillance is often referred to as the biological monitoring of health effects and, depending on the job exposure or demands, usually involves a number of activities, including biological monitoring, health questionnaires and examinations, and laboratory and other clinical measurements (e.g., chest x-ray examination, pulmonary function tests) involving similarly exposed workers. All data are analyzed and interpreted to develop a causal link between workplace exposure and adverse health outcomes. Thus, surveillance is designed for early detection of health impairments in order to reverse presumptive damage and prevent other individuals (who may be exposed but have yet to evidence clinical signs and symptoms) from developing disease through appropriate control strategies. Early detection before the development of symptoms will lead to a more favorable health outcome than will detection after the development of symptoms (Cohen, 1984; Garry, 1984; Papp & Miller, 2000; Schilling, 1986; Terry & Ryan, 1998; Travers, 1989; Walter, 1993).

These types of programs have been historically and traditionally termed *medical surveillance,* implying that surveillance activities require a medical intervention, with *medical* referring to the practice of medicine or treatment of disease. However, the term *health surveillance* is more accurate and reflective of the nature of the activity than is *medical surveillance.* Surveillance activities may encompass taking an occupational health history, evaluating employee health data through health assessments, or performing screening tests (e.g., blood pressure, pulmonary function test [PFT]), all of which are in the realm of occupational and environmental health nursing practice (Rogers, 1996). In addition, surveillance activities are often directed, managed, and implemented by occupational and environmental health nurses. This concept is supported by a study that examined the contributions of occupational health nurses in screening, prevention, and surveillance activities (Rogers & Livsey, 2000). The study examined the scope of independent and interdependent practice by occupational health nurses related to these activities and found that 71% of occupational health professionals—nurses (51%) and nurse practitioners (20%)—had overall responsibility for program management, and that most performed surveillance, screening, and prevention functions as independent practice. Direct physician supervision for any of these activities ranged from 0% to 8% in reporting. The results of this study validate the independent functioning in scope of occupational health nursing practice related to surveillance, screening, and prevention activities while recognizing the contributions all providers make to healthy workforce. Tables 10-1 and 10-2 provide data about the scope and degree of independent, collaborative, or medically supervised practice of occupational health nurses with regard to occupational health surveillance and screening/prevention activities. These data reflect a high degree of independent functioning in most of these areas, with at least 60% of occupational health nurse respondents reporting independent functioning in more than three fourths of the activities identified. This percentage of respondents increased to at least 90% when considering independent and collaborative practice together. As expected, independent functioning by occupational health nurse practitioners was increased substantially in all activities identified.

Management of the health/medical surveillance program should be under the direction of a health professional who is qualified by education, experience, and training to evaluate workers and workplace exposures, detect adverse health outcomes, and design strategies to eliminate or reduce risks (AAOHN, 2001; Rogers & Livsey, 2000). This will be the most cost-effective, quality-driven approach to a successful program.

Surveillance Activities

The most effective means of protecting workers from adverse workplace exposures include, in order of preference, those which accomplish the following:

1. Prevent or contain hazardous workplace emissions at their source (such as product substitution);
2. Remove the emissions from the pathway between the source and the worker (such as local exhaust ventilation);
3. Control the exposure of the worker with barriers between the worker and the hazardous work environment (e.g., the use of respirators) (Matte et al., 1990).

Health/medical surveillance programs should only be considered as an adjunct to worker health hazard protection, never a substitute.

When developing a health/medical surveillance program, several areas should be considered; among these are the population at risk,

TABLE 10-1 Occupational Health Nurses' Responsibility for Health Surveillance Activities				
HEALTH SURVEILLANCE ACTIVITIES	**PERCENT WHO PROVIDE OR COULD PROVIDE INDEPENDENTLY**	**PERCENT WHO PROVIDE OR COULD PROVIDE IN COLLABORATION WITH A PHYSICIAN**	**PERCENT WHO REQUIRE OR WOULD REQUIRE DIRECT PHYSICIAN SUPERVISION**	**PERCENT OF BLANK RESPONSES**
Occupational health history	94	5	0	1
Worksite risk assessment/hazard identification	80	17	1	2
Hearing conservation/protection	79	18	1	3
Recommendation/evaluation of control and prevention strategies for risk reduction	76	20	1	3
Referral to physician or other health care provider (e.g., psychologist) for intervention, consultation	76	20	4	1
Evaluation of surveillance program effectiveness	75	21	1	3
Counseling/notification of employee of work-related adverse health effects and effective control strategies	74	23	1	1
Respiratory protection surveillance	69	27	1	3
Physical assessment of ill/injured worker(s)	68	27	3	2
Bloodborne pathogen exposure investigation and follow-up	64	30	4	2
Intervention to reduce risk when positive finding noted	64	31	2	3
Employee travel health surveillance	63	28	2	6
Recommendation for job modification or removal	60	31	6	3
Exposure assessment and follow-up of ill/injured worker(s)	55	42	2	2
Evaluation of test results for follow-up, intervention, or referral	51	41	4	4
OSHA-mandated biological monitoring	49	37	5	9
Site-specific exposure detection and surveillance, (e.g., toxic chemicals-lead, benzene)	40	46	6	8

Percentages many not add up to 100% due to rounding.

workplace/health hazard assessment, determination of health effects, and selection of appropriate surveillance measures including the availability and reliability of tests, testing procedures and frequency, and interpretation of surveillance data examining trends and patterns that might relate any adverse health end point to an exposure. Implementation of program procedures can help detect aberrant control strategies or particular occupations related to the health effect. All cate-

TABLE 10-2   Occupational Health Nurses' Responsibility for Screening and Prevention Activities

Screening/Prevention Activities	Percent who provide or could provide independently	Percent who provide or could provide in collaboration with a physician	Percent who require or would require direct physician supervision	Percent of blank responses
Health education for lifestyles changes (e.g., smoking cessation, diet)	96	2	0	2
Chronic disease screening/ monitoring (e.g., blood pressure)	90	7	1	2
Cardiovascular risk factors screening/ monitoring (e.g., blood pressure, cholesterol)	86	11	1	2
Health risk appraisal	83	13	1	3
Tuberculosis screening (skin testing)	78	16	2	4
Immunization management	76	21	1	2
Return to work/job transfer evaluation	60	30	7	3
Cancer screening (e.g., breast, colon, skin)	60	31	4	5
Preplacement examination	59	32	6	3
Periodic examination (fit for duty)	55	34	8	3

gories of hazards should be assessed (Box 10-3). OSHA has developed a quick reference guide that provides a general overview of screening and surveillance requirements for OSHA standards (Appendix 10-1). However, the appropriate OSHA standard must be consulted for specific compliance directives.

An effective health/medical surveillance program demands a thorough assessment of all occupations, work processes and related hazards, and work areas and conditions in order to identify employees potentially at risk. As previously discussed, the occupational and environmental health nurse will need to recognize the workforce at risk of adverse health hazards through a full understanding of job tasks, demands, requirements, and worker capabilities. In addition to the worksite walk-through discussed in Chapter 7, environmental monitoring, although limited, can yield exposure levels that can then be measured against existing standards.

The purposes of environmental monitoring are to determine the level of ambient exposure of workers to harmful agents, assess the need for control measures, and ensure the efficiency of control measures in use (WHO, 1986). This type of monitoring is aimed at early exposure detection so that controls can be instituted to protect the worker before human harm occurs. Ambient monitoring for workplace chemicals assesses the health risk by monitoring the external exposure to the chemical such as its concentration in air, food, and water. The risk is estimated by reference to environmental exposure limits (e.g., threshold limit values or time-weighted averages) (Smith & Schneider, 2000).

Environmental monitoring such as air sampling for airborne contaminants is usually done by an industrial hygienist. Included in the assessment are (1) a determination of all routes of exposure (inhalation, skin absorption, ingestion) by degree and scope, (2) a determination of mixed exposures that may have synergistic, interactive, or antagonistic effects, (3) detailed knowledge of job demands and worker capabilities, such as the rate and extent of physical exertion, which may

---

Box 10-3   Categories of Potential or Actual Occupational Hazards

Biological/infectious hazards are infectious/biological agents, such as bacteria, viruses, fungi, or parasites, that may be transmitted via contact with infected patients or contaminated body secretions/fluids.

Chemical hazards are various forms of chemicals, including medications, solutions, and gases, that are potentially toxic or irritating to the body system.

Enviromechanical hazards are factors in the work environment such as poor equipment or lifting devices, slippery floors, deficient workstations, that cause or potentiate accidents, injuries, strain, or discomfort.

Physical hazards are agents within the work environment, such as radiation, electricity, extreme temperatures, and noise, that can cause tissue trauma from agent energy transfer.

Psychosocial hazards are factors and situations encountered or associated with one's job or work environment that create or potentiate stress, emotional strain, and/or interpersonal problems.

---

increase the uptake of chemical substances in the body and thus decrease the safety margin of applicable standards, and (4) compliance with control measures (see Chapter 7).

Control of exposure is accomplished most effectively through the application of industrial hygiene principles. Exposure control may take the form of (1) ventilation engineering control approaches, such as installing ventilation exhaust systems that remove hazardous dusts, (2) elimination of a hazardous substance, (3) substitution of a nonhazardous substance for a hazardous one, such as synthetic fibers for asbestos, or (4) isolation of the offending agent through construction of barriers. In addition to these controls, work practice and administrative controls may be implemented, which include training and education, using safe work practices, job rotation, and task rescheduling. Work practice is another control strategy, but it must be used in conjunction with the aforementioned control strategies. Examples of this would be the use of needle disposal boxes, handwashing, and management of hazardous spill (blood) contaminant. Use of protective gloves and clothing as with implementation of the

Bloodborne Pathogen Standard is another control strategy. Moreover, attention must be focused on selecting PPE that is specific to the work hazards and does not compromise the users' ability to work. For example, respirators must be fit to the workers to afford adequate protection, gloves must prevent penetration of harmful substances, and protective clothing must be appropriately selected to provide protection from exposure (AAOHN, 2001). Control measures are discussed in more detail in Chapter 7.

In conjunction with workplace hazard assessment a determination of the types of adverse health effects or end-organ toxicities that might be expected in exposed workers should be made. Health complaints from exposed workers should be evaluated within the context of workplace exposures. For example, headache, dizziness, drowsiness, and nausea and vomiting symptoms consistent with toxic exposure to carbon monoxide should trigger health surveillance testing of all exposed workers regardless of the absence of obvious complaints.

Workers should be encouraged to report signs or symptoms of illness that develop gradually or occur intermittently so adverse effects can be detected early and the problem ameliorated. Workers must feel free to respond to questions without fear of retribution. Through regular health surveillance activities job modification can also be recommended to enable a worker to remain in the job. However, if health deterioration is evident, removal may be necessary. Surveillance activities provide the occupational and environmental health nurse the opportunity to reinforce upon the employee the importance of symptom recognition and reporting and the need for safe work practices.

As part of the health/medical surveillance program physical examinations may be required as appropriate to detect adverse health effects. Examinations should be performed by individuals competent to perform such appraisals. When an employee is placed in a health surveillance program, a baseline examination may suggest that an employee may be at increased risk of adverse health effects due to a potential exposure (e.g., asthmatic reaction from chemical exposure). This needs to be discussed in depth with the employee so that informed decisions regarding appropriate job placement can be made.

Periodic health/medical surveillance examinations should be carried out at regular intervals based on the expected timing of health effects in relation to the exposure. The scope and periodicity of the examination should be relative to the type and degree of risk involved; thus, a total, complete examination may not be warranted, especially if overt signs and symptoms of illness are absent. The examination should emphasize the body system most likely to be affected by the hazardous agents in the work environment. For example, for workers exposed to lead, such as those working in foundries or battery manufacturing operations, special emphasis should be placed on the gastrointestinal, hematopoietic, nervous, and renal systems during the examination. Workers exposed to manganese in iron and steel industries and those involved in the production of dry cell batteries and welding rods should have special attention paid to the nervous and respiratory systems.

Although the latency period—the period between exposure to a toxic agent and manifestation of adverse health effects—is a major consideration in scheduling the frequency of examinations, it often is unknown. Screening before the adverse health effect can be made apparent by the designated test is inefficient and ineffective. However, examinations should be given at short enough intervals to detect health problems early on. Because of individual biovariation and susceptibility and variations in exposures over time, early detection of adverse health effects may not be ensured. Thus, periodic health/medical surveillance examinations should be scheduled to maximize the chances of detecting a toxic effect. If signs or symptoms of exposure toxicity occur prior to the scheduled periodic examination, an examination should be performed immediately.

BIOLOGICAL MONITORING OF EXPOSURE

Health/medical surveillance programs often utilize biological monitoring as an assessment of exposure through measurement of agents or their metabolites in biological specimens (Rosenberg & Rernpel, 1990). Biological monitoring evaluates the health risk by monitoring the internal dose of the chemical—that is, the amount of chemical absorbed by the body (Bernard & Lauwerys, 1986). The rationale is that the estimate of the internal dose is likely to yield a better prediction of potential toxic effects than ambient air measure-

ment. Yodaiken (1986) states that the objective of monitoring is to anticipate any disease before it occurs, avoid any pathological consequence, and abort any irreversible tissue change. The intent of biological monitoring is to detect potentially toxic exposures before their effects become manifest as adverse health endpoints. Biological monitoring is aimed at adverse effects prevention, whereas health/medical surveillance is aimed at adverse health effects detection (Figure 10-2). However, if a quantitative relationship is established between internal dose and adverse effects (i.e., dose-effect or dose-response relationships), biological monitoring allows for a direct health risk assessment and thus for effective prevention of adverse effects (Bernard & Lauwerys, 1986).

Biological monitoring integrates the exposure of all routes, sources, use of personal protective devices, differences in physical activity, working habits, personal hygiene, and nonoccupational exposure, which is not accounted for in environmental monitoring. This is usually done through the evaluation of blood, urine, or exhaled air. For example, carbon monoxide exposure may be detected by measuring carboxyhemoglobin blood concentration, whereas trichloroethylene may be measured as metabolites in the urine by spectrophotometry. Pulmonary function testing is often used to detect the degree of functional lung impairment from dust exposure. The measurement of zinc protoporphyrin from lead exposure and blood cholinesterase from organophosphate pesticide exposure are other examples of blood biological monitoring.

Urine is the most common medium used for biological monitoring, because it is noninvasive, usually easy to collect, and is more suitable for measurement of most exposures, particularly those with short half-lives. The normal standardized values obtained on healthy individuals are needed in order to comparatively evaluate the significance of the values observed in exposed workers. Here again, individual baseline data are important to obtain because these provide a basis for comparison of data throughout the worker's work life. Examples of substances measured through biological monitoring are shown in Table 10-3.

Whatever samples are obtained, collection should occur at specific times relative to the substance under investigation, such as at the end of the workshift. Variation in test results due to mul-

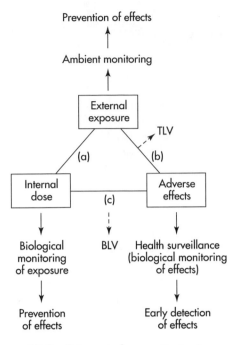

Figure 10-2   Schemata for monitoring in occupational or environmental health protection. *(From "Present Status and Trends in Biological Monitoring of Exposure to Industrial Chemicals," by A. Bernard and R. Lauwerys, 1986,* Journal of Occupational Medicine, 28, *558-562.)*

tiple factors including diet, medications, alcohol, cigarette smoking, timing of specimen collection, and specimen contamination must be considered limitations when interpreting results. Interpretation of measurement results is usually done by comparing the observed result against an established parameter such as the Biological Exposure Indices (BEI), established by the American Conference of Governmental Industrial Hygienists. The BEI is defined as an index chemical that appears in a biological fluid or in exhaled air following an exposure to a workplace chemical (Lowry, 1986). The BEI is a warning of exposure rather than an indicator of a health effect and thus can serve as a preventive monitor prior to disease onset. The BEI is intended to correlate with ambient threshold monitoring limit values. Because biological monitoring is in its developmental stages, few indices are available. Evaluations may then be made from indirect estimates, such as dose-response relationships or ambient levels and toxic effects.

SURVEILLANCE DATA INTERPRETATION AND NOTIFICATION

Interpretation of test results is determined by comparing the observed value (from the exposed worker) against an appropriate reference measure determined statistically from a reference population of healthy, unexposed individuals. When demographic characteristics affect the test results (as with spirometric testing), reference values from the appropriate demographic group should be used when available. A reference value is usually what is considered within a normal range, and whatever falls outside that range may be indicative of a toxic effect.

As previously mentioned, baseline examinations are very important because they serve as a comparative reference point for future examination data. Accurate information about the reliability and precision of the test is essential in order to account for any variation in change from baseline results. For example, a 3% decline in forced expiratory volume [FEV] over a 1-year period may be considered normal variation. However, if this degree of annual decline persisted over several years, pulmonary impairment would be indicated.

After the health surveillance examination and testing have been completed, all results should be reviewed and any deviations exceeding the accepted threshold should be evaluated by the occupational and environmental health nurse and the physician. Consultation from other health professionals, such as the industrial hygienist, may be in order when clinical data are evaluated in reference to an ambient exposure or in concert with sampling data. If an abnormal test result is observed, test errors might be a potential explanation, and test confirmation should be considered. Once confirmed, a definitive medical diagnosis should be made by the physician, and further evaluation, testing, or referral to a medical specialist may be in order.

Employees should be notified in writing of test results by the appropriate health care practitioner according to company policy. Information provided to the employee should include the actual test results, the potential significance of abnormal test results, any risk from continued exposure to the work environment, the recommended changes in work practices

TABLE 10-3	Biologic Monitoring for Selected Chemicals
CHEMICAL DETERMINANT	**MEDIA (UNITS)**
INORGANICS: METALS	
Arsenic	Urine (μg/L)
Cadmium	Urine (μg/g Cr)
	Blood (μg/L)
Chromium	Urine (μg/g Cr)
Lead	Blood (μg/dl)
	Urine (μg/g Cr)
Zn protoporphyrin (ZPP)	Blood (μg/dl)
Mercury (inorganic)	Urine (μg/L)
Nickel	Urine (μg/L)
	Plasma (μg/dl)
Selenium	Plasma (μg/dl)
	Urine (μg/g Cr)
Vanadium	Urine (μg/g Cr)
INORGANICS: OTHER	
Carbon disulfide (TTCA [2 thiothiazoline 4-carboxylic acid])	Urine (mg/g Cr)
Carbon monoxide COHb	Blood (%)
Cyanide	
Thiocyanate	Urine (mg/24 h)
Fluorides	Urine (mg/L)
ORGANICS: ALIPHATICS AND ALICYCLICS	
Acetone	Urine (mg/g Cr)
	Blood (mg/dl)
	Alveolar air (mg/m^3)
Ethylene glycol	Urine (mg/g Cr)
Oxalic acid	
Methanol	Urine (mg/L)
Formic acid	Urine (mg/g Cr)
Methyl ethyl ketone	Urine (mg/L)
Propylene glycol monoethyl air ether (PGME)	End-exhaled air (ppm)
ORGANICS: AROMATIC	
Benzene	Mixed-exhaled air (ppm)
	Blood (ug/dl)
Benzene total phenol	Urine (mg/L)
Ethyl benzene	Urine (g/g Cr)
Mandelic acid	Urine (g/g Cr)
Phenol	Urine (mg/g Cr)
Styrene	Urine (g/g Cr)
Mandelic acid	Urine (g/g Cr)
Styrene	Mid-exhaled air (ppm)
	Blood (mg/L)
Toluene	
Hippuric acid	Urine (g/g Cr)
	Urine (mg/min)

Cr, creatinine.

Continued

TABLE 10-3   Biologic Monitoring for Selected Chemicals—cont'd

CHEMICAL DETERMINANT	MEDIA (UNITS)
Toluene	Blood (mg/L)
	End-exhaled air (ppm)
Xylene	
Total methylhippuric acid	Urine (g/g Cr)
	Urine (mg/min)
Xylene	Blood (mg/L)
ORGANICS: HALOGENATED	
Methyl bromide	Blood (mg/L)
Methylene chloride	
COHb	End-exhaled air (ppm)
	Blood (mg/dl)
Methylene chloride	Blood (mg/dl)
Perchloroethylene	Blood (mg/dl)
Polychlorinated biphenyl	
Total chlorobiphenyl	Blood (μg/dl)
Trichloroethylene	End-exhaled air (ppm)
Free trichloroethanol	Blood (mg/L)
ORGANICS: NITROGEN-CONTAINING	
Aniline	
p-Aminophenol	Urine (mg/L)
Methemoglobin	Blood (%)
Dinitrobenzene	Blood (%)
Nitrobenzene	
p-Nitrophenol and p-aminophenol	Urine (mg/g Cr)
Methemoglobin	Blood (%)
ORGANICS: PESTICIDES	
Organophosphates	
RBC cholinesterase	Blood (% depression)
Parathion	
RBC cholinesterase	Blood (% depression)
p-Nitrophenol	Urine (mg/L)
Carbamates	
RBC cholinesterase	Blood (% depression)
Carbaryl	
RBC cholinesterase	Blood (% depression)
1-Naphthol	Urine (mg/g Cr)
Chlordane	Blood (g/L)
Dieldrin	Blood (g/L)
Hexachlorobenzene	Blood (mg/L)

and personal habits, any medical follow-up or treatment indicated, the legal implications of the notification (e.g., workers' compensation), and the need for ongoing testing and surveillance (Matte et al., 1990).

After an adverse health indicator or effect has been established from a workplace exposure, the work environment must be reassessed for hazardous exposure (through, for example, environmental sampling or observation), and appropriate modifications and control measures must be instituted to reduce or eliminate the exposure. The employee may need to be removed if sufficient workplace changes cannot be made to protect the affected employee. This removal may be only temporary until exposures are controlled. In addition, careful monitoring and surveillance of unaffected employees should be a priority. Employers must be appropriately notified; however, only information relevant to the exposure and modifications needed should be given, not confidential health and medical data.

After workplace modifications are made and the affected employee is returned to the job, continuing surveillance is necessary to ensure adequate protection. Accurate records must be kept and should include sampling measurements, examination and testing results, data interpretation, employee and employer notification, workplace reassessment and recommended modifications, and actions regarding those recommendations.

In addition to individual monitoring and surveillance, periodic health surveillance data are usually collected on groups of potentially exposed workers. Depending on the test measure used to detect biological or health effects, preexposure data can be compared with postexposure data. This can provide valuable information in determining if any statistically significant changes have occurred over time. In addition, individual test results can be compared to group data to find significant departures from group results. Nonsignificant data, however, should not be discounted, particularly in the face of clinically apparent symptoms. The emphasis in data interpretation must be placed on evaluating the relationship among exposure, test results, and biophysiological effects, not just on whether the test results are normal or abnormal (Tyler & Last, 1992).

While some periodic health surveillance programs are mandated by the Occupational Safety and Health Administration, workers' participation in workplace health surveillance programs is voluntary and will be enhanced by providing employees with information about the purposes of the programs, how the test results will be used, and issues pertaining to confidentiality of health data. Workers must decide for themselves if they choose to participate. Voluntary nonparticipation should be documented.

RECORDKEEPING

Maintenance of health records is essential to an effective health surveillance program and includes individual records on the type of surveillance activities performed, their results, and the follow-up provided. These records should be kept for the period of time specified by OSHA regulations in order to compare future test results or further investigate exposure situations. In addition, group records related to exposure data should be maintained and should include the number of employees monitored; types of potential exposures observed; environmental, biological, and other health/medical screening and diagnostic measures performed; written protocols and procedures for the surveillance activities implemented; data interpretation; and recommendations and actions taken for exposure abatement.

Information obtained from health surveillance activities should be treated confidentially and should not be released without the written consent of the employee, except as required by law. Employers should be given information related to surveillance activities when it requires workplace modifications or removal of an affected employee from an exposure situation to protect the worker's health and safety. Confidentiality must be safeguarded, and details of the worker's medical or health condition should not be disclosed (Papp & Miller, 2000; Rogers, 2001).

Summary

Occupational and environmental health nurses have a major role in the assessment, surveillance, and monitoring of worker health and safety. Occupational and environmental health nurses perform many of the health assessment and monitoring activities of workers and make judgments and decisions regarding their health status. Nurses must be knowledgeable about the work-related demands, potential associated hazards, signs and symptoms of acute and chronic exposure, and the need for appropriate and prompt follow-up care to be provided if a health problem develops. The development of a diagnosis and plan of care to facilitate worker placement, as well as to promote and protect worker health and safety, is essential.

The occupational health professional needs to be thoroughly involved in the development and management of any health/medical surveillance program. Collaborative efforts, utilizing a team approach, are critical to the initiation and maintenance of a successful program, which includes but is not limited to the following:

- Acquisition of resources for an effective health/medical surveillance program
- Development of policies and procedures for management and administration of the program
- Coordination of the health/medical surveillance program, including identification of high-risk workers and work areas
- Identification of work areas needing monitoring
- Development, implementation, and evaluation of health/medical surveillance protocols related to specific exposures
- Documentation, interpretation, and communication of health/medical surveillance data and health/medical hazard risks to workers, and appropriate maintenance of confidentiality
- Identification and institution of appropriate control measures
- Education and counseling of workers and management regarding effective strategies for health/medical promotion and protection
- Research and investigation of work-related health/medical problems and recommendations for alteration or modification of risk situations
- Maintenance of knowledge about work-related hazards and strategies for risk reduction

Provision of a safe and healthful work environment is the responsibility of the employer, and measures should be implemented to achieve this goal. Workplace health assessment and surveillance programs are designed to aid in identifying hazardous exposures and in recommending risk reduction strategies; however, these programs should never be considered a substitute for active, progressive workplace hazard prevention.

References

American Association of Occupational and Environmental Health Nurses. (2001). *Core curriculum in occupational and environmental health nursing.* Atlanta: Author.

Ashford, N. A., Spadafor, C. J. Hattis, D. B., & Caldart, C. C. (1990). *Monitoring the worker for exposure and diseases.* Baltimore, MD: Johns Hopkins University Press.

Bernard, A., & Lauwerys, R. (1986). Present status and trends in biological monitoring of exposure to industrial chemicals. *Journal of Occupational Medicine, 28*(8), 558-562.

Brown, M. L. (1981). *Occupational health nursing.* New York: Springer.

Burkeen, O., & Cooper, G. (1985). Preplacement health assessment: The occupational health nurse's role. *AAOHN Update Series, 1*(15), 1-8.

Cassidy, C. (1993). Taking the employee's history of the present problem. *AAOHN Update Series, 5*(7), 1-7.

Cohen, R. (1984). Medical surveillance—Which tests? *Occupational Health Nursing, 32*(5), 244-247.

Felton, J. S. (1990). *Occupational medical management.* Boston: Little, Brown & Company.

Freeman, C. (1983). Importance of pre-employment physicals. *Occupational Health Nursing, 31*(5), 35-37.

Garry, M. (1984). The nurse's role in medical surveillance. *Occupational Health Nursing, 32*(5), 248-250.

Ginetti, J., & Greig, A. (1981, December). The occupational health history. *Nurse Practitioner,* 12-13.

Goldman, R., & Peters, J. (1981). The occupational and environmental health history. *Journal of the American Medical Association, 246*(24), 2831-2836.

Guidotti, T., Cowell, J., & Jamieson, G. (1989). *Occupational health services: A practical approach.* Chicago: American Medical Association.

Halperin, W., Ratcliff, J., Frazier, T., Wilson, L., Becket, S., & Schulle, P. (1986). Medical screening in the workplace: Proposed principles. *Journal of Occupational Medicine, 28*(8): 547-552.

Hayes, W. (1993). Health screening and medical surveillance: Program development and implementation considerations. *AAOHN Update Series, 5*(8), 1-7.

Jarvis, C. (1996). *Physical examination and health assessment.* Philadelphia: Saunders.

Kelsey, J. J., & White, A. A. (1980). Epidemiology and impact of low back pain. *Spine,* 5, 133-139.

Kemerer, S., & Raniere, T. (1990). Cost-effective job placement physical examinations. *AAOHN Journal, 38*(5), 236-242.

LaDou, L. (2000). *Occupational medicine.* Norwalk, CT: Appleton & Lange.

Levy, B. & Wegman, D. (2000). *Occupational health: Recognizing and preventing work-related disease.* Boston: Little, Brown & Company.

Lowry, L. (1986). Biological exposure index as a complement to the TLV. *Journal of Occupational Medicine, 28*(8): 578-582.

Matte, T., Fine, L., Meinhardt, T., & Baker, E. (1990). Guidelines for medical screening in the workplace. *Occupational Medicine: State of the Art Reviews, 5*(3), 439-456.

McCunney, R. (2002). *Handbook of occupational medicine.* Boston: Little, Brown & Company.

Meservy, D., Bass, J., & Toth, W. (1997). Health surveillance: Effective components of a successful program. *AAOHN Journal, 45*(10), 500-511.

Miller, A. (1986). Synthesis of papers on biological monitoring, case studies in screening, and social and economic issues. *Journal of Occupational Medicine, 28*(8), 782-788.

Occupational Safety and Health Administration. *Screening and surveillance: A guide to OSHA standards.* (1999). http://www.OSHA.gov.

Ordin, D. (1992). Surveillance, monitoring and screening in occupational health. In J. M. Last and R. B. Wallace (Eds.), *Maxcy-Rosenau-Last public health and preventive medicine* (13th ed.). Norwalk, CT: Appleton & Lange.

Papp, E. M., & Miller, A. S. (2000). Screening and surveillance: OSHA's medical surveillance provisions. *AAOHN Journal, 48*(2): 59-72.

Peters, P. (1990). Successful return to work following a musculoskeletal injury. *AAOHN Journal, 38*(6), 264-270.

Pimentel, R. (1995). *The return to work process.* Chatsworth, CA: Milt Wright.

Pimentel, R., Bissonnette, D., & Lotito, M. S. (1992). *What managers and supervisors need to know about the ADA.* Chatsworth, CA: Milt Wright.

Randolph, S., & Dalton, P. (1989). Limited duty work: An innovative approach to early return to work. *AAOHN Journal, 37*(11): 446-453.

Rernpel, D. (1990). Medical surveillance in the workplace. *Occupational Medicine: State of the Art Reviews, 5*(3), 435-438.

Rogers, B. (2001). Confidentiality and genetic information. *AAOHN Journal, 49,* 321-322.

Rogers, B., & Livsey, K. (2000) Occupational health and surveillance, screening, and prevention activities in occupational health nursing practice. *AAOHN Journal, 48*(2), 92-99.

Rosenberg, J., & Rernpel, D. (1990). Biologic monitoring. *Occupational Medicine: State of the Art Reviews, 5*(3), 491-498.

Rosenstock, L., & Cullen, M. (1994). *Clinical occupational medicine.* Philadelphia: W. B. Saunders.

Schilling, R. (1986). The role of medical examinations in protecting worker health. *Journal of Occupational Medicine, 28*(8), 553-557.

Smith, T. J., & Schneider, T. (2000). Occupational hygiene. In B. Levy and D. Wegman (Eds.), *Occupational health* (pp. 161-171). Philadelphia: Lippincott Williams & Wilkins.

Terry, T. M., & Ryan, G. (1998). Making sense of OSHA standards with medical requirements: Part I. *Applied Occupational and Environmental Hygiene, 13*(3), 144-148.

Travers, P. (1989). OSHA notice of proposed rulemaking on medical surveillance programs. *OEM Report, 3*(5), 34-36.

Tyler, C., & Last, J. (1992). Epidemiology. In J. M. Last and R. B. Wallace (Eds.), *Maxcy-Rosenau-Last public health and preventive medicine* (13th ed.). Norwalk, CT: Appleton & Lange.

U.S. Preventive Services Task Force. (1996). *Guide to clinical preventive services.* Baltimore, MD: Williams & Wilkins.

Walter, E. (1993). The role of the primary care physician in occupational medicine. In C. Zenz (Ed.), *Occupational medicine.* Chicago: Year Book.

Weeks, J., Levy, D., & Wagner, G. (1991). *Preventing occupational disease and injury.* Washington, DC: American Public Health Association.

World Health Organization. (1986). *Early detection of occupational diseases.* Geneva, Switzerland: Author.

Yodaiken, R. (1986). Surveillance, monitoring, and regulatory concerns. *Journal of Occupational Medicine, 28*(8), 569-571.

10-1 Screening and Surveillance: A Guide to OSHA Standards

Standard Requirements	Acrylonitrile* 1910.1045(N)/ 1926.1145/ 1915.1045	Arsenic (Inorganic)* 1910.1018(N)/ 1926.1118/ 1915.1018	Asbestos (General Industry) 1910.1001(L)
Preplacement examination	Yes[1]	Yes[1]	Yes[1,3]
Periodic examination	Yes—annual[1]	Yes[1]	Yes—annual[1]
Emergency/exposure examination and tests	Yes	Yes	No
Termination examination	Yes—if no examination within 6 months of termination	Yes—if no examination within 6 months of termination	Yes—within ± 30 days of termination
Examination includes special emphasis on these body systems	Respiratory, gastrointestinal[1], thyroid, skin, neurological (peripheral and central)	Skin, nasal	Respiratory, cardiovascular, gastrointestinal
Work and medical history	Required for all examinations[2]	Required for all examinations[2] with focus on respiratory symptoms, including smoking history	Required for all examinations[2]. Standardized form required, see standard Appendix D
Chest x-ray	Yes	Yes	Yes[1]—B reader, board eligible/certified radiologist or physician with expertise in pneumoconioses required. See standard Appendix E for x-ray interpretation and classification requirements
Pulmonary function test (PFT)	No	No	Forced Vital Capacity (FVC), Forced Expiratory Volume (FEV_1)
Other required tests	Fecal occult blood[1]	No	No
Evaluation of ability to wear a respirator	Yes	Yes	Yes
Additional tests if deemed necessary	Yes	Yes	Yes
Written medical opinion	Yes—physician to employer, employer to employee	Yes—physician to employer, employer to employee	Yes—physician to employer, employer to employee
Employee counseling in relation to examination results and conditions of increased risk	Yes—by physician	Yes—by physician	Yes—by physician; includes informing employee of increased risk of lung cancer from combined effect of smoking and asbestos exposure
Medical removal plan	No	No	No

Continued

STANDARD REQUIREMENTS	ASBESTOS (CONSTRUCTION AND SHIPYARDS) 1926.1101(M)/ 1915.1001	BENZENE* 1910.1028(I)/ 1926.1128/ 1915.1028	BLOODBORNE PATHOGENS 1910.1030(F)
Preplacement examination	Yes[1,3]	Yes[1,3,4]	No—must offer Hepatitis B (HBV) vaccine unless already immune or vaccine contraindicated
Periodic examination	Yes—annual[1] or more frequently if determined by physician	Yes—annual[1,4]	No
Emergency/exposure examination and tests	No	Yes[1,4]—includes urinary phenol test	Specific postexposure monitoring for employee and source; HBV vaccine. See standard
Termination examination	No	No	No
Examination includes special emphasis on these body systems	Pulmonary and gastrointestinal	Hemopoietic; add cardiopulmonary if respiratory protection used at least 30 day/year (initially, then every 3 years)	No
Work and medical history	Required for all examinations[2]; special emphasis on pulmonary, cardiovascular, gastrointestinal; standardized form required. See standard Appendix D	Required for initial and periodic examinations (preplacement examination requires special history)[2]	No
Chest x-ray	Yes[1]—B reader, board eligible/certified radiologist or physician with expertise in pneumoconioses required. See standard Appendix E for x-ray interpretation and classification requirements	No	No
Pulmonary function test	FVC, FEV$_1$	Initially and every 3 years if respiratory protection used 30 days/year; specific tester requirements	No
Other required tests	No	CBC, differential, other specific blood tests; repeated as required. See standard	Yes—postexposure incident. Follow USPHS postexposure protocols.
Evaluation of ability to wear a respirator	Yes	Yes—if respirators are used	No
Additional tests if deemed necessary	Yes	Yes	Yes—for postexposure incident. Follow USPHS postexposure protocols
Written medical opinion	Yes—physician to employer, employer to employee	Yes—physician to employer, employer to employee	Yes—licensed health care professionals to employer, employer to employee
Employee counseling in relation to examination results and conditions of increased risk	Yes—by physician, includes informing employee of increased risk of lung cancer from combined effect of smoking and asbestos exposure	Yes—by physician	Yes—by licensed health care professional; counseling in relation to HBV vaccine and postexposure follow-up. See standard
Medical removal plan	No	Yes	No

Standard Requirements	1,3-Butadiene* 1910.1051(k)/ 1926.1151	Cadmium* 1910.1027(L)/ 1926.1127/ 1915.1027/ 1928.1027	Carcinogens (Suspect)* 1910.1003-1016(g)/ 1926.1103/ 1915.1003-1016
Preplacement examination	Yes[1,3,4]	Yes[1,3,4]	Yes
Periodic examination	Yes[1,4]	Yes[1,4]	Yes—annual
Emergency/exposure examination and tests	Yes[1,4]—within 48 hours of exposure	Yes[1,4]	Yes[1]—special medical surveillance begins within 24 hours
Termination examination	Yes[4]—if 12 months have elapsed since last examination	Yes[3]—see standard for time frame and other specifics	No
Examination includes special emphasis on these body systems	Liver, spleen, lymph nodes, skin	Respiratory, cardiovascular (blood pressure), urinary, and for men older than age 40 prostate palpation[1]	Determination for increased risk (e.g., treatment with steroids or cytotoxic agents, reduced immunological competence, pregnancy, or cigarette smoking)
Work and medical history	Required annually and for all examinations[2]; standardized form or equivalent; includes comprehensive occupational and health history. See standard Appendixes F and C	Required for preplacement and periodic exams[2]; standardized form required	Required for all examinations, includes family and occupational history, and genetic and environmental factors
Chest x-ray	No	Yes	No
Pulmonary function test	No	FCV, FEV[1]	No
Other required tests	CBC with differential and platelet count, annually; also within 48 hours after exposure in an emergency situation and repeated monthly for 3 more months	Annually[1], cadmium in urine, beta-2 microglobulin in urine, cadmium in blood, CBC, BUN, serum creatinine, urinalysis. See standard	No
Evaluation of ability to wear a respirator	Yes—if respirators are used	Yes	Yes—as specified in the respiratory protection standard 1910.134(e), if respirators are used
Additional tests if deemed necessary	Yes	Yes	Yes
Written medical opinion	Yes—physician or other licensed health care professional to employer and employee	Yes—physician to employer, employer to employee	Yes—physician to employer
Employee counseling in relation to examination results and conditions of increased risk	Yes—by physician or other licensed health care professional	Yes—by physician; includes explanation of results, treatment, and diet and discussion of decisions related to medical removal. See standard for details	No
Medical removal plan	No	Yes	No

Continued

STANDARD REQUIREMENTS	COKE OVEN* EMISSIONS 1910.1029(J)	COMPRESSED AIR ENVIRONMENTS 1926.803(B)	COTTON DUST 1910.1043(H)
Preplacement examination	Yes[1]	Yes	Physical examination not specified; other tests required
Periodic examination	Yes[1]	Yes[1]	Physical examination not specified; other tests required[1,4]
Emergency/exposure examination and tests	No	No	No
Termination examination	Yes—if no examination within 6 months of termination	No	No
Examination includes special emphasis on these body systems	Skin	Not specified	Not specified
Work and medical history	Required for all examinations[2]; includes smokinig history and presence and degree of respiratory symptoms	No	Medical history; standardized questionnaire required. See standard Appendix B-1[1,2,4]
Chest x-ray	Yes	No	No
Pulmonary function test	FVC, FEV$_1$	No	FVC, FEV$_1$, FEV$_1$/FVC Employees with specific abnormalities are referred to specialists[1,4,5]
Other required tests	Weight, urine cytology, urinalysis for sugar, albumin, hematuria	No	No
Evaluation of ability to wear a respirator	Yes	No	Yes
Additional tests if deemed necessary	Yes—see standard Appendix B	No	No
Written medical opinion	Yes—physician to employer, employer to employee	No	Yes—physician to employer, employer to employee
Employee counseling in relation to examination results and conditions of increased risk	Yes—by physician, also employer must inform employee of possible health consequences if employee refuses any required medical examination	No	Yes—by physician in relation to results of examination and any medical conditions requiring further examination or treatment
Medical removal plan	No	No	Yes—for inability to wear a respirator (6 months)

STANDARD REQUIREMENTS	DBCP* 1910.1044(M)/ 1926.1144/ 1915.1044	ETHYLENE OXIDE* 1910.1047(L)/ 1926.1147	FORMALDEHYDE* 1910.1048(L)/ 1926.1148/ 1915.1048
Preplacement examination	Yes	Yes[1]	Yes[1,4]
Periodic examination	Yes[1]	Yes—annual[1]	Yes[1,4]
Emergency/exposure examination and tests	Yes—male reproductive, repeat in 3 months	Yes[1]	Yes[4]
Termination examination	No	Yes[1]	No
Examination includes special emphasis on these body systems	Reproductive, genitourinary. See standard for details	Pulmonary, skin, neurologic, hematologic, reproductive, eyes	Evidence of irritation or sensitization of skin, respiratory system, eyes, shortness of breath
Work and medical history	Required for all examinations[2], includes reproductive history. See standard Appendix C	Required for all examinations, includes reproductive history and special emphasis on some body systems. See standard	Required for all examinations[2], questionnaire required. See standard Appendix D
Chest x-ray	No	No	No
Pulmonary function test	No	No	FVC, FEV$_1$, FEF should be evaluated if respiratory protection is used
Other required tests	Sperm count, FSH, LH, Total estrogen (women). See standard Appendix C for guidelines	CBC, white cell count with differential, hematocrit, hemoglobin, red cell count; if requested by employee, pregnancy testing and fertility testing (women/men) will be added to the examination as deemed appropriate by physician	No
Evaluation of ability to wear a respirator	Yes	Yes	Yes
Additional tests if deemed necessary	Yes	Yes	Yes
Written medical opinion	Yes—physician to employer, employer to employee	Yes—physician to employer, employer to employee	Yes—physician to employer, employer to employee
Employee counseling in relation to examination results and conditions of increased risk	Yes—by physician	Yes—by physician	Yes—by physician, includes information on whether medical conditions were caused by past exposures or emergency exposures
Medical removal plan	No	No	Yes

Continued

STANDARD REQUIREMENTS	HAZWOPER* 1910.120(F)/1926.65	HAZARDOUS CHEMICALS IN LABORATORIES 1910.1450(G)
Preplacement examination	Yes[1]	When required by other standards
Periodic examination	Yes—annually or at physician's discretion[1]	When required by other standards
Emergency/exposure examination and tests	Yes[1]	Yes[1]
Termination examination	Yes—if no examination within 6 months of termination/reassignment	No
Examination includes special emphasis on these body systems	Determined by physician. See standard Appendix D, reference 10 for guidelines	Not specified
Work and medical history	Yes—with emphasis on symptoms related to handling hazardous substances and health hazards, fitness for duty, and ability to wear PPE[2]	When required by other standards
Chest x-ray	No—unless determined by physician	When required by other standards
Pulmonary function test	No—unless determined by physician	When required by other standards
Other required tests	No—unless determined by physician	When required by other standards
Evaluation of ability to wear a respirator	Yes	Yes—When required by other standards
Additional tests if deemed necessary	Yes	When required by other standards
Written medical opinion	Yes—physician to employer, employer to employee	Yes—physician to employer
Employee counseling in relation to examination results and conditions of increased risk	Yes—by physician	Yes—by physician
Medical removal plan	No	No

Standard Requirements	Lead* 1910.1025(j)/ 1926.62	Methylenedianiline 1910.1050(m)	Methylene Chloride* 1910.1052(j)/ 1926.1152
Preplacement examination	Yes[1,4] except in construction industries; construction requires initial blood tests only	Yes[1,3,4]	Yes[1,4]
Periodic examination	Yes[1,4]	Yes—annual[1,4]	Yes[1,4]
Emergency/exposure examination and tests	Yes[1,4]	Yes[1,4]	Yes[4]—see standard for specifics
Termination examination	No	No	Yes—if no examination within 6 months of termination
Examination includes special emphasis on these body systems	Teeth, gums, hematologic, gastrointestinal, renal, cardiovascular (blood pressure), neurological; pulmonary status if respiratory protection used	Skin, hepatic	Lungs, cardiovascular (including blood pressure and pulse), liver, nervous, skin; extent of examination determined by examiner based on employee's health status, and work and medical history
Work and medical history	Required for all examinations[2], includes reproductive history, past lead exposure, both work/nonwork, and history of specific body systems. See standard	Required for all examinations[2], includes past work with MDA and other specific items. See standard	Required for all examinations; example of work and medical history form provided in standard Appendix B
Chest x-ray	No	No	No
Pulmonary function test	No—unless deemed necessary by physician	No	No—unless deemed necessary by physician or other licensed health care professional
Other required tests	Hemoglobin, hematocrit, ZPP, BUN, serum creatinine, urinalysis with microscopic examination, blood lead levels, peripheral smear morphology, red cell indices[1,5]. If requested by employee, pregnancy testing and fertility testing (women/men)	Liver function tests, urinalysis	Laboratory surveillance may include tests as determined by examiner including "before and after shift tests." See standard Appendix B
Evaluation of ability to wear a respirator	Yes	Yes	Yes—as specified under the respiratory protection standard 1910.134(e)
Additional tests if deemed necessary	Yes	Yes	Yes
Written medical opinion	Yes—physician to employer, employer to employee	Yes—physician to employer, employer to employee	Yes—physician or other licensed health care professional to employer and employee
Employee counseling in relation to examination results and conditions of increased risk	Yes—by physician, includes advising the employee of any medical condition, occupational or nonoccupational, requiring further medical examination or treatment	Yes—by physician	Yes—by physician or other licensed health care professional
Medical removal plan	Yes	Yes	Yes

Continued

STANDARD REQUIREMENTS	NOISE 1910.95(G)/ 1926.52†	RESPIRATORY PROTECTION* 1910.134(E)/ 1926.103	VINYL CHLORIDE* 1910.1017(K)/ 1926.1117
Preplacement examination	No physical examination but audiometric testing required	Evaluation questionnaire or examination; follow-up examination when required[5]	Yes[1]
Periodic examination	No physical examination but audiometric testing required	Yes—in specific situations[5]	Yes[1]
Emergency/exposure examination and tests	No	No	Yes
Termination examination	No physical examination but audiometric testing required	No	No
Examination includes special emphasis on these body systems	No	Yes[5]—see standard Appendix C	Special attention to detecting enlargement of the liver, spleen or kidneys, or dysfunction of these organs and abnormalities in skin, connective tissue, and pulmonary system. See standard, Appendix A
Work and medical history	No	Yes[2]—see standard Appendix C	Required for initial and periodic examinations[2], includes alcohol intake, history of hepatitis, exposure to hepatotoxic agents, blood transfusion, hospitalizations, and work history
Chest x-ray	No	As determined by physician or other licensed health care professional	No
Pulmonary function test	No	As determined by physician or other licensed health care professional	No
Other required tests	Initial and annual audiometric testing[1,4,5]. See standard related to specific qualifications for the test administrator	As determined by physician or other licensed health care professional	Blood test for total bilirubin, alkaline phosphatase, SGOT, SGPT and gamma glutamyl transpeptidase
Evaluation of ability to wear a respirator	No	Yes	Yes
Additional tests if deemed necessary	Yes	Yes	Yes
Written medical opinion	No	Yes—physician or other licensed health care professional to employer and employee	Yes—physician to employer, employer to employee

Standard Requirements	Noise 1910.95(G)/ 1926.52†	Respiratory Protection* 1910.134(E)/ 1926.103	Vinyl Chloride* 1910.1017(K)/ 1926.1117
Employee counseling in relation to examination results and conditions of increased risk	Yes—if standard threshold shift or suspected ear pathology'	Yes—by physician or other licensed health care professional	No
Medical removal plan	No	No	Yes

From *Screening and Surveillance: A Guide to OSHA Standards,* by Occupational Safety and Health Administration, 1999, Washington, DC: Author.

[1] Preplacement and periodic examinations are dependent on specific factors cited in the standard such as airborne concentrations of the substance and/or years of exposure, biological indexes, age of employee, amount of time exposed per year. In addition, some standards require periodic examinations to be conducted at varying time intervals. Refer to standard for complete details.

[2] Standard requires medical and work history focused on special body systems, symptoms, personal habits, and/or specific family, environmental, or occupational history. Refer to standard for complete details.

[3] No examination required if previous examination completed within specified time frame (e.g., 6 months or 12 months) and provisions of standard met. Refer to standard for details.

[4] Additional physician review: Some standards have provisions for referring employees with abnormalities to a specialist as deemed necessary by examiner. Other standards have provisions for multiple physician review. See specific standard for details.

[5] Standard requires specific protocol. See standard for details.

* These Maritime and Construction standards are identical to 29 CFR 1910, General Industry standards.

† 1926.52 requires an effective and continued hearing conservation program. OSHA has interpreted this to include audiograms when feasible. See letter of interpretation dated August 4, 1992.

Note: "See standard, Appendix X" refers the reader to the standard listed in the corresponding column heading; the appendix will be found within that standard. "B reader" is a physician certified by NIOSH to detect pneumoconiosis on x-rays using International Labour Office guidelines.

BP, Blood pressure; *BUN,* blood urea nitrogen; *CBC,* complete blood count; *DBCP,* 1,2-dibromo-3-chloropropane; *ETO,* ethylene oxide; *FEF,* forced expiratory flow; *FEV$_1$,* forced expiratory volume one second; *FSH,* follicle stimulating hormone; *FVC,* forced vital capacity; *HAZWOPER,* hazardous waste operations and emergency response; *HBV,* hepatitis B virus; *LH,* luteinizing hormone; *MDA,* methylenedianiline; *PPE,* personal protective equipment; *PHS or USPHS,* United States Public Health Service; *SGOT,* serum glutamic oxalacetic transaminase; *SGPT,* serum glutamic pyruvic transaminase; *ZPP,* zinc protoporphyrin.

CHAPTER 11

Clinical Practice in Occupational and Environmental Health Nursing

In most work settings the occupational and environmental health nurse is the sole provider of health care to worker populations and is responsible for the clinical management of many occupational and nonoccupational health-related problems. This may include direct care provided by the nurse on-site or through contractual arrangements with community health care providers within the context of policies, procedures, and guidelines or protocols for practice. As discussed in Chapter 13, health promotion, health protection, and health maintenance are major areas of focus in the nurse's practice; however, the provision of primary care, management of emergencies, monitoring of chronic diseases, implementation of urgent/critical health interventions occurring as a result of work-related incidents, and counseling related to occupational and nonoccupational health problems are central to health care delivery. The nurse's interventions focus on the individual's response to altered functioning and require critical thinking about the types of nursing activities that are appropriate, efficient, and effective. This chapter will focus on the importance of direct care provision, the development of clinical nursing guidelines for occupational health nursing practice (with several examples presented), and the counseling and employee assistance programming in the occupational health setting.

Direct clinical care provided in a work setting or as part of the occupational health program is dependent on several factors including the following (Burgel, 2001):

- Company philosophy about direct care services for employees

- Demographics of the workforce (e.g., number, age, gender of employees)
- Occupational and nonoccupational illness and injury data of employees
- Hazard profile of the company
- Geographic proximity to the nearest emergency facility
- Health services benefit coverage
- Financial and personnel resources

The occupational and environmental health nurse will want to examine each of these factors to determine both the feasibility of providing care and the types of services to be offered to employees and, in some settings, to dependents and retirees. The nurse will also want to consider the accessibility and availability of community health care providers and the likely acceptability of specific on-site services provided for both occupationally and nonoccupationally related illnesses and injuries. The scope of direct care services may include the following:

- Clinical care for occupational and nonoccupational conditions
- First-aid and emergency care
- Minor acute care
- Chronic disease monitoring
- Prenatal care
- Prevention and surveillance services, such as immunizations and preplacement/screening examinations (discussed in Chapter 10)
- Physical therapy
- Case management
- Home health care
- Counseling

Depending on the setting, the actual list of services may be more or less expansive than that just provided; the scope of services will be determined by employee/employer needs and company philosophy and resources as previously mentioned. Consequently the occupational and environmental health nurse will need to be keenly aware of health care determinants and policy and financial implications related to health service delivery.

Direct on-site clinical services offer the following benefits:

- Greater convenience for employees as a result of less down-time from absence due to sickness and visits to off-site health care providers
- Greater opportunity for case management to monitor quality, outcomes, and cost of care
- Fast and accurate determination of work-related cause or aggravation of the symptom or disease
- Accommodations, if needed, that are made by on-site providers who are knowledgeable about the worksite
- Opportunity to reinforce safe work practices with each employee encounter
- Ability to tailor direct care services to the risk profile of the company and complement/maximize the health benefit plan
- Cost savings that are realized by controlling duplicate health care services and reducing absence resulting from sickness
- Opportunity to reinforce a self-care approach to health (Burgel, 2001)

In providing direct care services, the occupational and environmental health nurse will need to have good communication skills to obtain health history information and occupational exposure data and also the ability to conduct physical examinations or contract for examinations to be done. These elements are discussed in depth in Chapter 10.

OCCUPATIONAL HEALTH NURSING GUIDELINES FOR PRACTICE

As nursing has expanded its scope of practice, new tools are being developed and utilized to help delineate parameters of care and management. Guidelines for clinical nursing practice for certain health-related entities specify nursing actions within the legally defined limits of practice, and these guidelines are particularly helpful in occupational settings, where the occupational and environmental health nurse largely practices autonomously. For many health care problems seen in the occupational health unit, independent nursing strategies are appropriate. In these situations the nurse is not dependent on the physician's medical diagnosis but rather looks to the individual's response as a directive for nursing interventions. However, because of the interdependent nature of nursing and medicine, collaborative strategies are often appropriate and may necessitate physician referral (Rogers et al., 2002). In addition, some nursing activities are medical interventions prescribed by the physician and delegated to the nurse (Bates, 1995; Burgel, 1998; Glasgow, 1990). Standing orders from the physician should be used appropriately and within the legal scope of nursing practice.

Clinical nursing guidelines used within a model of collaborative practice in occupational settings can help foster and clarify communication among occupational and environmental health nurses and physicians and other health care providers with respect to appropriate and consistent procedures and parameters for clinical management and referral. In addition, the use of standardized clinical guidelines for nursing practice can help in the following ways:

- Provide for goal-directed outcomes;
- Guide the systematic collection of data;
- Enhance critical thinking and clinical management skills;
- Maximize clinical decision making;
- Improve the quality and consistency of nursing care based on scientific evidence;
- Reduce interdisciplinary and intradisciplinary practice variation;
- Guide the development of evaluative criteria, including quality assurance approaches;
- Foster best practices and cost-effective management approaches;
- Promote professional accountability (Rogers et al., 2002).

The quality and consistency of nursing care will be improved by standardizing care. Diagnostic labels help the nurse to develop a concept of focus for the particular health problem within the context of the health state of the individual and to make assessments to identify the problem, including problem characteristics (signs and symptoms) manifested by the individual. These standardized approaches of nursing interventions provide for a definitive goal-directed outcome with specific results rather than a hit-or-miss approach (Kosinski, 1998; USDHHS, 2000). Although the individualization of each (person's) plan of care is pivotal to effective nursing care, certain problems are common to many people. This commonality provides an opportunity to develop creative but consistent strategies that can be applied to meet the clinical needs of a given patient population (Akers, 1991). However, care of individuals is a dynamic process, and challenges for which the health care professional should be alert may appear without warning. Clinical nursing care guidelines and/or protocols enable the nurse to help individuals maintain health and to treat those with chronic or acute self-limiting illnesses and injuries, both occupational and nonoccupational (AAOHN, 1997).

In the delivery of effective health care at the worksite, the ability to exercise sound clinical judgment is contingent upon the diagnostic reasoning strategies of the occupational and environmental health nurse clinician. Gathering and organizing employee health data in a systematic manner is essential to the delivery of safe and competent care. This process is demonstrated by skilled actions or interventions designed to achieve a favorable outcome and involves the following:

1. Recognizing the problem, associated adverse health effects, and exposure linkages
2. Using diagnostic reasoning through skills, abilities, and knowledge (e.g., history taking examinations, laboratory analysis, clinical protocol/guidelines) to establish a working diagnosis
3. Setting a specific goal to effect the change or outcome
4. Choosing the appropriate intervention to meet the goal
5. Considering situational and psychosocial factors prior to implementing the interventions
6. Implementing the interventions with skill based on knowledge
7. Knowing the parameters for medical intervention and referral
8. Documenting care and care effectiveness

Always of importance is the ability to communicate effectively with the employee and other appropriate parties and to advocate for quality care.

When developing clinical guidelines or protocols, a literature review should be conducted for each clinical entity to obtain information on the most current and appropriate assessment techniques, management modalities, and follow-up approaches. Consultation with medical and other nursing professionals, such as the state occupational health nurse consultant, should be utilized when needed. Clinical nursing guidelines and protocols are helpful in the decision making process because they provide a series of clear, step-by-step recommendations to help delineate the problem and intervene appropriately. However, they are not intended to take the place of critical thinking and active nursing judgment; rather, they serve as a reference of essential elements for management of a specific problem. For example, if an employee reports having a headache, there should always be room for a healthy suspicion of chemical exposure, especially if a cluster effect or a temporal relationship between workplace exposure and symptom onset is apparent. Thus, clinical assessment needs to be complete and appropriately documented.

Based on an assessment of the health problems and conditions in the workforce, clinical nursing practice guidelines or protocols that reflect the health needs of that particular population can be easily developed through a review of employee health records and logs. The occupational and environmental health nurse, in collaboration with other health care professionals such as the physician or the physical therapist or both, can then develop or obtain guidelines or protocols specific to the needs of the workforce and in the format determined to be most useful.

Nursing clinical guidelines or protocols may be developed by diagnostic category or presenting problem and generally follow a specific format such as an algorithm or the SOAP format, which is patterned to identify *s*ubjective and *o*bjective data and arrive at an *a*ssessment and a *p*lan of action. A narrative or some other standard format that best meets the needs of the practitioner also may be utilized. The algorithm format specifies a logic or decision tree approach wherein decision points direct further investigation and action.

Box 11-1	**Sample Protocol: Narrative SOAP Format**

ACUTE SINUSITIS

Definition	A condition in which the mucous membrane lining of the paranasal sinuses is inflamed, causing obstruction of normal sinus drainage and subsequent bacterial infection.
Etiology	Commonly occurs following an upper respiratory infection; common causative agents are group A strep, *Haemophilus influenza, Staph. aureus,* and *Pneumococcus.* Bacterial sinusitis commonly occurs as a complication of viral nasopharyngitis.
Demographics	Most often affects persons who currently or recently have had an upper respiratory tract infection with marked inflammation of the paranasal sinuses. Less frequently may afflict persons who have recently sustained local injuries to the area within or surrounding the paranasal sinuses.
S (Subjective)	Present History: Client may complain of nasal congestion, sneezing, headache, and sore throat—symptoms of common cold. May also complain of pain and tenderness over affected sinuses, such as forehead and/or maxillary area. If sphenoidal sinuses are involved, the client may complain of pain at base of skull. Involvement of ethmoidal sinus commonly evokes complaint of pain in temples and around the eyes. Headache/pain may be worse in the early morning or at night and may vary with change in position. Complaints of purulent nasal discharge, postnasal drip, and sore throat may be elicited. The client may report fever, feeling of tiredness, and a night cough.
O (Objective)	Vital signs Temp.: Mild fever (101°F or 38.2°C). Pulse, Resp., and B/P: May be slightly elevated for clients according to age, intensity of pain, and level of anxiety. HEENT Viral: Findings congruent with those of common cold. Bacterial: May note edema and redness of nasal mucous membrane and yellow mucopurulent nasal discharge beneath the superior or middle turbinates. (If occlusion of the passage from the sinus to the nasal cavity occurs, discharge may be absent). Tenderness over involved sinus may be elicited on palpation and percussion; transillumination decreased over the involved sinus. Lab: None indicated in the absence of mucopurulent nasal discharge. (Culture if present.)
A (Assessment) Diagnosis	
Nursing	Alteration in comfort due to bacterial infection of the paranasal sinus(es).
Medical	Acute sinusitis.
P (Plan)	Consult with physician regarding client management (if bacterial sinusitis present, x-ray will show cloudiness of involved sinus) or if unsure of diagnosis. Refer any clients who are acutely or severely ill, those with chronic or recurrent bacterial sinusitis, or those with any signs of orbit or CNS involvement (any protrusion of the eyeball or neurological changes).
Therapeutic:	1. Tylenol and aspirin may be prescribed as needed for fever and pain. 2. Decongestants such as Chlortrimeton or Sudafed may be prescribed to reduce congestion and promote sinus drainage. 3. For bacterial sinusitis Ampicillin 500 mgm p.o. every 6 hours for 10 days; *if allergic to penicillin,* use Tetracycline 250 mgm p.o. every 6 hours for 10 days (prescribed). Note: Tetracycline is contraindicated in pregnant women and young children. 4. Increase oral fluid intake and use humidifier to promote liquefying of sinus drainage. 5. Follow-up: Call or return to clinic in 3 days if no improvement or condition worsens; if bacterial, return for HEENT exam 1 week following completion of antibiotics.

Box 11-1	**Sample Protocol: Narrative SOAP Format—cont'd**

Education

1. Explain the underlying etiology, the rationale for treatment, and the importance of taking entire course of medications, particularly if on antibiotics.
2. Alert client to signs/symptoms of complications (increasing fever, chills, epistaxis, or change in level of consciousness). If any of these occur, client should return to clinic or nearest emergency room immediately.
3. Encourage the client to rest as much as possible.
4. Provide the client with information regarding treatment regimen and potential side effects of drugs; include written instructions.
5. Inform client of side effects of:
   a. Aspirin: G.I. distress, nausea, vomiting, and increased bleeding tendency.
   b. Tylenol: G.I. distress, nausea, and vomiting.
   c. Decongestants: Mild nervousness, restlessness, and dry mouth.
      Note: Decongestants should be used with caution if high blood pressure, diabetes, heart disease, or thyroid disease are present.
   d. Antibiotics: Discuss how and when to take medication. (Take 1 hour before or 2 hours after meals).
   e. Amoxicillin: Skin rash, nausea, vomiting, and diarrhea, sneezing or wheezing should be reported immediately.
6. If Tetracycline is recommended:
   a. Instruct regarding side effects of drug: nausea, vomiting, diarrhea, and skin rash.
   b. Advise that drug may cause photosensitivity (increased sensitivity to sun).
   c. Advise that milk and milk products (e.g., cheese, yogurt, ice cream) and antacids should not be taken at the time the drug is ingested.

Modified from *Adult Health Management: Guidelines for Nurse Practitioners,* by C. E. Thompson, J. M. Jones, A. R. Cox, and E. Y. Levy, 1984, Reston, VA: Reston.

Examples of these types of formats are demonstrated in Box 11-1 and in Figures 11-1 and 11-2.

In 1992 another type of guideline format, now in its third edition, was developed by Rogers et al. (2003). The intent of these guidelines is to provide a format that defines and characterizes the clinical problem, gives direction as to a policy perspective, identifies assessment needs and specific interventions, delineates conditions requiring medical referral, and specifies follow-up actions. Based on needs assessments of practicing occupational and environmental health nurses, specific clinical entities related to common occupational health problems and needs have been identified for which clinical nursing guidelines have been developed. Ten examples of these guidelines are given in Appendix 11-1. For the complete inventory (of more than 125 guidelines) see Rogers et al. (2003).

Once developed, the guidelines or protocols should be reviewed by clinical experts for accuracy, modification, or refinement. Guidelines/protocols should be dated and maintained in the occupational health unit and other satellite settings where they are used; they also should be reviewed by the health care providers regularly, usually once a year, for currency and updated as appropriate. In the development and implementation of clinical nursing guidelines or protocols, the legal requirements as specified by individual state nurse practice acts must be observed and maintained. In addition, nurses must be cognizant of other legal parameters that may affect nursing practice, such as the state pharmacy and medical practice acts and regulations. Direct health care providers must be competent to perform activities required, and the nurse must be fully aware of all limitations of nursing practice in the state in which she or he practices.

Regardless of the problem, timely and targeted interventions are needed to effect a positive outcome (American College of Occupational and Environmental Medicine, 1998). Although clinical nursing guides or protocols cannot guarantee a positive outcome, they can provide a consistent care approach appropriate to the clinical problem.

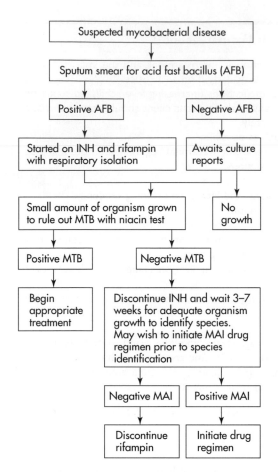

Figure 11-1   Example of algorithmic format. (From "Recognizing and Managing Mycobactefial Diseases in Clients with AIDS," by M. O'Grady and J. Frasier, 1992, *Nurse Practitioner, 17.*)

Clinical nursing guidelines provide the nurse with a foundation for decision making that is critical to preventing, detecting, and minimizing complications and contributes to better clinical management (Akers, 1991). In addition, these guides can be effective teaching aids, provide the occupational and environmental health nurse with cues to enhance clinical assessment and management skills, foster accountability, improve critical thinking, and reduce health and safety-related costs through early intervention. No one approach to clinical nursing management is always appropriate, and individualization, given the situational and personal variables at hand, must always be considered. Conditions requiring medical intervention must be recognized and referred.

COUNSELING AND EMPLOYEE ASSISTANCE

Employee counseling is offered as an integral component of the occupational health service. In providing health care to workers, the occupational and environmental health nurse is involved with counseling employees not only about prevention and management of work-related illnesses and injuries but also about interpersonal or situational problems that are nonoccupational in origin. The nurse may provide counseling about any number of issues, such as nutrition, exercise, substance abuse, marriage and divorce, birth and death, or other health-related events, including breast cancer, HIV/AIDS, or parenting, issues that may affect not only the employee but also family members or significant others. For example, counseling employees regarding chronic diseases, such as cancer, may include a discussion of knowledge of risk factors; methods for early cancer detection, treatment, and coping strategies; financial implications; cultural influences; return to work issues; and end-of-life decisions. These are counseling points with which the occupational and environmental health nurse may be involved (Mood, 1996; Weekes, 1998; Worden, 1995). Hood (2000) discusses issues surrounding latex exposure particularly to health care workers. The importance of education and counseling of staff using a multidisciplinary team approach is emphasized so that avenues related to health issues, product safety, and coworker safety are addressed. The author points out that all aspects of the exposure and topic need to be discussed, including pathogenesis of latex allergy, food cross-reaction, various types of exposures, avoidance of exposure issues, and treatment options.

Stenberg and Gammon (1995) point out that the workplace is a major arena within which societal tensions are played out; it creates enormous challenges to prevent and redress age, ethnic, and gender discrimination as well as sexual harassment. In addition, individual workers must balance the sometimes conflicting demands of work and family. How all these conflicts are resolved has substantial implications for job design, employee morale and productivity, marital stability, chil-

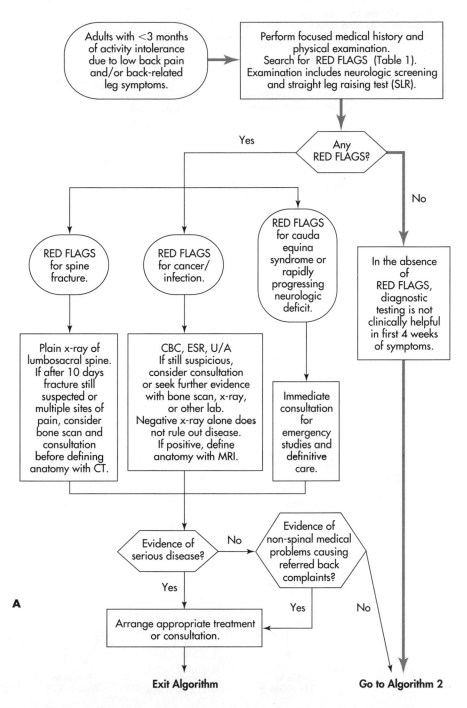

Figure 11-2   A, Algorithm 1: Initial evaluation of acute low back problem. *(From "Acute Low Back Problems in Adults: Assessment and Treatment," by S. Bigos, et al, 1994, in* Clinical Practice Guideline No. 14 *(AHCPR Publication No. 95-0642), Washington, DC: U.S. Department of Health and Human Services, AHCPR.)*

Continued

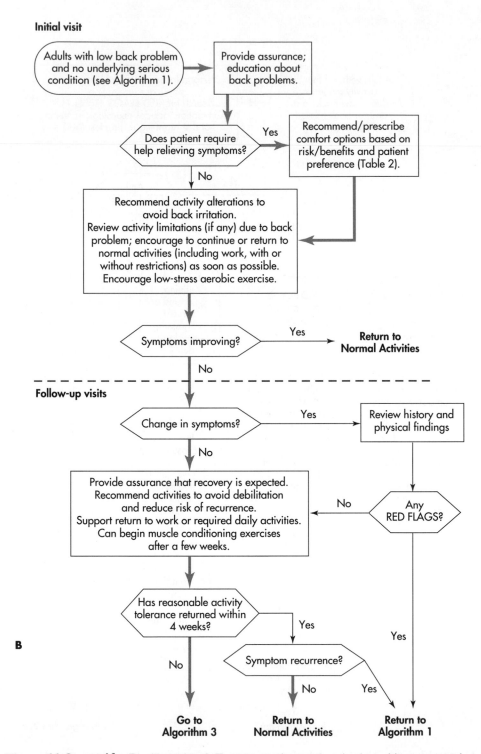

Figure 11-2, cont'd B, Algorithm 2: Treatment of acute low back problem on initial and followup visits. *(From "Acute Low Back Problems in Adults: Assessment and Treatment," by S. Bigos, et al, 1994, in* Clinical Practice Guideline No. 14 *(AHCPR Publication No. 95-0642), Washington, DC: U.S. Department of Health and Human Services, AHCPR.)*

drearing, and elder care. These, in turn, have profound impacts on the communities in which these people live.

Diagnosable mental illnesses exact a major toll in the workplace. Anxiety and depression are the two most common psychiatric disorders in the United States. Anxiety disorders have a lifetime prevalence of about 25% of the population; depressive disorders affect about 15% of males and 24% of females with increasing frequency and more than 11 million people in the United States annually. Depressive episodes also have a 50% rate of reoccurrence. Psychoses such as schizophrenia and other thought disorders, although occurring less often than anxiety and depression, can dramatically impair a worker's ability to function on the job and affect the will to work as well as cognitive skills such as concentration, problem solving, abstract reasoning, and judgment. Personality disorders are more prevalent than psychotic disorders and can affect an individual's ability to relate to others. Workers with personality disorders can be difficult to manage, due to the likelihood of conflicts with coworkers and supervisors (Cheng et al., 2000; Stenberg & Gammon, 1995).

An employee may appear in the occupational health unit with symptoms of depression (e.g., fatigue, decreased energy, loss of appetite, sleep dysfunction). The employee must be assessed in order to define an appropriate plan of care or intervention, and this requires communication and empathetic listening in an unhurried manner. Isaacs (1998) provides several assessment questions that may be useful in making an initial assessment (Box 11-2). In discussing the situation with an employee, the nurse determines the probable reason for depressive symptoms is a grief reaction due to loss of a family member. The nurse can proceed to offer support to the employee and also asks the employee if she or he desires therapy intervention. The nurse can probably assume this is a normal grief reaction but should continue to monitor the employee and offer support. If the depression worsens, or if self-harm (i.e., suicidal ideation) is evident, a referral for immediate intervention, such as to an employee assistance program or the employee's private physician, is needed. When counseling employees, the occupational and environmental health nurse should arrange for space or facilities that provide for adequate privacy. The nurse must be supportive;

Box 11-2 Assessment Questions for Depression

- Can you describe your mood for me?
- How long have you felt this way?
- What is the feeling of depression like for you?
- Have you noticed changes in your level of interest in normal activities?
- How would you rate your feeling of depression on a 1-to-10 scale?
- How do you explain your depression?
- Have you experienced any losses or changes in your life?
- If you could change one thing about your current situation, what would it be?
- What do you think would make you feel better?
- If you have had a problem with depression before, what helped you at that time?
- Are you experiencing thoughts of suicide?
- Do you have a plan for suicide? How would you go about it?

From "Depression and Your Patient," by A. Isaac, 1998, *American Journal of Nursing, 98,* 26-31.

---

demonstrate a sensitive, nonjudgmental, and caring attitude; and communicate respect for the employee.

These are but a few examples of counseling situations in which the occupational and environmental health nurse may be involved. Some of these problems may interfere with the worker's ability to perform the job, and the employee will probably benefit from some form of intervention, such as listening, support, or referral if indicated. The nurse's role is to help the employee find a solution to an immediate presenting problem or refer the employee for appropriate assistance or both. The role the nurse plays should not be confused with that of a therapist, unless the nurse is specifically trained and credentialed in this area. Thus, the nurse must be able to recognize problems, intervene, and refer as required. The nurse will need to have specific knowledge and skills, as identified by Csiemik (1990) (Box 11-3) in order to effectively provide assistance to the employee.

It is also important to recognize behavioral signs and symptoms that may indicate a troubled employee. Csiemik (1990) and Felton (1990) identify behavioral indicators suggestive of emo-

---

Box 11-3 Checklist of Knowledge and Skills for Occupational and Environmental Health Nurses Involved in Employee Assistance Counseling

KNOWLEDGE OF

1. Various problems associated with abuse of substances
2. Other health and personal problems
3. Personal attitudes, skills, and limitations
4. Counseling and crisis intervention
5. Intervention strategies to help employees
6. Referral approaches
7. Follow-up approaches
8. Community agencies and resources

SKILL IN

1. Building of a helping relationship (initiating, intervening, contracting, building rapport)
2. Interpersonal communication (active listening, verbal and nonverbal skills, attending, paraphrasing, and feedback)
3. Assessment and referral
4. Case management
5. Adult education (teaching and consulting)

From "An EAP Intervention Protocol for Occupational Health Nurses," by R. P. Csiemik, 1990, *AAOHN Journal, 38*, 381-384.

Box 11-4 Some Behavioral Indicators Suggestive of Emotional Distress

- Increased or chronic absenteeism and more frequent absence on Mondays, Fridays, and days after payday
- Sleeping at work or increased general fatigue
- Increased number of injuries or accidents at work
- Increased errors/decreased ability to concentrate and to complete tasks
- Decreased interpersonal and/or communication relationships with coworkers, peers, managers
- Increased criticism of others
- Change in mood or appearance or both
- Physical symptoms of stress disorder (e.g., weight loss, gastritis) and other complaints or signs (e.g., headache, pharyngitis, petechiae)
- Substance abuse problems and excessive use of prescribed meditations

---

tional distress or impairment (Box 11-4). If signs of behavioral changes or stress appear (which the occupational and environmental health nurse observes directly or the employee's supervisor or a coworker reports), the nurse can initiate contact with the employee to determine if assistance is needed or desired. Although employees may not share feelings and thoughts with fellow workers or their supervisors, they frequently will discuss their problems with the occupational and environmental health nurse or their physician if a trusting and confidential relationship has been established. As mentioned previously, employees may be referred to the Employee Assistance Program (EAP) for treatment or further referral or both. According to Stenberg and Gammon (1995), EAPs operate on the principle that both the employer's and the employee's best interests are served when people whose personal or family problems might affect job performance get help as soon as possible. EAP counselors serve as the li-

aison between companies and the broad range of professional and self-help treatment options available by helping link individuals with appropriate resources. Specific clinical services offered usually include assessment and referral. Increasingly, EAP programs are providing short-term counseling, 24-hour telephone crisis counseling, case tracking, and program evaluation.

The nurse also must identify employees at risk for psychiatric emergencies, such as suicidal, homicidal, or psychotic behavior, and have preidentified community resources and referral options available if emergency hospitalization or care is required (Hughes, 1991). In these instances the employee may be too incapacitated to handle the situation, and the occupational and environmental health nurse must be prepared to initiate appropriate action.

Stenberg and Gammon (1995) point out that for any counseling services to be effective, whether performed in-house or through referral to an EAP, the employee must feel that the program is a safe environment where problems are dealt with confidentially and in a professional manner with protection against job loss, criminal sanctions, or embarrassment. However, the EAP is not a safe haven in which employees may escape appropriate discipline for poor performance, nor are employees disciplined or terminated because they fail to comply with the EAP. Decisions about those matters are based on employee's workplace behavior (Stenberg & Gammon, 1995). Accurate documentation is extremely important, and all data collected must remain confidential. When providing aggregate information to management, care should be taken to delete demographic descriptions that could identify a client/employee.

STRESS

Stress in the work environment is pervasive and insidious and may be characterized by physical, psychological, and behavioral manifestations (Box 11-5). NIOSH (1999) defines occupational stress as the harmful physical and emotional responses that occur when the requirements of the job do not match the capabilities, resources, or needs of the worker. Job stress can lead to poor health and even injury. This is not meant to imply that highly challenging jobs are bad—quite the contrary. Challenge energizes workers both psychologically and physically and motivates workers to learn and acquire new skills. However, when challenge turns into job demands that cannot be met, exhaustion, fatigue, feelings of being overwhelmed, and stress can set in (NIOSH, 1999). Studies on the scope of job stress in the United States indicate the following:

- One fourth of employees view their jobs as the number one stressor in their lives (Northwestern National Life Insurance Company, 1991).
- Three fourths of employees believe the worker has more on-the-job stress than the worker a generation ago (Princeton Survey Research Associates, 1997).
- Problems at work are more strongly associated with health complaints than are any other life stressor—more so than even financial problems or family problems (St. Paul Fire and Marine Insurance Company, 1992).

NIOSH (1999) points to several job conditions that may lead to job stress; among these are poor task design, ineffective management styles, poor interpersonal relationships at the job, conflicting work roles, career concerns, and unpleasant environmental conditions. These closely match the model presented in Figure 11-3, which shows sev-

---

Box 11-5 Stress-related Symptoms and Disorders

Physical	Psychological	Behavioral
Fatigue	Irritability	Smoking
Headaches	Anger	Overeating
Musculoskeletal	Depression	Substance
disorders	Apathy	abuse
Hypertension	Anxiety	Insomnia
Heart disease	Worry	Hostility
Gastrointestinal	Withdrawal	Burnout
problems		Absenteeism
Infection		

---

eral workplace factors that influence the stress state and generally fall into six broad areas.

Personal factors are related to individual characteristics or conditions that affect personal motivation; these include health status, personality, performance ability, coping and communication skills, value systems, and conflict between demands of the job and home life. More widely recognized than ever before as sources of stress are the multiple roles women find themselves in, such as mother, worker, and student.

Situational/interpersonal factors are related to events or conditions of the job, such as quality of social support systems; conflicts with managers, peers, or colleagues; or lack of respect. Social support systems at work influence psychological well-being, job satisfaction, health status, and work absenteeism.

Organizational factors are related to policy and operational controls such as workload, role ambiguity, poor communication, ineffective organizational and managerial leadership, inadequate resources, job depersonalization, lack of shared decision making when job demands exceed worker control, and lack of opportunity provided for professional growth. Workers may be faced with too many demands and vigilant tasks without enough help or adequate, state-of-the-art equipment and supplies. The politics of the institution in terms of corporate culture and level of productivity expected may also result in varying degrees of stress.

Shiftwork deserves special mention. Studies of shiftworkers have shown that shiftwork, especially night and rotating shiftwork, has a negative impact on the worker's general well-being and per-

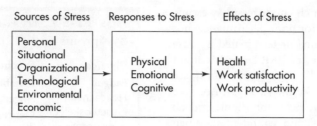

Figure 11-3 Psychosocial stress and work.

formance because of the constant disruption of the individual's circadian rhythms. Loss of sleep, alterations in eating habits, headaches, stomach problems, and disturbances in elimination and relaxation patterns have been reported. Other physiological and psychological complaints include "feeling tired and worn out," feeling like a "nervous wreck," "being quickly angered," and experiencing anxiety and depression (NIOSH, 1997). Rotating shifts and working night shifts also affect the worker's interactions with family and friends.

Technological factors are related to new or advanced systems for delivery of services, such as handling of sophisticated equipment, task design, interaction with computers and communication networks, and complex advances in high technology fields (e.g., engineering, medicine). Grout (1980) reviewed literature on air traffic controllers and drew an analogy between this type of work and the nursing profession. Both professions were seen as demanding, performing critical and managing complex tasks crucial to the lives of others.

Environmental factors are concerned with the quality of the work setting. This category includes the physical design of the work station, ergonomic controls, stimuli (e.g., lights, noise, and odors), dangerous environmental location, air pollution, crowding, and general tension level in the environment.

Economic factors can cause considerable stress, particularly when the worker's economic security is in jeopardy, such as with company downsizing or reduction in pay or benefits. In addition, when a person spends more than what she or he earns in order to maintain a certain standard of living, financial crises can ensue.

These various sources of stress can result in one or more clinical manifestations, including physi-

cal, emotional, or cognitive disruption, and can cause health dysfunction or a decrease in work satisfaction and performance or both. It may be anticipated that even larger numbers of people in the future will be at risk for stress responses and stress outcomes, such as chronic fatigue, loss of interest, and alcoholism or drug abuse, which also interfere with their work productivity.

The effects of job stress on chronic diseases are difficult to see because chronic diseases take a long time to develop and can be influenced by many factors other than stress. Nonetheless, evidence is rapidly accumulating to suggest that stress plays an important role in several types of chronic health problems—especially cardiovascular disease, musculoskeletal disorders, and psychological disorders. Strategies to deal with stress in the workplace and the offering of employee assistance programs to aid in counseling must be encouraged.

Employees may come to the occupational health unit with stress-related symptoms. The occupational and environmental health nurse can assist the employee through individual counseling about the specific stress-producing situation and ways to manage stress through enhanced coping skills, relaxation skills, and lifestyle modification such as physical fitness skills. However, this approach is very limited because it focuses on the worker and not the environment, even if the environment is the cause of stress. The occupational and environmental health nurse will want to work with management to create a more satisfying organizational climate through supervisory training programs and more functional policies and structures, such as the establishment of flexible work schedules, encouraging of participative management, provision of social support and feedback, team building, improved career development, redesign of work tasks and demands, and shared rewards. This approach deals more directly with the root causes of stress at work. NIOSH suggests several steps toward stress prevention at work that include the following:

Step 1: Identify the Problem
- Hold group discussions with employees.
- Design an employee survey.
- Measure employee perceptions of job conditions, stress, health, and satisfaction.
- Collect objective data.
- Analyze data to identify problem locations and stressful job conditions.

Step 2: Design and Implement Interventions
- Target the source of stress for change.
- Propose and prioritize intervention strategies.
- Communicate planned interventions to employees.
- Implement interventions.

Step 3: Evaluate Interventions
- Conduct both short-term and long-term evaluations.
- Measure employee perceptions of job conditions, stress, health, and satisfaction.
- Include objective measures.
- Refine the intervention strategy and return to Step 1.

The process should be seen as continuous to redefine or redirect the intervention strategy.

Summary

In the occupational setting assessment and management of clinical problems and counseling of employees regarding work-related and nonoccupational health and related concerns is a central component within the scope of occupational and environmental health nursing practice. Employees will come to the occupational health unit with various complaints of a physical, emotional, or psychological nature, and the occupational and environmental health nurse must be skilled in making assessments and judgments regarding necessary care and appropriate referral. The development and use of clinical nursing guidelines will help provide a systematic approach to nursing care; however, individual judgments are always required. The nurse must always practice within the legal limits of state nurse practice acts and utilize appropriate and current resources to provide safe and effective care.

References

Akers, P. (1991). An algorithmic approach to clinical decision making. *Oncology Nursing Forum, 18,* 1159-1163.

American Association of Occupational Health Nurses. (1997). *Developing clinical guidelines or protocols for practice: AAOHN advisory.* Atlanta, GA: AAOHN.

American College of Occupational and Environmental Medicine. (1997). *Occupational medicine practice guidelines* (J. S. Harris, Ed.). Beverly, MA: OEM Press.

Bates, B. (1995). *A guide to clinical thinking.* Philadelphia: Lippincott.

Burgel, B. J. (1998). Tendonitis. In G. Collins-Bride & J. M. Saxe, (Eds.), *Nurse practitioner/physician collaborative practice: Clinical guidelines for ambulatory care.* San Francisco: UCSF Nursing Press.

Burgel, B. J. (2001). Direct care. In AAOHN (Eds.), *Core curriculum in occupational and environmental health nursing.* Philadelphia: Saunders.

Cheng, Y., Kawachi, I., Coakley, E. H., Schwartz, J., Colditz, G. (2000). Association between psychosocial work characteristics and health functioning in American women: Prospective study. *British Medical Journal, 320,* 1432-1436.

Csiemik, R. P. (1990). An EAP intervention protocol for occupational health nurses. *AAOHN Journal, 38*(8), 381-384.

Felton, J. (1990). *Occupational medical management.* Boston: Little, Brown & Company.

Glasgow, G. (1990). Quality of care in occupational health through nursing diagnosis. *AAOHN Journal, 38,* 105-109.

Grout, J. W. (1980). Stress and the nurse: Selected bibliography. *Journal of Nursing Education, 19,* 58-63.

Hood, J. (2000). Is "latex safe" possible? *AAOHN Journal, 48,* 291-296.

Hughes, K. H. (1991). Psychiatric emergencies in the workplace. *AAOHN Journal, 39*(6), 265-269.

Isaacs, A. (1998). Depression and your patient. *American Journal of Nursing, 98,* 26-31.

Kosinski, M. (1998). Effective outcomes management in occupational and environmental health. *AAOHN Journal, 46*(10), 500-509.

Mood, D. W. (1996). The diagnosis of cancer: A life transition. In R. McCorkle, M. Grant, M. Frank-Stromborg, & S. B. Baird (Eds.), *Cancer nursing: A comprehensive textbook* (2nd ed., pp. 298-314). Philadelphia: W. B. Saunders.

National Institute for Occupational Safety and Health. (1997). *Plain language about shiftwork.* Cincinnati, OH: U.S. Department of Health and Human Services.

National Institutes for Occupational Safety and Health. (1999). *Stress . . . at work.* Cincinnati, OH: U.S. Department of Health and Human Services.

Northwestern National Life Insurance Company (1991). *Employee burnout: America's newest epidemic.* Minneapolis, MN: Author.

Princeton Survey Research Associates. (1997). *Labor day survey: State of workers.* Princeton, NJ: Author.

Rogers, B., Randolph, S., & Mastroianni, K. (2003). *Occupational health nursing guidelines for primary clinical conditions.* Boston: OEM Press.

St. Paul Fire and Marine Insurance Company. (1992). *American workers under pressure technical report.* St. Paul, MN: Author.

Stenberg, C. R., & Gammon, P. J. (1995). Occupational mental health. *North Carolina Medical Journal, 56,* 228-233.

U.S. Department of Health and Human Services. (2000). *Healthy People 2010: Conference edition,* (Vols. 1 and 2). Washington, DC: U.S. Government Printing Office. (Available online at http://www.health.gov/healthy-people.)

Weekes, D. P. (1998). Cultural influences on the psychosocial experience. In R. M. Carroll-Johnson, L. M. Gorman, & N. J. Bush (Eds.), *Psychosocial nursing care along the cancer continuum* (pp. 61-69). Pittsburgh, PA: Oncology Nursing Press.

Worden, W. (1995). Bereavement care. *Seminars in Oncology, 12,* 472-475.

11-1 Examples of Clinical Nursing Guidelines for Common Occupational Health Problems

Abrasion or Laceration

Amputation

Burn: Thermal

Contusion

Convulsion or Seizure

Eye Injury: Flash Burn (Nonwelding)

Fracture: Open

Fracture: Closed

Medical Waste Disposal

Sunburn

Copyright Bonnie Rogers, 2002.
From *Occupational Health Nursing Guidelines for Primary Clinical Conditions,* by B. Rogers, S. Randolph, and K. Mastroianni, 2003, Boston: OEM Press. See this reference for additional guidelines.

Abrasion or Laceration

Definition	An *abrasion* is a superficial wound caused by a rubbing or scraping trauma resulting in a break in the skin and removal of epidermis. A *laceration* is a slice or tear in the skin or mucosa and can range from superficial to deep. Trauma usually occurs from contact with sharp objects and machinery or from falls. An *avulsion* is a piece of skin torn loose with part of the tissue still attached.
Characteristics	Abrasions often are painful and might be embedded with foreign matter. Bleeding usually is minimal. Lacerations can have sharp or jagged edges. Tissue, nerves, or blood vessels might be involved and significant bleeding can be present. Any break in the skin involves the risk of infection and contamination with the tetanus organism.
Policy	Evaluate employee in the occupational health unit to determine degree and severity of the injury. **Always** assess the employee's immunization status against tetanus when an abrasion or laceration has occurred.

OBJECTIVES	CLINICAL ASSESSMENTS AND INTERVENTIONS	REFERRAL FOR MEDICAL ACTION
Determine the extent and location of the injury and control any bleeding.	• Apply firm pressure to injury site; if needed, elevate extremity and use pressure points. • Cleanse area with mild antiseptic solution and water and rinse. • Approximate edges of laceration with Steri-strips if indicated.	• Any wound over flex/ stress point or area where steristrips would not provide for closure. • Gaping or jagged edges. • Embedded material. • A cut producing a flap. • A serious cut to fingers, hands, toes, feet, or over joints. • Human or animal bite. • Facial laceration. • Functional disturbance. • Uncontrolled bleeding. • Gross contamination.
Prevent infection.	• Apply antibiotic ointment per standing order. • Apply nonadherent dry sterile dressing (e.g., Telfa, Jellnet); minor abrasions can be left undressed. • Assess immunization status for tetanus and proceed as outlined in guideline 13, Tetanus Prophylaxis. If required, administer immunizations within 24 hours. • Counsel employee regarding care of the wound on and off the job (e.g., hygiene and avoiding a repeat injury). • Advise keeping the dressing clean and dry to prevent infection and changing the dressing daily for observation of wound. • Instruct regarding signs and symptoms of infection (redness at site, warmth at site, tenderness, swelling, pain, or fever).	**FOLLOW-UP ACTIONS** • Evaluate wound for infection and healing. • If wound is infected, refer employee for medical evaluation. • Evaluate worksite for potential hazards and recommend prevention strategies.

Amputation

Definition	Severance of a body part, most frequently caused by heavy machinery (such as farm machines) or heavy industrial equipment.
Characteristics	Bone and other body tissues are exposed. Bleeding and shock can be apparent, with complications of infection and disability.
Policy	Give employee immediate treatment in the occupational health unit or use emergency response personnel. Preserve the severed part and take steps to enhance its viability. Arrange for immediate transport to the hospital.

OBJECTIVES	CLINICAL ASSESSMENTS AND INTERVENTIONS	REFERRAL FOR MEDICAL ACTION
Institute emergency action.	• Assure airway patency. • Control bleeding by applying firm pressure, and elevate extremity and use pressure points as needed. • Give oxygen as indicated. • Support and immobilize the affected part in a functional position and keep employee at rest. • Cleanse and irrigate wound with sterile saline or tap water. • Cover the wound with sterile gauze or ABD pads. • Arrange for immediate transport of employee and the severed part to the hospital. • Notify health care transporters if suspected foreign bodies are in the wound. • **Do not compromise employee's life to save the part.**	• Need for immediate medical evaluation and treatment (i.e., transport to hospital).
Preserve severed part.	• Clean off any gross foreign matter. • Wrap the severed part in a sterile gauze or towel (a clean sheet for large limb). • Wet the wrapping with sterile normal saline or lactated Ringer's solution. Do not immerse the part in any solution. • Place the part in a waterproof bag or container and seal. • Maintain anatomical position of the part. • Place the bag or container inside another ice-filled container. Do not freeze the part. • Record the time the affected part was severed.	**FOLLOW-UP ACTIONS** • Counsel employee regarding safety measures, rehabilitation, disability management, and return to work. • Provide support and referral to employee assistance program if needed.

Burn: Thermal

Definition	Injury to the tissues as a result of heat or flame exposure or contact with hot substance (e.g., scalding water). Severity is determined by the amount of body surface area (BSA) involved and the burn depth. First-degree burns involve the epithelial layer (erythema); second-degree burns include a partial thickness of the dermal skin layer (erythema with blister); and third-degree burns involve full thickness of the dermal skin layer (white or leathery, with no blisters and charred appearance), and can extend to muscle and bone (sometimes called *fourth-degree burns).*
Characteristics	*First-degree burns* usually are superficial and result initially in reddening of the skin and in pain. *Second-degree burns* (partial thickness) are accompanied by severe pain, erythema, latent blister formation, and cell fluid loss. In *third-degree burns,* the area can appear black, white, or leathery. Excessive fluid loss can cause shock.
Policy	Remove employee from the heat or fire. Immediately evaluate at the scene or in the occupational health unit any employee who sustains a thermal burn. Depending on degree and extent of burn, hospital transport might be required.

OBJECTIVES	CLINICAL ASSESSMENTS AND INTERVENTIONS	REFERRAL FOR MEDICAL ACTION
Remove employee from burn source, determine status, and stabilize.	• At the scene, remove employee from the heat source and extinguish the fire. • Ensure patent airway. • Anticipate airway obstruction if inhalation injury. • Assess extent and degree of burns (see Rule of Nines). • Inspect face and neck for early swelling, soot in the mouth, and sputum (if employee can cough). • Apply oxygen if needed. • Examine employee for other injuries. • Obtain vital signs.	• Burn involving hands, face, eyes, feet, or perineum. • Electrical or inhalation burn. • Burn with associated major trauma. • Second-degree burn > 10% of BSA or third-degree burn. • Elderly employee or employee with chronic disease.

Burn: Thermal—cont'd

Treat major burn immediately, while preparing for hospital transport.	• Cool burned area with tap water to no more than 20% of BSA for 10 minutes. **Do not apply ice.** • Do not remove adherent clothing. • Remove nonadherent burned clothing that is smoldering and retaining heat, and jewelry. • Cover burned area with dry, sterile clean material. • Check for signs of smoke inhalation (e.g., soot in nostrils, singed hair, hoarseness, drooling, stridor, cough, mouth burns). • Initiate intravenous lactated Ringer's solution per standing order, if needed. • Elevate burned extremity to decrease fluid loss and swelling. • Do not break blisters or apply ointments, creams, or topical anesthetics. • Prevent shock (see guideline 103, Shock). • Transport to hospital.	**FOLLOW-UP ACTIONS** • Advise employee about signs and symptoms of infection. • Advise keeping burned site elevated for at least 24 hours. • Counsel regarding safety precautions. • Change dressing as needed. • Observe wound for infection. • Evaluate worksite for thermal hazard and associated risk.
Treat and provide symptom relief for minor burn (usually mild to moderate).	• Remove smoldering material. • Initiate cooling efforts (saline-soaked dressings). • Minimize local sensitivity depending on the degree and extensiveness of the burn (may require medical treatment). • Leave blisters intact. • Administer medications (i.e., antimicrobial agents, analgesics) per standing order. • Apply dry, sterile dressing. • Keep affected part elevated to reduce edema. • Assess tetanus immunization status per guideline 13, Tetanus Prophylaxis. Administer immunization accordingly.	

Burn: Rule of Nines

THE BODY IS DIVIDED INTO MULTIPLES OF NINE

Head and neck	9%
Each upper extremity, 9% (i.e., 9 × 2)	18%
Each lower extremity, 18% (i.e., 18 × 2)	36%
Each anterior and posterior trunk surface, 18% (i.e., 18 × 2)	36%
Perineum and genitalia	1%
	100%

9%

18% Front

9%   18% Back   9%

1%

18%   18%

Contusion

Definition	Injury to soft tissue in which the skin is not broken (a bruise), caused by blunt force, blow, kick, or fall.
Characteristics	Clinical manifestations include hemorrhage into injured parts (ecchymosis), pain, swelling, and discoloration.
Policy	Evaluate employee in the occupational health unit.

OBJECTIVES	CLINICAL ASSESSMENTS AND INTERVENTIONS	REFERRAL FOR MEDICAL ACTION
Determine extent of injury.	• Inspect contusion and surrounding area. • Assess neurovascular status distal to injury, looking for digital cyanosis, and assess for peripheral nerve damage.	• Persistent soreness or disability.
Provide symptom relief.	• Elevate affected part. • Apply cold compresses to area for 10 minutes, remove for 5 minutes, then reapply 3-4 times to reduce edema formation. • Apply elastic or elastic adhesive pressure bandage to reduce swelling and edema.	
		FOLLOW-UP ACTIONS
	• Apply warm moist heat as needed to affected area after swelling is reduced, usually after 48 hours. • Administer analgesics per standing order.	Advise employee to: • Continue cold compresses or ice packs periodically during first 24 hours or until swelling is relieved. • Keep affected part at rest and elevated. • Apply heat once swelling has stopped. • Report persistent soreness or disability.

Convulsion or Seizure

Definition	Paroxysms of involuntary muscular contractions and relaxations. They can be caused by epilepsy, meningitis, acute infectious disease, heat cramps, brain lesions, eclampsia, hypoglycemia (related to diabetes), or poisoning from camphor, cyanides, strychnine, or other chemical agents.
Characteristics	Intermittent contractions and relaxations of muscles, periodic lapses of consciousness, and incontinence.
Policy	Evaluate employee in the occupational health unit and refer for medical care.

OBJECTIVES	CLINICAL ASSESSMENTS AND INTERVENTIONS	REFERRAL FOR MEDICAL ACTION

Determine status of employee and keep safe from injury during seizure.	• Assess employee status.
	• Keep employee lying down.
	• Maintain open airway after seizure, turn employee to prone or semiprone position, and turn head to side.
	• Monitor vital signs.
	• Record the following:
	  – Time of onset of convulsion or seizure.
	  – Duration of seizure.
	  – Origin of convulsion (i.e., certain area of body or generalized).
	  – Type of contractions.
	  – Incontinence.
	  – Injury to head or other areas.
	  – Abnormal breath odor.
	• Arrange for medical care.
		• Any occurrence of seizure activity.
		
		FOLLOW-UP ACTIONS
		
		• Collaborate with personal physician regarding follow-up treatment plan
		• Educate employee regarding importance of taking medication as directed.
		• Counsel regarding communicating procedures for seizures.
		• Monitor appropriate placement of worker to ensure safety.

Eye Injury: Flash Burn (Nonwelding)

Definition	Injury to eye tissue from intense heat. Generally both eyes are affected.
Characteristics	Acute pain, photophobia, inflammation, swelling, and marked tearing.
Policy	Evaluate employee in the occupational health unit.

OBJECTIVES	CLINICAL ASSESSMENTS AND INTERVENTIONS	REFERRAL FOR MEDICAL ACTION
Determine extent and severity of injury.	• Assess injury to eye and surrounding areas. • Check eye for contact lens and remove it. • Inspect eye for foreign body.	• Need for immediate medical evaluation and treatment.
Provide symptom relief.	• Apply cold compresses for 5-minute periods until swelling is reduced. • Give analgesic per standing order. • Determine employee visual acuity. • Provide for medical care as needed.	**FOLLOW-UP ACTIONS** • Determine visual acuity. • Instruct regarding use of eye protection. • Discuss signs and symptoms of further injury. • Provide follow-up care as indicated per medical order. • Conduct worksite assessment to identify potential hazards and prevention strategies

Fracture: Open

Definition	Interruption in the continuity of a bone. Any bone in the body can be fractured if sufficient stress is applied; however, some bones (e.g., the wrist) are more prone to fracture because of their location. Open or compound fractures are associated with an open wound penetrating to the area of the injured bone or a bone end that has pierced through the skin, causing damage to the surrounding tissues.
Characteristics	An open fracture carries a higher risk for complications than does a closed fracture because contamination of the wound can lead to infection. Characteristics include localized pain, deformity or unnatural position or movement, shortening of the injured limb, tenderness to touch, swelling, ecchymosis, loss of range of motion, open wound (possibly with protruding bone or bone fragments), and a guarding or protective position. Femur fractures can result in substantial, unrecognized blood loss leading to hypovolemia and shock.
Policy	Provide initial stabilization of employee and arrange immediate medical care.

OBJECTIVES	CLINICAL ASSESSMENTS AND INTERVENTIONS	REFERRAL FOR MEDICAL ACTION
Determine extent and severity of injury.	• Determine and maintain airway, breathing, and circulation. • Assess site of fracture for swelling and obvious deformity. • Assess pulses, sensation, and motion distal to the injury and record them.	• Suspected fracture requiring immediate medical referral.
Stabilize employee in preparation for transport.	• Maintain universal precautions and aseptic technique to control bleeding. • **Do not attempt** to push exposed bone back beneath the skin. If bone fragment is protruding, cover the entire wound with large sterile bandage, compress, or pads. • Immobilize the injury by splinting the joint proximal and distal to fracture site in position found, if at all possible. Ensure the splint is sufficiently long and generously padded. • Reassess pulses and sensation. • Assess and treat for shock. If hypovolemia is suspected, start IV per standing order and monitor vital signs every 5 minutes. • Apply cold or ice packs to the area. • Give nothing to eat or drink. • Elevate the limb after splinting if there are no contraindications, such as suspected pelvic fractures, spinal injury, or skull fractures. • If pelvic fracture is suspected, prevent movement and avoid log-rolling. • Arrange immediate medical care with employee's personal physician or transport to hospital.	**FOLLOW-UP ACTIONS** • Arrange incident investigation to identify and eliminate cause of injury. • Provide safety education for employee and coworkers to prevent recurrence. • Counsel regarding return to work, restricted duty, or job transfer as indicated. • Assess status regarding return to work.

Fracture: Closed

Definition	Interruption in the continuity of a bone. Any bone in the body can be fractured if sufficient stress is applied; however, some bones (e.g., the tibia) are more prone to fracture because of their location. A closed or simple fracture does not cause a break or open wound on the surface of the body. Fractures are classified according to their appearance on x-ray and can be transverse, greenstick, oblique, spiral, impacted, or comminuted. Neighboring muscles and other tissues can remain largely undamaged.
Characteristics	Localized pain, deformity or unnatural position or movement, shortening of the injured limb, tenderness to touch, swelling, ecchymosis, loss of range of motion, and a guarding or protective position. Femur fractures might cause substantial internal bleeding, causing hypovolemic shock. With hip or pelvic fractures, the thigh might be rotated internally and adducted. Suspect a spinal injury if there has been enough force to cause a pelvic fracture.
Policy	Provide initial stabilization of employee and arrange immediate medical care.

OBJECTIVES	CLINICAL ASSESSMENTS AND INTERVENTIONS	REFERRAL FOR MEDICAL ACTION
Determine extent and severity of injury.	• Determine and maintain airway, breathing, and circulation. • Assess site of fracture for swelling and obvious deformity. • Assess pulses, sensation, and motion distal to the injury and record them.	• Suspected fracture requiring immediate medical referral.
Stabilize employee in preparation for transport.	• Immobilize the injury by splinting the joint proximal and distal to fracture site in position found, if at all possible. Ensure the splint is sufficiently long and generously padded. • Reassess pulses and sensation. • Assess and treat for shock. If hypovolemia is suspected, start IV per medical order and monitor vital signs every 5 minutes. • Apply cold or ice packs to the area. • Give nothing to eat or drink. • Elevate the limb after splinting if there are no contraindications, such as suspected pelvic fractures, spinal injury, or skull fractures. • Protect cervical spine as appropriate. • If pelvic fracture is suspected, prevent movement and avoid log-rolling. • Arrange immediate medical care with the employee's personal physician or transport to hospital.	**FOLLOW-UP ACTIONS** • Arrange incident investigation to identify and eliminate cause of injury. • Provide safety education for employee and coworkers to prevent recurrence. • Counsel on return to work, restricted duty, or job transfer as indicated. • Assess status prior to return to work.

Medical Waste Disposal

Definition and Purpose

Hazardous waste is discarded material that can be harmful to human health or the health of the environment, owing to the quantity or concentration or physical, chemical, or toxic characteristics. Elements from chemical spills, chemical release, and biological release are examples. This guideline is specific to medical waste generated in the occupational health unit. For information regarding other types of waste disposal or emergency response to hazardous materials, refer to the Resource Conservation and Recovery Act of 1976 (RCRA), Comprehensive Environmental Response Compensation and Liability Act of 1980 (CERCLA), SuperFund Amendments and Reauthorization Act of 1986 (SARA), and Hazardous Waste Operations and Emergency Response Standard of 1990 (HAZWOPER).

Program Objectives and Elements

Occupational health unit personnel should develop a written plan for medical waste disposal based on current federal and state laws and on company policy regarding such disposal. The following principles and practices should be addressed:

1. Proper management of regulated medical waste per regulatory ordinances.
2. Prevention of exposures to staff, employees, and the environment.
   - Place sharps in a container that is rigid, leak-proof, and puncture-resistant; do not compact prior to off-site shipping; and handle in a manner that avoids human contact with the sharps.
   - Label contaminated sharps containers appropriately with the biohazard symbol.
   - Package medical waste in a minimum of one plastic bag placed in a rigid fiberboard box or drum to prevent leakage of contents. (The plastic bag should be impervious to moisture and strong enough to preclude ripping or bursting under normal handling conditions.)
   - Place liquid medical waste in a capped bottle or similar container.
   - Store waste for a limited time in an area with limited access and in a manner that maintains the integrity of the packaging at all times.
3. Adherence to company policies and regulations.
   - Label medical waste with a water-resistant universal biohazard symbol and label the storage area.
   - Contain medical waste from the point of origin to the point at which they are no longer infectious.
   - Treat medical waste or contract with a company specializing in the treatment and disposal of medical waste according to

Medical Waste Disposal—cont'd

local, state, and federal regulations.
- Selection of treatment methods according to type of waste, company policy, and regulations. Treatment methods include steam sterilization, incinerations, gas or vapor sterilization, chemical disinfection, thermal inactivation, and irradiation. After treatment the medical waste can be buried in sanitary landfills or ashes and liquids can be discharged into sanitary sewer systems.

Interdisciplinary Interactions and Collaboration

The occupational health nurse (OHN) should use available corporate resources when developing procedures for handling medical waste. In addition, available community resources should be consulted, including local or state health departments, the Environmental Protection Agency, OHNs in the area, and the company physician. Interdisciplinary collaboration can assist the OHN in developing effective waste management strategies and control procedures and can include the following:
- Referral of any exposure to blood or other infectious body fluid immediately to the company physician (see *Universal Precautions* guidelines).
- Periodic review of the waste disposal plan with other professionals to ensure proper compliance with procedures.
- Collaboration with other OHNs in the area and medical providers to discuss medical waste disposal options.

Nursing Roles

In addition to developing the policy and procedures for handling and disposing of medical waste, the OHN should educate housekeeping staff or janitors and first-aid response team members. Specific procedures should be developed for these employees to follow when a medical emergency occurs and the health unit is closed. The OHN often is involved with educating employees regarding hazardous spill prevention and control and waste disposal.

Sunburn

Definition	Excessive exposure to ultraviolet (UV) light that results in injury to the superficial dermis of the skin.
Characteristics	Locally, there is dilation of the capillaries, erythema, tenderness, edema, and occasional blister formation. Systemically, sunburn can involve large areas of the body and can cause headache, nausea, chills, fever, and photosensitivity.
Policy	Evaluate employee in the occupational health unit.

OBJECTIVES	CLINICAL ASSESSMENTS AND INTERVENTIONS	REFERRAL FOR MEDICAL ACTION
Obtain history of sun exposure.	• Obtain information regarding duration of recent sun exposure, type of protection used, and use of photosensitive drugs that cause an exaggerated burn after exposure to sun (refer to table photosensitizing drugs).	• Signs and symptoms of infection. • Second-degree burn > 10% of body surface area or third-degree burn. • Abnormal moles or lesions.
Assess skin.	• Assess skin type. • Assess skin area for redness, tenderness, blistering, and abnormal moles and lesions.	
Provide symptom relief.	• If pain persists, puncture large blisters with a sterile needle or surgical blade, leaving the roof of the blister intact to serve as a pain-reducing biological dressing. • Administer analgesics for skin tenderness per standing order.	**FOLLOW-UP ACTIONS** Advise employee to: • Recognize harmful effects of UV light, such as sunburn and skin cancers. • Avoid concentrated sun exposure between 10 AM and 3 PM.
Recommend symptom relief procedures to be used at home.	• Recommend cool baths, soothing lotions (e.g., Rhuli gel, aloe vera lotion, or Noxzema), and a colloidal oatmeal bath (one cup of Aveeno oatmeal to lukewarm or cool bath water) for 20 minutes for extensive burn.	• Avoid tanning salons, sun lamps, and tanning promoters. • Use sunscreen* with high sun protection factor that blocks both UVB and UVA rays.

	Sunburn—cont'd

	FOLLOW-UP ACTIONS—CONT'D
	• Apply sunscreen 30 minutes before exposure to sun and routinely reapply every 2 hours after bathing, and after heavily perspiring.
	• Apply sunscreen to cover ears, lips, nose, and other areas prone to sun burning.
	• Wear protective clothing (e.g., broad-brimmed hat and long-sleeved shirt) and use an umbrella.
	• Avoid direct sunlight exposure if taking photosensitizing drug (see table on next page).
	• Instruct employee about skin self-examination to observe for abnormal moles or lesions.

Sunscreen chemically reacts with UV light when it comes in contact with the skin, changing it to heat that evaporates from the surface. *Sunblock* (i.e., zinc oxide, titanium dioxide, talc) physically blocks out (scatters, reflects) the light.

Drugs That Can Cause Photosensitivity

ANTIDEPRESSANTS

Amitriptyline (Elavil)
Amoxapine (Asendin)
Clomipramine (Anafranil)
Desipramine (Norpramin, Pertofrane)
Doxepin (Adapin, Sinequan)
Imipramine (Tofranil)
Isocarboxazid (Marplan)
Maprotiline (Ludiomil)
Nortriptyline (Aventyl, Pamelor)
Protriptyline (Vivactil)
Trimipramine (Surmontil)

ANTIHISTAMINES

Cyproheptadine (Periactin)
Diphenhydramine (Benadryl)

ANTIMICROBIALS

Ciprofloxacin (Cipro)
*Demeclocycline (Declomycin)
Doxycycline (Vibramycin)
Griseofulvin (Fulvicin)
Minocycline (Minocin)
*Nalidixic acid (NegGram)
Norfloxacin (Noroxin)
Oxytetracycline (Terramycin)
Sulfasalazine (Azulfidine)
*Sulfonamides (Septra, Gantrisin, Bactrim)
Tetracyclines

ANTIPARASITICS

*Bithionol (Bitin)
Chloroquine (Aralen)
Mefloquine (Lariam)
Pyrvinium pamoate (Povan, Vanquin)
Quinine

ANTIPSYCHOTICS

Chlorprothixene (Taractan, Tarasan)
Haloperidol (Haldol)
*Phenothiazines (Compazine, Mellaril, Stelazine, Phenergan, Thorazine)

CARDIOVASCULARS

*Amiodarone (Cordarone)
Captopril (Capoten)
Disopyramide (Norpace)
Enalapril (Vasotec)
Quinadine (Quinaglute)

DIURETICS

Acetazolamide (Diamox)
Amiloride (Midamor)
Furosemide (Lasix)
Metolazone (Diulo, Zaroxolyn)
*Thiazides (HydoDiuril, Naturetin)

*HYPOGLYCEMIC SULFONYLUREAS

Acetohexamide (Dymelor)
Chlorpropamide (Diabinese)
Glipizide (Glucotrol)
Glyburide (DiaBeta, Micronase)
Tolazamide (Tolinase)
Tolbutamide (Orinase)

NONSTEROIDAL ANTI-INFLAMMATORY DRUGS

All nonsteroidal anti-inflammatory drugs (ibuprofen [Motrin], naproxen [Anaprox, Naprosyn], Orudis, Feldene, Voltaren)

MISCELLANEOUS

Benzocaine
Carbamazepine (Tegretol)
Coal tar (Tegrin, Zetar)
Contraceptives, oral
*Etretinate (Tegison)
Gold salts (Myochrysine, Ridaura, Solganol)
Hexachlorophene (pHisoHex)
*Isotretinoin (Accutane)
*Perfume oils (bergamot, citron, lavender, sandalwood, cedar, musk)
*Psoralens
Selegiline (Deprenyl, Eldepryl)
*Tretinoin (Retin-A, Vitamin A Acid)

*Items more likely to cause photosensitivity reactions. Overall, the drugs in this table cause reactions in fewer than 1% of users. However, persons receiving any of the drugs in this table should be counseled so that they are made aware of the possibility of a reaction. If they get an unusual sunburn or an allergic or eczematous reaction in skin areas exposed to light, they should let their pharmacist or physician know.

12 Case Management

Case management services are not new to nursing. In the United States in the late 1800s public health nurses coordinated health care services often through visiting nurses associations and the establishment of settlement houses that became the hub for health care and social welfare programs. The most well known of these houses, the Henry Street Settlement House, established by Lillian Wald and Mary Brewster, later became the Visiting Nurse Service of New York City. In 1909 Lillian Wald also established the first community health nursing program cooperative with the Metropolitan Life Insurance Company to provide health care services to policyholders. The intent was to provide coordinated care in a cost-effective manner to reduce morbidity and premature mortality (Dieckmann, 2000). Throughout the twentieth century insurance companies have developed in-house case management services using nurses and social workers to coordinate multidisciplinary health care and focus on cost containment.

Case management is defined by the Case Management Society of America (CMSA) as a collaborative process that assesses, plans, implements, coordinates, monitors, and evaluates the options and services required to meet an individual's health needs and uses communication and available resources to promote quality and cost-effective outcomes (Case Management Society of America [CMSA], 1995). Thus, the goal of case management is to work with and through various health care service systems to deliver quality health care by utilizing cost-effective strategies. The case manager establishes a provider network, recommends treatment plans that ensure quality and efficacy while controlling costs, monitors outcomes, and maintains a strong communication link among all the parties (AAOHN, 1994; Commission for Case Manager Certification [CCM], 1995; Powell & Ignatavicius, 2001).

As described by Leahy (1994), knowledge domains essential to case management practice include the following (Chan et al., 1999):

1. *Coordination and service delivery.* This content area emphasizes the medical knowledge needed to manage the injury/disease process, including the expected length of recovery and treatment options available, the ability to integrate a variety of assessment data to develop treatment goals, and the skills to effectively communicate with all team members to facilitate cost-effective case care that maintains client confidentiality.
2. *Physical and psychosocial aspects factors.* This content area emphasizes knowledge of and among medical, psychological, sociological, and behavioral components of injury/illness and how they affect client health and health outcomes.
3. *Benefit systems/cost-benefit analysis.* This content area emphasizes knowledge of health and health-related benefit system coverage and evaluation methods for services and cost containment opportunities, including maximum patient benefit.
4. *Case management concepts.* This content area emphasizes the basic knowledge required to function effectively as a case manager and includes understanding the role of the case manager; determining effective approaches to problems solving; planning, coordinating, directing, and organizing the case management process; and providing results-oriented, cost-effective services.

5. *Community resources.* This content area emphasizes knowledge of health and disability-related legislation, community resources, and the services needed to address vocational accommodation and support needs of clients.

Elements in each of these core component areas are shown in Box 12-1.

In the occupational health arena the occupational health nurse case manager coordinates the client employee's health care services from the onset of illness or injury through a safe return to work or optimal alternative (AAOHN, 1994). This means helping employees understand what choices exist within a complex health care system in order to facilitate health care control and avoid

---

Box 12-1 **Knowledge Domains Essential to Case Management Practice**

COORDINATION AND SERVICE DELIVERY
- Understands legal and ethical issues pertaining to confidentiality
- Understands medical terminology
- Understands restrictions on the release of confidential information
- Knows how to obtain an accurate history
- Establishes treatment goals that meet the client's health care needs and the referral source's requirements
- Assesses clinical information to develop treatment plans
- Communicates case objectives to those who know them

PHYSICAL AND PSYCHOLOGICAL FACTORS
- Identifies cases with potential for high-risk complications
- Acts as an advocate for an individual's health care needs
- Understands methods for assessing an individual's present level of health care needs
- Understands the physical characteristics of illness
- Understands the psychological characteristics of disabling conditions
- Understands the psychological characteristics of illness
- Assists individuals with the development of short- and long-term health goals
- Understands the psychological characteristics of wellness

BENEFIT SYSTEMS AND COST-BENEFIT ANALYSIS
- Evaluates the quality of necessary medical services
- Understands requirements for prior approval by payer

- Identifies cases that would benefit from alternative care
- Evaluates necessary medical services for cost containment
- Analyzes data necessary to determine cost of care
- Understands home health resources
- Understands health care delivery systems

CASE MANAGEMENT CONCEPTS
- Understands the role of the case manager
- Documents case management services
- Applies problem-solving techniques to the case management process
- Understands case management philosophy and principles
- Knows how to evaluate the effectiveness of case management
- Understands planning and goal development techniques
- Understands liability issues for case management activities
- Develops case management plans that address the individual's needs

COMMUNITY RESOURCES
- Understands interviewing techniques
- Knows how to explain services and available resources (including limitations) to individuals with disabilities
- Knows how to establish a client's support system
- Understands assistive devices needed by individuals with disabilities
- Understands the Americans With Disabilities Act
- Understands federal legislation affecting individuals with disabilities
- Understands the client's need for vocational services

Data from *CMM Certification Guide,* by Commission for Case Manager Certification, 1995, Little Rock, AR: Author.

delayed recovery. This includes benefiting people with acute and chronic illnesses and serious injuries that may be occupational or nonoccupational in origin and accommodating ill or injured employees upon return to the workplace as soon as they are fit for duty without harm to themselves or others.

Occupational health case and disability management programs have increased dramatically in the last few years, driven mostly by increased economic costs as a result of rising disability claims, increased lost time, and decreased productivity. Cost associated with illness or injury-related absence may arise from the following (Denton & Leinart, 2001; Dyck, 2000):

- Paid employee sick leave, weekly indemnity, and/or short term disability
- Salary for replacement workers' recruitment and training of replacement workers
- Health care benefits
- Extended supplementary health care benefits
- Rising Workers' Compensation rates
- Long-term disability premium rates and costs
- Lowered productivity

The purposes of occupational health case management programs include the following:

1. Identify appropriate cases for occupational health case management services;
2. Provide access to quality health care services that are cost-effective and outcome-effective;
3. Prevent fragmented health care and delayed recovery;
4. Return the employee to as optimal work performance as possible whether through full, transitional, or modified duty.

The focus in providing occupational health case management services is on the best care, in the most appropriate setting, that results in the best outcome.

THE CASE MANAGEMENT PROCESS

In general, the case management process involves the following stages (Powell, 2000):

- Case selection
- Assessment/problem identification
- Development and coordination of the case plan
- Implementation of plan
- Evaluation and follow-up
- Continuous monitoring, reassessing, and reevaluating

CASE SELECTION

The process of case selection, the first step in the case management process, is used to evaluate individuals to determine the need for case management services based on established criteria. Early identification of cases requiring intervention is critical for case management to be effective. Individuals who may require a case manager include those with complex medical problems such as chronic diseases (e.g., diabetes), high risk conditions (e.g., AIDS, high risk infants), or work-related conditions when the injury has the potential for disability or high cost. Box 12-2 identifies examples of indications useful to trigger a case management investigation. The use of routine methods for case selection may overlook critical cases, and the occupational health nurse needs to remain vigilant in identifying unusual situations for case management services.

One valuable method for case selection determination is to review past data and trends available from worker's compensation systems, group health claims, and disability systems in order to examine high cost, high volume cases. For example, working with an employee newly diagnosed with migraine headache in order to facilitate the therapeutic regime and work capacity and reduce the need for work loss is appropriate for case management intervention. This will involve maintaining employee contact during and after the health care provider evaluation, facilitating the understanding of the treatment plan and options, providing the employee with educational information and resources, communicating with health care providers about treatment effectiveness, and working with management on appropriate accommodations (e.g., need for quiet space if headache approaches) within the parameters of client confidentiality. With regard to possible indicators for case selection, common indicators such as extended length of stay and high dollar amounts exclude the possibility of early case management; that is, early nursing case management may in fact reduce the length of stay and reduce health care costs (Powell, 2000).

Box 12-2   Indicators for Early Case Identification for Case Management Services

Repeat surgery or complications
Multiple hospital admissions
Poor compliance with treatment regimen
Continuous symptoms/medication
Attorney involvement
Injured employee near retirement
Problem with supervisor or coworkers
Multiple diagnoses
Psychiatric diagnosis and history of an emotional problem
Significant life change events (e.g., death in family, job move)
Alteration in body image
Victim or perpetrator of violence
Prior claims history
Fraud
Multiple or severe trauma
Severe genetic anomalies
Debilitating or terminal illness
Several treating health care providers and/or agencies

"Doctor shopping"
Poor work performer
Age (extremes of age range [e.g., over age 65] increase need for case management)
Potential secondary gains associated with injury/illness
Financial difficulties
Lives alone or with someone with a disability
Hospital readmission within 15 days
Overdose
Eating disorder
Alzheimer's dementia
Homelessness
Poor living environment
No known social or family support system
Admission from an extended care facility or sheltered living arrangement
Need for transitional care in an extended care facility or sheltered living arrangement
No or inadequate health insurance
Dependent in activities of daily living

ASSESSMENT/PROBLEM IDENTIFICATION

After an employee has been identified as potentially needing case management services, thorough and comprehensive assessment must be done to determine the client's physical and functional status and physical, social, financial, and psychosocial needs (Dees & Anderson, 1996; Maldonado & Quinn, 1999). Early support for the ill or injured employee must be established so all lines of communication are open. Assessment is the critical foundation piece around which the case management process revolves. Inadequate data assessment can result in chaos and unstable, inaccurate care plans.

There are several sources of assessment data, and the client or employee is the primary contributor of information. The family and employer may also be important information sources, and surrogate data sources (e.g., spouse, children, parents) may need to be used if the employee is incapable of interviewing. Sources for medical information include the treating health care provider, family physician, and numerous health care records, including hospital, office-based, home care, and dental. The employer may also provide

helpful functional capacity data before the illness or injury occurrence. General assessment data to be collected include the following:

- Health history and demographics
- Current medical status/medication status
- Nutritional status
- Financial status
- Functional ability
- Psychosocial status
- Cultural/religious diversity
- Community resources
- Employer/employee responsibilities

Box 12-3 provides examples of each of these assessment elements.

In completing the assessment, the occupational and environmental health nurse may find assessment tools already developed that cover most of the areas targeted in the assessment (Powell, 2000). These tools can be modified to address specific needs identified. In addition, screening tools such as health risk assessment can be used to help predict health problems such as lifestyle health risk factors (e.g., smoking, lack of exercise). The Health Status Survey is another self-assessment tool

---

Box 12-3 Example of Assessment Elements in Case Management

Health History and Demographics
- Age
- Ethnicity
- Marital status
- Children
- Employment
- Education level
- Religion
- Language
- Medical history, including all hospitalizations and diseases
- Noncompliance issues
- Family history
- Alternative therapies

Current Medical Status/Medication Status
- Complete health assessment
- Diagnoses
- Treatment modalities
- Medications (all) + compliance
- Allergies
- Understanding of health status
- Understanding of medications use, dose, adverse effects, lab monitoring

Nutritional Status
- Food intake: adequacy/appropriateness
- Financial issues
- Social issues
- Dental issues
- Acute/chronic disease

Financial Status
- Insurance coverage
- Ability to pay co-payments
- Equipment/supplies cost
- Basic financial obligations

Functional Ability
- Safety issues
- Performance of activities of daily living (ADLs)
- Home environment
    Telephone, stairs, sanitation, transportation
- Balance/wheelchair use

Psychosocial Status
- Coping skills
- Family relationships
- Hobbies/recreational outlets
- Mental status/cognitive ability
- Dependency needs
- Support systems

Cultural/Religious Diversity
- Traditions
- Language
- Spiritual beliefs, including health care relationship
- Dietary practices

Community Resources
- Voluntary agencies
- Accessibility availability
- Transportation
- Equipment
- Social services/clergy

Employer/Employee Responsibilities
- Job functions/demands
- Return to work policies
- Accommodations
- Health care provision/compliance

---

that can be used (by individuals) to indicate health status perception in eight domains of quality of life functioning. The eight domains include the following:

1. *Physical functioning* assesses a range of physical activities such as performing self-care, walking, climbing stairs, and performing vigorous activities.
2. *Role physical* assesses the effects of physical health on the patient's life roles and regular daily activities.
3. *Bodily pain* assesses the severity of bodily pain and its interference with work inside or outside the home.
4. *General health* assesses perception of general health, health outlook, and resistance to illness.
5. *Vitality* assesses the frequency of feeling tired versus energetic.
6. *Social functioning* assesses the extent and frequency of limitations in social activities due to health problems.
7. *Role emotional* assesses the effects of emotional problems on the patient's life roles and regular daily activities.
8. *Mental health* assesses anxiety, depression, and loss of behavioral/emotional control versus psychological well-being (Powell, 2000).

DEVELOPMENT AND COORDINATION OF CARE PLAN

Through the process of assessment the case manager has amassed and analyzed many pieces of data and information to identify strengths, weaknesses, and gaps and develop and coordinate a plan of care consistent with the client's needs. In order to have an effective and realistic plan of care, the case manager must understand the medical condition, problems, management, and focus of the treatment plans prescribed by each provider and understand the care plan objectives and expected outcomes. The case manager must develop a plan of care with the client and other team members significant in the care plan implementation. This will include the physician, family, payer, and others such as physical therapist, speech therapist, or rehabilitation specialist. For the plan to be successful, the client (and family) must actively participate in all decisions that affect areas such as diet preparation or medication noncompliance. The team must decide the following:

- What needs to be done?
- How and where services will be provided?
- Who will provide necessary services?
- What is the timetable for accomplishment of both short-term and long-term goals/objectives?

The next step is to prioritize the goals and objectives in terms of what is the most pressing client need while recognizing that at times what the client identifies as important may be in conflict with what the case manager identifies as important. Education and negotiation will be needed to help resolve this type of conflict. For example, an employee may want to return to work too soon after an injury that the case manager believes requires more recovery time. As a progressive plan, it may be that certain aspects of the work could be done at home that would not jeopardize the recovery process but would fulfill the employee's needs to maintain work productivity. Other issues may center around financial and resource allocations and limitations (Wolfe, 1998); that is, the insurance company may refuse to pay for a certain piece of equipment or medication, which both the employee and case manager believe are needed. Again here, negotiations may be needed to justify the expenditures.

In the planning and coordinating of care function, the occupational and environmental health nurse case manager will need to have knowledge of company resources available to meet employee needs and external public and private organizations that may be helpful in the case management process (Boseman, 2001; Wassell et al., 2000). This will require that the nurse have a good understanding of employee benefit plans and options including special provider arrangements (i.e., preferred provider organizations, health maintenance organizations, point of service), be able to acquire and coordinate service providers needed for care management, and participate in disability plan design and policy development. As the case manager, the occupational and environmental health nurse will need to recognize the unique features of each case in service planning and coordination in terms of the types and degrees of intervention needed. In some cases limited therapy and education are all that are needed but in other situations skilled nursing home visits for a period of time may be in order.

The occupational and environmental health nurse will need to be cognizant of the changing needs of the client and recognize that care plan alterations may be in order. This will need to be communicated to all parties involved in the case management to make certain that all treatment plans are integrated and are in alignment with each other.

IMPLEMENTATION OF THE PLAN

Implementation of the plan means putting the plan into action. In this stage the occupational and environmental health nurse case manager links the employee with the most appropriate private and community resources to meet the employee's targeted needs and fill identified gaps in health care service. Although in general the occupational and environmental health nurse case manager does not provide the direct hands-on care needed, the nurse acts as a liaison with health care professionals to help coordinate clinical care management while always mindful of expected outcomes (Alliotta, 1999). This coordinated effort can include the following:

- Monitoring medical stability
- Educating about treatment plan coordination and compliance

- Arranging for home care and equipment needs
- Providing a list of community agencies and contact information
- Reviewing short-term and extended benefit coverage to reduce the occurrence of coverage gaps
- Monitoring satisfaction with treatment plan, provider, and services
- Implementing early return to work, modified, and transitional work programs
- Facilitating rehabilitation and job accommodation
- Communicating accurate information to employee, family, and providers as appropriate

The occupational and environmental health nurse case manager must act as an advocate for the employee and in some instances may need to speak on behalf of the employee (and family) who may be fearful of or confused by a complex health care system. This is true for both the physical and psychological aspects of injury and illness care, regardless of whether the illness or injury is catastrophic, such as a spinal cord injury or cancer, or a more self-limiting condition. A carpenter who loses the use of his hand, a dancer who suffers a permanent foot injury, or a construction worker with a permanent back disability are examples that may not be considered by most to be catastrophic, yet each individual has suffered a serious and painful event that can result in a lost career and income. The case manager must consider the impact of any injury beyond the employee's physical capabilities and examine limitations, disabilities, employment issues, and psychological effects.

EVALUATION AND FOLLOW-UP

The stage of evaluation and follow-up are continuous and dynamic to make certain that the interventions and strategies implemented are indeed working and that the employee will be ready to return to work when indicated (McClinton, 2000; Mullahy, 1998; Salazar et al., 1999). This means that the occupational and environmental health nurse case manager evaluates the care plan for effectiveness and timeliness and evaluates the employee in terms of continued progress. Follow-up contact can provide the employee with an opportunity to ask questions, clarify and reclarify issues or concerns, and discuss revisions in care or alternate options, and it can aid in preventing compli-

cations or eliminating unnecessary care that may be ineffective. Follow-up may be in person or telephone/electronic depending on the situation.

The occupational and environmental health nurse case manager will need to evaluate if the goals and objectives were met, and if not, why. For example, the case manager will want to ask, Was the treatment realistic and affordable? Were services delivered by appropriately trained providers? Was equipment available and delivered? Did the employee understand the treatment regime? In addition, the case manager will need to evaluate if the achievement of anticipated outcomes, such as if the employee returned to work within the expected four weeks after evaluation was initiated. Another aspect of outcome evaluation is from a cost-effectiveness view indicating if the case manager's intervention helped to reduce care cost and/or return the worker to productive work rather than unnecessarily extend disability or absence.

CONTINUOUS MONITORING, REASSESSING, AND REEVALUATING

The process of continuous monitoring, reassessing, and reevaluating continues until the case is closed. The case is not closed until goals and objectives are reached. Case stability and complexity will determine the frequency of monitoring and evaluating activities.

Generally, the case manager will want to closely monitor the following:

- Changes in the employee's health/medical status that varies from the prescribed improvement path, which may indicate a need to alter the care plan
- Changes in functional capacity and mobility that indicate recovery is not progressing on target
- Changes in satisfaction of the employee and/or family with regard to treatment and/or service providers—changes that may indicate that the employee's needs for recovery or return to work are not being met or even that the employee needs reassurance as to progression toward recovery

The occupational and environmental health nurse case manager will need to monitor and in some instances modify the return to work plan to ensure a smooth transition and facilitate recovery without further injury or setback. Once the employee has reached maximum recovery, the case manager will need to terminate services. Most employees and families will be appreciative of the professional care and services rendered, and the employer will also appreciate the cost-effective approach used in achieving the desired outcome.

RETURN TO WORK

In occupational health case management a key focus is to assist the returning worker to safe and productive work at the earliest possible medically feasible time. Return to work programs begin with early intervention at the time the worker's illness or injury occurs. This includes prompt notification of supervisors, transportation of the worker to health care treatment, accident or hazard investigation, and reporting of the illness or injury to the insurance carrier (Wassel, 2000). Early intervention fosters appropriate and timely care; helps the employee meet physical, psychological, and vocational needs; facilitates successful rehabilitation and early return to work; and integrates cost-effective health care intervention and approaches. Return to work programs should promote full-time, transitional, or modified work assignments in order to match the job to the work capacity of the employee. To do this, employers will need to accurately assess each job and complete a job analysis for each job category (discussed in Chapter 7). The job analysis should provide a clear picture of the essential physical and psychosocial functions of the job and be made available to treating health care professionals to assist in making a determination about work capacity, job accommodation, and work return dates.

The return to work plan may range from the employee doing the original job with no restrictions to a completely new job outside the organization. This hierarchy of return to work options is depicted in Figure 12-1 (Dyck, 2000). Return to work assignments that are other than full-duty must be reviewed at regular intervals in the context of evaluating the affected worker's health progress, transitional duty progression to full-time or original job duties, or options for perma-

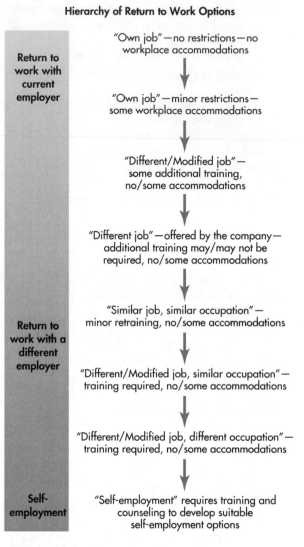

Figure 12-1 Hierarchy of return to work options. *(Data from* Disability Management: Theory, Strategy, and Industry Practice, *by D. Dyck, 2000, Toronto: Butterworths.)*

nent accommodation, modified work, or alternative position (Shrey & Lacerte, 1997). In addition, the permanence of worker recovery should be determined within a defined period of time. If job accommodations are needed, they should be viewed in terms of how to best support the worker and employer in creating opportunities for productive work. One tool that can assist with this type of decision making is the Job Accommodation Network (JAN), which provides numerous publications and guidelines related to worksite accommodations for individuals with disabilities. An example of a worksite accommodation for those with cancer is shown in Appendix 12-1.

CASE MANAGEMENT INTEGRATION

Understanding the purposes and processes in case management is key to a sound and comprehensive framework for case management service delivery. Case managers must base the case management plan on information that is obtained in the assessment stage; accurately depicts the current status of the employee's illness or injury; examines the treatment components, alternatives, and regimens of care agreed on; and recognizes the need for a care plan that reduces fragmentation. The occupational and environmental health nurse case manager plays a critical role in facilitating a coordinated care plan that includes continuous monitoring for quality care, making certain that progress is being made in achieving stated objectives, fostering treatment compliance or determining if the treatment regimen is ineffective, and devising care changes that are needed in a timely manner to effect decided outcomes. Utilization of relevant resources will be important to a successful effort. Several resource organizations are listed in Appendix 12-2.

The case manager must be an advocate for the employee; this is at the heart of the process, which entails understanding the needs and wants of the employee and family, communicating that information to all parties involved in the care, ensuring that needs are met through appropriate intervention and referral, and providing continuous follow-up.

Summary

Case management in occupational health is a natural role for and major component of practice of the occupational and environmental health nurse. The occupational and environmental health nurse case manager works with the employee (and family) and health care providers to provide cost-effective, quality-driven health care services and a coordinated approach to health care service delivery in order to facilitate optimal health recovery and timely return to work. Employees and employers alike will benefit from this integrated process.

References

Alliotta, S. (1999). Patient adherence outcome indicators and measurement in case management and health care. *Care Management, 5*(4), 24-81.

American Association of Occupational Health Nurses. (1994). *Case management advisory.* Atlanta, GA: Author.

Boseman, J. (2001). Disability management: Application of a nurse-based model in a large corporation. *AAOHN Journal, 49*(4),176-186.

Case Management Society of America. (1995). *Standards of practice for case managers.* Little Rock, AR: Author.

Chan, F., Leahy, M. J., McMahon, B. T., Mirch, M., & DeVinney, D. (1999). Foundational knowledge and major practice domains of case management. *Journal of Care Management, 5*(1),12-30.

Commission for Case Manager Certification. (1995). *CMM certification guide.* Rolling Meadows, IL: Author.

Dees, J. P., & Anderson, N. L. (1996). Case management. *AAOHN Journal, 44*(9), 385-390.

Denton, V. Y., & Leinart, N. J. (2001). Absence monitoring: A case management perspective. *AAOHN Journal, 49*(10), 465-470.

Dieckmann, J. (2000). History of public health and public change. In M. Stanhope. and J. Lancaster (Eds.), *Community and public health nursing* (5th ed., pp. 20-41). St. Louis, MO: Mosby.

Dyck, D. (2000). *Disability management: Theory, strategy, and industry practice.* Toronto: Butterworths.

Leahy, M. J. (1994). *Validation of essential knowledge dimensions in case management* (Technical Report). Rolling Meadows, IL: Foundation for Rehabilitation Education and Research.

Maldonado, D., & Quinn, C. (1999). *A case manager's study guide.* Gaithersburg, MD: Aspen.

McClinton, D. H. (2000, January). How case management can impact health care in the next millennium. *Continuing Care,* 19-25.

Mullahy, C. M. (1998). *The case manager's handbook* (2nd ed.). Gaithersburg, MD: Aspen.

Powell, S. K. (2000). *Case management: A practical guide to success in managed care.* Philadelphia: Lippincott.

Powell, S. K. & Ignatavicius, D. (2001). *Core curriculum for case management.* Philadelphia: Lippincott.

Salazar, M. K., Graham, K. Y., & Lantz, B. (1999). Evaluating case management services for injured workers: Use of a quality assessment model. *AAOHN Journal, 47*(8), 348-354.

Shrey, D. E., & Lacerte, M. (1997). *Principles and practices of disability management in industry.* Boca Raton, FL: CRC Press.

Wassell, M. L., Randolph, J., Stepler, K. B., & Winzeller, S. (2001). Disability case management. In AAOHN (Ed.), *Core curriculum for occupational and environmental health nursing* (2nd ed. pp. 271-292). Philadelphia: W.B. Saunders.

Wolfe, G. S. (1998). Cost savings and case management. *Care Management, 4*(5), 5.

12-1 Worksite Accommodation Ideas for Individuals Who Have Cancer

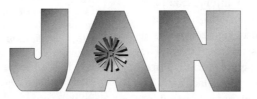

JOB ACCOMMODATION NETWORK

1-800-526-7234 (V/TTY)

http://www.jan.wvu.edu

A service of the U.S. DOL Office of Disability Employment Policy

By Beth Loy, Ph.D. and Linda Carter Batiste, MS

PREFACE

Worldwide there are over 6 million new cancer cases and more than 4 million cancer deaths each year. One in four deaths are caused by cancer; only cardiovascular diseases account for a higher percentage. In 2001 in the United States 553,400 people are expected to die of cancer; more than 1,500 people a day. Nearly 5 million lives have been lost to cancer since 1990, and the National Cancer Institute estimates that approximately 8.9 million Americans alive today have a history of cancer. The American Cancer Society predicts that about 33% of Americans will eventually develop some form of the disease. Skin cancer is the most prevalent cancer in both men and women, followed by prostate cancer in men and breast cancer in women. Lung cancer, however, causes the most deaths in both men and women, and

leukemia is the most common type of cancer in children.

Today millions of people in the workforce have a history of cancer. Therefore, employers are seeing incidents of cancer among their employees. This, coupled with the requirements of the Americans With Disabilities Act (ADA), shows why knowing about workplace accommodations for people with cancer is important. When considering accommodations for people with cancer, the accommodation process must be conducted on a case-by-case basis. Symptoms caused by cancer vary; so when determining effective accommodations, the person's individual abilities and limitations should be considered and problematic job tasks must be identified. Therefore the person with cancer should be involved in the accommodation process.

Not all people with cancer will need accommodations to perform their jobs, and many others may need only a few accommodations. For those who need accommodation, the following pages provide basic information about common limitations, symptoms, useful questions to consider, and accommodation possibilities. The following is only a sample of possibilities to consider; numerous other solutions and considerations may exist. Also included in this publication is a list of resources for additional information.

CANCER

The following information regarding cancer was edited from several sources, including many of the resources listed in the resource section of this publication and especially the American Cancer Society. The information is not intended to be medical advice. If medical advice is needed, appropriate medical professionals should be consulted.

What is cancer? Cancer is a group of many related diseases. All forms of cancer involve out-of-control growth of abnormal cells. Normal body cells grow, divide, and die in an orderly fashion. During the early years of a person's life normal cells divide more rapidly until the person becomes an adult. Then normal cells divide only to replace dying cells and to repair injuries. Cancer cells, however, continue to grow and divide, spreading to other parts of the body and accumulating to form tumors that destroy normal tissue. If cells break away, they can travel through the bloodstream or the lymph system to other areas of the body where they may settle and form "colony" tumors. In their new location the cancer cells continue growing and spread to a new site, metastasis. When cancer spreads, it is still named after the part of the body where it started. Different types of cancer vary in their rates of growth, patterns of spread, and responses to different types of treatment.

What are the symptoms of cancer? Some generalized symptoms and signs such as unexplained weight loss, fever, fatigue, or lumps may be seen in several types of cancer; however, other signs and symptoms are relatively specific to a particular type of cancer.

What causes cancer? Cancer is caused by both external (chemicals, radiation, and viruses) and internal (hormones, immune conditions, and inherited mutations) factors. Different cancers have different risk factors. Causal factors may act together or in sequence to initiate or promote cancer. Risk factors may increase a person's risk but do not always "cause" the disease. Many people with one or more risk factors never develop cancer, while others with this disease have no known risk factors. Ten or more years can pass between exposures or mutations and detectable cancer.

Who gets cancer? The chance of getting cancer increases as individuals age; most cases affect middle aged or older individuals. In the U.S., men have a one in two lifetime risk of developing cancer, women one in three. Risk factors vary: smokers are 10 times more likely to develop lung cancer than nonsmokers, and women with a first-degree family history are 2 times more likely to develop breast cancer than women who do not have a family history of the disease.

How is cancer staged? Staging is the process of describing the extent of the disease or the spread of cancer from the site of origin. Staging is essential in determining the choice of therapy and assessing prognosis. A cancer's stage is based on information about the primary tumor's size and location in the body and whether or not it has spread to other areas of the body. A number of different staging systems are currently being used to classify tumors. The TNM staging system assesses tumors in three ways: extent of the primary tumor (T), absence or presence of regional lymph node involvement (N), and absence or presence of distant metastases (M). Once the T, N, and M are determined, a stage of I, II, III, or IV is assigned with summary staging of "in situ," local, regional, or distant. If cancer cells are present only in the layer of cells they developed in and they have not spread to other parts of that organ or elsewhere in the body, then the stage is "in situ." If cancer cells have spread, the cancer is considered invasive and falls in the summary staging of local, regional, or distant.

How is cancer treated? Treatment options may include surgery, radiation, chemotherapy, hormone therapy, and immunotherapy. Surgery is the oldest form of cancer treatment; 60% of people with cancer will have surgery. Radiation therapy uses high-energy waves, such as x-rays or gamma rays, to destroy cancer cells. Chemotherapy is the use of drugs to treat cancer. Systemic chemotherapy uses anticancer drugs that are usually given into a vein or by mouth to enter the bloodstream and reach all areas of the body. Hormone therapy is treatment with hormones, drugs that interfere with hormone production. Immunotherapy is the use of treatments that promote or support the body's immune system response to a disease such as cancer.

Questions to Consider When Determining Accommodations

What symptoms or limitations are being experienced by the individual with cancer?

How do the individual's symptoms or limitations affect the person and the person's job performance?

What specific job tasks are problematic as a result of the individual's symptoms and limitations?

What accommodations are available to reduce or eliminate the problem job tasks? Are all possible resources being used to determine possible accommodations for the individual with cancer?

Has the employee with cancer been consulted regarding possible accommodations?

Once accommodations are in place, would it be useful to meet with the person with cancer to evaluate the effectiveness of the accommodations and to determine whether additional accommodations are needed?

Do supervisory personnel and employees need training regarding cancer, etiquette, other disability areas, or the ADA?

Accommodation Considerations for People With Cancer

(Note: People with cancer will develop some of these limitations/symptoms but seldom develop all of them. Limitations will vary among individuals. Also note that not all people who have cancer will need accommodations to perform their jobs and many others may need only a few accommodations. The following is only a sample of the possibilities available. Numerous other accommodation solutions exist as well.)

Fatigue/Weakness

- Reduce or eliminate physical exertion and workplace stress.

- Allow a flexible work schedule and flexible use of leave time.
- Allow work from home.
- Implement ergonomic workstation design.
- Provide a scooter or other mobility aid if walking cannot be reduced.
- Provide parking close to the worksite.
- Install automatic door openers.
- Make sure materials and equipment are within reach range.
- Move workstation close to other work areas, office equipment, and break rooms.
- Reduce noise with sound absorbent baffles/partitions, environmental sound machines, and headsets.
- Provide alternate work space to reduce visual and auditory distractions.

Medical Treatment Allowances

- Provide flexible schedules.
- Provide flexible leave.
- Allow a self-paced workload with flexible hours.
- Allow employee to work from home.
- Provide part-time work schedules.

Respiratory Difficulties

- Provide adjustable ventilation.
- Keep work environment free from dust, smoke, odor, and fumes.
- Implement a "fragrance free" workplace policy and a "smoke free" building policy.
- Avoid temperature extremes.
- Use fan/air conditioner or heater at the workstation.
- Redirect air-conditioning and heating vents.

Skin Irritations

- Avoid infectious agents and chemicals.
- Avoid invasive procedures (activities that could be harmful to a person's skin condition).
- Provide protective clothing.

Stress

- Develop strategies to deal with work problems before they arise.
- Provide sensitivity training to coworkers.
- Allow telephone calls during work hours to doctors and others for support.
- Provide information on counseling and employee assistance programs.

Temperature Sensitivity

- Modify worksite temperature.
- Modify dress code.
- Use fan/air conditioner or heater at the workstation.
- Allow flexible scheduling and flexible use of leave time.
- Allow work from home during extremely hot or cold weather.
- Maintain the ventilation system.
- Redirect air conditioning and heating vents.
- Provide an office with separate temperature control.

Products

There are numerous products that can be used to accommodate people with limitations. JAN's Searchable Online Accommodation Resource (SOAR) at http://www.jan.wvu.edu/soar is designed to let users explore various accommodation options. Many product vendor lists are accessible through this system; however, JAN provides these lists and many more that are not available on the Web site upon request. Contact JAN directly if you have specific accommodation situations, are looking for products, need vendor information, or are seeking a referral.

Example Accommodations for People With Cancer

- An engineer working for a large industrial company had to undergo radiation treatment for cancer during working hours. She was provided a flexible schedule in order to attend therapy and also continue to work full-time.
- A machine operator who was undergoing radiation therapy for cancer was accommodated by having his workstation moved. The move transferred the individual to an area of the plant where no radiation exposure existed.
- A warehouse worker whose job involved maintaining and delivering supplies was having difficulty with the physical demands of his job due to fatigue from chemotherapy treatment. The individual was accommodated with a three-wheeled scooter to reduce walking. The warehouse was also rearranged to reduce the individual's climbing and reaching.
- A secretary with cancer was having difficulty working full-time due to fatigue from chemothearapy. Her employer accommodated her by allowing her to work part-time and allowing her to take frequent rest breaks while working.
- A psychiatric nurse with cancer was experiencing difficulty dealing with job-related stress. He was accommodated with a temporary transfer and was referred to the employer's employee assistance program for emotional support and stress management tools.
- A lawyer with cancer was experiencing lapses in concentration due to the medication she was taking. Her employer accommodated her by giving her uninterrupted time to work. She was also allowed to work at home two days a week.

Resources

This is a noninclusive list.

JOB ACCOMMODATION NETWORK
A Service of the U.S. DOL Office of Disability Employment Policy
West Virginia University
PO Box 6080
Morgantown, WV 26506-6080
(800) 526-7234 & 800-ADA-WORK (V/TTY)
(304) 293-7186 (Local Line, V/TTY)
http://www.jan.wvu.edu

OFFICE OF DISABILITY EMPLOYMENT POLICY
1331 F St. NW
Washington, DC 20004-1107
(202) 376-6200 (Voice)
(202) 376-6205 (TT)
http://www.dol.gov/dol/odep/

AMERICAN CANCER SOCIETY
1599 Clifton Rd. NE
Atlanta, GA 30329
(800) ACS-2345
http://www.cancer.org
The American Cancer Society is the nationwide community-based voluntary health organization dedicated to eliminating cancer.

AMERICAN INSTITUTE FOR CANCER
   RESEARCH
1759 R. St., NW
Washington, DC 20009
(800) 843-8114/(202) 328-7744
http://www.aicr.org
The American Institute for Cancer Research is the
   nation's leading charity in the field of diet, nutrition, and cancer prevention.

CANCER CARE, INC.
1180 Avenue of the Americas
New York, NY 10036
(800) 813-HOPE
http://www.cancercare.org
Cancer Care, Inc. provides counseling, information, and support services to people with any
   type of cancer at any stage of illness.

CANCER INFORMATION SERVICE
Building 31, Room 10A31
31 Center Dr., MSC 2580
Bethesda, MD 20892
(800) 4-CANCER/(800) 332-8615 (TTY)
http://www.nci.nih.gov/info/what.htm
The Cancer Information Service (CIS) is a nationwide network of 19 regional offices supported
   by the National Cancer Institute, the federal
   government's primary agency for cancer research. Through its toll free phone service, the
   CIS provides accurate, up-to-date information
   on cancer to patients and their families, health
   professionals, and the general public. Through
   the outreach program, the CIS serves as a resource for state and regional organizations by
   providing printed materials and technical assistance to cancer education, media campaigns,
   and community programs. The CIS offices are
   located at NCI-designated cancer centers and
   other health care institutions.

CENTERS FOR DISEASE CONTROL
   AND PREVENTION (CDC)
1600 Clifton Rd.
Atlanta, GA 30333
(800) 331-3435
http://www.cdc.gov

The CDC promotes health and quality of life by
   preventing and controlling disease, injury, and
   disability.

CANCER HOPE NETWORK
2 North Rd., Suite A
Chester, NJ 07930
(877) HopeNet
Cancer Hope Network is a program of personal
   support and encouragement offered to people
   undergoing chemotherapy or radiation therapy
   by persons who have experienced therapy
   themselves. A visit between a support person
   and the patient is arranged on a one-to-one basis and persons are matched according to their
   similarity of treatment.

NATIONAL BONE MARROW TRANSPLANT
   LINK
20411 W 12 Mile Rd., Suite 108
Southfield, MI 48034
(800) LINK-BMT
http://comnet.org/nbmtlink
The National Bone Marrow Transplant Link is a
   reference for bone marrow transplantation, finances and medical insurance, information
   about peer support, and survivor stories.

NATIONAL CANCER INSTITUTE
Building 31, Room 10A31
31 Center Drive, MSC 2580
Bethesda, MD 20892-2580
(800) 4-CANCER/(800) 332-8615 (TTY)
http://www.nci.nih.gov
The National Cancer Institute is the nation's primary agency for cancer research.

NATIONAL COALITION FOR CANCER
   SURVIVORSHIP
1010 Wayne Avenue, Suite 770
Silver Spring, MD 20910
(301) 650-9127/(877) NCCS-YES
http://www.cansearch.org
The National Coalition for Cancer Survivorship
   (NCCS) is a grassroots network of individuals
   and organizations working on behalf of people
   with all types of cancer.

NATIONAL MARROW DONOR PROGRAM
Suite 500, 3001 Broadway St., NE
Minneapolis, MN 55413
(800) MARROW-2
http://www.marrow.org

The National Marrow Donor Program is an organization helping patients through stem cell transplantation.

NATIONAL ORGANIZATION FOR RARE
  DISORDERS
PO Box 8923

New Fairfield, CT 06812-8923
(800) 999-6673/(203) 746-6518
http://www.rarediseases.org

The National Organization for Rare Disorders (NORD) is a unique federation of voluntary health organizations dedicated to helping people with rare "orphan" diseases and assisting the organizations that serve them. NORD is committed to the identification, treatment, and cure of rare disorders through programs of education, advocacy, research, and service.

12-2 Case Management Web Resources

4anything.com
www.4arthritis.com

Agency for Healthcare Research and Quality
http://www.ahcpr.gov/

American Academy of Physical Medicine and
  Rehabilitation
http://www.aapmr.org

American Association of Legal Nurse Consultants
http://www.aalnc.org/

American Association of Managed Care Nurses
http://www.aamcn.org/

American Association of Nurse Attorneys
http://www.taana.org/

American Association of Occupational Health
  Nurses
http://www.aaohn.org/

American Board of Independent Medical
  Examiners
http://www.abime.org/

American Board of Occupational Health
  Nursing
http://www.abohn.org/

American Cancer Society
http://www.cancer.org/

American College of Allergy, Asthma, and
  Immunology
http://www.allergy.mcg.edu/

American College of Rheumatology
http://www.rheumatology.org

American Diabetes Association
http://www.diabetes.org/

American Lung Association
http://www.lungusa.org/

American Medical Association
http://www.ama-assn.org/

American Nurses Association
http://www.ana.org/

American Occupational Therapy Association
http://www.aota.org

Arthritis
http://www.arthritis.com

Arthritis Foundation
http://www.arthritis.org/

Arthritis National Research Foundation
http://www.curearthritis.org

Books on Arthritis
http://www.wellnessbooks.com/arthritis

Association of Rehabilitation Nurses
http://www.rehabnurse.org/

Attorney Find
http://www.attorneyfind.com/

Case Management Society of America
http://www.cmsa.org/

Centers for Disease Control—CDC
http://www.CDC.GOV/

Center Watch
http://www.centerwatch.com

Certification of Disability Management Specialist
Commission—CDMSC
http://www.cdms.org/

Commission for Case Management
Certification
http://www.ccmcertification.org/

Department of Health and Human Services
http://www.dhhs.gov/

Department of Labor
http://www.dol.gov/

Department of Transportation
http://www.dot.gov/

Doctor's Guide to the Internet
http://pslgroup.com

Education for Latex Allergy/Support Team &
Information Coalition (ELASTIC)
http://www.latex-allergy.org/

Equal Employment Opportunity Commission
http://www.eeoc.gov/

Foundation for Accountability
http://www.facct.org/

Health Care Financing Administration
http://www.hcfa.gov

Health Care Report Cards
http://www.healthgrades.com

Health Grades
http://www.healthgrades.com/

Healthfinders Information Web Site
http://www.healthfinder.org/

Health Insurance Association of America
http://www.hiaa.org/

Job Accommodation Network
http://janweb.icdi.wvu.edu/

Johns Hopkins Arthritis Center
http://www.hopkins-arthritis.som.jhmi.edu

Joint Commission on Accreditation of
Healthcare Organizations—JCAHO
http://www.jcaho.org/

Inter Qual Products Group
http://www.interqual.com/

Kids on the Block
http://www.kotb.com

Latex Allergy Information Resource
http://www.anesth.com/lair/lair.html

Law Log-Case Management
http://www.lawlog.com/

LawNet Info Network
http://www.lawnetinfo.com/

Legal Eagle Eye Newsletter for Nursing
http://www.nursinglaw.com/

Medicare Beneficiaries Information
http://www.medicare.gov

MedWeb: Rheumatology
http://www.medweb.emory.edu

Milliman & Robertson (M&R) Actuaries and
Consultants
http://www.milliman.com/

National AIDS Clearinghouse
http://www.cdcnpin.org/

National Arthritis and Musculoskeletal and
Skin Diseases Information Clearing House
(NAMSIC)
http://www.nih.gov/niams

National Committee for Quality Assurance—
NCQA
http://www.ncqa.org
National Council on Disability
http://www.ncd.gov/

National Institute for Occupational Safety and
Health—NIOSH
http://www.cdc.gov/niosh/homepage.html

National Practitioner Data Bank
http://www.npdb.com/

Nursing Ethics
http://www.arnoldpublishers.com/Journals/
    Journpages/09697330.htm

Occupational Safety and Health Administration
http://www.osha.gov/
OEM Health Information
http://www.oempress.com

Rehabilitation Nursing Certification Board
http://rehabnurse.org/index5.htm

Research on Arthritis
http://drkoop.com/conditions/Arthritis

Social Security Administration
http://www.ssa.gov/

Spina Bifida Association of America
http://www.sbaa.org/

Washington Business Group on Health
http://www.wbgh.org/

Helping people stay healthy and optimize health is the prime goal of health promotion initiatives and services. Historically, this focus extends from the epidemiological revolution of the nineteenth century in which the reduction of morbidity and mortality was brought about through social and environmental reforms that improved hygiene, housing, sanitation, and working conditions (Burnham, 1984). The concept of health promotion and disease prevention has evolved over time to focus efforts aimed at enhancing optimal health levels. Legislative acts such as the Health Maintenance Organization Act of 1973 and the National Health Planning and Resource Development Act of 1974 have stressed the importance of preventive health and health education efforts to improve health in the United States. In addition, more emphasis has been placed on developing positive rather than risky health behaviors, having individuals recognize their responsibility for their health, and engaging families and communities in health promotion and disease prevention efforts.

Although preventive interventions have resulted in overall health improvements, preventable illness and injury continue to affect health, quality of living, and health-related costs. This is true worldwide. For example, according to the World Health Organization (Global Strategy on Occupational Health for All, 1999):

- Each year, work-related injuries and diseases kill an estimated 1.1 million people worldwide (Figure 13-1), which roughly equals the annual number of deaths worldwide from malaria.
- About 300,000 fatalities from 250 million accidents happen in the workplace annually. Many of these accidents lead to partial or complete incapacity to work and generate income.
- Annually, an estimated 160 million new cases of work-related diseases occur worldwide, including respiratory and cardiovascular diseases, cancer, hearing loss, musculoskeletal and reproductive disorders, and mental and neurological illnesses.
- An increasing number of workers in industrialized countries complain about psychological stress and overwork. These psychological factors have been found to be strongly associated with sleep disturbance, depression, and elevated risks of cardiovascular diseases, particularly hypertension.
- Only 5% to 10% of workers in developing countries and 20% to 50% of workers in industrialized countries (with a few exceptions) are estimated to have access to adequate occupational health services. In the United States, for example, 40% of the workforce of some 130 million people do not have such access.
- Even in advanced economies a large proportion of worksites is not regularly inspected for occupational health and safety.

The health status of the workforce in every country has an immediate and direct impact on national and world economies. Total economic losses due to occupational illnesses and injuries are enormous. Such losses are a serious burden on economic development. Thus, apart from health considerations the improvement of working conditions is a sound economic investment (Global Strategy on Occupational Health for All, 1999) for the following reasons:

- The International Labour Organization (ILO) has estimated that in 1997 the overall economic losses resulting from work-related diseases and injuries were approximately 4% of the world's gross national product.

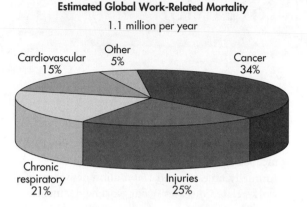

Estimated Global Work-Related Mortality

1.1 million per year

Cardiovascular 15%

Other 5%

Cancer 34%

Chronic respiratory 21%

Injuries 25%

Figure 13-1 Estimated global work-related mortality. Other diseases include pneumoconioses and nervous system and renal disorders. *(From The XVth World Congress on Occupational Safety and Health,* Introductory Report. *Copyright © 1999, International Labour Organization.*

- In 1992 in European Union countries the direct cost paid out in compensation for work-related diseases and injuries reached 27 billion EUR (at time of publication 1 EUR = 0.97 USD).
- In 1994 the overall cost of all work accidents and work-related ill health to the British economy was estimated between £6 billion and £12 billion.
- In 1992 total direct and indirect costs associated with work-related injuries and diseases in the United States were estimated to be $171 billion, surpassing those of AIDS and on par with those of cancer and heart disease.
- In the United States, health care expenditures are increased nearly 50% for workers who report high levels of stress at work.

In 1996 the WHO, through its *Global Strategy on Occupational Health for All,* proposed the following 10 objectives for workers' health:

1. Strengthen international and national policies for health at work and develop the necessary policy tools.
2. Develop healthy work environments.

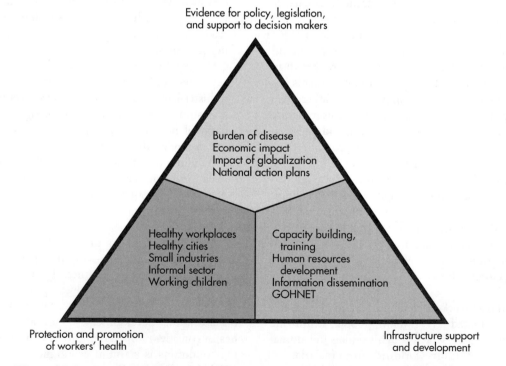

Evidence for policy, legislation, and support to decision makers

Burden of disease
Economic impact
Impact of globalization
National action plans

Healthy workplaces
Healthy cities
Small industries
Informal sector
Working children

Capacity building, training
Human resources development
Information dissemination
GOHNET

Protection and promotion of workers' health

Infrastructure support and development

Figure 13-2 Focus of WHO global activities in occupational health. *(From* The Global Occupational Health Network Newsletter (1), *by World Health Organization, 2000, Geneva, Switzerland: Author.)*

3. Develop healthy work practices and promotion of health at work.
4. Strengthen occupational health services.
5. Establish support services for occupational health.
6. Develop occupational health standards based on scientific risk assessment.
7. Develop human resources for occupational health.
8. Establish registration and data systems, develop information services for experts, ensure effective transmission of data, and raise public awareness through public information.
9. Strengthen research.
10. Develop collaboration in occupational health and with other activities and services.

This will be discussed further in Chapter 18.

In addition, the WHO is developing a program to focus on the three following main areas of activities (Figure 13-2):

1. *Evidence for policy, legislation, and support to decision makers.* This requires the development of a sound database on the global burden of diseases resulting from occupational risk factors and an estimation of its economic impact.

2. *Protection and promotion of workers' health.* Emphasis is to be placed on small industries, the informal sector, and the problems associated with working children.
3. *Infrastructure support and development.* Required infrastructures and human resources, as well as information dissemination and exchange, must be supported, developed, or strengthened through the preparation of educational materials and practical guidance documents, technical cooperation, and the creation of the Global Occupational Health Network (GOHNET).

These statements from the WHO clearly emphasize health promotion and health protection at the worksite and beg for programs and interventions that support healthy workplaces and workforces.

In the United States health care costs have risen from 5.1% of the gross domestic product in 1960 ($26.9 billion) to 13.8% in 1998 ($1.149 trillion) (Anderson, 1998; Health Care Financing Administration, 2000). These costs are of particular concern to employers because they bear a large share of the expense, rising from 17% in 1960 to 29% in 1999 (Koretz, 2000).

In an important study, Goetzel (1998) provided data on the relationship between health care costs and health risk factors (Table 13-1). Depression

TABLE 13-1   Medical Care Costs Associated With Risk Factors

Risk Factor	Mean Cost With Risk Factor ($)	Mean Cost Without Risk Factor ($)	Percent Difference (Unadjusted)	Percent Difference *(Adjusted)
Depression	3,189	1,679	90	70
Stress	2,287	1,579	45	46
Blood glucose	2,598	1,691	54	35
Body weight	2,318	1,571	48	21
Tobacco (former)	1,950	1,503	25	20
Tobacco (current)	1,873	1,503	30	14
Blood pressure	2,123	1,716	24	12
Exercise	2,011	1,567	28	10
Cholesterol	1,962	1,678	17	−1
Alcohol use	1,431	1,726	−17	−3
Nutrition	1,498	1,772	−15	−9

From "Relationship Between Modifiable Health Risks and Health Care Expenditures," by R. Goetzel, *Journal of Occupational and Environmental Medicine, 40,* 10-18. 1998.
*The adjusted differences are the differences between those with and without each risk factor that persisted after adjusting for all the other risk factors in a multivariate analysis.

TABLE 13-2 Medical Care Costs Associated With Clusters of Risk Factors, United States

RISK FACTOR CLUSTER	WITH RISK FACTORS ($)	WITHOUT RISK FACTORS ($)	PERCENT DIFFERENCE
Heart disease risks	3,804	1,158	228
Stroke risks	2,349	1,272	85
Psychosocial risks	3,368	1,368	147
No risk factors		1,166	

From "Relationship Between Modifiable Health Risks and Health Care Expenditures," by R. Goetzel, *Journal of Occupational and Environmental Medicine, 40*, 10-18. 1998.

TABLE 13-3 *Healthy People 2010* Objective Focus Areas

OBJECTIVE FOCUS AREA	GOAL
1. Access to quality health services	Improve access to comprehensive, high quality health care services.
2. Arthritis, osteoporosis, and chronic back conditions	Prevent illness and disability related to arthritis and other rheumatic conditions, osteoporosis, and chronic back conditions.
3. Cancer	Reduce the number of new cancer cases as well as the illness, disability, and death caused by cancer.
4. Chronic kidney disease	Reduce new cases of chronic kidney disease and its complications, disability, death, and economic costs.
5. Diabetes	Through prevention programs reduce the disease and economic burden of diabetes and improve the quality of life for all persons who have or are at risk for diabetes.
6. Disability and secondary conditions	Promote the health of people with disabilities, prevent secondary conditions, and eliminate disparities between people with and without disabilities in the U.S. population.
7. Educational and community-based programs	Increase the quality, availability, and effectiveness of educational and community-based programs designed to prevent disease and improve health and quality of life.
8. Environmental health	Promote health for all through a healthy environment.
9. Family planning	Improve pregnancy planning and spacing and prevent unintended pregnancy.
10. Food safety	Reduce foodborne illnesses.
11. Health communication	Use communication strategically to improve health.
12. Heart disease and stroke	Improve cardiovascular health and quality of life through the prevention, detection, and treatment of risk factors; early identification and treatment of heart attacks and strokes; and prevention of recurrent cardiovascular events.
13. HIV	Prevent HIV infection and its related illness and death.
14. Immunization and infectious diseases	Prevent disease, disability, and death from infectious diseases, including vaccine-preventable diseases.
15. Injury and violence prevention	Reduce injuries, disabilities, and deaths due to unintentional injuries and violence.

TABLE 13-3	*Healthy People 2010* Objective Focus Areas—cont'd
OBJECTIVE	**GOAL**
16. Maternal, infant, and child health	Improve the health and well-being of women, infants, children, and families.
17. Medical product safety	Ensure the safe and effective use of medical products.
18. Mental health and mental illness	Improve mental health and ensure access to appropriate, quality mental health services.
19. Nutrition and overweight	Promote health and reduce chronic disease associated with diet and weight.
20. Occupational safety and health	Promote the health and safety of people at work through prevention and early intervention.
21. Oral health	Prevent and control oral and craniofacial diseases, conditions, and injuries and improve access to related services.
22. Physical fitness and activity	Improve health, fitness, and quality of life through daily physical activity.
23. Public health infrastructure	Ensure that federal, tribal, state, and local health agencies have the infrastructure to provide essential public health services effectively.
24. Respiratory diseases	Promote respiratory health through better prevention, detection, treatment, and educational efforts.
25. Sexually transmitted diseases	Promote responsible sexual behaviors, strengthen community capacity, and increase access to quality services to prevent sexually transmitted diseases (STDs) and their complications.
26. Substance abuse	Reduce substance abuse to protect the health, safety, and quality of life for all, especially children.
27. Tobacco use	Reduce illness, disability, and death related to tobacco use and exposure to secondhand smoke.
28. Vision and hearing	Improve the visual and hearing health of the nation through prevention, early detection, treatment, and rehabilitation.

From *Healthy People 2010: Understanding and Improving Health,* by U.S. Department of Health and Human Services, Washington, DC: U.S. Government Printing Office. 2001.

and stress were the most costly risk factors, with costs 70% higher for those with depression and 46% higher for those with stress than for workers without those risk factors. In addition, employees with clusters of risk factors (e.g., heart disease) had even higher costs (Table 13-2). Further investigations have found that health care costs decrease a median average of $153 with every decrease in the number of risk factors and increase a median average of $350 with every increase in the number of risk factors (Edington, 2000). These data and related intervention studies support the need for health promotion and risk reduction programs (Aldana, 1998).

On a national level efforts to address preventable causes of disease, disability, and premature mortality are addressed in *Healthy People 2010: Understanding and Improving Health* (USDHHS, 2001). *Healthy People 2010* is designed to achieve the two following overarching goals:

• Increase quality and years of healthy life.
• Eliminate health disparities.

These two goals are supported by 467 specific objectives in 28 focus areas, with a target to be achieved by the year 2010. The 28 focus areas are shown in Table 13-3. (Readers should refer to *Healthy People 2010* for a complete description and the detailed objectives.) This effort emphasizes health promotion and protection and disease prevention and reflects the scientific advances that have taken place over the past 20 years in

TABLE 13-4	Percent of Employers Offering Health Promotion Programs at the Worksite		
EMPLOYER SIZE	**1999 (%)**	**1992 (%)**	**1985 (%)**
50-99	86	75	NA*
100-249	92	86	NA*
250-749	96	90	NA*
750+	98	99	NA*
All employees	**90**	**80**	**66**

From *National Worksite Health Promotion Survey,* Association for Worksite Health Promotion & W. M. Mercer, Northbrook, IL: Association of Worksite Health Promotion, U.S. Department of Health and Human Services. 2000.
*The 1985 survey did not measure program prevalence by employer size.

preventive medicine, disease surveillance, vaccine and therapeutic development, and information technology; it also mirrors the changing demographics of our country, the changes that have taken place in health care, and the growing impact of global forces on our national health status. Many people in the United States have embraced the health promotion philosophy, as demonstrated by efforts to become better informed about health problems and to change lifestyle behaviors to improve their health and quality of life (Breslow, 1999). In addition, employers are also investing in worksite health promotion programs, with approximately 90% of all workplaces offering some type of health promotion activity at the worksite (Table 13-4) (Association for Worksite Health Promotion, 2000).

Healthy People 2010 formulates a comprehensive blueprint or nationwide health promotion and disease agenda to combat the leading preventable diseases and health-related problems and improve the health of all the people in the United States. For the first time a set of Leading Health Indicators (Box 13-1) has been developed to assist individuals and communities to target actions to improve health. The Leading Health Indicators reflect the major public health concerns in the United States and were chosen based on their ability to motivate action, the availability of data to measure their progress, and their relevance as broad public health issues. The Leading Health Indicators illuminate individual behaviors, physical and social environmental factors, and important health systems issues that greatly affect the health of individuals and communities. They are intended to help everyone more easily understand the importance of health promotion and disease prevention and to encourage wide participation in improving health in the next decade. Developing strategies and action plans to address one or more of these indicators can have a profound effect on increasing the quality of life and the years of healthy life and on eliminating health disparities, all of which create healthy people in healthy communities.

For each of the Leading Health Indicators, specific objectives derived from *Healthy People 2010* will be used to track progress. This small set of measures will provide a snapshot of the health of the nation. Tracking and communicating progress on the Leading Health Indicators through national- and state-level report cards will spotlight achievements and challenges in the next decade. The Leading Health Indicators serve as a link to the 467 objectives in *Healthy People 2010* and can become the basic building blocks for community health initiatives. Efforts to achieve these priorities will require a commitment on the part of society and its members to promote and adopt healthy lifestyles and behaviors conducive to optimal health and by business, government, and other organizations to develop the strategies, opportunities, and resources required to support the behavioral and environmental changes needed.

The importance of a comprehensive approach to worker health promotion and protection must be emphasized and facilitated by using the

Box 13-1   Leading Health Indicators

PHYSICAL ACTIVITY

Regular physical activity is associated with lower death rates for young adults of any age, even when only moderate levels of physical activity are performed. Regular physical activity decreases the risk of death from heart disease, lowers the risk of developing diabetes, and is associated with a decreased risk of colon cancer. Regular physical activity helps prevent high blood pressure and helps reduce blood pressure in persons with elevated levels.

OVERWEIGHT AND OBESITY

Overweight and obesity substantially raise the risk of illness from high blood pressure, high cholesterol, type 2 diabetes, heart disease and stroke, gallbladder disease, arthritis, sleep disturbances and problems breathing, and certain types of cancer. Obese individuals also may suffer from social stigmatization, discrimination, and lowered self-esteem.

TOBACCO USE

Smoking is a major risk factor for heart disease, stroke, lung cancer, and chronic lung diseases—all leading causes of death. Smoking during pregnancy can result in miscarriages, premature delivery, and sudden infant death syndrome. Other effects of smoking result from injuries and environmental damage caused by fires.

SUBSTANCE ABUSE

Alcohol and illicit drug use are associated with child and spousal abuse; sexually transmitted diseases, including HIV infection; teen pregnancy; school failure; motor vehicle accidents; escalation of health care costs; low worker productivity; and homelessness. Alcohol and illicit drug use also can result in substantial disruptions in family, work, and personal life. Alcohol abuse alone is associated with motor vehicle crashes, homicides, suicides, and drowning—leading causes of death among youth. Long-term heavy drinking can lead to heart disease, cancer, alcohol-related liver disease, and pancreatitis. Alcohol use during pregnancy is known to cause fetal alcohol syndrome, a leading cause of preventable mental retardation.

RESPONSIBLE SEXUAL BEHAVIOR

Unintended pregnancies and sexually transmitted diseases (STDs), including infection with the human immunodeficiency virus that causes AIDS, can result from unprotected sexual behaviors. There has been an increasing abstinence among all youth. In addition, condoms, if used correctly and consistently, can help prevent both unintended pregnancy and STDs.

MENTAL HEALTH

Approximately 20% of the U.S. population is affected by mental illness during a given year; no one is immune. Of all mental illnesses, depression is the most common disorder. More than 19 million adults in the United States suffer from depression. Major depression is the leading cause of disability and is the cause of more than two thirds of suicides each year. Depression is associated with other medical conditions, such as heart disease, cancer, and diabetes as well as anxiety and eating disorders. Depression also has been associated with alcohol and illicit drug abuse. An estimated 8 million persons age 15 to 54 years had coexisting mental and substance abuse disorders within the past year.

INJURY AND VIOLENCE

More than 400 Americans die each day from injuries due primarily to motor vehicle crashes, firearms, poisonings, suffocations, falls, fires, and drowning. The risk of injury is so great that most persons sustain a significant injury at some time during their lives. Motor vehicle crashes are the most common cause of serious injury. In 1998 there were 15.6 deaths from motor vehicle crashes per 100,000 persons. Because no other crime is measured as accurately and precisely, homicide is a reliable indicator of all violent crime. In 1998 the murder rate in the United States fell to its lowest level in three decades—6.5 homicides per 100,000 persons.

ENVIRONMENTAL QUALITY

An estimated 25% of preventable illnesses worldwide can be attributed to poor environmental quality. In the United States air pollution alone is estimated to be associated with 50,000 premature deaths and an estimated $40 billion in health-related costs annually. Two indicators of air quality are ozone (outdoor) and environmental tobacco smoke (ETS) (indoor). Poor air quality

Continued

Box 13-1 Leading Health Indicators—cont'd

contributes to respiratory illness, cardiovascular disease, and cancer. For example, asthma can be triggered or worsened by exposure to ozone and ETS. The overall death rate from asthma increased 57% between 1980 and 1993, and for children it increased 67%.

IMMUNIZATION

Many once common vaccine-preventable diseases are now controlled. Smallpox has been eradicated, poliomyelitis has been eliminated from the Western Hemisphere, and measles cases in the United States are at a record low. Immunizations against influenza and pneumococcal disease can prevent serious illness and death. Pneumonia and influenza deaths together constitute the sixth leading cause of death in the United States. Influenza causes an average of 110,000 hospitalizations and 20,000 deaths annually;

pneumococcal disease causes 10,000 to 14,000 deaths annually.

ACCESS TO HEALTH CARE

Strong predictors of access to quality health care include having health insurance, a higher income level, and a regular primary care provider or other source of ongoing health care. Use of clinical preventive services, such as early prenatal care, can serve as indicators of access to quality health care services. In 1997 83% of all persons under age 65 years had health insurance. In 1998 87% of persons of all ages had a usual source of health care. Also in that year 83% of pregnant women received prenatal care in the first trimester of pregnancy. More than 44 million persons in the United States do not have health insurance, including 11 million uninsured children.

From *Healthy People 2010: Understanding and Improving Health,* by U.S. Department of Health and Human Services, 2001, Washington, DC: U.S. Government Printing Office.

national health objectives as foundational elements. This can best be accomplished through developing a concept of health at the worksite and operationalizing this concept through program planning, implementation, and evaluation. This includes not only a corporate and company-wide commitment to health but a combination of educational, organizational, economic, or other environmental supports rather than only appeals for changes in specific behaviors.

The occupational and environmental health nurse is uniquely positioned to facilitate a worksite health concept and establish worksite health promotion programs. In so doing, these nurses should be at the forefront in developing interactive health promotion/education programs, counseling efforts, and behavioral interventions. Recognizing that breakthroughs in understanding the human genome have the potential to markedly enhance health and prevent disease and that in the next decade molecular prevention will become a reality, nurses will be pivotal in helping clients to combine knowledge about personal genetic makeup, genetic prevention techniques, and behavior change strategies to prevent illness for which they are at high risk (Pender et al., 2002).

PREVENTION AND HEALTH

In 1922 the American Medical Association recommended that a routine physical examination accompanied by a battery of laboratory tests be performed annually on all patients as a preventive medical service (American Medical Association, 1947), and this remained a common practice for decades. Over time controversy developed about the relative value of conducting annual physical examinations in healthy or asymptomatic individuals with respect to the efficacy and cost-effectiveness of such evaluations. Experience now indicates that, although routine visits with the primary health care clinician are important, performing the same interventions on all individuals and performing them as frequently as every year are not the most clinically cost-effective approaches to disease prevention. Rather, both the frequency and the content of preventive or periodic health examinations need to be tailored to the unique health risks of the individual and should take into consideration the quality of the evidence that specific preventive services are clinically effective. This approach to the periodic visit was endorsed by the American Medical

Association in 1983 in a policy statement that withdrew support for a standard annual physical examination. However, this does not diminish the benefits of preventive or periodic health evaluations related to specific epidemiological characteristics of the population, related risk factors, morbidity, and mortality experiences in the early detection of disease. For example, with the widespread use of Papanicolaou testing to detect cervical dysplasia, invasive cervical cancer has been reduced by more than 90% when screening is done at recommended levels of every 3 years (U.S. Preventive Services Task Force, 1996).

In 1979 the Canadian Task Force on Periodic Health Examination published its findings after an extensive study of the usefulness or value of annual/periodic health evaluations. Recommendations centered on offering health protection pack-ages tied to targeted conditions and selected demographic characteristics (e.g., age-group) (Canadian Task Force on Periodic Health Examination, 1979). In 1977 Breslow and Sommers proposed a Lifetime Health Monitoring Program (LHMP), which uses epidemiologic data to delineate schedules and parameters for health monitoring according to a person's age and known risk factors. The LHMP offers a sound approach to periodic health evaluation that is unlikely to miss preventable diseases or conditions identifiable by the screening elements selected (Guidotti et al., 1989). Occupational health professionals can collaboratively construct a monitoring program schedule to match the specifics of their industry population (e.g., age, sex, risk factor profile). Parameters to consider in constructing such a monitoring program are shown in Table 13-5.

TABLE 13-5   **Conditions/Parameters to Consider When Modifying a Lifetime Health Monitoring Program in Healthy Adults***

PROCEDURE	FACTOR	MODIFICATION
Complete history	Family history of cancer in several members; possible genetic risk	Increase frequency of history and physical examination to annually if appropriate.
History of alcohol intake	Family history of alcoholism, pattern of heavy use	Increase frequency of history of alcohol intake; refer for education or counseling.
History of tobacco use	Heavy smoker	Increase frequency of history of smoking; use spirometry as opportunity to counsel patient on cessation.
Sexual history	Multiple partners; homosexual lifestyle	Evaluate frequency of Papanicolaou smear, VDRL, rectal examinations.
Occupational history	Exposure on job to hazardous substances, continuing or antecedent	Increase frequency of occupational history, considering appropriate surveillance strategy.
Complete physical	Family history suggestive of elevated risk	Modify frequency of screening elements accordingly.
Blood pressure	Race—black; family history of essential hypertension	Increase frequency to annually and every visit in between.
Breast examination	Family history of breast cancer; female	Increase frequency to annually before age 40; reinforce need for self-examination.

From *Occupational Health Services: A Practical Approach,* by T. Guidotti, J. Cowell, and G. Jamieson, Chicago: American Medical Association. 1989.
*These recommendations apply only to asymptomatic individuals. Positive findings, known preexisting conditions, and unusual exposure opportunities alter the subject risk profile and impose additional requirements for surveillance or monitoring.

Continued

TABLE 13-5	Conditions/Parameters to Consider When Modifying a Lifetime Health Monitoring Program in Healthy Adults—cont'd	
PROCEDURE	**FACTOR**	**MODIFICATION**
Pelvic examination	Family history of malignancy	Increase frequency to annually before age 40; see Papanicolaou smear.
Rectal examination	Family history of malignancy	Consider increase in frequency.
Stool occult blood	Family history of malignancy	Increase frequency to annually before age 50.
Serum glucose	Family history of juvenile-onset diabetes	Increase frequency to annually.
Serum lipids	Family history of cardiovascular disease	Consider increasing frequency; emphasize cardiovascular examination.
VDRL	Homosexual or heterosexual lifestyle with multiple partners	Consider increasing frequency.
Papanicolaou smear[†]	Multiple sexual partners; proclivity to noncompliance	Consider increasing frequency to annually.
Proctosigmoidoscopy	Family history of malignancy	Increase frequency.
Mammography	Family history of breast cancer, female	Consider increasing frequency before age 50; emphasize need for breast self-examination.
HIV antibody	Men who have sex with other men, intravenous drug users, partners of those in high-risk groups	Evaluate frequency.

From *Occupational Health Services: A Practical Approach*, by T. Guidotti, J. Cowell, and G. Jamieson, Chicago: American Medical Association. 1989.
[†]The American Medical Association recommends periodic Pap smears for women starting at age 18 or at time of first sexual intercourse.

In 1984 the U.S. Preventive Services Task Force, composed of 20 nonfederal panel members, was commissioned by the U.S. Department of Health and Human Services to develop recommendations by age-group on the appropriate use of preventive interventions based on evidence of clinical effectiveness. Extensive work of the U.S. Preventive Services Task Force included defining the services to be examined and the review process, adopting specific criteria for recommending certain preventive services, conducting extensive literature searches and reviewing quality studies, adopting guidelines for clinical practice, and having recommendations reviewed extensively by more than 300 international experts. The first report has now been updated, and its recommendations include the following (U.S. Preventive Services Task Force, 1996):

1. Interventions that address patients' personal health practices are vitally important.
2. The clinicians and the patient should share in decision making.
3. Clinicians should be selective in ordering and providing preventive services.
4. Clinicians must take every opportunity to deliver preventive services, especially to people with limited access to care.
5. For some health problems community-level interventions may be more effective than clinical preventive services.

Interventions are identified for the prevention of 53 targeted conditions, with content specific for periodic health evaluations by age-group. These recommendations are based on the recognition that the leading causes of illness and injury in populations are age-, sex-, and risk factor-specific. These recommendations are accompanied by counseling interventions for 11 conditions and immunization and chemoprophylaxis recommendations.

The health care professional must consider the leading causes of mortality and morbidity within each age-group to target specific interventions appropriate to these groups and set priorities for preventive health services. The Task Force's recommendations for preventive care or periodic health evaluations in age-specific populations are presented in Box 13-2. The services recommended are carefully defined to be performed on asymptomatic persons within the context of routine health care. Interventions listed are not exhaustive; rather they reflect preventive services (as examined in the report) as having satisfactory evidence of clinical effectiveness. The reader is encouraged to read the Task Force's report in its entirety for a more detailed description of the preventive services examined.

LEVELS OF PREVENTION

Leavell and Clark (1965) first described the concept of levels of prevention within the medical context of preventing or halting disease (see Chapter 3). Shamansky and Clausen (1980) further explicated the concept to provide for a nursing application. While Leavell and Clark (1965) describe health promotion activities within the context of primary prevention, Pender et al. (2002) distinguish health promotion from health protection/illness prevention and argue that underlying conceptual differences for each exist related to the motivation for the behavior on the part of individuals and aggregates. Pender et al. (2002) note that health promotion is neither illness- nor injury-specific whereas health protection is; that health promotion is "approach" motivated while health protection is "avoidance" motivated; and that health promotion seeks to expand positive potential for health, while health protection seeks to thwart the occurrence of insults to health and well-being. Both health promotion and health protection are considered complementary processes aimed at enhancing the quality of life or altering person-environment interactions.

Pender et al. (2002) define *health promotion* as "behavior motivated by a desire to increase well-being and actualize health potential. *Health protection* (italic added) is behavior motivated by a desire to actively avoid illness, detect it early, or maintain functioning within the constraints of illness" (p. 7). Health promotion behaviors are described as continuing activities that must be an integral part of a person's lifestyle and include examples such as engaging in physical exercise or healthy, nutritional eating practices directed at maximizing optimal health. For example, some individuals may exercise and/or reduce their cholesterol and fat intake because they are at risk for cardiovascular disease (health protection motivation), whereas others engage in the same type of activities primarily to improve health (health promotion motivation).

Pender uses the terms *health-protecting behavior* and *preventive health behavior* interchangeably. In the classic article by Shamansky and Clausen (1980) *prevention* is best described as health-protecting behavior because primary emphasis is placed on guarding or defending an individual or group against specific illness or injury. *Primary prevention* activities are aimed at eliminating or reducing the risk of disease through specific protective actions. Effective primary prevention measures include providing worksite immunizations to control infectious disease onset; counseling and education about at-risk behaviors such as physical inactivity and unhealthy food choices; mandatory seat belt usage to protect against motor vehicle accident injury; and training regarding the appropriate use of personal protective equipment for health hazard reduction.

Secondary prevention is directed at early detection and case finding and diagnosis of individuals with disease to institute prompt interventions to halt the further progression of the disease and limit disability. For employees and employee groups secondary prevention activities involve screening examinations (e.g., preplacement, periodic assessments) and medical and health surveillance efforts to identify illness or injury from potential hazardous exposures and initiate measures to eliminate the problem. For example, through reviewing Material Safety Data Sheets, the occupational and environmental health nurse may become aware of the potential for health effects related to specific chemicals used in a work process. This would support the design and implementation of health surveillance programs/measures for early detection of harmful effects. Health surveillance programs or activities for regulatory compliance related to

Text continued on p. 396

Box 13-2   Periodic Health Examination and Age-Specific Charts

BIRTH TO 10 YEARS

Interventions Considered and Recommended for the Periodic Health Examination

Leading Causes of Death

Conditions originating in perinatal period
Congenital anomalies
Sudden infant death syndrome (SIDS)

Unintentional injuries (nonmotor vehicle)
Motor vehicle injuries

Interventions for the General Population

Screening
Height and weight
Blood pressure
Vision screen (age 3 to 4 years)
Hemoglobinopathy screen (birth)[1]
Phenylalanine level (birth)[2]
T_4 and/or TSH (birth)[3]

Counseling
Injury Prevention
Child safety car seats (age <5 years)
Lap-shoulder belts (age ≥5 years)
Bicycle helmet, avoid bicycling near traffic
Smoke detector, flame retardant sleepwear
Hot water heater temperature <120° to 130° F
Window/stair guards, pool fence
Safe storage of drugs, toxic substances, firearms, and matches
Syrup of ipecac, poison control phone number
CPR training for parents/caretakers

Diet and Exercise
Breast-feeding, iron-enriched formula and foods (infants & toddlers)

Limit fat & cholesterol, maintain caloric balance, emphasize grains, fruits, vegetables (age ≥2 years)
Regular physical activity*

Substance Use
Effects of passive smoking*
Antitobacco message*

Dental Health
Regular visits to dental care provider*
Floss, brush with fluoride toothpaste daily*
Advice about baby bottle tooth decay*

Immunizations
Diphtheria-tetanus-pertussis (DTP)[4]
Oral poliovirus (OPV)[5]
Measles-mumps-rubella (MMR)[6]
H. influenza type b (Hib) conjugate[7]
Hepatitis B[8]
Varicella[9]

Chemoprophylaxis
Ocular prophylaxis (birth)

[1]Whether screening should be universal or targeted to high-risk groups will depend on the proportion of high-risk individuals in the screening area and other considerations.
[2]If done during first 24 hours of life, repeat by age 2 weeks.
[3]Optimally between days 2 and 6, but in all cases before newborn nursery discharge.
[4]2, 4, 6, and 12 to 18 months; once between ages 4 to 6 years (DtaP may be used at 15 months and older).
[5]2, 4, and 6 to 18 months; once between ages 4 to 6 years.
[6]12 to 15 months and 4 to 6 years.
[7]2, 4, 6 and 12 to 15 months; no dose needed at 6 months if PRP-OMP vaccine is used for first two doses.
[8]Birth, 1 month, 6 months; or 0 to 2 months, 1 to 2 months later, and 6 to 18 months. If not done in infancy: current visit, and 1 and 6 months later.
[9]12 to 18 months; or any child without history of chickenpox or previous immunization. Include information on risk in adulthood, duration of immunity, and potential need for booster doses.
*The ability of clinician counseling to influence this behavior is unproven.

Interventions for High-Risk Populations

POPULATION	POTENTIAL INTERVENTIONS (See detailed high risk definitions)
Preterm or low birth weight	Hemoglobin/hematocrit (HR1)
Infants of mothers at risk for HIV	HIV testing (HR2)
Low income; immigrants	Hemoglobin/hematocrit (HR1); PPD (HR3)

From *Guide to Clinical Preventive Services* (2nd ed.), by U.S. Preventive Services Task Force, 1996, Baltimore, MD: Williams & Wilkins.

Box 13-2   Periodic Health Examination and Age-Specific Charts—cont'd

POPULATION	POTENTIAL INTERVENTIONS (See detailed high risk definitions)
TB contacts	PPD (HR3)
Native Americans/Alaska Natives	Hemoglobin/hematocrit (HR1); PPD (HR3); hepatitis A vaccine (HR4); pneumococcal vaccine (HR5)
Travelers to developing countries	Hepatitis A vaccine (HR4)
Residents of long-term care facilities	PPD (HR3); hepatitis A vaccine (HR4); influenza vaccine (HR6)
Certain chronic medical conditions	PPD (HR3); pneumococcal vaccine (HR5); influenza vaccine (HR6)
Increased individual or community lead exposure	Blood lead level (HR7)
Inadequate water fluoridation	Daily fluoride supplement (HR8)
Family history of skin cancer; nevi; fair skin, eyes, hair	Avoid excess/midday sun, use protective clothing* (HR9)

*The ability of clinician counseling to influence this behavior is unproven.

High-Risk Definitions

HR1 = Infants age 6 to 12 months who are living in poverty; black, Native American, or Alaska Native, immigrants from developing countries; preterm or low birth weight infants; or infants whose principal dietary intake is unfortified cow's milk.

HR2 = Infants born to high-risk mothers whose HIV status is unknown. Women at high risk include past or present injection drug use; persons who exchange sex for money or drugs, and their sex partners; injection drug-using, bisexual, or HIV-positive sex partners currently or in past; persons seeking treatment for STDs; blood transfusion during 1978 to 1985.

HR3 = Persons infected with HIV, close contacts of persons with known or suspected TB, persons with medical risk factors associated with TB, immigrants from countries with high TB prevalence, medically underserved low-income populations (including homeless), residents of long-term care facilities.

HR4 = Persons ≥2 years living in or traveling to areas where the disease is endemic and where periodic outbreaks occur (e.g., countries with high or intermediate endemicity; certain Alaska Native, Pacific Island, Native American, and religious communities). Consider for institutionalized children aged ≥2 years. Clinicians should also consider local epidemiology.

HR5 = Immunocompetent persons ≥2 years with certain medical conditions, including chronic cardiac or pulmonary disease, diabetes mellitus, and anatomic asplenia. Immunocompetent persons ≥2 years living in high-risk environments or social settings (e.g., certain Native American and Alaska Native populations).

HR6 = Annual vaccination of children >6 months who are residents of chronic care facilities or who have chronic cardiopulmonary disorders, metabolic diseases (including diabetes mellitus), hemoglobinopathies, immunosuppression, or renal dysfunction.

HR7 = Children about age 12 months who (1) live in communities in which the prevalence of lead levels requiring individual intervention, including residential lead hazard control or chelation, is high or undefined; (2) live in or frequently visit a home built before 1950 with dilapidated paint or with recent or ongoing renovation or remodeling; (3) have close contact with a person who has an elevated lead level; (4) live near lead industry or heavy traffic; (5) live with someone whose job or hobby

Continued

Box 13-2 Periodic Health Examination and Age-Specific Charts—cont'd

involves lead exposure; (6) use lead-based pottery; or (7) take traditional ethnic remedies that contain lead.

HR8 = Children living in areas with inadequate water fluoridation (<0.6 ppm).

HR9 = Persons with a family history of skin cancer, a large number of moles, atypical moles, poor tanning ability, or light skin, hair, and eye color.

AGES 11-24 YEARS

Interventions Considered and Recommended for the Periodic Health Examination

Leading Causes of Death

Motor vehicle/other unintentional injuries
Homicide
Suicide
Malignant neoplasms
Heart diseases

Interventions for the General Population

Screening
Height and weight
Blood pressure[1]
Papanicolaou (Pap) test[2] (females)
Chlamydia screen[3] (females <20 years)
Rubella serology or vaccination hx[4] (females >12 years)
Assess for problem drinking

Counseling
Injury Prevention
Lap/shoulder belts
Bicycle/motorcycle/ATV helmets*
Smoke detector*
Safe storage/removal of firearms*

Substance Use
Avoid tobacco use
Avoid underage drinking and illicit drug use*
Avoid alcohol/drug use while driving, swimming, boating, etc.*

Sexual Behavior
STD prevention: abstinence*; avoid high-risk behavior*; condoms/female barrier with spermicide*
Unintended pregnancy: contraception

Diet and Exercise
Limit fat and cholesterol; maintain caloric balance; emphasize grains, fruits, vegetables
Adequate calcium intake (females)
Regular physical activity*

Dental Health
Regular visits to dental care provider*
Floss, brush with fluoride toothpaste daily*

Immunizations
Tetanus-diphtheria (Td) boosters (11 to 16 years)
Hepatitis B[5]
MMR (11 to 12 years)[6]
Varicella (11 to 12 years)
Rubella[4] (females >12 years)

Chemoprophylaxis
Multivitamin with folic acid (females planning/capable of pregnancy)

From *Guide to Clinical Preventive Services* (2nd ed.), by U.S. Preventive Services Task Force, 1996, Baltimore, MD: Williams & Wilkins.[1]Periodic BP for persons aged ≥21 years.
[2]If sexually active at present or in the past: q ≤3 years. If sexual history is unreliable, begin Pap tests at age 18 years.
[3]If sexually active.
[4]Serologic testing documented vaccination history, and routine vaccination against rubella (preferably with MMR) are equally acceptable alternatives.
[5]If not previously immunized: current visit, 1 and 6 months later.
[6]If susceptible to chickenpox.
*The ability of clinician counseling to influence this behavior is unproven.

Box 13-2   Periodic Health Examination and Age-Specific Charts—cont'd

Interventions for High-Risk Populations

POPULATION	POTENTIAL INTERVENTIONS (See detailed high-risk definitions)
High-risk sexual behavior	RPR/VDRL (HR1); screen for gonorrhea (female) (HR2), HIV (HR3), chlamydia (female) (HR4); hepatitis A vaccine (HR5)
Injection or street drug use	RPR/VDRL (HR1); HIV screen (HR3); hepatitis A vaccine (HR5); PPD (HR6); advice to reduce infection risk (HR7)
TB contacts; immigrants; low income	PPD (HR6)
Native Americans/Alaska Natives	Hepatitis A vaccine (HR5); PPD (HR6); pneumococcal vaccine (HR8)
Travelers to developing countries	Hepatitis A vaccine (HR5)
Certain chronic medical conditions	PPD (HR6); pneumococcal vaccine (HR8); influenza vaccine (HR9)
Settings where adolescents and young adults congregate	Second MMR (HR10)
Susceptible to varicella, measles, mumps	Varicella vaccine (HR11); MMR (HR12)
Blood transfusion between 1978 and 1985	HIV screen (HR3)
Institutionalized persons; health care/lab workers	Hepatitis A vaccine (HR5); PPD (HR6); influenza vaccine (HR9)
Family history of skin cancer; nevi; fair skin, eyes, hair	Avoid excess/midday sun, use protective clothing* (HR13)
Prior pregnancy with neural tube defect	Folic acid 4.0 mg (HR14)
Inadequate water fluoridation	Daily fluoride supplement (HR15)

*The ability of clinician counseling to influence this behavior is unproven.

High-Risk Definitions

HR1 = Persons who exchange sex for money or drugs, and their sex partners; persons with other STDs (including HIV); and sexual contacts of persons with active syphilis. Clinicians should also consider local epidemiology.

HR2 = Females who have two or more sex partners in the last year; a sex partner with multiple sexual contacts; exchanged sex for money or drugs; or a history of repeated episodes of gonorrhea. Clinicians should also consider local epidemiology.

HR3 = Males who had sex with males after 1975; past or present injection drug use; persons who exchange sex for money or drugs, and their sex partners; injection drug-using, bisexual, or HIV-positive sex partner currently or in the past; blood transfusion during 1978 to 1985; persons

seeking treatment for STDs. Clinicians should also consider local epidemiology.

HR4 = Sexually active females with multiple risk factors including history of prior STD, new or multiple sex partners, age under 25, nonuse or inconsistent use of barrier contraceptives, cervical ectopy. Clinicians should consider local epidemiology of the disease in identifying other high-risk groups.

HR5 = Persons living in, traveling to, or working in areas where the disease is endemic and where periodic outbreaks occur (e.g., countries with high or intermediate endemicity; certain Alaska Native, Pacific Island, Native American, and religious communities); men who have sex with men; injection or street drug users. Vaccine may be considered for institutionalized persons and

Continued

Box 13-2 Periodic Health Examination and Age-Specific Charts—cont'd

workers in these institutions, military person-nel, and day care, hospital, and laboratory workers. Clinicians should also consider local epidemiology.

HR6 = HIV positive, close contacts of persons with known or suspected TB, health care work-ers, persons with medical risk factors associated with TB, immigrants from countries with high TB prevalence, medically underserved low income populations (including homeless), alco-holics, injection drug users, and residents of long-term care facilities.

HR7 = Persons who continue to inject drugs.

HR8 = Immunocompetent persons with certain medical conditions, including chronic cardiac or pulmonary disease, diabetes melli-tus, and anatomic asplenia. Immunocompetent persons who live in high-risk environments or social settings (e.g., certain Native American and Alaska Native populations).

HR9 = Annual vaccination of residents of chronic care facilities; persons with chronic cardiopulmonary disorders, metabolic diseases (including diabetes mellitus), hemoglo-binopathies, immunosuppression, or renal dys-function; and health care providers for high-risk patients.

HR10 = Adolescents and young adults in settings where such individuals congregate (e.g., high schools and colleges), if they have not previously received a second dose.

HR11 = Healthy persons aged ≥13 years without a history of chickenpox or previous immunization. Consider serologic testing for presumed susceptible persons aged ≥13 years.

HR12 = Persons born after 1956 who lack evidence of immunity to measles or mumps (e.g., documented receipt of live vaccine on or after the first birthday, laboratory evidence of immunity, or a history of physician-diagnosed measles or mumps).

HR13 = Persons with a family or personal history of skin cancer, a large number of moles, atypical moles, poor tanning ability, or light skin, hair, and eye color.

HR14 = Women with prior pregnancy affected by neural tube defect who are planning pregnancy.

HR15 = Persons aged <17 years living in areas with inadequate water fluoridation (<0.6 ppm).

AGES 25-64 YEARS
Interventions Considered and Recommended for the Periodic Health Examination

Leading Causes of Death

Malignant neoplasms
Heart diseases
Motor vehicle and other unintentional injuries

Human immunodeficiency virus (HIV) infection
Suicide and homicide

Interventions for the General Population

Screening
Blood pressure
Height and weight
Total blood cholesterol (men ages 35 to 65, women ages 45 to 65)
Papanicolaou (Pap) test (women)[1]

Fecal occult blood test[2] and/or sigmoidoscopy (≥50 years)
Mammogram ± clinical breast exam[3] (women 50 to 69 years)
Assess for problem drinking
Rubella serology or vaccination history[4] (women of childbearing age)

From *Guide to Clinical Preventive Services* (2nd ed.), by U.S. Preventive Services Task Force, 1996, Baltimore, MD: Williams & Wilkins.
[1]Women who are or have been sexually active and who have a cervix: q ≤3 years.
[2]Annually
[3]Mammogram q1 to 2 years, or mammogram q1 to 2 years with annual clinical breast examination.
[4]Serologic testing, documented vaccination history, and routine vaccination (preferably with MMR) are equally acceptable.

Box 13-2 Periodic Health Examination and Age-Specific Charts—cont'd

Counseling
Substance Use
Tobacco cessation
Avoid alcohol/drug use while driving,
  swimming, boating, etc.*

Diet and Exercise
Limit fat & cholesterol; maintain caloric
  balance; emphasize grains, fruits,
  vegetables
Adequate calcium intake (women)
Regular physical activity*

Injury Prevention
Lap/shoulder belts
Motorcycle/bicycle/ATV helmets*
Smoke detector*
Safe storage/removal of firearms*

Dental Health
Regular visits to dental care provider*
Floss, brush with fluoride toothpaste daily*

Sexual Behavior
STD prevention: avoid high-risk behavior*;
  condoms/female barrier with spermicide*
Unintended pregnancy: contraception

Immunizations
Tetanus-diphtheria (Td) boosters
Rubella[4] (women of childbearing age)

Chemoprophylaxis
Multivitamin with folic acid (women planning
  or capable of pregnancy)
Discuss hormone prophylaxis (perimeno-
  pausal and postmenopausal women)

*The ability of clinician counseling to influence this behavior is unproven.

Interventions for High-Risk Populations

POPULATION	POTENTIAL INTERVENTIONS (See detailed high-risk definitions)
High-risk sexual behavior	RPR/VDRL (HR1); screen for gonorrhea (female) (HR2), HIV (HR3), chlamydia (female) (HR4); hepatitis B vaccine (HR5); hepatitis A vaccine (HR6)
Injection or street drug use	RPR/VDRL (HR1); HIV screen (HR3); hepatitis B vaccine (HR5); hepatitis A vaccine (HR6); PPD (HR7); advice to reduce infection risk (HR8)
Low income; TB contacts; immigrants; alcoholics	PPD (HR7)
Native Americans/Alaska Natives	Hepatitis A vaccine (HR6); PPD (HR7); pneumococcal vaccine (HR9)
Travelers to developing countries	Hepatitis B vaccine (HR5); hepatitis A vaccine (HR6)
Certain chronic medical conditions	PPD (HR7); pneumococcal vaccine (HR9); influenza vaccine (HR10)
Blood product recipients	HIV screen (HR3); hepatitis B vaccine (HR5)
Susceptible to measles, mumps, or varicella	MMR (HR11); varicella vaccine (HR12)
Institutionalized persons	Hepatitis A vaccine (HR6); PPD (HR7); pneumococcal vaccine (HR9); influenza vaccine (HR10)
Health care/lab workers	Hepatitis B vaccine (HR5); hepatitis A vaccine (HR6); PPD (HR7); influenza vaccine (HR10)
Family history of skin cancer; fair skin, eyes, hair	Avoid excess/midday sun, use protective clothing* (HR13)
Previous pregnancy with neural tube defect	Folic acid 4.0 mg (HR14)

*The ability of clinician counseling to influence this behavior is unproven.

Continued

Box 13-2   Periodic Health Examination and Age-Specific Charts—cont'd

High-Risk Definitions

HRI = Persons who exchange sex for money or drugs, and their sex partners; persons with other STDs (including HIV); and sexual contacts of persons with active syphilis. Clinicians should also consider local epidemiology.

HR2 = Women who exchange sex for money or drugs or who have had repeated episodes of gonorrhea. Clinicians should also consider local epidemiology.

HR3 = Men who had sex with men after 1975; past or present injection drug use; persons who exchange sex for money or drugs, and their sex partners; injection drug-using, bisexual, or HIV-positive sex partner currently or in the past; blood transfusion during 1978 to 1985; persons seeking treatment for STDs. Clinicians should also consider local epidemiology.

HR4 = Sexually active women with multiple risk factors including history of STD, new or multiple sex partners, nonuse or inconsistent use of barrier contraceptives, cervical ectopy. Clinicians should also consider local epidemiology.

HR5 = Blood product recipients (including hemodialysis patients), persons with frequent occupational exposure to blood or blood products, men who have sex with men, injection drug users and their sex partners, persons with multiple recent sex partners, persons with other STDs (including HIV), travelers to countries with endemic hepatitis B.

HR6 = Persons living in, traveling to, or working in areas where the disease is endemic and where periodic outbreaks occur (e.g., countries with high or intermediate endemicity; certain Alaska Native, Pacific Island, Native American, and religious communities); men who have sex with men; injection or street drug users. Consider for institutionalized persons and workers in these institutions, military personnel, and day care, hospital, and laboratory workers. Clinicians should also consider local epidemiology.

HR7 = HIV positive, close contacts of persons with known or suspected TB, health care workers, persons with medical risk factors associated with TB, immigrants from countries with high TB prevalence, medically underserved low-income populations (including homeless), alcoholics, injection drug users, and residents of long-term care facilities.

HR8 = Persons who continue to inject drugs.

HR9 = Immunocompetent institutionalized persons aged ≥50 years and immunocompetent persons with certain medical conditions, including chronic cardiac or pulmonary disease, diabetes mellitus, and anatomic asplenia. Immunocompetent persons who live in high-risk environments or social settings (e.g., certain Native American and Alaska Native populations).

HR10 = Annual vaccination of residents of chronic care facilities; persons with chronic cardiopulmonary disorders, metabolic diseases (including diabetes mellitus), hemoglobinopathies, immunosuppression, or renal dysfunction; and health care providers for high-risk patients.

HR11 = Persons born after 1956 who lack evidence of immunity to measles or mumps (e.g., documented receipt of live vaccine on or after the first birthday, laboratory evidence of immunity, or a history of physician-diagnosed measles or mumps).

HR12 = Healthy adults without a history of chickenpox or previous immunization. Consider serologic testing for presumed susceptible adults.

HR13 = Persons with a family or personal history of skin cancer, a large number of moles, atypical moles, poor tanning ability, or light skin, hair, and eye color.

HR14 = Women with previous pregnancy affected by neural tube defect who are planning pregnancy.

From *Guide to Clinical Preventive Services* (2nd ed.), by U.S. Preventive Services Task Force, 1996, Baltimore, MD: Williams & Wilkins.

Box 13-2   Periodic Health Examination and Age-Specific Charts—cont'd

AGE 65 AND OLDER

Interventions Considered and Recommended for the Periodic Health Examination

Leading Causes of Death

Heart diseases
Malignant neoplasms (lung, colorectal, breast)
Cerebrovascular disease

Chronic obstructive pulmonary disease
Pneumonia and influenza

Interventions for the General Population

Screening
Blood pressure
Height and weight
Fecal occult blood test[1] and/or
  sigmoidoscopy
Mammogram ± clinical breast exam[2]
  (women ≤69 years)
Papanicolaou (Pap) test (women)[3]
Vision screening
Assess for hearing impairment
Assess for problem drinking

Counseling
Substance Use
Tobacco cessation
Avoid alcohol/drug use while driving,
  swimming, boating, etc.*

Diet and Exercise
Limit fat and cholesterol; maintain caloric
  balance; emphasize grains, fruits,
  vegetables
Adequate calcium intake (women)
Regular physical activity*

Injury Prevention
Lap/shoulder belts
Motorcycle and bicycle helmets*
Fall prevention*
Safe storage/removal of firearms*
Smoke detector*
Set hot water heater to <120° to 130° F
CPR training for household members

Dental Health
Regular visits to dental care provider*
Floss, brush with fluoride toothpaste daily*

Sexual Behavior
STD prevention: avoid high-risk sexual
  behavior*; use condoms*

Immunizations
Pneumococcal vaccine
Influenza[1]
Tetanus-diphtheria (Td) boosters

Chemoprophylaxis
Discuss hormone prophylaxis (women)

[1]Annually.
[2]Mammogram q1 to 2 years or mammogram q1 to 2 years with annual clinical breast examination.
[3]All women who are or have been sexually active and who have a cervix. Consider discontinuation of testing after age 65 years
  if previous regular screening with consistently normal results.
*The ability of clinician counseling to influence this behavior is unproven.

Interventions for High-Risk Populations

POPULATION	POTENTIAL INTERVENTIONS (See detailed high-risk definitions)
Institutionalized persons	PPD (HR1); hepatitis A vaccine (HR2); amantadine/rimantadine (HR4)
Chronic medical conditions; TB contacts; low income; immigrants; alcoholics	PPD (HR1)
Persons ≥75 years; or ≥70 years with risk factors for falls	Fall prevention intervention (HR5)
Cardiovascular disease risk factors	Consider cholesterol screening (HR6)
Family history of skin cancer; nevi; fair skin, eyes, hair	Avoid excess/midday sun, use protective clothing* (HR7)

Continued

Box 13-2 Periodic Health Examination and Age-Specific Charts — cont'd

POPULATION—cont'd	POTENTIAL INTERVENTIONS—cont'd
Native Americans/Alaska Natives	Hepatitis A vaccine (HR2); hepatitis B vaccine (HR8)
Travelers to developing countries	HIV screen (HR3); hepatitis B vaccine (HR8)
Blood product recipients	Hepatitis A vaccine (HR2); HIV screen (HR3); hepatitis B vaccine (HR8); RPR/VDRL (HR9)
High-risk sexual behavior	PPD (HR1); hepatitis A vaccine (HR2); HIV screen (HR3); hepatitis B vaccine (HR8); RPR/VDRL (HR9); advice to reduce infection risk (HR10)
Injection or street drug use	PPD (HR1); hepatitis A vaccine (HR2); amantadine/rimantadine (HR4); hepatitis B vaccine (HR8)
Health care/lab workers	PPD (HR1); hepatitis A vaccine (HR2); amantadine/rimantadine (HR4); hepatitis B vaccine (HR8)
Persons susceptible to varicella	Varicella vaccine (HR11)

*The ability of clinician counseling to influence this behavior is unproven.

High-Risk Definitions

HR1 = HIV positive, close contacts of persons with known or suspected TB, health care workers, persons with medical risk factors associated with TB, immigrants from countries with high TB prevalence, medically underserved low income populations (including homeless), alcoholics, injection drug users, and residents of long-term care facilities.

HR2 = Persons living in, traveling to, or working in areas where the disease is endemic and where periodic outbreaks occur (e.g., countries with high or intermediate endemicity; certain Alaska Native, Pacific Island, Native American, and religious communities); men who have sex with men; injection or street drug users. Consider for institutionalized persons and workers in these institutions, and day care, hospital, and laboratory workers. Clinicians should also consider local epidemiology.

HR3 = Men who had sex with men after 1975; past or present injection drug use; persons who exchange sex for money or drugs, and their sex partners; injection drug-using, bisexual, or HIV-positive sex partner currently or in the past; blood transfusion during 1978 to 1985; persons seeking treatment for STDs. Clinicians should also consider local epidemiology.

HR4 = Consider for persons who have not received influenza vaccine or are vaccinated late; when the vaccine may be ineffective due to major antigenic changes in the virus; for unvaccinated persons who provide home care for high-risk persons; to supplement protection provided by vaccine in persons who are expected to have a poor antibody response; and for high-risk persons in whom the vaccine is contraindicated.

HR5 = Persons age 75 years and older; or age 70 to 74 with one or more additional risk factors including use of certain psychoactive and cardiac medications (e.g., benzodiazepines, antihypertensives); use of ≥4 prescription medications; impaired cognition, strength, balance, or gait. Intensive individualized home-based multifactorial fall prevention intervention is recommended in settings where adequate resources are available to deliver such services.

HR6 = Although evidence is insufficient to recommend routine screening in elderly persons, clinicians should consider cholesterol screening on a case-by-case basis for persons ages 65 to 75 with additional risk factors (e.g., smoking, diabetes, or hypertension).

HR7 = Persons with a family or personal history of skin cancer, a large number of moles,

From *Guide to Clinical Preventive Services* (2nd ed.), by U.S. Preventive Services Task Force, 1996, Baltimore, MD: Williams & Wilkins.

Box 13-2   Periodic Health Examination and Age-Specific Charts—cont'd

atypical moles, poor tanning ability, or light skin, hair, and eye color.

HR8 = Blood product recipients (including hemodialysis patients), persons with frequent occupational exposure to blood or blood products, men who have sex with men, injection drug users and their sex partners, persons with multiple recent sex partners, persons with other STDs (including HIV), travelers to countries with endemic hepatitis B.

HR9 = Persons who exchange sex for money or drugs, and their sex partners; persons with other STDs (including HIV); and sexual contacts of persons with active syphilis. Clinicians should also consider local epidemiology.

HR10 = Persons who continue to inject drugs.

HR11 = Healthy adults without a history of chickenpox or previous immunization. Consider serologic testing for presumed susceptible adults.

PREGNANT WOMEN

Interventions Considered and Recommended for the Periodic Health Examination

Interventions for the General Population

Screening
First Visit
Blood pressure
Hemoglobin/hematocrit
Hepatitis B surface antigen (HBsAg)
RPR/VDRL
Chlamydia screen (<25 years)
Rubella serology or vaccination history
D(Rh) typing, antibody screen
Offer CVS (<13 weeks)[1] or amniocentesis
   (15 to 18 weeks)[1] (age ≥35 years)
Offer hemoglobinopathy screening
Assess for problem or risk drinking
Offer HIV screening[2]
Follow-up visits
Blood pressure
Urine culture (12 to 16 weeks)
Offer amniocentesis (15 to 18 weeks)[1]
   (age ≥35 years)

Offer multiple marker testing[1]
   (15 to 18 weeks)
Offer serum a-fetoprotein1 (16 to 18 weeks)

Counseling
Tobacco cessation; effects of passive
   smoking
Alcohol/other drug use
Nutrition, including adequate calcium intake
Encourage breastfeeding
Lap/shoulder belts
Infant safety car seats
STD prevention: avoid high-risk sexual
   behavior*; use condoms*

Chemoprophylaxis
Multivitamin with folic acid[3]

[1]Women with access to counseling and follow-up services, reliable standardized laboratories, skilled high-resolution ultrasound, and, for those receiving serum marker testing, amniocentesis capabilities.
[2]Universal screening is recommended for areas (states, counties, or cities) with an increased prevalence of HIV infection among pregnant women. In low prevalence areas the choice between universal and targeted screening may depend on other considerations.
[3]Beginning at least 1 month before conception and continuing through the first trimester.
*The ability of clinician counseling to influence this behavior is unproven.

Interventions for High-Risk Populations

POPULATION	POTENTIAL INTERVENTIONS (See detailed high-risk definitions)
High-risk sexual behavior	Screen for chlamydia (first visit) (HR1), gonorrhea (first visit) (HR2), HIV (first visit) (HR3); HBsAg (third trimester) (HR4); RPR/VDRL (third trimester) (HR5)

Continued

Box 13-2 Periodic Health Examination and Age-Specific Charts—cont'd	
Blood transfusion 1978 to 1985	HIV screen (first visit) (HR3)
Injection drug use	HIV screen (HR3); HBsAg (third trimester) (HR4); advice to reduce infection risk (HR6)
Unsensitized D-negative women	D(Rh) antibody testing (24 to 28 weeks) (HR7)
Risk factors for Down syndrome	Offer CVS[1] (first trimester), amniocentesis[1] (15 to 18 weeks) (HR8)
Prior pregnancy with neural tube defect	Folic acid 4.0 mg3; offer amniocentesis[1] (15 to 18 weeks) (HR9)

[1]Women with access to counseling and follow-up services, reliable standardized laboratories, skilled high-resolution ultrasound, and, for those receiving serum marker testing, amniocentesis capabilities.

High-Risk Definitions

HR1 = Women with history of STD or new or multiple sex partners. Clinicians should also consider local epidemiology. Chlamydia screen should be repeated in third trimester if at continued risk.

HR2 = Women under age 25 with two or more sex partners in the last year or whose sex partner has multiple sexual contacts; women who exchange sex for money or drugs; and women with a history of repeated episodes of gonorrhea. Clinicians should also consider local epidemiology. Gonorrhea screen should be repeated in the third trimester if at continued risk.

HR3 = In areas where universal screening is not performed due to low prevalence of HIV infection, pregnant women with the following individual risk factors should be screened: past or present injection drug use; women who exchange sex for money or drugs; injection drug-using, bisexual, or HIV-positive sex partner currently or in the past; blood transfusion during 1978 to 1985; persons seeking treatment for STDs.

HR4 = Women who are initially HBsAg-negative, who are at high risk due to injection drug use, suspected exposure to hepatitis B during pregnancy, multiple sex partners.

HR5 = Women who exchange sex for money or drugs, women with other STDs (including HIV), and sexual contacts of persons with active syphilis. Clinicians should also consider local epidemiology.

HR6 = Women who continue to inject drugs.

HR7 = Unsensitized D-negative women.

HR8 = Prior pregnancy affected by Down syndrome, advanced maternal age (≥35 years), known carriage of chromosome rearrangement.

HR9 = Women with previous pregnancy affected by neural tube defect.

From *Guide to Clinical Preventive Services* (2nd ed.), by U.S. Preventive Services Task Force, 1996, Baltimore, MD: Williams & Wilkins.

specific chemical exposures are also secondary prevention efforts.

Screening for hypertension or cancer (e.g., mammography) are examples of other types of traditional early detection screening activities that may be performed at the worksite. The provision of health care and prompt treatment to ill and injured employees, whether for occupational or nonoccupational health problems, to interrupt the disease process and limit further deterioration, are also considered secondary prevention activities. Screening

programs and early referral or treatment provide educational opportunities for employees and a measure of cost-containment for the employer through reduction in progressive morbidity and premature mortality.

Tertiary prevention comes into play when a health problem or disability is fixed, stabilized, or irreversible. Tertiary prevention activities are directed at minimizing residual disability from disease and rehabilitating and restoring individuals to an optimal level of health and functioning within

---

Box 13-3   Examples of Health Promotion-Health Protection-Prevention Activities

PRIMARY PREVENTION		SECONDARY PREVENTION	TERTIARY PREVENTION
Health ←→ Promotion	Risk Reduction/ Prevention		
Nutrition enhancement	Immunization	Preplacement, periodic examination	Disability/case management
Exercise/fitness	Stress management	Health surveillance	Early return to work
Reproductive health	Smoking cessation	Screening programs	Chronic illness monitoring/education
Health motivation enhancement	Risk factor appraisal (e.g., weight, smoking, sun exposure)	Monitoring health/illness trend data	Substance abuse rehabilitation
	Seat belt use	Nutrition education for illness control (e.g., diabetes, hypertension)	
	Worksite walk-throughs		
	Personal protective equipment use		

---

the constraints of their health problem or disability (Shamansky & Clausen, 1980; Wachs, 1991). The occupational and environmental health nurse can help ill or injured workers return to limited- or full-duty work as soon as feasible, so they may continue to function as productive members of the work-force. The nurse can be involved in the counseling and rehabilitative processes and programs, such as with an employee following a stroke, to help mini-mize any residual disability and work with commu-nity agencies to optimize resources available to the worker and her or his family. In addition, the nurse can work with management to develop, where nec-essary, policy initiatives with respect to job modifi-cations or restructuring to accommodate an em-ployee with a residual disability.

Chronic disease monitoring, including educa-tion and counseling about and reinforcement of the medical regimen, enables workers to exercise more control over their disease and remain on the job. The occupational and environmental health nurse can work to assure continuity of health care and provide the employee with information regarding signs and symptoms of exacerbation of a health problem. Cardiac rehabilitation pro-grams and employee substance abuse programs that emphasize lifestyle changes and occupational and environmental modifications are excellent examples of tertiary prevention programs. Several examples of health promotion and protection/prevention activities are shown in Box 13-3.

▌DEFINITIONS AND MODELS

Definitions for the concepts of health promotion and disease prevention or health protection have been provided by experts in the field. Several of these definitions are presented in Box 13-4. In addition, models to identify conceptual linkages to support measures for health promotion and health protection program planning and strat-egies for risk reduction have also been delineated. Several definitions and models will be briefly presented; however, the reader is referred to the reference source for an in-depth description and discussion.

O'Donnell (1989, 2002) provides the following definition of health promotion:

Health promotion is the science and art of helping people change their lifestyle to move toward a state of optimal health—that is, a balance of physical, emotional, social, spir-itual, and intellectual health. Lifestyle change can be facilitated through a combi-nation of efforts to enhance awareness, change behavior, and create environments that support good health practices. Of these three, supportive environments will prob-ably have the greatest impact in producing lasting change. (p. 49)

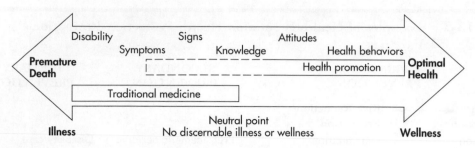

Figure 13-3 Health Continuum Model. *(From "Definitions of Health Promotion," by M. P. O'Donnell, 1986, American Journal of Health Promotion, 1, 4-5.)*

Box 13-4 Definitions of Health Promotion

- Health promotion is behavior motivated by a desire to increase well-being and actualize human health potential. Health protection is behavior motivated by a desire to actively avoid illness, detect it early, or maintain functioning within the constraints of illness. (Pender et al., 2002, p. 7).

- Health promotion is the combination of educational and ecological supports for actions and conditions of living conducive to health. *Combination* refers to the necessity of matching the multiple determinants of health with multiple interventions or sources of support. *Educational* refers to health education as any combination of learning experiences designed to facilitate voluntary actions conducive to health, including matching the multiple determinants of behavior with multiple learning experiences or educational interventions. *Ecological* refers to the social, political, economic, organizational, policy, regulatory, and other environmental circumstances

interacting with behavior in affecting health. (Green and Kreuter, 1999, p. 56).

- Health promotion is the science and art of helping people change their lifestyle to move toward a state of optimal health. Optimal health is defined as a balance of physical, emotional, social, spiritual, and intellectual health. Lifestyle change can be facilitated through a combination of efforts to enhance awareness, change behavior, and create environments that support good health practices. Of these three, supportive environments will probably have the greatest impact in producing lasting changes. (O'Donnell, 2002, p. 49).

- Health promotion is the process of enabling individuals and communities to increase control over their health. Furthermore, health promotion encompasses the principles that underlie a series of strategies that seek to foster conditions that allow populations to be healthy and make healthy choices. (WHO, 1988).

O'Donnell (1986) presents the Health Continuum Model (Figure 13-3) adapted from the work of John Travis, M.D. The extreme left end represents a state of severe illness or premature death, the midpoint represents a neutral point of no discernible illness, and the right end depicts a state of optimal wellness. O'Donnell points out that (1) traditional medicine has focused on the far left side of the continuum by

treating patients with chronic disabilities and disease and moving them toward the continuum's midpoint of a healthy state or a state where the disease process can be managed and controlled and (2) health promotion has traditionally focused on the right side of the continuum to support strategies/behaviors aimed at optimum health. These strategies are focused on changing, modifying, or enhancing health-

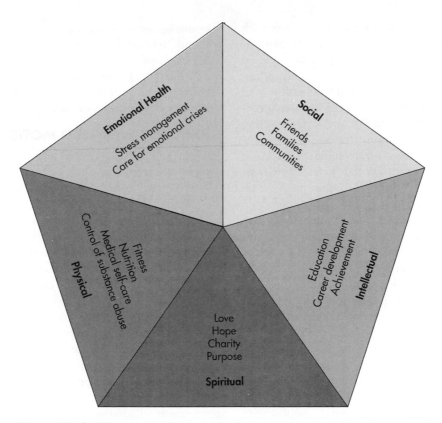

Figure 13-4   Dimensions of optimal health. *(From "Definition of Health Promotion," by M. P. O'Donnell, 1986,* American Journal of Health Promotion, 1, *6-9.)*

related behaviors and lifestyle practices of individuals who are presumed healthy but may be at risk of consequences damaging to health. O'Donnell (2002) further emphasizes that, to promote lifestyle changes that facilitate recovery and enhance health, health promotion activities also should be directed at individuals who may be in a process of rehabilitation. In this definition health promotion and health protection are not explicitly differentiated.

DIMENSIONS OF OPTIMAL HEALTH

O'Donnell (2002) indicates that employee health is affected by many dimensions of their lives—not just physical parameters—that are both modifiable and nonmodifiable (Figure 13-4). For example, an employee who practices healthy lifestyle behaviors (i.e., does not smoke, exercises regularly, eats healthy) may be overwhelmed and overloaded at work, creating a perfect stress-laden situation. Still another worker may appear to be

doing well professionally but may be a substance abuser. O'Donnell identifies five dimensions of optimal health (pp. xx-xxi):

1. *Physical* health refers to the physiological condition of a person's body, including the impacts from lifestyle behaviors such as smoking, physical activity, alcohol, and nutrition. Genetic and environmental influences may also play a role. Many worksite health promotion programs address these areas.
2. *Emotional* health refers to one's mental state of being. It encompasses the stresses in a person's life, how one reacts to those stresses, and the ability to relax and devote time to leisure. Increasing evidence links emotional health to health care utilization, susceptibility to disease, and unhealthy lifestyle practices. Worksite health promotion programs designed to address this area include stress management, employee assistance programs, and recreation and leisure programs.

3. *Social* health is the ability to get along with others, including family members, friends, professional colleagues, and neighbors. Social support has been shown to be very important in facilitating recovery and rehabilitation from disease, reducing the impact of stress on physical and emotional health, and even lowering disease and mortality rates. Additionally, social norms have a tremendous impact on lifestyle behaviors. Social health programs might include child and frail parent care programs; support groups; peer leadership development opportunities; culture change efforts; group recreation and sports teams; and skill development programs in communication, parenting, and assertiveness. Incorporating social health programs into workplace health promotion may represent the greatest opportunity available to us for improving the impact of our efforts.

4. *Spiritual* health is the condition of one's spirit, including having a sense of purpose in life, the ability to give and receive love, and feeling charity and goodwill toward others. For some people, religion will be a central component of spiritual health programs; for others it will not. Programs might include life planning workshops, service to voluntary and charitable organizations, and cooperative programs with religious groups. Research in this area is limited but growing.

5. *Intellectual* health is related to achievements in life, which can occur through work, school, community service, hobbies, or cultural pursuits. Intellectual health manifests its impact on overall health through relationships between education and healthy lifestyle practices; unemployment and disease; socioeconomic status and medical care utilization; and self-esteem, self-efficacy, and health practices. Psychoneuroimmunology and neuropsychology are beginning to help us understand these relationships. Intellectual health programs are unusual in workplace health promotion but in the future might include programs to enhance self-esteem and career planning and development efforts. Some of these might be best coordinated by training departments.

It is important to note that these areas should be complimentary rather than competing. For example, workaholics may sacrifice family and friend relationships for the sake of career advancement. Each area is important to optimal health, and O'Donnell emphasizes the need for a balance in all of these areas rather than sacrificing one area to achieve excellence in another.

PRECEDE-PROCEED MODEL

Green and Kreuter (1999) offer as a definition of health promotion "the combination of educational and ecological supports for actions and conditions of living conducive to health" (p. 56). The actions or behaviors in question may be those of individuals, groups, communities, policymakers, employers, teachers, or others whose actions control or influence the determinants of health. The authors discuss the lifestyle construct and place caution on the use of the term. They describe lifestyle as a complex of related practices and behavioral patterns, in a person or group, that is maintained with some consistency over time and, when considered within the context of health-related behaviors and practices, can be viewed as having consequences that either promote or damage health. In addition to individual responsibility for health, lifestyle changes require a multifaceted approach, including attention to cultural, socioeconomic, and environmental influences and regulatory, policy, and organizational initiatives. While Green and Krueter (1999) point out that changing lifestyle behaviors requires a long-term commitment involving complex health promotion strategies, they support the idea that actions and practices that affect even one determinant of health, such as smoking cessation or getting an immunization, should be emphasized within the context of health promotion program planning.

Green and Kreuter offer the comprehensive multiphase PRECEDE-PROCEED Model (Figure 13-5), designed through the use of specific data benchmarks and analyses, to help the health promotion planner (e.g., occupational and environmental health nurse) develop programs with targeted objectives, interventions, and evaluation processes. The PRECEDE framework considers the factors that shape health status (e.g., health, lifestyle, environment) and focuses on those targets for intervention through development of specific objectives and criteria for evaluation. PRECEDE is an acronym for *pre*disposing, *r*einforcing, and *e*nabling *c*onstructs in

PRECEDE

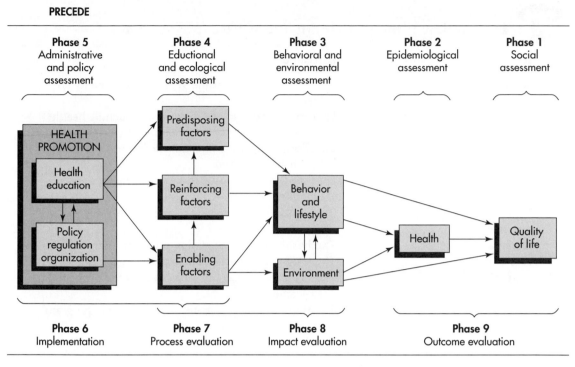

Figure 13-5   PRECEDE-PROCEED: A health promotion planning and evaluation model.
(Modified from Health Promotion Planning: An Educational & Environmental Approach, *by L. Green and M. Kreuter, 1999, Mountain View, CA: Mayfield. Reproduced with permission of the McGraw Hill companies.)*

educational/ecological *d*iagnosis and *e*valuation. The PRECEDE model, which is an acronym for *p*olicy, *r*egulatory, and *o*rganizational content in *e*ducational and *e*cological *d*evelopment, continues with the development of additional steps for policy formulation and the initiation of implementation and evaluation processes. Brief descriptions of the model phase elements are described here and in Table 13-6; however, the reader is referred to the reference for an in-depth discussion of the model and its application.

The PRECEDE model includes phases 1 through 5 and begins with Phase 1, which is a social assessment of the quality of life or health concerns of the target population within the context of the community or organizational environments in which people live and work. To have a successful program, the perceptions of health and related problems of the target group must be analyzed; otherwise, programs developed apart from group input and understanding may not succeed. Within the context of social assessment

in the occupational setting, the occupational and environmental health nurse should consider an inventory of concerns regarding occupational health exposures and problems, issues of productivity and morale, and safety (e.g., absenteeism, medical claims, injuries, substance abuse, violence) from both the workers' and management's perception.

Phase 2 involves epidemiologic assessment of data in preparation for planning a health promotion program and includes assessment of morbidity and mortality disability patterns and trends and other relevant health information, such as population risk factors, in order to target and prioritize specific health problems needing intervention. In addition, an epidemiologic assessment should consider which behavioral and environmental factors might contribute to the health problems. Programmatic goals and objectives in terms of mortality/morbidity reduction can then be developed. In the work setting a determination of the incidence and prevalence of work-related

TABLE 13-6   **Description of the PRECEDE-PROCEED Model Phases**

PHASES	DESCRIPTION
Social assessment	The social concerns of the group or community are identified.
Epidemiological assessment	Epidemiological data are examined to identify health problems.
Behavioral and environmental assessment	Behavioral and environmental risk factors that affect health are identified.
Educational and ecological assessment	Predisposing, reinforcing, and enabling factors are identified.
Administrative and policy assessment	Factors supporting or hindering program initiatives are examined.
Implementation	The health practice/education program is implemented.
Process evaluation	The program process is evaluated in an ongoing fashion.
Impact evaluation	The immediate effects or objectives of the program are evaluated.
Outcome evaluation	The short-term and long-term effects of the program are evaluated.

From *Health Promotion Planning: An Educational & Environmental Approach.*, by L. Green, and M. Kreuter, Mountain View, CA: Mayfield. 1999. *Reproduced with permission of the McGraw Hill companies.*

diseases and health problems, such as hearing loss, high blood pressure, stress, musculoskeletal disorders, or reproductive disorders, which may be aggravated by working conditions or family problems or both, will be beneficial in helping the occupational and environmental health nurse target interventions to reduce risk. Further, morbidity and premature mortality may be ultimately reduced through screening programs for early detection.

Phase 3 involves a systematic assessment of the behavioral and environmental links related to the health problems targeted in Phase 2. For example, controllable risk factors such as smoking, elevated cholesterol, obesity, and lack of exercise are related to cardiovascular diseases. An inventory of specific behavioral and environmental risks can be developed, which will then lead to the development of objectives to promote behavioral/environmental changes. In the work setting behavioral actions might include use of personal protective equipment, compliance with safety programs, and participation in voluntary health programs. Environmental influences relate to industrial monitoring, control of safety and

hygiene conditions, and issues of working conditions such as work schedules, work organization, and security.

Phase 4 involves the educational and ecological assessment of approaches likely to be employed in a health promotion program to bring about behavioral and environmental changes that are linked to health concerns. These include predisposing, reinforcing, and enabling factors. Predisposing factors include a person's knowledge, attitudes, beliefs, values, and perceptions that facilitate or hinder motivation to change. Reinforcing factors are rewards and/or positive feedback used to encourage or discourage continuation of the behavior. These include social support, peer influences, or a feeling of well-being (or pain) from exercise. Enabling factors are those skills or resources that facilitate or hinder the performance of the desired behavioral and environmental changes, such as the ability to physically participate in a fitness program.

The occupational health professional will find it helpful to examine factors that influence an individual's willingness, desire, or ability to participate in an educational intervention. For example, participation in a worksite skin cancer screening program could be influenced by predisposing factors such as knowledge and awareness of the risks associated with sun exposure; personal experience, such as having a relative with skin cancer; and/or the perceived value of early detection. Reinforcing factors that influence motivation to continue to participate in the program might include management's support, attitude and role modeling performance related to program participation, timely feedback about results of screening, and assured maintenance of confidentiality of the findings. Enabling factors include influences such as program accessibility and convenience. For example, offering the screening program on company time at the worksite can greatly influence participation. In addition, the ease or lack of discomfort related to the method of examination, such as skin observation in this example; the company-borne cost of the screening; and perhaps an incentive for participation, such as giving sunblock lotion, would be considered enabling factors.

Phase 5 is an assessment of organizational and administrative capabilities and resources needed for the development and implementation of a program. Issues related to personnel, space, equipment, money, and policy initiatives to support worker health and safety, such as release or flex time, are important to determine. In addition, the nurse will want to identify barriers, such as lack of commitment, negative attitude, or limitations on resources, to develop strategies to deal with these hindrances. For example, if a goal is to establish a smoke-free work environment, a determination needs to be made regarding the resources available to conduct or offer smoking cessation programs and the viability of establishing policy directives to support the change.

The PROCEED model segment includes phases 6 through 9. It begins with the implementation component, Phase 6, and employs a combination of methods and strategies, including staffing and marketing techniques appropriate to the intervention. The implementation phase may follow the following steps:

1. Introduction of the overall program to management
2. Announcement of the program to the employees
3. Recruitment and organization of a worker-management committee
4. In-house communication planning
5. Employee interest and risk factor surveys
6. Formation of subcommittees for each risk factor
7. Exploration of community risk factor reduction programs
8. Committee review and program selection
9. Development of a program proposal
10. Discussion of the proposal with management
11. Promotion of programs and recruitment of employees
12. Scheduling of programs
13. Program implementation, modification, and maintenance

The final phases, 7 through 9, include the evaluation components that will be dependent upon the objectives established during the initial phases of program development. Evaluation should target the effectiveness of available educational and organizational resources, program satisfaction, and behavioral and environmental changes made. For example, in a worksite skin cancer screening program, performance variables to measure knowledge/skill development and utilization might include doing a self-skin assessment, avoiding sun exposure, and using sunscreens. In addition, the evaluation of health-related outcomes such as increased productivity, improved performance, enhanced well-being, reduced morbidity and premature mortality, and improved quality of life will be important indicators to measure. The occupational and environmental health nurse may find this model helpful in the overall assessment, diagnosis, implementation, and evaluation of health promotion and protection programs, and this model can provide a comprehensive framework to guide practice options and evaluate findings in order to improve programming efforts.

HEALTH BELIEF MODEL

The Health Belief Model (HBM) is one of the models most widely used to explain why people do or do not take preventive health actions (Nemcek, 1990). The HBM was first developed in the early 1950s by Hochbaum (1958) and further explicated by Kegeles et al. (1965) and Rosenstock

(1966) to determine causes for nonparticipation in preventive measures, such as Pap smears and tuberculosis screening. Becker et al. (1974) and Becker et al. (1977) later modified the model (Figure 13-6) to include the influence of health motivation. The model also was viewed as potentially useful in suggesting interventions that might increase the predisposition of resistant individuals to engage in health promoting behaviors (Pender, 2002).

The HBM comprises three primary components, including individual perceptions, modifying factors, and factors affecting the likelihood of initiating or engaging in an action. Individual perceptions relate to beliefs about perceived susceptibility and the perceived seriousness of a specific illness to produce the degree of threat of that illness. Perceived susceptibility reflects an individual's feelings of personal understanding of a specific

health problem, and perceived seriousness reflects a person's degree of concern created by the thought of disease or problems associated with a given health condition. Perceived threat is the combined impact of perceived susceptibility and perceived seriousness.

Modifying factors include a variety of demographic, sociopsychological, and structural factors that predispose a person to take preventive action, and cues to action are factors that purport to trigger preventive health actions, depending on the person's level of readiness to engage in such activities. Examples of modifying factors are included in Figure 13-6.

The likelihood-of-action component of the model is driven by the positive difference between perceived benefits and perceived barriers (Becker et al., 1977). Perceived benefits are beliefs about the effectiveness of recommended preventive

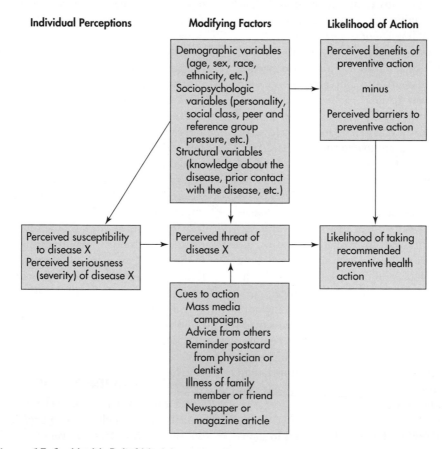

Figure 13-6 Health Belief Model. *(From "A New Approach to Explaining Sick-Role Behavior in Low Income Populations," by M. H. Becker, R. H. Drachman, and J. P. Kirscht, 1974,* American Journal of Public Health, 64*(3), 205-216.)*

health actions such as the ability of a screening test to detect a health problem. Perceived barriers are possible blocks or hindrances to engaging in preventive behaviors and include such factors as cost, inconvenience, and discomfort.

Several studies both support and negate the various constructs of the HBM. Rundull (1979) surveyed 500 senior citizens regarding taking the swine flu inoculation. While perceived susceptibility, benefits, and barriers were significantly correlated with obtaining the vaccination, perceived seriousness was not. However, vaccination studies conducted by Cummings et al. (1979) and Larson et al. (1979) found all four constructs to be significantly correlated.

Serxner et al. (2001) examined the relationship between behavioral health risks and worker absenteeism. Data on absenteeism and on 10 behavioral health risk areas (alcohol use, back care, driving, eating, exercise and activity, mental health, self-care, smoking/tobacco use, stress, and weight control) were collected from 35,451 employees. The authors examined whether higher health risks are associated with higher absenteeism and whether a reduction in health risks translates into a reduction in absenteeism. Results revealed that a significant relationship existed between health risks and absenteeism in all but 2 (alcohol use and self-care) of the 10 risk areas examined.

Several investigators have used the HBM to examine breast self-examination practices (BSE). The model proposes that women who practice BSE regularly will exhibit positive beliefs with respect to perceived susceptibility, seriousness, benefits, and health motivation. Perceived barriers are predicted to be minimal or absent. Champion (1999) studied women regarding BSE practices and found that perceived barriers to preventive actions, followed by health motivation, were the most important variables in explaining BSE behavior. The variables of perceived susceptibility, seriousness, and benefits were not significant. Masey (1986) found that perceived susceptibility and the demographic variables of younger age and higher education correlated positively with the frequency of BSE practice in a sample of 225 women.

Studies such as these suggest that certain demographic characteristics and beliefs regarding health and illness influence an individual's use of preventive health measures. The occupational and environmental health nurse can use this model to identify factors in the worker population that can facilitate or hinder compliance with health and safety programs. Programs and strategies can then be developed to meet specific workforce needs to increase participation in health promotion/protection activities.

The HBM offers some insight into utilization of preventive health; however, concern exists that the model lacks specificity in defining relationships between variables and lacks consistency in operationalizing and measuring variables across studies (Strecher & Rosenstock, 1997). Thus, further research is needed to test and refine the constructs to increase the validity of the model in order to fully operationalize health promotion programming efforts at the worksite. The occupational and environmental health nurse can help in this process through collecting and analyzing data when using the model for preventive health programming.

HEALTH PROMOTION MODEL

Pender (2002) indicates that the HBM is a model for health protecting (preventive) behaviors and is directed at decreasing the probability of experiencing illness by active protection of the body against pathological stressors or detection of illness in the asymptomatic stage. Pender suggests the Health Promotion Model (HPM) as a complementary counterpart that is directed at increasing the level of well-being and self-actualization of an individual or group. Health promoting behaviors are viewed as proactive rather than reactive.

The HPM was initially developed in the early 1980s and has since been revised (Figure 13-7) (Pender, 2002). It is structurally similar to the HBM; however, the HPM is a competence or approach-oriented model and does not include fear or threat as sources of motivation for health behavior. Pender indicates that although immediate threats to health have been shown to motivate action, threats in the distant future lack the same motivational strength. Thus, avoidance-oriented models of health behavior are of limited use in motivating overall healthy lifestyles, particularly in children, youths, and young adults, who often perceive themselves to be invulnerable to illness. Because the HPM does not rely on personal threat as a primary source of health

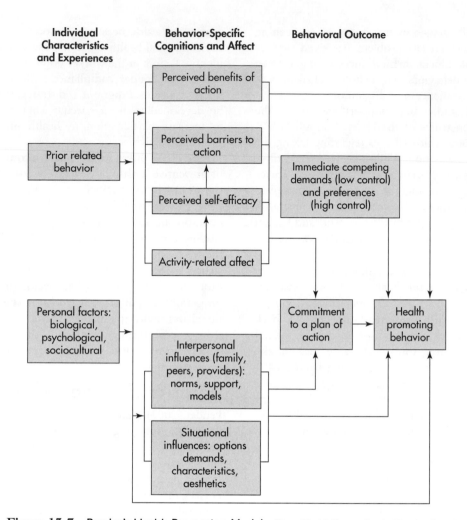

Figure 13-7 Pender's Health Promotion Model. *(From* Health Promotion in Nursing Practice *[4th ed.], by N. Pender, 2002. Reprinted by permission of Pearson Education, Inc., Upper Saddle River, NJ.)*

motivation, this model has potential applicability across the life span. In reality the sources of health behavior motivation for any given individual have a combination of unique properties, from predominantly health promotion or approach-oriented motives, through mixed motives of both approach and avoidance, to predominantly avoidance-oriented or protective motives. The HPM is applicable to any health behavior in which threat is not proposed as a major source of motivation for the behavior. The HPM is composed of three major components: individual characteristics and experiences, behavior-specific cognitions and affect, and behavioral outcome. Individual characteristics and experiences include the following:

- *Prior related behavior.* The likelihood of engaging in health promoting behaviors based on previous experience/actions
- *Personal factors.* Biological, psychological, and sociocultural factors that are amenable to modification

Behavior-specific cognitions and affect include the following:

- *Perceived benefits of actions.* Positive outcomes that influence the increased frequency of and continued participation in health promotion behaviors
- *Perceived barriers to actions.* The influence of barriers (e.g., inconvenience, discomfort) in

reducing engagement in health promoting behaviors

- *Perceived self-efficacy.* The ability of the individual to implement behavioral skills to enhance health
- *Activity-related affect.* The likelihood of an individual initiating and repeating an action/behavior, positive or negative (e.g., behaviors producing negative feelings are unlikely to be repeated)
- *Interpersonal influences.* Expectations or supports (or both) of significant others and health care professionals, and family patterns of health care
- *Situational influences.* Environmental or situational conditions or options that enhance or hinder health promoting alternatives (e.g., availability of vending machines with low nutrient or nonnutrient foods)

Behavioral outcome includes the following:

- *Health-promoting behavior.* The behavior or action directed toward positive health outcomes

According to the model, participation in health promoting behavior is concerned with the likelihood of implementing health promoting actions as viewed by a commitment to a plan of action. This involves identification of specific strategies for carrying out and reinforcing the behavior. In addition, the HPM recognizes that individuals have competing demands and preferences that must be acknowledged and resisted (e.g., choosing high fat foods). Strong commitment to a reasonable plan of action will help sustain dedication to complete the behavioral intent.

As an example, Lusk et al. (1999) tested a training intervention to increase the use of hearing protectors among construction workers. The constructs of perceived self-efficacy (mastery in using the hearing protection devices), interpersonal influences (role models using hearing protection devices), situational influences (discussion of environmental factors), and perceived barriers (successfully coping with using the devices) were tested. Results indicated a 20% increase in hearing protection use when evaluated after 10 months.

In a randomized trial, Buller et al. (1999) tested the effectiveness of a peer nutrition education program in increasing fruit/vegetable intake. At the end of the intervention and at the 6-month follow-up, the effects of the peer education program were seen in increases of the total daily serv-

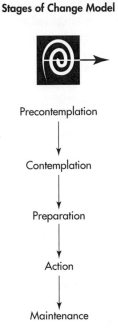

Stages of Change Model

Precontemplation

↓

Contemplation

↓

Preparation

↓

Action

↓

Maintenance

Figure 13-8   Stages of Change Model. *(From "Transtheoretical Therapy: Toward a More Integrative Model of Change," by J. O. Prochaska and C. C. DiClemente, 1982,* Psychotherapy: Theory, Research, and Practice, 19, *276-288.)*

ings measured by intake recall and food frequency questions. The 6-month follow-up survey revealed a persistent effect of the peer education program in increases of the total daily servings measured by intake recall. Findings in this study demonstrated that peer education influenced the dietary changes of populations of culturally diverse employees at workplaces, and these findings are consistent with the effects of interpersonal influences presented in the model.

The occupational and environmental health nurse can use the HPM model to evaluate facilitators and barriers that either enhance or negate preventive health activities. Programs can then be designed to effectively reduce the barriers to participation (e.g., cost, time) and increase strategies that support health improvement.

TRANSTHEORETICAL MODEL (STAGES OF CHANGE MODEL)

Another popular model is the Transtheoretical Model, also called the Stages of Change Model (Figure 13-8), which was developed by Prochaska and DiClemente (1982). Early on this model was applied to smoking cessation among adults. The model describes behavioral change actions and has since been applied to numerous health problems and behaviors, including eating behaviors, birth control practices, medication compliance, and mammography screening (Prochaska & Velicer, 1997). This model attempts to explain a five stage process through which individuals change their behavior:

1. *Precontemplation.* Individuals have no intention of changing behavior in the near future, typically defined as 6 months (i.e., generally unaware a problem exists).
2. *Contemplation.* Individuals recognize their problem and are considering changing the behavior in the next 6 months (e.g., thinking about stopping smoking).
3. *Preparation.* Individuals intend to change the behavior in next month or have engaged in recent sporadic behavior changes (e.g., tried to quit smoking).
4. *Action.* Individuals are actively engaged in behavior change (e.g., have stopped smoking for 6 months).
5. *Maintenance.* Individuals sustain behavior change for more than 6 months.

Prochaska and Diclemente (1982) identify 10 processes of change that are appropriate at different stages of behavior change and categorize these processes as either experiential (consciousness-raising, dramatic relief, self-reevaluation, environmental reevaluation, self-liberation, and social liberation) or behavioral (counter-conditioning, reinforcement management, stimulus control, and helping relationships). The nurse can identify the stage of change and utilize appropriate processes to help the employee move through the stages. In addition, an important element to consider—one that is significant in most attempts to change behavior—is relapse.

Marlatt and Gordon (1985) propose a model of relapse prevention for addictive behaviors such as alcoholism, smoking, obesity, and drug dependency, which have a high rate of recidivism. It is important to distinguish between lapse and relapse. A lapse is a slip that results in a single repeat of the addictive behavior, whereas a relapse is a return to the addictive behavior,

often with increased vigor. Marlatt and Gordon indicate that by allowing room for mistakes to occur but providing clients with preparatory training (coping responses) to deal with these lapses, relapses can be prevented. For example, the client in a weight loss program has an occasion of eating high fat foods (e.g., potato chips, cake). If taught appropriate coping responses, this may be a single event, and the individual feels competent at being able to return to sensible eating practices. According to the theory, this should result in a decreased probability of experiencing relapse. In contrast, the individual who lapses and has no coping responses to draw upon is likely to experience decreased self-efficacy for eating healthy, positive effects from return to unhealthy foods, and feeling guilty and "out of control."

Marlatt and Gordon propose that individuals experience enhanced self-efficacy and personal control from maintaining desired behavior. Perceived control will continue to strengthen but can be threatened by a high-risk situation defined as one that threatens self-control and can potentially trigger relapse. Three categories of events associated with high rates of relapse are negative emotional states (anger, frustration, depression, boredom); social situations (negative situations, such as interpersonal conflict, or positive situations, such as partying or relaxing with friends); and physical craving (withdrawal symptoms and physical response to cues). In these situations use of coping responses such as self-monitoring and relaxation training that have been learned and rehearsed as part of relapse-prevention training can prevent a lapse from becoming a relapse.

HEALTH PROMOTION PROGRAM PLANNING

Worksite health promotion programs are designed to reduce health risk and enhance employee well-being and movement toward a state of optimal health. Health promotion encompasses various activities such as physical fitness, weight and stress management, smoking cessation, good eating habits, self-care, substance abuse reduction, and maintenance of a work/life balance in order to improve the quality of life (Pelletier, 1996, 1999).

O'Donnell (2002) indicates that health promotion (and protection) programs should be targeted at three levels: awareness, lifestyle behavioral change, and supportive environments. Awareness programs are targeted at individuals and groups to increase their understanding of health and related risk factors. Awareness programs are most appropriate for those who need to increase their knowledge and reflect on attitudes and/or beliefs in order to effect a behavior change. These types of programs can be used as direct feeders to lifestyle change programs.

Lifestyle change programs go a step beyond awareness programs and help individuals make behavioral changes such as starting and sustaining exercise, eating nutritious foods, and enhancing communication and coping skills. Lifestyle change programs are most successful if they use a multistep process (i.e., introducing one or two programs/activities at a time), include a combination of educational and behavioral modification experiences, and take place over time. Lifestyle changes require stamina to sustain the change effort; relapse, as previously discussed, often occurs. Thus, supportive environment programs will better foster long-term changes (Allen & Allen, 1999).

Supportive environments seek to create an environment in the work setting that encourages a healthy lifestyle. An example of this would be a smoke-free work environment that makes it difficult to smoke at work. Families, friends, organizational/work cultures, coworkers, communities, and regulations can also help shape these environments (e.g., no smoking in the building, availability of jogging trails, or on-site exercise classes at work). Fostering a supportive environment or changing an environment to encourage a concept of health will go a long way in improving ultimate health behavior and outcomes. This will include changing the physical setting, company policies, and corporate culture; implementing health protection programs; and fostering employee ownership of health promotion events. Occupational and environmental health nurses are well-positioned to design programs that will help meet these aims and promote healthy behaviors and wellness (Selleck et al., 1989).

HEALTH PROMOTION PROGRAM MODEL

The Health Promotion Program Model (Figure 13-9) (Rogers, 1994, 2003) can be used by the occupational and environmental health nurse as a guide or framework for health promotion program development. The framework comprises four phases: assessment, planning/development, implementation, and evaluation.

Assessment

The health promotion program assessment phase includes a determination of the following components: corporate commitment and support, needs assessment, and availability of internal and external programs/services. Determining and obtaining commitment and support from top and middle management is essential to the success of any health promotion program. The occupational and environmental health nurse needs to assess management's attitude regarding employee health and safety, the company's corporate image, the cost-effectiveness of health programming, and personal attitudes about health promotion and protection activities. In addition, the nurse will want to determine what the organization is willing to contribute in terms of financial and physical support (space, equipment), personnel support, and employee off-duty participation. A management survey such as that shown in Appendix 13-1 can be useful in making this determination.

The occupational and environmental health nurse may find it necessary to persuade management of the benefits of health promotion, wellness, and health protection programs. This will often entail providing a review of the health indices of the employee population and related health care costs—which may be obtained from the insurance carrier—for specific employee illnesses and injuries. For example, comparing health care costs of smokers and nonsmokers and related absenteeism and productivity, providing benchmark data examples of successful programs from other companies, and being prepared to discuss different types of programs (educational, screening, behavior and environmental change) and cost options will lend support to the health promotion initiative. It is important that management's commitment be demonstrated through operational, strategic, and personnel resource

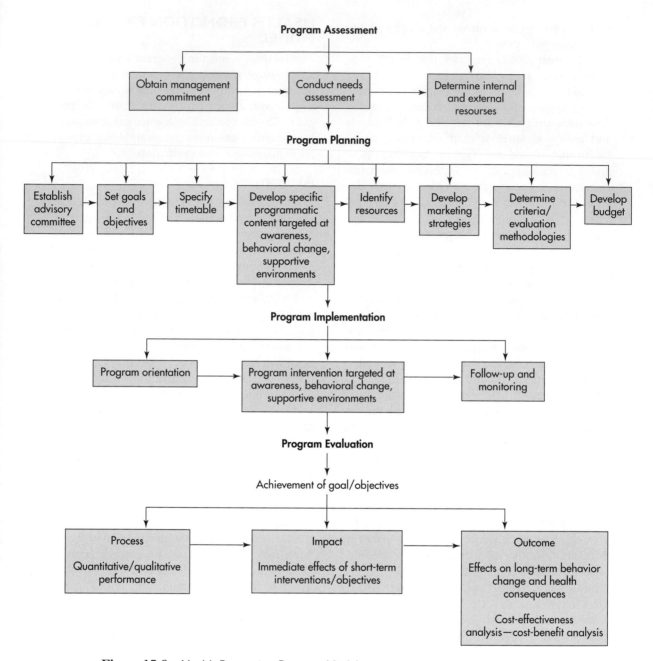

Figure 13-9 Health Promotion Program Model. *(Copyright 2003 by Bonnie Rogers.)*

allocation and managerial participation in program planning and visibility.

The second component of the assessment phase involves performing an employee needs assessment, which will help identify employee goals and interests. This information will help the occupational and environmental health nurse plan a more effective health promotion program and involve employees in the decision making for programming. In conducting the needs assessment, the nurse must know the following:

- Characteristics of the participants
- Any knowledge requirements

- Job and hazard analysis issues
- Regulatory requirements
- Health status indicators
- Interests/input of participants

A health interest survey that can be distributed to all employees or to a targeted group has several advantages, including the following:

- Gathering program ideas
- Fostering employee ownership of the program
- Providing some health education awareness
- Reducing resistance to future program participation
- Evaluating program impact

Numerous health interest surveys are available from various resources, and several examples from the Wellness Councils of America (1990) are included in Appendix 13-2. The occupational and environmental health nurse can also design a simple health interest survey specific to the company style and employee profile. Whatever format is used, the survey form should (1) be limited in length, (2) be graphically attractive, (3) ask relevant questions that are sensitive in tone and give the nurse useful information regarding health risks and needs, (4) include a variety of topics from which the employee can choose, (5) allow space for employees to write comments, and (6) indicate by which date and to whom the survey form should be returned.

A cover letter should accompany the survey, explain the concept of health promotion and wellness, and point out potential benefits. Emphasis should be placed on anonymity to ensure employee confidentiality of responses (Chapman, 1999b). A letter of support from the company manager or CEO that accompanies the survey may also help increase survey participation. After completing the needs assessment, employees should be provided with feedback about the survey results, which will be linked to program implementation.

Another tool to consider using when conducting the needs assessment is a health risk appraisal (HRA). General HRA forms cover many topics such as smoking, substance abuse, eating/nutrition habits, exercise and fitness, stress, safety, and other preventive health activities (e.g., mammography, BSE). HRAs may also be more specific and address each of these areas as singular topics or may be population-focused such as with women's health. By focusing on health behaviors, HRAs can enhance employee awareness of health risks and thus encourage thinking directed at making lifestyle changes. For employers, if HRAs disclose major health risks in the employee aggregate, the information can be very useful in program planning for targeted activities.

HRAs are usually self-administered either in paper and pencil format or via computer software packages. Scoring can be done on-site by the occupational and environmental health nurse, or the completed questionnaires (or computer discs) can be submitted to the vendor or HRA source, who scores the HRAs and then returns both individual and group results. Consideration of the best time for administering the HRA and informing employees about the process for education of the appraisal will help enhance participation. Many HRA forms come with an instruction manual that serves as a guide to present the questionnaire to participants and to interpret the responses. Individual counseling and referral regarding risk factors should be provided as appropriate.

Although aggregate data can be shared with management for program planning purposes, strict confidentiality of individual employee responses should be maintained so that only the employee and appropriate health professionals have access to the data. Demographic information about employees (e.g., age, sex, race, type of job), and past history of claims and payments for health insurance, workers' compensation, and disability, if accessible, can provide additional data about actual and potential health problems within the workplace (Selleck et al., 1989).

The Centers for Disease Control and Prevention, in conjunction with the Carter Center at Emory University, initially developed and distributed the HRA form in the late 1980s through 1991. That work continues through the Healthier People Network in Decatur, Georgia (Appendix 13-3). In addition, *healthfinder,* published by the Office of Disease Prevention and Health Prevention, Public Health Service, of the U.S. Department of Health and Human Services, provides numerous resources related to health promotion topics, including HRAs, which can be found at http://www.healthfinder.gov/.

Determining the availability and capabilities of existing internal and external programs and services is the third component of the assessment phase. The occupational and environmental health nurse will want to meet with other department managers such as food service and environment and safety to complete an inventory of programs and services currently offered to employees. This will also help determine the need for new programs or modification or expansion of existing programs and may enhance opportunities for health promotion program support and collaboration.

Making a determination about a supportive environment is part of the internal assessment. For example, is lighting adequate in work areas? Are ergonomics addressed? Do desk chairs cause back problems? Other examples of signs of support for a healthy environment include nonsmoking areas, vending machines stocked with healthful foods, nonalcoholic alternatives at company functions, rooms set aside for exercise classes, availability of shower facilities or bicycle racks, and appropriate security. It is also important to assess the types of space available for holding seminars, conferences, and/or exercise classes; the types of equipment available for specific program implementation (e.g., fitness equipment, scales, hematological instruments); and the methods used for communication of information (e.g., audiovisual, bulletin boards). Other areas such as a seat belt policy for company vehicles, an absenteeism policy that offers incentives for job attendance (and days off for illness), and flexible hours to attend to health and wellness needs can all add up to an environment that shows the company's commitment to good health.

Community resources can provide an enormous array of programs for employees, thus providing a more cost-effective and efficient approach to health promotion programming. The occupational and environmental health nurse can conduct an assessment of external nonprofit organizations such as the American Heart Association, American Lung Association, American Cancer Society, and American Red Cross to determine the types of educational materials or packaged programs available for cosponsoring with the company. Churches, temples, and community centers often have recreational facilities available to use for free or at

a low cost. Universities may have students in academic training programs such as nursing, nutrition, or exercise physiology who may be interested in participating in a health promotion program/service as part of a curricular learning requirement. In addition, communication and collaboration with other occupational and environmental health nurses and local nursing societies, and exploration of other available resources such as professional journals, newsletters, library references, and telephone directories may provide valuable information. The Internet provides information about and access to thousands of resources the occupational and environmental health nurse may choose in the planning and implementation of health promotion and protection programs (Machels, 1988), several of which are identified by Campbell and Ebert (2001). In addition, a listing of selected health promotion resources produced by the Federal Health Information Centers and Clearinghouses can be found in Appendix 13-4. Utilization of existing internal and external resources will prove beneficial not only in cost containment but also in collaborative initiatives and sharing of ideas and resources.

Planning and Development

The health promotion planning phase is critical to a successful effort and includes the following:

- Forming an advisory committee
- Setting goals and measurable objectives
- Setting a timeline for implementation and completion of activities
- Developing specific programmatic content and delivery strategies
- Identifying program resources
- Developing marketing strategies
- Identifying employee benefits
- Determining evaluation criteria methodologies
- Developing a budget

A successful health promotion program requires a high level of employee and employer participation. Thus, forming a health promotion planning and advisory committee can help foster both employee and management ownership of the program and encourage an environment supportive of health behavior change. Committee members should include the occupational and environmental health nurse and other appropriate health care professionals (e.g., the physician or industrial hygienist), respected employee leaders, representatives from management who can provide company support, line supervisors, individuals responsible for other program areas (e.g., compensation/benefits, employee assistance, dietary), and union representatives, if appropriate. The worksite health promotion manager, who often is the nurse, should be responsible for coordinating and providing leadership and direction for programmatic activities.

The advisory committee is usually involved with reviewing all pertinent aggregate data relative to health promotion activities, obtaining information about successful health promotion programs in other companies, and reviewing historical information about the successes and failures of previously tried program activities. Specific determinations can then be made about the types and extent of program activities to be developed. In addition, committee members can serve as a sounding board for ideas prior to their implementation, help market the program to employees, and provide feedback on program operation (Allen & Allen, 1999).

Goals and objectives set the framework for measuring program successes. Program goals and objectives are based on priorities identified through employee needs assessment and other available data; however, the prudent planner will pay particular attention to employee interests that scored high on the surveys and supplement them with information from HRAs and other data sources. Goals are broad statements that provide the overall direction for the intended activity, and objectives are measurable statements of the intended outcome derived from the goals. For example, the goal might be to increase the employees' understanding of HIV/AIDS. Objectives would be stated as programmatic, a statement of activity to be carried out by the program, or behavioral, a statement of desired individual change, or both; these objectives would include a knowledge, behavior, or biomedical parameter such as the following:

1. Provide information on HIV transmission and prevention (programmatic).
2. By the end of the program session the employee will be able to state the routes of transmission of HIV (behavioral).

Box 13-5 Objectives Terminology	
BEHAVIORAL TERMS TO USE	**NONBEHAVIORAL TERMS TO AVOID**
To record	To know
To write	To think
To list	To learn
To state	To stipulate
To name	To perceive
To compare	To understand
To match	To appreciate
To identify	To comprehend
To explain	To be familiar with
To select	To develop an
To define	appreciation of
To demonstrate	To develop conceptual
	thinking
	To view

When setting goals and objectives, expected outcomes must be considered because one approach will promote health awareness while another will be more supportive of behavior change as previously described. Box 13-5 shows examples of both behavioral terms, which are clear and amenable to measurement, and nonbehavioral terms, which are broad and ambiguous, represent a process rather than an outcome, and are more difficult to measure than behavioral terms.

Setting a timetable for health promotion program development will help foster a logical flow of activities. For most organizations the best strategy for program implementation is timely or organized planning through which programs can be gradually phased in. This often begins with one or two programs and later develops into a more comprehensive approach to health and wellness. In addition, organizing programs or activities around national campaigns such as the Great American Smokeout or National Safety Week may add impetus to employee participation. An example of a timeline for program planning development is shown in Box 13-6.

Program content development will be based on the goals and objectives set forth in the plan and will be targeted at awareness and education, behavioral change, and development of supportive environments. A comprehensive approach to worksite

---

Box 13-6   Timeline for Organizing Health and Wellness Programs/Activities

Following are some general rules of thumb concerning when to schedule wellness programs:

- Good times to launch wellness programs are in the fall (September), at the new year (January), and any time in the spring (March, April, and May).
- Workshop series should be planned for the same day and time each month.
- Aerobics should be planned for lunch time if showers are available, and at the end of the workday if showers are not available. Eliminate summer scheduling of indoor aerobics because people usually like to be outside in the summer.
- Schedule multiple offerings of the same type of activity. For example, schedule several sessions of a stress management workshop, with an evening session offered for spouses and second-shift workers.
- Plan a health and fitness testing activity to take place right before you offer programs such as smoking cessation and weight management so that people have a logical follow-up to the testing process.

- Start out with "lunch and learn" sessions on employees' time. Then later offer activities that are scheduled on work time.
- Publish an article in the employee newsletter on the personal side of a wellness topic and then follow up with a workshop or program.
- Don't plan too much at one time. Spread the program offerings out over the year so that every couple of weeks some event or wellness issue comes to the attention of employees.
- Tag along with national campaigns such as the Great American Smokeout in November of each year or National Employee Health and Fitness Day (held annually in May). Brochures, posters, table tents, fact sheets, and press releases are usually free for the asking. Your Wellness Council can keep you supplied with materials and ideas.
- Start your program and build it slowly. That way you can assure that the quality will be good. Employees will recognize that the wellness program will be around for the long haul.

From *Healthy, Wealthy, Well and Wise,* by Wellness Councils of America, 1990, Omaha, NE.: Author.

---

health promotion and health protection should fit with the company's commitment and philosophy toward health and wellness and employee needs and may include a variety of programs focusing on such areas as exercise, nutrition, weight loss, smoking cessation, stress management, coping enhancement, and risk factor screening (Campbell, 1991; Wachs & Parker-Conrad, 1990). Numerous and specific types of programs, such as back care or prenatal education, can be offered, but which ones to offer will depend on an analysis of workforce needs (Bigbee & Jonsa, 1991). The occupational and environmental health nurse may develop health promotion/protection programs for groups of employees based on aggregate interests or identified needs and may provide individual counseling about selected risk factors or health problems. The nurse will want to determine awareness, knowledge, and behavior of the employee(s) so that appropriate counseling and education interventions can be initiated. In addition, the program

content and delivery will also depend on the objectives, budget, and whether the program is developed in-house or provided by an external contractor.

Several factors, including age, gender, ethnicity, perception, and social and family support, will influence participation in health promotion programs. These factors need to be taken into account when planning any programs. For example, studies show that women are more likely than men to engage in preventive health programs and that family and other forms of social support help strengthen efforts in the modification of lifestyle health habits (Rose, 1989; Sandroff et al., 1990). In addition, health promotion activities at the worksite help create an atmosphere that supports and rewards health-promoting behaviors. The occupational and environmental health nurse will want to consider these factors when planning programs.

After reviewing available resources, the nurse can then develop a program in-house or use an external source program. The latter is often a prepackaged program, from which there are several to choose. If the nurse decides to develop a specific health promotion educational program in-house, several considerations need to be explored related to course design and content delivery methods.

Course design should include the following:

1. Content
   a. Information to achieve learning objectives
      Based on current literature, scientific principles
   b. Subject matter expertise
   c. Regulatory requirements
2. Instructional materials
   a. Audio-visual aids
   b. Handouts
   c. Resources
   d. Maturity, interests
3. Time allocation
   a. Meeting of objectives
   b. Sequence of content
      1) Simple to complex
      2) Familiar to unknown
      3) Concrete to abstract
   c. Interaction with participants
   d. Number of participants
   e. Teaching strategies

Content delivery methods should include the following:

1. On the Job Training (OJT)
2. Lecture
3. Discussion
4. Computer-based training
5. Group exercises
6. Distance learning
7. Demonstrations
8. Simulations
9. Independent study
10. Practice makes perfect

As an example, one option for planning and developing a nutrition program will be discussed.

The decision to develop and offer a nutrition program should take into account the previous factors discussed, such as employee interests and needs, available resources, and management's commitment to the program. Adequate nutrition is essential to healthy living and also plays a part in the prevention and control of many types of diseases, such as cardiovascular disorders, cancer, diabetes, obesity, and hypercholesterolemia. Convenience foods constitute a significant portion of the U.S. diet, and many of these types of food are high in fat, salt, and refined carbohydrates and are low in fiber. It is important to establish baseline information about what employees' concerns and knowledge are about nutrition and eating practices.

Glanz et al. (1996) suggest that the most effective health promotion programs involve many approaches at varying levels, including employee awareness, employee knowledge, behavior change, and supportive workplace environments. Nutrition awareness is the first step in promoting healthy food choices and working with employees to further their understanding about the nature of different food groups and their relationship to healthy and unhealthy states. What is taught or discussed will be dependent on the employees' needs. However, general topics for discussion might include the basics of good nutrition, the consequences of poor nutrition, and the role of exercise as a contributing practice. Other awareness activities might include distributing literature or pamphlets on a certain topic such as cholesterol, posting information on bulletin boards, or publishing information in the company newsletter.

Increasing employee knowledge, which is a higher level activity, is the next step designed to help employees begin to make behavioral change and expands on information generated through awareness activities. The occupational and environmental health nurse may consider asking a registered dietitian to help plan and/or participate in the program activities or teaching. This level of program planning and development might include the following:

1. Planning a Nutrition Awareness Month
2. Developing an extended nutrition educational seminar series over a period of 6 to 10 weeks (Box 13-7), which would involve increased employee participation, such as sharing of experiences
3. Inviting family members to participate in nutrition activities
4. Involving employees in developing newsletter publications through, for example, contributing healthy recipes or providing healthy cooking tips

---

Box 13-7 **Suggested Topics for a 10-Week Nutrition Management Program**

WEEK 1: ORIENTATION AND ASSESSMENT

- Program goals, methods, and content
- Individual assessment and goal setting
- Nutrition and exercise—weekly participation

WEEK 2: BASICS OF GOOD NUTRITION

- The role of nutrition in prevention
- Nutrient and caloric density
- Important nutrients
- Food-drug interactions
- Establishing a healthy eating pattern-nutrient balance
- Review food diary, calorie regulation

WEEK 3: FACTORS INFLUENCING EATING BEHAVIOR

- Biological factors
- Psychological factors
- Sociocultural factors
- Environmental factors
- Sharing experiences

WEEK 4: REVIEW OF EXERCISE AND NUTRITION AND SELF-MONITORING TECHNIQUES

- Exercise theory and recommendations
- Exploring variety in exercise
- Exercise activity record
- Food diary relationship

WEEK 5: MEAL PLANNING

- Shopping strategies
- Menu planning
- Low fat cooking techniques (microwave, stir-fry)

WEEK 6: BEHAVIORS AND ATTITUDES ABOUT NUTRITION MANAGEMENT

- Behavior modification and stress management techniques
- Review of nutrition weight-management myths
- Effects of personal relationships

WEEK 7: BODY IMAGE

- Effect of genetics on body size and shape
- Making peace with your body

WEEK 8: SPECIAL EATING SITUATIONS

- Eating in restaurants
- Holiday (party/celebration) situations
- Traveling

WEEK 9: RELAPSE PREVENTION

- Coping with problem times
- Support systems

WEEK 10: MAINTAINING MOTIVATION

- Motivational techniques—highlights of nutrition/exercise
- Review of personal goals
- Overview of weight maintenance theory

---

5. Obtaining physiological measurements of height and weight for comparative purposes

It is important to remember that planning for behavioral changes will require more intense participation by employees, the occupational health professionals, and others responsible for the program (MacStravic, 1999). Nutrition education must remain an integral part of the program so that employees can develop an understanding of the adverse physical and psychological effects of fad and quick weight loss diets. Strategies need to be developed to include family members in any nutritional education/behavior modification efforts because family members significantly influence dietary practices. Examples of activities designed to promote behavioral changes include the following:

1. Self-monitoring of eating practices and habits (e.g., food/behavior diaries)
2. Using self, family, or significant other reward reinforcement strategies
3. Contracting for nutrition/eating practice changes
4. Participating in group sessions
5. Engaging in regular physical activity

Each of these activities will need to be discussed in the planning/development phase as to where focused efforts should be directed. In addition, planning for strategies to deal with potential obstacles that may interfere with the behavior change, such as with nutrition behavior, might include changing eating behaviors, reaching a plateau, prematurely ceasing new

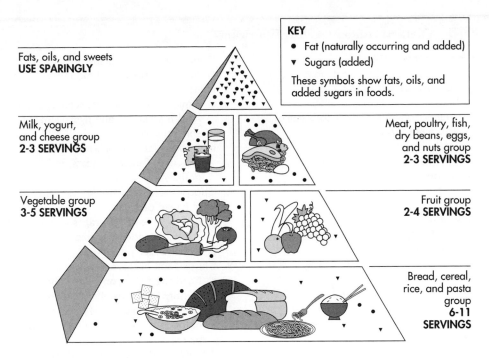

Figure 13-10   Food Guide Pyramid: A guide to daily food choices.   *(From* Food Guide Pyramid: A Guide to Daily Food Choices, *by U.S. Department of Agriculture, U.S. Department of Health and Human Services, 1992, Washington, DC: Author.)*

behaviors, rewarding weight loss with food treats, or having interpersonal difficulties with significant others because of physical changes (Pender, 2002). Having a supportive environment is of paramount importance in the program's success. This will usually require enhanced commitment on the part of management in further resource allocation and supporting environmental changes. Examples of environmental strategies include providing the following:

1. Company-sponsored cooking classes for employees and family members
2. Nutritious foods in the cafeteria with caloric, sodium, and cholesterol content displayed
3. Nutritious foods in vending machines
4. Space/equipment for exercise or developing a walking/jogging trail

The next step is to identify resources needed for the program, which again will vary depending on the program focus (e.g., awareness, behavioral change). However, for any health promotion effort numerous print and interactive media are widely available. Locating government and private vendor resources on the Internet will be very useful, as will be obtaining assistance from a health sciences library. For example, for the nutrition program, using the "Food Guide Pyramid: A Guide to Daily Food Choices" (Figure 13-10), accompanied by a discussion of dietary guidelines developed by the U.S. Department of Agriculture (Box 13-8), will be a valuable visual tool; these can be obtained from the government source via the Internet. Also, in any training session the information presented must be accurate and delivered in ways that can be understood without being boring. The qualifications of any program trainer must be assessed so as to affect content delivery. Criteria for evaluating a trainer should include subject matter expertise, training delivery skills, and continuing knowledge.

Marketing the health promotion program is critical to program success. Marketing strategies are designed to attract individuals into the program and provide sufficient benefits, incentives, or challenges to maintain commitment to

---

Box 13-8 **Dietary Guidelines for Americans**

1. Aim for a healthy weight.
   a. Evaluate your weight. Avoid weight gain or lose weight to improve your health.
   b. Get regular physical activity to balance calories from food.
2. Be physically active each day.
   a. Engage in at least 30 minutes of moderate physical activity each day.
   b. Stay active throughout your life.
3. Let the pyramid guide your food choices.
   a. Build your eating pattern on a variety of plant foods, including whole grains, fruits, and vegetables.
4. Eat a variety of grains daily, especially whole grains.
   a. Make a variety of grain products a foundation of your diet.
   b. Eat six or more servings of grain products daily.
5. Choose a variety of fruits and vegetables daily.
   a. Enjoy five a day.
   b. Choose fresh, frozen, or canned forms and a variety of colors and kinds.
6. Keep foods safe to eat.
   a. Keep clean. Wash hands and surfaces often.
   b. Cook foods to a safe temperature. Refrigerate perishable foods.
7. Choose a diet that is low in saturated fat and cholesterol and moderate in fat.
   a. Limit use of solid fats, such as butter, hard margarines and hydrogenated shortenings.
   b. Choose fat-free or low fat dairy products, fish, lean meats, and poultry.
8. Choose beverages and foods to moderate your intake of sugar.
   a. Limit intake of beverages and foods that are high in added sugars.
   b. Drink water often.
9. Choose and prepare foods with less salt.
   a. Read the Nutrition Facts Label to identify foods lower in sodium.
   b. Use herbs, spices, and fruits to flavor food, and cut the amount of salt by half.
10. IF YOU DRINK ALCOHOLIC BEVERAGES, DO SO IN MODERATION.
    a. Limit alcoholic beverages to one per day for women and two per day for men.
    b. Some persons should not drink: women who are pregnant or trying to become pregnant; persons who cannot moderate their alcohol intake; persons using certain prescription and over-the-counter medications.

From *Nutrition and Your Health: Dietary Guidelines for Americans,* by U.S. Department of Agriculture and U.S. Department of Health and Human Services, 2000, Washington, DC: Author.

---

participation. Some strategies for in-house marketing might include the following:

- Inviting employees to a healthy breakfast to introduce the program
- Distributing a letter from the CEO that promotes the wellness concept and related programs to employees
- Using posters and fliers to advertise the programs
- Publishing a calendar of events to give employees an advance preview
- Capturing photos of the programs and displaying them on a poster in the lunchroom, break room, or employee entrance for viewing
- Disseminating information about the program and any results in the company newsletter

In addition, promoting a positive company image is also important to the health promotion effort, and this can be done through use of media public service announcements. Marketing activities should be scheduled several weeks in advance of the health promotion program, building from week to week, thus providing a continued stimulus for sustained interest in the program (Kizer, 1987; O'Donnell, 2002).

Incentives, which are offered to stimulate employee motivation for program participation, may be considered as part of the overall marketing design. Incentives are viewed as something the employee values in exchange for a prescribed action or behavior, which may range from program attendance to a sustained lifestyle change, such as quitting smoking (Wellness Councils of America, 1990). Incentives may be offered for program participation, program completion, and behavioral change. Examples include the following:

For program participation
- Door prizes for those attending wellness events
- Discount fees for early registration
- "Bring a buddy" bonus
- Free or subsidized lunches
- Health snacks
- Beverages for brown baggers

For program completion
- Bonuses for perfect attendance
- Prize drawings for near perfect attendance
- Formal certificates for attendance
- T-shirts, sportswear, and other material goods for high attendance

For behavioral changes
- Write-up in newsletter of an employee who makes a major health habit change
- Fee rebate for sustained weight loss or completing a course
- Day off after 1 year of successful, sustained, behavior change

Although the formal evaluation strategy is conducted after the program implementation, an evaluation plan should be determined in the planning phase. As discussed by Selleck et al. (1989), evaluation need not be costly or conducted by experts. The main purposes for evaluating programs are to determine that program objectives were met and ensure that funds for program planning were used appropriately, efficiently, and effectively. Evaluation development includes the creation of any forms that will be necessary to gather appropriate data for evaluation. Evaluation methods are developed to measure employee and employer benefits that accrue from the health promotion program, including cost/benefits, reduction in data claims and accidents, and cost-effectiveness. Measures for evaluation from participants should be derived from the program objectives. Thus an evaluation plan for a weight loss program may call for the collec-

tion and analysis of preintervention and postintervention data on dietary knowledge and dietary choices, weight loss, and cost elements.

According to Chapman (1999a), program evaluation is important for the following reasons:

1. To verify what improvements should be made in the program
2. To document the effects of the program on behavior, risk factors, quality of life, and economic variables
3. To respond to the concerns of critics
4. To penetrate blind spots in programming
5. To contribute to the knowledge base in occupational and environmental health nursing
6. To help secure future funding
7. To provide an opportunity for career visibility

In developing the evaluation plan, the following questions will need to be addressed (Chapman, 1999a; O'Donnell, 2002):

1. Why should programs be evaluated?
2. What should be evaluated?
3. Should the focus be on a few or many outcome measures?
4. How much program activity actually reached employees?
5. How many employees participated in the program?
6. How many employees completed the program?
7. What difference in individual health risk factors were achieved?
8. How many employees actually made the desired behavior change?
9. How much did the program cost?
10. What effect did the program have on illness, injury, and risk reduction?
11. What effect did the program have on employee health benefit costs?
12. What was the net economic effect (cost/benefit) of the program?
13. What improvements should be made in the program for next year?
14. Why do health promotion programs fail?
15. Can results be generalized from one program to another?

Elements in evaluation will be discussed later.

In planning for the program, a budget will need to be developed. When developing the budget, several points should be considered, such as whether a singular or more comprehensive program will be offered; what external resources will be utilized with associated costs anticipated (e.g., consultants, HRAs, educational materials, instructors); the number of employees expected to participate in the program(s); and how costs will be paid—that is, will the company pay all costs (e.g., screening programs) or will cost for some programs (e.g., smoking cessation) be shared?

Determining resources and developing the budget entails reviewing, from the assessment phase, what currently exists within the company in terms of such quantities as human resources, space, equipment, and supplies, and what is available from external community resources. Based on this review, determinations can be made about additional resources needed for new or expanded programs within the context of the goals, objectives, and feasible budget allocations.

In general, when planning for health promotion programs, the following operational costs should be considered: utilization of company personnel such as graphic artists from other departments; additional professional staff such as consultants, instructors, technicians, and support staff; equipment and supplies; audiovisual aids and educational materials, such as pamphlets, slides, and video tapes; refreshments; incentives, marketing materials, and printing; off-site space and travel; and program evaluation. Indirect costs related to employee off-duty time may also need to be factored in, particularly when determining program cost-effectiveness. Every effort should be made to develop a realistic budget that allows for implementation of the programmatic objectives, and each objective specified should be incorporated into the budget.

Implementation

The implementation phase of the health promotion program is the actual action phase of the overall program. The implementation phase flows from the planning phase and should run smoothly, assuming planning has been adequate and realistic.

Implementation is concerned with carrying out the steps outlined in the plan—that is, putting the plan into action. This involves program orientation, conducting the program or intervention, and follow-up and monitoring. Program enrollment and orientation provide the participant the opportunity to understand the purpose of the program and the expected outcome. Here, the occupational health professional will want to discuss the overall meaning of the program or intervention, explain each objective and how it will be implemented and evaluated, and indicate expected outcomes related to the objectives and how and when the outcomes will be measured (i.e., short-term, long-term).

The next step is the actual implementation of the program or intervention targeted at awareness, behavioral change, or supportive environmental change or some combination of each of these elements. As previously described, awareness approaches are major strategies used in worksite health promotion programs. *Awareness strategies* are defined by O'Donnell (2002) as "a variety of communication dissemination and information transfer activities that are intended to enhance the knowledge levels of individuals, help catalyze and reinforce behavior change, while intentionally leading to improved individual health and productivity" (p. 166).

Awareness strategies are intended to do the following:

- Communicate relevant information to help prepare the individual for behavior change;
- Help empower and enable the individual to devise a plan to use the information received;
- Help the individual gain practical access to information that can assist in the reinforcement of the specific behavior.

Examples of awareness communication methods are shown in Box 13-9. There are several implementation approaches that can help increase the effectiveness of awareness strategies for adult learning, (Chapman, 1996) including the following:

1. *Showing, discussion, application.* Participants are shown the information in ways they can understand; the information is discussed so that it can be assimilated, and finally the

---

Box 13-9   **Awareness Communication Methods**

TRADITIONAL	NONTRADITIONAL	TECHNOLOGY-BASED
Announcements during meetings	Information-based puzzles, acrostics, or limericks	Electronic mail
Written individual notices	Self-quizzes	Proactive telephone contact
Bulletin board notices	Health risk appraisals	Computer-based multimedia presentations
Printed pamphlets	Mail-requested vehicles	Interactive voice response
Payroll inserts	Trigger cards	Tailored messaging
Marquees and electronic billboards	Electronic bulletin boards	Interactive informational kiosk
Face-to-face individual information sessions	Fax networks	Internet websites
Group information sessions	Online telephone support	Virtual reality applications
Audio presentations		Adaptive survey technology
Audiovisual presentations		
Video presentations		

---

information is applied by the participants to their particular situation.

2. *Repetitive exposure.* Multiple repetitions of unfamiliar material are offered to make the information familiar.

3. *Experiential learning.* This powerful learning strategy places participants in the position of actually implementing a given strategy, such as content teaching or participation in the conducting of health risk appraisals.

4. *Incremental information introduction.* Information should be introduced in small doses so as not to overwhelm participants with too much information, which might not then be assimilated. By exceeding the participants' capacity for learning, it is possible to cause a "freeze-up" in the learning process, resulting in a halt to learning progression.

5. *Value-added approach.* Information is presented that demonstrates the benefits or value to the participant. Information not viewed as relevant is more difficult for the participant to internalize than is information viewed as relevant.

Behavioral change flows from an elevated awareness of the target problems or behavior needing modification. In approaching behavioral change, it is important to first understand the basis of the behavior and then introduce strategies that will help the individual change the unhealthy behavior to a healthy behavior. Earlier in this chapter

Box 13-10   **Health Behavior Change Strategies**

- Readiness to change
- Referent power
- Goal setting and self-monitoring
- Reinforcement/incentives
- Behavior contract
- Social supports

a variety of health promotion models were discussed. These can be used as frameworks for understanding why certain behaviors occur, and then appropriate strategies can be introduced to assist in behavioral change.

Many common strategies can be used to assist individuals to consider, adopt, and adhere to healthy behavior changes (Box 13-10). A full discussion of each of these is beyond the scope of this text; however, each is mentioned here.

- *Readiness to change.* Assessing the individual's willingness to entertain behavioral change is important. As pointed out in Prochaska's Stages of Change theory, individuals in the precontemplation stage have no immediate intent to change behavior. Determining behavior change readiness can be done by asking individuals to enroll in health promotion activities (enrollment = readiness) or distributing questionnaires about willingness or readiness (e.g., using a Likert-type scale: 1 = *very ready* to 5 = *not at all ready*) to determine readiness interest. This can then help determine if behavioral change is a likelihood.

- *Referent power.* Individuals may be motivated to change their behavior because another person influences the desire to change (Janis, 1983). Here, the "helper" builds motivation by helping the individual self-disclose the problem and supports this with his/her own self-disclosure and offering positive encouragement; next, the helper uses motivational power to effect the desired change through endorsing specific actions, eliciting commitment and responsibility for the action, and providing positive feedback; and finally, the helper promotes the individual's internalization of the change through giving reassurances of continued maintenance of the change, giving reminders of the individual's commitment to and responsibility for the behavior, and building the individual's self-confidence about succeeding.

- *Goal setting and self-monitoring.* This is the process of helping the individual set appropriate and specific behavioral change goals that are defined, achievable, and measurable. Individual goals should be self-determined or negotiated with the health care professional or some combination of both. In general, goals of specific behavioral change (e.g., reduce the number of fat grams consumed per day to 25 or less) is more useful than goals for specific outcomes (e.g., lose 20 pounds in 8 weeks) (O'Donnell, 2002). Self-monitoring is fairly straightforward and involves self-observation by the individual for the specific behavior, such as monitoring caloric intake. The behavior can then be modified accordingly. Being successful in goal achievement in small increments will be beneficial and encouraging. This can also be complemented by having the individual observe model behavior in peers. Self-efficacy, or the belief that one can make the change, is crucial in initiating any change in behavior.

- *Reinforcement/incentives.* A variety of reinforcement strategies, such as reward and positive feedback to help the individual stay on target, can be used to promote healthy behavioral changes. Incentives can take on many forms, such as public recognition, directed monetary payment or gifts, or credits given toward larger rewards. Gradually, external reinforcements are phased out over time, with internal intrinsic rewards substituting as the benefit.

- *Behavior contract.* The individual contracts in writing, usually with a health care professional, about specific behavioral changes intended and agreed upon, with dates for change included. The intent is to foster a higher degree of commitment to the behavioral change.

- *Social supports.* Most people need the support of at least one other individual to make a behavioral change. This support can be from family, friends, coworkers, or peers. Individuals can identify the supporters, and in that way support can enhance the behavior change. Human behavior is multidimensional and is often similar to figuring out a puzzle when it comes to understanding what makes someone change a specific behavior. No one simple strategy will fit all or even one individual, but a combination of strategies will most likely be useful.

Supportive cultural environments at the worksite are aimed at enhancing and fostering healthy behaviors of workers. This means that the organization itself adopts approaches to facilitate its employees' behavioral change processes. This includes designing and organizing strategies to promote health, such as putting in place health friendly policies like no smoking at the worksite, encouraging health fitness by providing exercise programs or jogging trails, and offering healthy food choices whether in the cafeteria or through vending machines. In addition, participating in teams with peer support in aggregate wellness program initiatives, identifying role modeling behaviors, working through relapse, monitoring behavior, participating in support group endeavors, and celebrating the successes of achievements will be particularly helpful in supportive worksite climates.

In the work environment a sense of community, shared vision, and positive outlook will be foundational to a supportive environment (O'Donnell, 2002). This starts with the leadership's commitment to a healthy work environment, a commitment that fosters positive work practices, healthy lifestyles, and environments conducive to healthy behaviors. Examples of supportive environments are shown in Box 13-11.

Follow-up and monitoring completes the implementation phase. Follow-up is done with employees to determine if there are issues of clarification that need to be addressed, and if any questions need to be answered; to offer continued support, encouragement, and motivation; and to determine barriers to effective achievement of the employee's goals. In the case of screening programs offered as a prevention strategy, follow-up is particularly important when a referral has been made for an abnormal finding such as elevated cholesterol or elevated blood pressure.

Monitoring includes implementing a tracking program to maintain contact with program participants to monitor both short-term and long-term progress toward achievement of behavioral change. The monitoring system itself should be planned and developed prior to implementation. Results of monitoring should be evaluated during this phase.

EVALUATION

The final phase of the health promotion program is program evaluation. Evaluation, which actually begins in the planning phase, denotes the extent to which the program has met preestablished goals and objectives and desired program outcomes. O'Donnell (2002) identifies potential benefits of worksite health promotion programs to both employees and employers (Box 13-12). These benefits should be considered when developing an evaluation plan. Although individuals have responsibility for certain health-related behaviors such as smoking and diet, strong social pressures, particularly in some work groups, can condone or encourage smoking, or the cafeteria or vending machines may not offer sufficient

---

Box 13-11   **Examples of Supportive Environments**

- Physical environment conducive to health/safety
- Healthy food offerings
- No cigarette vending machines
- Health/safety policies
- Safety hazard controls
- Healthy organizational structure

- Cultural role models that support health/safety
- Health/wellness commitment
- Employee partnership in decision making
- Employee assistance programs
- Employee health leadership involvement

Box 13-12   **Major Benefits to Employers From Health Promotion Programs**

IMPROVED PRODUCTIVITY

Reduced absenteeism
Improved morale
Conserved operating costs
Improved ability to perform
Development of higher quality staff

REDUCED BENEFITS COSTS

Reduced health insurance costs
Lowered life insurance costs
Reduced workers' compensation claims
Provision of welfare benefits

REDUCED HUMAN RESOURCES AND DEVELOPMENT COSTS

Decreased recruiting costs
Decreased costs for educating and training new employees

IMPROVED IMAGE OF THE ORGANIZATION

General visibility
Concerned and responsible employers

From *Health Promotion in the Workplace* (3rd ed.), by M. P. O'Donnell, 2002, New York: Delmar.

healthful food choices (Katz & Showstack, 1990). In addition, social networks, family, community, and institutional policies often influence individual behavior, yet these factors are often neglected both in developing objectives and in the evaluation component.

Green and Kreuter (1999) define three levels of evaluation: process, impact, and outcome. *Process* evaluation focuses on the actual process of the program and includes materials, resources, space, quantitative adequacy and qualitative performance of staff, and programmatic activities, including quantity and quality of programs or services. The quality of the process can be determined by evaluative evidence, which could include the completion of evaluation forms by employees to determine the degree of satisfaction and the quality of programs, instructors, teaching materials, facilities, or any other program components. Other measures frequently examined are the number of program attendees, the number of brochures distributed, and the number of referrals made for further monitoring as a result of the program.

Impact evaluation is concerned with the immediate effects of the program or intervention on meeting short-term or intermediate objectives or targeted behavior change, such as an increase in employee awareness or knowledge about a specific topic, attitudinal changes about health or related risk factors such as smoking, or a behavioral change such as seat belt usage or smoking reduction. This might be measured through a comparison of pretest and posttest measures of knowledge or attitudes, indications of change in the targeted behavior such as self-report of smoking reduction (number of cigarettes smoked) or smoking cessation, or physiological or biochemical changes such as reduction in blood pressure, weight, or cholesterol levels. In addition, the impact of family or social support systems as related to attitudinal or behavioral change could be examined.

Outcome evaluation determines the effects of the program on long-term behavioral change or health consequences, including sustained behavioral or lifestyle changes and improvements in quality of health, life, and supportive environments. These evaluations typically include measures of absenteeism, productivity, morbidity, sustained risk factor reduction for disease preven-

tion, and mortality. Some of these indicators might be measured in a 1 to 3 year span; however, long-term outcome measures are more difficult to determine because the time lag for health effects may be too long when considering employee attrition.

In addition to program evaluation strategies, determinations about cost analyses may be required. The primary reason for performing evaluations of health promotion programs is to be able to draw inferences about the effectiveness of the program, generally measured by the degree to which specific program activities are associated with desired outcomes. Health promotion programs in a business setting must also be evaluated as to whether the outcomes produced are worth the cost of implementation. For example, do enough employees quit smoking to justify the cost of the intervention (Russell et al., 1996)?

Walsh and Egdahl (1989) reported that the top reasons cited by executive level corporate managers for the establishment of health promotion programs included cost containment (the primary reason cited), increased productivity and morale, promotion of employee health, and enhancement of the corporate image. More recently, William M. Mercer, Inc. (1999) asked employers about reasons to implement a health management program, and this survey resulted in the following findings from 248 respondents:

High health benefit cost	57%
Enhancement of corporate image	54%
Attraction and retention of employees	28%
Pressure to cut costs	25%
Employer demand for services	19%
Pressure to improve productivity	9%

However, little empirical evidence exists regarding the cost-effectiveness of health promotion programs largely because most companies fail to conduct economic evaluations (O'Donnell, 2002) or because valid evaluation methods are not used. Several reasons have been cited with respect to the difficulty in determining the true cost analyses of health promotion programs, including lack of a consistent definition of worksite health promotion; varying degrees of employee participation in both in-house and off-site programs; wide differences in corporate resources and goals; poor definition of outcome measures; significant variation in target populations, program activities, and program continuation follow-up; absence of comparative baseline measures; and failure to deal with self-selection of program participants (Katz & Showstack, 1990). Although these problems need to be addressed, several programs have demonstrated cost-effective results; for example, an evaluation of the Johnson & Johnson Live for Life Program showed a decrease in the annual outpatient costs, hospital days, and admission rates for employees who participated in the healthy lifestyles program over a 5-year period (Johnson & Johnson Health Management, Inc., 1992). The program's objectives are to help contain illness costs attributable to unhealthy behavior and lifestyles that are amenable to modifications in the work setting while promoting improvements in quality of life, work performance, and attitudes of employees.

Two types of costs analyses used today include cost-effectiveness and cost-benefit analyses (Barry & DeFriese, 1990). The purpose of a cost-effectiveness analysis is to determine which activities or interventions, given alternative approaches, will achieve the program objective and yield the most value or greatest impact for the least cost (Eddy et al., 1989). Cost-effectiveness measures the resources consumed in monetary terms as related to planned outcomes, usually in terms of participant successes. For example, Erfurt et al. (1990) and Erfurt et al. (1991) examined the cost-effectiveness of a worksite wellness program in reducing cardiovascular disease risks of employees at four manufacturing sites. Worksites were randomly assigned by intervention strategy. Site 1, the control site, included advice only, where blood pressure screening was done followed by only one postscreening health education class, to provide advice and information; Site 2 offered media-focused health education, which included the use of promotional materials, at least two health education classes, and health foci; Site 3 included individualized support, encouragement, and assistance with problem solving with emphasis on one-on-one and follow-up counseling, in addition to activities offered at Site 2; and Site 4 involved organizational strategies including peer support groups, organized competition, and buddy systems, in addition to activities offered at Sites 2 and 3. For engaging employees in treatment/program par-

ticipation, Sites 3 and 4 were 9 to 10 times more cost-effective than Site 2, and for reducing risks/preventing relapse, Sites 3 and 4 were 5 to 6 times more cost-effective than Site 2. At Sites 3 and 4, the total direct cost per percent of risks reduced/relapse prevented was less than $1 (67¢ and 74¢, respectively) per employee per year.

Cost-benefit analysis is a technique whereby both costs and benefits or outcomes of a program are represented in monetary terms, thus permitting a comparison between unlike elements and yielding a benefit-to-cost ratio (Eley, 1989). For example, one can determine the benefit of a smoking cessation program in terms of reduction in per capita and aggregate health care costs. The cost of implementing a smoking cessation program for x number of employees can be compared to costs assigned to insurance, absenteeism, and productivity of employees who smoke. Cost-benefit validation studies have been discussed by Aldana (1998), who reviewed eight studies and found a cost savings ranging from $2.30 to $5.90, with an average of $3.35 for every dollar invested in health promotion practices.

ADULT LEARNING

In preparing to offer a health promotion or protection program, the occupational and environmental health nurse must be cognizant of the characteristics of the audience and the best methods to present the material. To be effective in teaching and communicating health promotion and protection strategies in the work environment, the occupational and environmental health nurse must be familiar with principles of adult education. Knowles (1984) extensively describes the differences between adult and child patterns of learning and emphasizes the importance of teaching adults based on a framework of andragogy (teaching of adults) rather than pedagogy (teaching of children). Knowles suggests that adults, because of their greater independence and more extensive backgrounds, bring more to the learning experience and that the instructor should serve as a facilitator and enhancer of the teaching-learning process (Table 13-7).

Knowles' principles of adult education focus on four areas: independent learning, usefulness of past experiences, readiness to learn, and problem-oriented learning.

TABLE 13-7 Role of the Teacher/Facilitator

Conditions of Learning	Principles of Teaching
The learners feel a need to learn.	1. Exposes students to new possibilities of self-fulfillment. 2. Helps each student clarify her or his own aspirations for improved behavior. 3. Helps each student diagnose the gap between her or his aspiration and present level of performance. 4. Helps the students identify the life problems they experience because of the gaps in their personal equipment.
The learning environment is characterized by physical comfort; mutual trust, respect, and helpfulness; freedom of expression; and acceptance of differences.	5. Provides physical conditions that are comfortable (as to seating, smoking, temperature, ventilation, lighting, decoration) and conducive to interaction (preferably, no person sitting behind another person). 6. Accepts each student as a person of worth and respects her or his feelings and ideas. 7. Seeks to build relationships of mutual trust and helpfulness among the students by encouraging cooperative activities and refraining from inducing competitiveness and judgmentalness. 8. Exposes own feelings and contributes resources as a colearner in the spirit of mutual inquiry.
The learners perceive the goals of a learning experience to be their goals.	9. Involves the students in a mutual process of formulating learning objectives in which the needs of the students, of the institution, of the teacher, of the subject matter, and of the society are taken into account.
The learners accept a share of the responsibility for planning and operating a learning experience and therefore have a feeling of commitment toward it.	10. Shares thinking about options available in the designing of learning experiences and the selection of materials and methods and involves the students in deciding among these options jointly
The learners participate actively in the learning process.	11. Helps the students to organize themselves (project groups, learning-teaching teams, independent study, etc.) to share responsibility in the process of mutual inquiry.
The learning process is related to and makes use of the experience of the learners.	12. Helps the students exploit their own experiences as resources for learning through the use of such techniques as discussion, role playing, case method, and so forth. 13. Gears the presentation of own resources to the levels of experience of her or his particular students. 14. Helps the students to apply new learning to their experience and thus to make the learning more meaningful and integrated.
The learners have a sense of progress toward their goals.	15. Involves the students in developing mutually acceptable criteria and methods for measuring progress toward the learning objectives. 16. Helps the students develop and apply procedures for self-evaluation according to these criteria.

From *The Adult Learner: A Neglected Species,* by M. Knowles, Houston, TX: Gulf. 1984.

1. *Independent learning.* Emphasis is placed on the importance of the health care professional respecting the independence of the learners and including them as active, self-directed participants rather than passive recipients. This can be done by finding out what they already know about a topic, what they need to know to do the job better and safer, or what more they would like to learn about the topic.

2. *Previous experience.* Puetz (1988) points out that adults have a wealth of life experiences on which to base new learning. For example, an employee may have a relative who has had a heart attack and may be able to share related information about the rehabilitation process. This also presents an opportunity to assess employee baseline knowledge and to focus on areas of special concern.

3. *Readiness to learn.* At certain times in life, such as during times of critical incidents or situations, adults are ready to learn or a teachable moment presents itself. For example, a woman who becomes pregnant may be more interested in learning about workplace hazards or the effects of related lifestyle hazards such as smoking, and an employee recently diagnosed with high blood pressure may be more interested in learning about dietary control strategies.

   Preventive information on topics such as AIDS or diabetes may not have a direct impact unless the employee knows someone affected. In addition, other changes or concerns in the individual's life, such as family or career issues, may take precedence over the learning event. The occupational and environmental health nurse will need to be aware of this and use this barrier as an opportunity for other teaching or counseling.

4. *Problem-oriented learning.* Knowles (1984) suggests that adults' learning is usually in response to a problem. For example, employees who have had difficulty in quitting smoking will probably consider it a health problem and thus be more amenable to a smoking cessation clinic or educational program. Adult education will be most effective when it responds as directly as possible to an individual's concerns.

Loos (2001) further points out that adult learners:

- Do not regard instruction as a means of reinforcing learning.
- Utilize instruction to construct knowledge.
- Learn best what they "discover" for themselves.

Therefore, instructing adults must be the following:

- An active process wherein the learner constructs knowledge rather than acquires it
- A process of supporting this construction rather than one of communicating knowledge

The occupational and environmental health nurse can use Knowles' framework as a guide to structure the teaching/learning process and facilitate the motivation to learn. Puetz (1988) suggests that the occupational and environmental health nurse concentrate motivational efforts on enhancing the beginning learning situation, stimulating sustained interest, and providing for skill/knowledge reinforcement. Motivational strategies directed at these aims may include the following:

- Providing visual marketing strategies such as photos and posters to stimulate interest
- Structuring simulated activities such as a mock disaster drill or having the participants actually learn to take blood pressures
- Being enthusiastic about the topic
- Using a variety of teaching methods (e.g., films, videos, discussions)
- Inviting the participants to share experiences
- Providing skill laboratory exercises
- Testing for skill/knowledge acquisition to provide for learning feedback
- Recognizing employee participation and program completion through, for example, newsletters and bulletin board photos

Knowles (1984) encourages mutual respect in the teaching/learning process. Applied to the occupational health setting, employees are seen as independent learners, and both the nurse and the employees learn from each other. Previous experiences are considered valuable and useful resources for teaching opportunities, and employee learning should be structured to be responsive to problems or concerns. The occupational and environmental health nurse can use this framework to help employees achieve learning goals rather than manipulate the learning experience. Using this approach, both the employees and the occupational and environmental health nurse will benefit.

Summary

Concepts and principles of health promotion and health protection are fundamental to occupational and environmental health nursing practice. In applying these concepts, the nurse will spend a good deal of her or his time in planning, developing, implementing, and evaluating strategies that will enhance worker health and productivity and reduce work-related and lifestyle risks. The models and approaches discussed in this chapter can offer a foundation for understanding issues regarding behavior and need for change when unhealthy behaviors are evident. The guide provided for developing health promotion and health protection programs that are worker-driven and cost-effective can help in the overall planning and delivery of health care programs and services. A healthy workforce within the framework of quality living and work is the goal.

References

Aldana, S. (1998). Financial impact of worksite health promotion and methodological quality of the evidence. *Art of Health Promotion. 2*(1), 1-8.

Allen, J., & Allen, R. F. (1999). From short-term compliance to long-term freedom: Culture-based health promotion by health professionals. *American Journal of Health Promotion, 1,* 39-47.

Allen, J., & Leutzinger, J. (1999). The role of culture change in health promotion. *Art of Health Promotion, 3*(1), 1-10.

American Medical Association. (1947). *Periodic health examination: A manual for physicians.* Chicago: Author.

Anderson, G. (1998). *Multinational comparisions of health care: Expenditures, coverage, and outcomes.* New York: Commonwealth Fund.

Association for Worksite Health Promotion, & W. M. Mercer. (2000). *National Worksite Health Promotion Survey.* Northbrook, IL: Association of Worksite Health Promotion, U.S. Department of Health and Human Services.

Barry, P. Z., & DeFriese, G. H. (1990). Cost-benefit and cost-effectiveness analysis for health promotion programs. *American Journal of Health Promotion, 4,* 448-452.

Becker, M. H., Drachman, R. H., & Kirscht, J. P. (1974). A new approach to explaining sick-role behavior in low-income populations. *American Journal of Public Health, 64,* 205-216.

Becker, M. H., Maiman, L. A., Kirscht, J. P., Haefner, D. P., & Drachman, R. H. (1977). The health belief model and prediction of dietary compliance: A field experiment. *Journal of Health and Social Behavior, 18,* 348-366.

Bigbee, J. L., & Jonsa, N. (1991). Strategies for promoting health protection. *Nursing Clinics of North America, 26,* 895-913.

Breslow, L. (1999). From disease prevention to health promotion. *Journal of the American Medical Association, 281,* 1030-1033.

Breslow, L., & Sommers, A. R. (1977). The lifetime health monitoring program: A practical approach to preventive medicine. *New England Journal of Medicine, 292,* 601-608.

Buller, D. B., Morrill, C., Taren, D., Sennot-Miller, L., Miller, L., Buller, M. K., Larkey, L., Alatorre, C., & Wentzel, T. M. (1999). Random trial testing the effect of peer education at increasing fruit and vegetable intake. *Journal of the National Cancer Institute, 91,* 1491-1500.

Burnham, J. C. (1984). Change in the popularization of health in the United States. *Bulletin of the History of Medicine, 58,* 183-197.

Campbell, K. (1991). Worksite health promotion: Prevention for the future. *AAOHN Update Series, 4*(19), 1-8.

Campbell, K. & Ebert, R. (2001). Conducting Research on the Internet—Part II. *AAOHN Journal, 49,* 273-275.

Canadian Task Force on the Periodic Health Examination. (1979). The periodic health examination. *Canadian Medical Journal, 121,* 1194-1254.

Champion, V. C. (1999). Use of the health belief model in determining frequency of breast self-examination. *Research in Nursing and Health, 8,* 373-379.

Chapman, L. (1996). *Worksite wellness: Presenting the business case.* Seattle, WA: Summex Corporation.

Chapman, L. (1999a). Evaluating your program. *Art of Health Promotion, 3*(3), 1-11.

Chapman, L. (1999b). Population health management. *Art of Health Promotion, 3*(2),1-10.

Cummings, K. M., Jette, A. M., Brock, B. M., & Haefner, D. (1979). Psychosocial determinants of immunization behavior in a swine influenza campaign. *Medical Care, 17,* 639-649.

Eddy, J. M., Gold, R. S., & Zimmerli, W. H. (1989). Evaluation of worksite health enhancement programs. *Health Values, 13,* 3-9.

Edington, D. (2000). *Changes in costs related to changes in psychological and social support risk factors.* Paper presented at the Arts and Sciences Health Promotion Conference, Colorado Springs, CO.

Eley, J. W. (1989). Analyzing costs and benefits of mammography screening in the workplace. *AAOHN Journal, 37,* 171-177.

Erfurt, J. C., Foote, A., & Heinrich, M. A. (1991). The cost-effectiveness of worksite wellness programs for hypertension control, weight loss, and smoking cessation. *Journal of Occupational Medicine, 33,* 962-970.

Erfurt, J. C., Foote, A., Heinrich, M. A., & Gregg, W. (1990). Improving participation in worksite wellness programs: Comparing health education classes, a menu approach, and follow-up counseling. *American Journal of Health Promotion, 4*(4), 270-278.

Glanz, K., Sorensen, G., & Farmer, A. (1996). The health impact of worksite nutrition and cholesterol programs. *American Journal of Health Promotion, 10,* 453-470.

Global Strategy on Occupational Health for All. (1999). Geneva, Switzerland: World Health Organization.

Goetzel, R. (1998). Relationship between modifiable health risks and health care expenditures. *Journal of Occupational and Environmental Medicine, 40,* 10-18.

Green, L., & Kreuter, M. (1999) *Health promotion planning: An educational & environmental approach.* Mountain View, CA: Mayfield.

Guidotti, T., Cowell, J., & Jamieson, G. (1989). *Occupational health services: A practical approach.* Chicago: American Medical Association.

Health Care Financing Administration. *National Health Care Expenditures, 2000,* Table 1. (2000). http://www.hcfa.gov/.

Hochbaum, G. M. (1958). *Public participation in medical screening programs: A sociopsychological study.* (Public Health Service Publication No. 572). Washington, DC: U.S. Government Printing Office.

Janis, I. L. (1983). *Short-term counseling: Guidelines based on recent research.* New Haven, CT: Yale University Press.

Johnson & Johnson Health Management, Inc. (1992). *Relationship between participation and cost: Results of LIVE FOR LIFE program results.* Unpublished manuscript. Santa Monica, CA.

Katz, P. P., & Showstack, J. A. (1990). Is it worth it? Evaluating the economic impact of worksite health promotion. *Occupational Medicine: State of the Art Reviews, 5,* 837-850.

Kegeles, S. S., Kirscht, J. P., & Haefner, D. P. (1965). Surveys of beliefs about cancer detection and taking Papanicolaou tests. *Public Health Reports, 80,* 815-823.

Kizer, W. M. (1987). *The healthy workplace: A blueprint for corporate action.* New York: John Wiley & Sons.

Knowles, M. (1984). *The adult learner: A neglected species.* Houston, TX: Gulf.

Koretz, G. (2000). Employers tame medical costs: But workers pick up a bigger share. *Business Week, 26,* 26.

Larson, E. B., Olsen, E., Cole, W., & Shortell, S. (1979). The relationship of health beliefs and a postcard reminder to influenza vaccination. *Journal of Family Practice, 89,* 1207-1211.

Leavell, H., & Clark, E. (1965). *Preventive medicine for the doctor in his community.* New York: McGraw-Hill.

Loos, G. (2001, July 25-26). *Education and training on life-long learning and information on demand.* Paper presented at NIOSH Conference, Cincinnati, OH.

Lukes, E. N. (1992). Program evaluation: Demonstrating cost savings. *AAOHN Update Series, 4*(12), 1-8.

Lusk, S. L., Hong, O. S., Ronis, D. L., Eakin, B. L., Kerr, M. J., & Early, M. R. (1999). Effectiveness of an intervention to increase construction workers' use of hearing protection. *Human Factors, 41,* 487-494.

Machles, D. (1998). Informatics: Using basic search tools on the Internet. *AAOHN Journal, 46,* 557-558.

MacStravic, S. (1999). Winning participant loyalty in health promotion programs. *Art of Health Promotion, 3*(4), 1-7.

Marlatt, G. A., & Gordon, J. R. (1985). *Relapse prevention: Maintenance strategies in the treatment of addictive behaviors.* New York: Guilford Press.

Masey, V. (1986). Perceived susceptibility to breast cancer and practice of breast self-examination. *Nursing Research, 35,* 183-185.

Nemcek, M. A. (1990). Health beliefs and preventive behavior. *AAOHN Journal, 38,* 127-138.

O'Donnell, M. P. (1986). Definition of health promotion. *American Journal of Health Promotion, 1,* 4-5.

O'Donnell, M. P. (1989). Definition of health promotion, Part II: Expanding the definition. *American Journal of Health Promotion, 3,* 5.

O'Donnell, M. P. (2002). *Health promotion in the workplace.* New York: Delmar.

Office of Disease Prevention and Health Promotion. (1987). *National survey of worksite health promotion activities.* Washington, DC: U.S. Department of Health and Human Services.

Pelletier, K. R. (1996). A review and analysis of the health and cost-effective outcome studies of comprehensive health promotion and disease prevention programs at the worksite: 1993-1995 update. *American Journal of Health Promotion, 10,* 380-388.

Pelletier, K. R. (1999). A review and analysis of the health and cost-effective outcome studies of comprehensive health promotion and disease prevention programs at the worksite: 1995-1998 update. *American Journal of Health Promotion, 13,* 333-345.

Pender, N., Murdaugh, C. L., & Parsons, M. A. (2002). *Health promotion in nursing practice* (4th ed.). Upper Saddle River, NJ: Prentice Hall.

Prochaska, J. O., & DiClemente, C. C. (1982). Transtheoretical therapy: Toward a more integrative model of change. *Psychotherapy: Theory, Research, and Practice, 19,* 276-288.

Prochaska, J. O., & Velicer, W. F. (1997). The Transtheoretical Model of health behavior change. *American Journal of Health Promotion, 12,* 38-48.

Puetz, B. E. (1988). Theories of adult education and their application to occupational health nursing. *AAOHN Update Series, 3*(19), 1-8.

Rose, M. A. (1989). Health promotion and risk prevention: Application for cancer survivors. *Oncology Nursing Forum, 16,* 335-340.

Rosenstock, I. M. (1966). Why people use health services. *Milbank Memorial Fund Quarterly, 44,* 94-127.

Rundull, T. G., & Wheeler, J. R. C. (1979). Factors associated with utilization of the swine flu vaccination program among senior citizens in Tompkins County. Medical Care 17, 191-200.

Russell, L., Siegel, J., Daniels, N., Gold, M., Luce, B., Mandelblatt, J. (1996). Cost-effectiveness analysis as a guide to resource allocation in health. In M. Gold, J. Siegel, L. Russell, and M. Weinstein (Eds.), Cost-effectiveness in health and medicine. New York: Oxford Press.

Sandroff, O. J., Bradford, S., & Guligan, V. F. (1990). Meeting the health promotion challenges through a mode of shared responsibility. *Occupational Medicine: State of the Art Reviews, 5,* 677-690.

Selleck, C. S., Sirles, A. T., & Newman, K. D. (1989). Health promotion at the workplace. *AAOHN Journal, 37,* 412-422.

Serxner, S. A., Gold, D. B., & Bultman, K. K. (2001). The impact of behavioral health risks on worker absenteeism. *Journal of Occupational and Environmental Medicine, 43,* 347-354.

Shamansky, S. L., & Clausen, C. L. (1980). Levels of prevention: Examination of the concept. *Nursing Outlook, 28,* 104-108.

Strecher, V. J., & Rosenstock, I. M. (1997). The Health Belief Model. In K. Glanz, F. M. Lewis, & B. K. Rimer, (Eds.), *Health behavior and heath education: Theory, research, and practice* (pp. 41-59). San Franscico: Jossey-Bass.

Taming the health cost monster. (1992, October). *Workplace Health, I,* 5.

U.S. Department of Health and Human Services. (2001). *Healthy people 2010: Understanding and improving health.* Washington, DC: U.S. Government Printing Office.

U.S. Preventive Services Task Force. (1996). *Guide to clinical preventive services* (2nd ed.). Baltimore, MD: Williams & Wilkins.

Wachs, J. E. (1991). Levels of prevention: A framework for cost-effective occupational health programs. *AAOHN Update Series, 4*(7), 1-8.

Wachs, J. E., & Parker-Conrad, J. E. (1990). Occupational health nursing in 1990 and the coming decade. *Applied Occupational and Environmental Hygiene, 5*(4), 200-203.

Walsh, D. C., & Egdahl, R. H. (1989). Corporate perspectives on worksite wellness programs: A report on the seventh Pew Fellows Conference. *Journal of Occupational Medicine, 31,* 551-556.

Wellness Councils of America. (1990). *Healthy, wealthy, well and wise.* Omaha, NE: Author.

William M. Mercer, Inc. *Mercer's fax facts survey: Health management.* (1999). http://www.wmmesces.com. Mercer's USA resource center: New releases.

World Health Organization. (1988). *WHO health promotion glossary.* Geneva, Switzerland: Author.

We are currently undertaking a study to determine the amount of interest and the kinds of feelings and assumptions that employees have about the development of a worksite health promotion program. Please answer the questions honestly. The survey is completely confidential. You do not need to give us your name.

AGREE OR DISAGREE?	Agree	Disagree
It is cheaper to prevent disease than to treat it after the fact.	☐	☐
People need accurate health information and education about their		
1. Health risks	☐	☐
2. Behaviors that create risks	☐	☐
3. Health care costs	☐	☐
4. Health choices	☐	☐
5. How to change their behaviors	☐	☐
People will choose to change their behavior if they are informed, motivated, and supported.	☐	☐
Healthy people do their best and are more productive on and off the job.	☐	☐
The people I associate with have an influence on my choices.	☐	☐
My work environment has an impact on my health, my behaviors, and my choices.	☐	☐

Because of the influence of the company's work environment, I have changed or I have seen coworkers change the following:

	T	F
1. Started and maintain a regular exercise program	T	F
2. Stopped or cut back on my smoking	T	F
3. Developed skills to manage the stress in my life	T	F
4. Adopted new eating habits to maintain healthy body weight	T	F
5. Adopted new eating habits to lower cholesterol	T	F

6. Avoid the overuse of caffeine, sugar, salt	T	F
7. Avoid the overuse or misuse of alcohol and/or drugs	T	F
8. Have regular medical and dental check-ups	T	F
9. Maintain healthy blood pressure	T	F
10. Understand the importance of and need for good mental and emotional health as well as physical health	T	F

What is your reaction to the prospect of a worksite health promotion program in our company?

Excited	☐
Moderately interested	☐
Neutral	☐
Slightly disinterested	☐
Opposed	☐

If a worksite health promotion program is implemented here, would you:

Personally participate in any programs or activities?	Y	N
Encourage the employees you supervise to participate?	Y	N

From *Wellness Councils of America: Healthy, Wealthy & Wise—Fundamentals of Workplace Health Promotion* (3rd ed.), by Wellness Council of The Midlands (WELCOM)-Omaha, 1993, Omaha, NE: Wellness Councils of America. By permission of Wellness Councils of America, Community Health Plaza, Suite 311, 7101 Newport Ave., Omaha, NE 68152, (402) 572-3590.

13-2 Health Interest Surveys

TABLE A: EMPLOYEE HEALTH PROMOTION SURVEY

From the following list of programs and activities, circle the number that shows your level of interest for each, "1" being the lowest level and "5" the highest.

Priority   **I. PROGRAMS**

Least				Highest	A. Understanding Personal Health
1	2	3	4	5	1. Nutrition
1	2	3	4	5	2. Healthy lifestyle
1	2	3	4	5	3. Physical fitness education
1	2	3	4	5	4. Alcohol and other drug control
1	2	3	4	5	5. Healthy back
1	2	3	4	5	6. Men's health issues
1	2	3	4	5	7. Women's health issues
1	2	3	4	5	8. Stress management
1	2	3	4	5	9. Blood pressure management

Least				Highest	B. Reducing Risks
1	2	3	4	5	1. Safety—accident prevention:
1	2	3	4	5	a. Home
1	2	3	4	5	b. Gun
1	2	3	4	5	c. Water
1	2	3	4	5	d. Automobile
1	2	3	4	5	e. Motorcycle
1	2	3	4	5	f. Other
1	2	3	4	5	2. Cancer risk reduction
1	2	3	4	5	3. Dental disease prevention
1	2	3	4	5	4. Heart attack risk reduction

Least				Highest	C. Developing Healthy Relations With Others
1	2	3	4	5	1. Caring for and understanding aging parents
1	2	3	4	5	2. Parenting issues: Caring for and understanding children
1	2	3	4	5	3. Dealing with difficult people
1	2	3	4	5	4. Positive mental attitude

Priority   **II. ACTIVITIES**

Least				Highest	A. Promoting Health Through Actions
1	2	3	4	5	1. Physical fitness activities (Circle the type(s) of physical fitness activities you would like to take part in.)
1	2	3	4	5	a. Aerobics—Exercises that bring the heart rate up to a certain level for a period of time.

1	2	3	4	5	b. Calisthenics—Exercises that increase strength, balance, coordination, and joint movement.
1	2	3	4	5	c. Flexibility and stretching—Exercises that increase blood supply to the muscles, improve range of motion.
1	2	3	4	5	d. Walking/jogging
1	2	3	4	5	e. Other
1	2	3	4	5	2. Smoking cessation
1	2	3	4	5	3. Weight management
1	2	3	4	5	4. Arthritis (help for self and family)
1	2	3	4	5	5. Blood pressure control (managing high blood pressure)

Least				*Highest*	**B. Screening for Specific Health Concerns**
1	2	3	4	5	1. Glaucoma
1	2	3	4	5	2. Cholesterol
1	2	3	4	5	3. Blood pressure
1	2	3	4	5	4. Cancer
1	2	3	4	5	5. Back problems

Least				*Highest*	**C. Developing Skills to Help Others**
1	2	3	4	5	1. CPR (cardiopulmonary resuscitation)
1	2	3	4	5	2. First aid

Would you attend one or more of the above programs if they were offered at a convenient time?
☐ Yes   ☐ No

III. ADDITIONAL CONSIDERATIONS

Would you prefer a health promotion program at the worksite or some other place? (If other, please write down the location you would prefer.)
☐ Worksite   ☐ Other, where? _____

Would your spouse and/or family take part in a health promotion program?
☐ Yes   ☐ No

Would you be willing to share in the cost for some programs?
☐ Yes   ☐ No

Would you take part in a weekend program?
☐ Yes   ☐ No

Would you take part in a lunch hour program?
☐ Yes   ☐ No

What hours do you work? _____ a.m./p.m. to _____ a.m./p.m.

What hours are best for you to take part in a health promotion program?
_____ a.m./p.m. to _____ a.m./p.m.

In the space below, let us know about any other health care or health promotion ideas or concerns that you may have.

_____

_____

_____

_____

Return survey to _____ by _____.

Thank You!

Used with permission from Milwaukee Wellness Council, 1442 North Farwell Ave., Suite 300, Milwaukee, WI 53202; phone: (414) 291-9355; fax: (414) 224-0243; e-mail: wcwi@wellnesscouncilwi.org.

TABLE B: HEALTH INTEREST SURVEY

Please circle the answer or answers that best fit the question.

1. Are you presently involved in some regular form of physical fitness?
   Yes   No
If yes, how often?
a. Three or more times per week   c. Once a month
b. Once a week
In what type of physical activity are you currently involved?
a. Running/walking   d. Tennis/racquetball
b. Weight/strength training   e. Team sports
c. Aerobics/jazzercize   f. Other _____
Would you use an on-site jogging/aerobic walking trail?
   Yes   No
Would you use exercise stations strategically placed along the trail?
   Yes   No

2. Which of the following would encourage your regular participation in physical fitness activities?
a. Par course   e. Weight/strength training
b. Bicycling   f. Tennis/racquetball
c. Swimming   g. Team sports
d. Indoor ski equipment   h. Other

3. Do you consider your diet a healthy one?
   Yes   No
Would you like to have information on:
a. Appropriate caloric intake   d. Special diets such as diabetic, sports diets,
b. Dietary salt, sugar, and fiber   bland ulcer diet
c. Healthy intake of cholesterol   e. Vitamin and mineral supplements
Are you overweight?
   Yes   No

4. Are you subject to daily stress?
   Yes   No
If yes, would you consider it:
a. High   c. Minimal
b. Medium
What is the likely source of your stress?
a. Marital/other relationship   d. Parenting
b. Financial   e. Other
c. Work-related

5. Do you smoke cigarettes?
   Yes   No
If yes, how many packs per day?
a. Less than one   c. Three or more
b. One to two
How long have you smoked?
a. Less than 1 year   d. 11-20 years
b. 2-5 years   e. Greater than 20 years
c. 6-10 years

Are you interested in quitting?
     Yes   No

6. Do you need information or assistance with coping with alcohol/drug abuse problems?
     Yes   No

7. Would information on the prevention of certain diseases such as cancer, heart disease, stroke, diabetes, and arthritis be helpful?
     Yes   No

Circle any activities you feel are important:
a. Availability of pamphlets and audiovisual materials
b. Learning of self-examination techniques, such as those for breast and testicular cancers
c. Presentation of worksite educational sessions
d. Worksite screening for blood sugar, cholesterol, and blood pressure

8. Would you complete a generalized HEALTH RISK APPRAISAL to advise you of your own health risk factors?
     Yes   No

9. Consider the following health promotion programs that could be offered at the workplace. Please rank them 1 through 7 in the order that you feel they should be offered.

Program rank (1-7)
a. High blood pressure workshop   _____
b. Stress management seminar   _____
c. Weight management program   _____
d. Smoking cessation program   _____
e. Fitness testing   _____
f. Nutrition program to encourage a healthy diet   _____
g. Neck and back pain prevention   _____

10. Other health-related information can also be important. For each item below, please indicate your level of interest by marking a "0" if no interest, a "1" if interested, and a "2" if extremely interested.
a. Sexually transmissible diseases (AIDS, herpes, etc.) _____
b. Prenatal care _____   g. Birth control _____
c. Parenting _____   h. Day care centers _____
d. Choosing the right doctor _____   I. "How to talk with your doctor" _____
e. Dental health _____   j. Cardiovascular fitness _____
f. Skin cancer _____   k. Food additives _____

Please complete the following information:
Age: _____   Sex: F _____ M _____
Educational level: _____
Position (circle): Clerical   Technical   Professional
Marital Status (circle): Married   Single   Divorced   Separated
Number of children _____ Ages: _____
Thank you for your participation.
Comments/Suggestions: _____
_____
_____
_____

Used with permission from Milwaukee Wellness Council, 1442 N. Farwell Ave., Suite 300, Milwaukee, WI 53202; phone: (414) 291-9355; fax: (414) 224-0234; e-mail: wcwi@wellnesscouncilwi.org.

TABLE C: EMPLOYEE HEALTH PROMOTION SURVEY

This information is for future program design purposes only. Please do not sign your name.

1. Please specify your work location: _____

_____

2. If the following health promotion programs were offered by [Company Name], please indicate in which programs, if any, you would participate. Please circle the programs of most interest to you and rank them in order of preference 1 through 10 with 1 of most importance to you, 2 is second, and 10 is of least importance.

_____ Physical fitness
_____ Weight management
_____ Nutrition
_____ Smoking cessation
_____ Stress management
_____ Blood pressure control
_____ Coping/interpersonal skills
_____ Home and auto safety
_____ Cardiac resuscitation and first aid
_____ Medical self-care and wiser use of medical services
_____ Other (specify) _____

3. Would you participate in the health promotion programs of interest you specified if they were offered after working hours?
_____ Yes _____ No

4. Which health practices are important to you for staying healthy? Check all that apply.

_____ Physical fitness
_____ Proper nutrition
_____ Ideal body weight
_____ Not smoking
_____ Stress management
_____ Having a good relationship with family

_____ Having a good relationship with coworkers
_____ Controlling blood pressure
_____ Safety on the job
_____ Using seat belts and child safety restraint devices
_____ Moderate use of alcohol

5. How often do you use seat belts?

_____ Every time
_____ Usually
_____ Half of the time

_____ Occasionally
_____ Never

6. If [Company Name] offered preventive health examinations periodically (e.g., every 3 years) would you participate?
_____ Yes _____ No

7. Do you think that people in good health are happier with their daily lives?
_____ Agree _____ Disagree _____ Neutral

8. Do you think people in good health are more productive?
_____ Agree_____ Disagree _____ Neutral

9. Do you think that you could improve your health by changing some habits or health practices?
_____ Agree _____ Disagree _____ Neutral

10. Would you consider the offering of screening and health promotion programs by [Company Name] a significant employment benefit?

_____ Agree_____ Disagree _____ Neutral

11. Do you favor providing smoking and nonsmoking areas in the workplace?

_____ Yes _____ No

12. Do you favor a no smoking policy when smokers and nonsmokers must meet in closed rooms?

_____ Yes _____ No

13. Do you favor a total no smoking policy at the workplace?

_____ Yes _____ No

14. Do you smoke now?

_____ Yes _____ No

15. Do you feel your job is stressful?

_____ Always _____ Much of the time _____ Occasionally _____ Rarely

16. Do you feel your life away from the job is stressful?

_____ Always _____ Much of the time _____ Occasionally _____ Rarely

17. Do you participate in an exercise program now?

_____ Yes _____ No

18. In what fitness activities do you participate?

_____ Jogging trail
_____ Swimming
_____ Racketball
_____ Aerobics
_____ Nautilus equipment
_____ Other _____(specify)

19. Your age is _____ (optional)

20. Are you: (circle one)

Salary Exempt   Salary Nonexempt   *or*   Hourly

Please make any additional comments you may have: _____

_____

_____

_____

_____

Used with permission from Milwaukee Wellness Council, 1442 N. Farwell Ave., Suite 300, Milwaukee, WI 53202; phone: (414) 291-9355; fax: (414) 224-0234; e-mail: wewi@wellnesscouncilwi.org.

TABLE D: HEALTH RISK INTEREST SURVEY

Please indicate in which of the following areas you have a need or interest by placing a check in the appropriate column that indicates the type of program that would best meet your needs or interests. This survey will help us determine the kinds of programs that will be offered.

If a health promotion program were made available to you, which of the following would you be most likely to attend?

	PLEASE CHECK ONE		
	Yes	**Yes, at a Small Cost**	**No**
1. Cardiovascular fitness/exercise	☐	☐	☐
2. Personal stress management	☐	☐	☐
3. Organizational stress management	☐	☐	☐
4. Smoking cessation	☐	☐	☐
5. Weight control and nutrition education	☐	☐	☐
6. High blood pressure management	☐	☐	☐
7. Medical self-care approaches	☐	☐	☐
8. Alcohol/drug use	☐	☐	☐
9. Mental/emotional problems (depression, nervousness)	☐	☐	☐
10. Parenting skills	☐	☐	☐
11. Marital problems	☐	☐	☐
12. Assertiveness training	☐	☐	☐
13. Educational/career planning	☐	☐	☐
14. Spiritual or philosophical values	☐	☐	☐
15. Interpersonal communication skills	☐	☐	☐
16. Home budgeting/financial planning	☐	☐	☐
17. Automobile safety	☐	☐	☐
18. Time management	☐	☐	☐

	After Work	**Lunch**	**Evenings**
19. When would you most likely attend a class or activity?	☐	☐	☐

	One Time	**6-8 Weeks**	**Either**
20. Would you be most likely to attend:	☐	☐	☐

	Yes		**No**
21. Would you be interested in programs that could include family members?	☐		☐

	Yes		**No**
22. Could changes be made in your work behaviors? (Example: choice of fruit and/or fruit juices as well as soft drinks and coffee) If Yes, please describe:	☐		☐

_____
_____
_____

	Yes		**No**
23. Would you be willing to assist in the planning and delivery of programs? If yes, give topics:	☐		☐

_____
_____

	Yes		**No**
24. Any suggestions for additional health promotion programs? If yes, suggestions:	☐		☐

_____
_____
_____

Thanks for your interest.

Name _____

Department _____

Telephone _____

From *Employee Health and Fitness Programs: A Guide for New Mexico Employers,* by New Mexico Department of Health, Public Health Division, Health Promotion Bureau, Albuquerque, NM: Author.

TABLE E: EMPLOYEE WELLNESS SURVEY

We are considering the development of an employee wellness program and would like to learn more about your interests in wellness and health-related activities. Your responses will be used in planning the program and deciding what types of activities should be included.

Please take a few minutes to complete this survey. Since we want to keep individual survey information confidential, please do not put your name on it.

1. Sex: _____ Male _____ Female

2. Age Group: _____ Under 21 _____ 21-30 _____ 31-40
   _____ 41-50 _____ 51-60 _____ Over 60

3. Check any of the following that apply regarding your current health habits:

   Yes   No

   Exercise
   _____ _____ I exercise vigorously for at least 20 minutes 3 times a week.
   _____ _____ I exercise once in a while.
   _____ _____ I rarely exercise.

   Eating
   _____ _____ I usually eat three nutritious meals daily.
   _____ _____ I often eat on the run, dropping meals.
   _____ _____ I avoid eating too much fat.
   _____ _____ I make an effort to eat enough high fiber foods.
   _____ _____ I like a lot of salt on my food.
   _____ _____ I eat breakfast every day.

   Weight
   _____ _____ I am about the right weight.
   _____ _____ I would like to lose weight.
   _____ _____ I am more than 20 pounds over my ideal weight.

   Sleep
   _____ _____ I usually get a good night's sleep.
   _____ _____ I average at least two nights of inadequate sleep per week.
   _____ _____ I often have trouble getting enough sleep.

   Smoking/Alcohol/Drugs
   _____ _____ I regularly smoke cigarettes.
   _____ _____ I have at least three drinks daily containing alcohol.
   _____ _____ I sometimes drive after drinking alcohol.
   _____ _____ I avoid drinking too many caffeinated drinks.
   _____ _____ I regularly use tranquilizers and similar drugs.

   Other
   _____ _____ I regularly practice some type of stress management.
   _____ _____ I have had lower back pain in the last 6 months.
   _____ _____ I usually consult a medical self-care book when I am sick.

4. List any health concerns you have about yourself or your family:

   _____
   _____

5. Would you like the organization to conduct a wellness program?
_____ Yes _____ No _____ Don't know

6. In which of the following activities would you consider participating?

Yes	Maybe		Yes	Maybe	
____	____	Aerobic exercise	____	____	Other exercise
____	____	Weight management	____	____	Health fair
____	____	Smoking cessation	____	____	Blood test for cholesterol
____	____	Confidential health screening	____	____	Cancer screening
____	____	Coping with stress	____	____	CPR training
____	____	Alcohol/drug abuse	____	____	Regular education wellness presentations
____	____	Safety/accident prevention	____	____	Retirement planning
____	____	Parenting	____	____	Back pain
____	____	Walking program	____	____	Medical self-care
____	____	Other, please specify _____			

7. When would you be most likely to participate? (Please check all that apply.)

_____ Monday	_____ Spring	_____ A.M., before work
_____ Tuesday	_____ Summer	_____ Lunchtime
_____ Wednesday	_____ Fall	_____ P.M., after work
_____ Thursday	_____ Winter	_____ Evening
_____ Friday	_____ Other, specify _____	

8. Where would you be most likely to participate? (Check as many as apply.)
_____ Worksite   _____ School
_____ YMCA/YWCA   _____ Private health club

9. Would you be willing to share the cost of participating in these programs?
_____ Yes   _____ No

10. Any additional comments? _____
Thank you for your help in completing this survey!

From Center for Health Promotion, Michigan Department of Public Health, Ann Arbor, Michigan.

TABLE F: NEEDS AND INTEREST SURVEY

The purpose of this survey is to obtain employee input for our health promotion program. It includes needs, interests, and other information to be used in deciding what programs to offer and when to offer them. There are no right or wrong answers. Please use an "X" to respond to questions. Your completion of the survey is completely voluntary. The surveys are completely anonymous; there is no identifying number on the form.

A. Tobacco Use

1. Do you chew or dip tobacco now?
_____ Yes   _____ No, but former user   _____ No, never used

2. Do you smoke a pipe or cigars?
_____ Yes   _____ No, but former user   _____ No, never used

3. How would you classify your current use of cigarettes?
_____ Current cigarette smoker (_____ cigarettes per day)
_____ Never smoked/smoked less than 100 cigarettes in my lifetime
_____ Ex-smoker, years quit _____ or _____ months if less than 1 year

B. Nutrition and Physical Activity

Please rate how often you do each of the following.

	Never	Seldom	Sometimes	Often	Very Often
1. Eat fresh fruits, vegetables, whole grain bread.	☐	☐	☐	☐	☐
2. Eat food high in cholesterol or fat, such as fatty meat, cheese, fried foods, or eggs?	☐	☐	☐	☐	☐
3. Eat foods at home that are already prepared (like TV dinners, pizzas, frozen main courses, canned soup).	☐	☐	☐	☐	☐
4. Eat food at a fast food outlet such as Kentucky Fried Chicken, McDonald's, or canteen trucks.	☐	☐	☐	☐	☐

5. Please check below the category that best describes your physical activity level for the previous year.
_____ No physical activity.
_____ Moderate to vigorous exercise 1 time/week for at least 20 minutes.
_____ Moderate to vigorous exercise 1-2 times/week for at least 20 minutes each time.
_____ Moderate to vigorous exercise 3 times/week for at least 20 minutes each time.
_____ Moderate to vigorous exercise 5 times/week for at least 30 minutes each time.

C. Health Screenings

Please indicate whether you have had the following screenings or examinations in the past year.

	Yes	No	Not Sure
6. Cholesterol check	☐	☐	☐
7. Blood sugar check	☐	☐	☐
8. Rectal exam	☐	☐	☐
9. Stool check	☐	☐	☐

Exams for women only (men skip to 13)
10. Breast physical exam by doctor   ☐   ☐   ☐
11. Mammogram (x-ray of breasts)   ☐   ☐   ☐
12. Pap smear during pelvic exam   ☐   ☐   ☐
Exam for men only (women skip to 14)
13. Prostate exam   ☐   ☐   ☐

D. Program Interests

Please indicate how likely you would be to participate in each of the following programs if they were offered at work during the next year.

	Extremely Likely	Somewhat Likely	Somewhat Unlikely	Extremely Unlikely
14. Nutrition and cancer	☐	☐	☐	☐
15. Cancer awareness for women	☐	☐	☐	☐
16. Cancer awareness for men	☐	☐	☐	☐
17. Smoking cessation	☐	☐	☐	☐
18. Walking program	☐	☐	☐	☐
19. Weight loss and nutrition program	☐	☐	☐	☐
20. Managing chronic health conditions (e.g., diabetes, hypertension)	☐	☐	☐	☐
21. Blood pressure screening	☐	☐	☐	☐
22. Cholesterol screening	☐	☐	☐	☐

Please indicate how likely you would be to participate in a health promotion program during the following times.

23. Before work	☐	☐	☐	☐
24. During lunch	☐	☐	☐	☐
25. After work	☐	☐	☐	☐

E. Demographic Information

What was your age on your last birthday? _____ years
What is your sex? _____ Male _____ Female
Your job category:
_____ Management/professional
_____ Clerical
_____ Technical
_____ Service/labor

Thank you for completing this survey

From *Health Promotion Team Leader's Guide* (3rd ed., pp. 22-23), by G. Sneden, W. Baun, N. Gottlieb, and D. Haydon, 1993, Austin, TX: American Cancer Society—Texas Division.

13-3 The Healthier People Network

Form C

The HEALTHIER PEOPLE NETWORK, Inc.

. . . linking science, technology, & education to serve the public interest . . .

IDENTIFICATION NUMBER

☐☐☐☐☐☐☐☐☐

The health risk appraisal is an educational tool, showing you choices you can make to keep good health and avoid the most common causes of death (for a person of your age and sex). This health risk appraisal is **not** a substitute for a check-up or physical exam that you get from a doctor or nurse; however, it does provide some ideas for lowering your risk of getting sick or injured in the future. It is NOT designed for people who already have HEART DISEASE, CANCER, KIDNEY DISEASE, OR OTHER SERIOUS CONDITIONS; if you have any of these problems, please ask your health care provider to interpret the report for you.

DIRECTIONS:

To get the most accurate results, **answer as many questions as you can.** If you do not know the answer, leave it blank.

The following questions __must__ be completed or the computer program cannot process your questionnaire:
1. SEX   2. AGE   3. HEIGHT   4. WEIGHT   15. CIGARETTE SMOKING

| Please write your answers in the boxes provided. ✏ (Examples: ⊠ or 98) |

1. **SEX**   1 ☐ Male   2 ☐ Female
2. **AGE**   ☐ Years
3. **HEIGHT**   (Without shoes)   ☐ Feet   ☐ Inches
                                   (No fractions)
4. **WEIGHT**   (Without shoes)   ☐ Pounds
                                   (No fractions)
5. Body frame size   1 ☐ Small
                                                                      2 ☐ Medium
                                                                      3 ☐ Large
6. Have you ever been told that you have diabetes (or sugar   1 ☐ Yes   2 ☐ No
   diabetes)?
7. Are you now taking medicine for high blood pressure?   1 ☐ Yes   2 ☐ No
8. What is your blood pressure now?   ☐ / ☐
                                                                      Systolic (high number)/Diastolic
                                                                      (low number)
9. If you do not know the number, check the box that   1 ☐ High
   describes your blood pressure.   2 ☐ Normal or Low
                                                                      3 ☐ Don't Know
10. What is your TOTAL cholesterol level (based on   ☐ mg/dl
    a blood test)?

11. What is your HDL cholesterol (based on a blood test)?
12. How many cigars do you usually smoke per day?
13. How many pipes of tobacco do you usually smoke per day?
14. How many times per day do you usually use
    smokeless tobacco?
    (Chewing tobacco, snuff, pouches, etc.)

☐ mg/dl
☐ cigars per day
☐ pipes per day
☐ times per day

15. **CIGARETTE SMOKING**
    How would you describe your cigarette smoking habits?

1 ☐ Never smoked   ☞ **Go to 18**
2 ☐ Used to smoke   ☞ **Go to 17**
3 ☐ Still smoke   ☞ **Go to 16**

16. **STILL SMOKE**
    How many cigarettes a day do you smoke?
    ☞ **GO TO QUESTION 18**

☐ cigarettes per day   ☞ **Go to 18**

17. **USED TO SMOKE**
    a. How many years has it been since you smoked
       cigarettes fairly regularly?
    b. What was the average number of cigarettes per day
       that you smoked in the 2 years before you quit?

☐ years

☐ cigarettes per day

18. In the next 12 months, how many thousands of miles
    will you probably travel by each of the following?
    (Note: U.S. average = 10,000 miles)
    a. Car, truck, or van:
    b. Motorcycle:

☐ ,000 miles
☐ ,000 miles

19. On a typical day, how do you USUALLY travel?
    (Check one only)

1 ☐ Walk
2 ☐ Bicycle
3 ☐ Motocycle
4 ☐ Subcompact or compact car
5 ☐ Mid-size or full-size car
6 ☐ Truck or van
7 ☐ Bus, subway, or train
8 ☐ Mostly stay home

20. What percent of time do you usually buckle your safety
    belt when driving or riding?

☐%

21. On the average, how close to the speed limit do you
    usually drive?

1 ☐ Within 5 mph of limit
2 ☐ 6-10 mph over limit
3 ☐ 11-15 mph over limit
4 ☐ More than 15 mph over limit

22. How many times in the last month did you drive or ride
    when the driver had perhaps too much alcohol to drink?

☐ times last month

23. How many drinks of an alcoholic beverage do you have
    in a typical week?

(Write the number of each type of drink)
☐ Bottles or cans of beer
☐ Glasses of wine
☐ Wine coolers
☐ Mixed drinks or shots of liquor

☞ *MEN GO TO QUESTION 33*

WOMEN ONLY

24. At what age did you have your first menstrual period?   ☐ years old

25. How old were you when your first child was born?   ☐ years old   (If no children, write 0)

26. How long has it been since your last breast x-ray (mammogram)?

    1 ☐ Less than 1 year ago
    2 ☐ 1 year ago
    3 ☐ 2 years ago
    4 ☐ 3 or more years ago
    5 ☐ Never

27. How many women in your natural family (mother and sisters only) have had breast cancer?   ☐ women

28. Have you had a hysterectomy operation?

    1 ☐ Yes
    2 ☐ No
    3 ☐ Not sure

29. How long has it been since you had a pap smear test?

    1 ☐ Less than 1 year ago
    2 ☐ 1 year ago
    3 ☐ 2 years ago
    4 ☐ 3 or more years ago
    5 ☐ Never

30. How often do you examine your breasts for lumps?

    1 ☐ Monthly
    2 ☐ Once every few months
    3 ☐ Rarely or never

31. About how long has it been since you had your breasts examined by a physician or nurse?

    1 ☐ Less than 1 year ago
    2 ☐ 1 year ago
    3 ☐ 2 years ago
    4 ☐ 3 or more years ago
    5 ☐ Never

32. About how long has it been since you had a rectal exam?

    1 ☐ Less than 1 year ago
    2 ☐ 1 year ago
    3 ☐ 2 years ago
    4 ☐ 3 or more years ago
    5 ☐ Never

☛ *WOMEN GO TO QUESTION 34*

MEN ONLY

33. About how long has it been since you had a rectal or prostate exam?

    1 ☐ Less than 1 year ago
    2 ☐ 1 year ago
    3 ☐ 2 years ago
    4 ☐ 3 or more years ago
    5 ☐ Never

☛ *MEN CONTINUE ON QUESTION 34*

34. How many times in the last year did you witness or become involved in a violent fight or attack where there was a good chance of a serious injury to someone?

    1 ☐ 4 or more times
    2 ☐ 2 or 3 times
    3 ☐ 1 time or never
    4 ☐ Not sure

35. Considering your age, how would you describe your overall physical health?

    1 ☐ Excellent
    2 ☐ Good
    3 ☐ Fair
    4 ☐ Poor

36. In an average week, how many times do you engage in physical activity (exercise or work which lasts at least 20 minutes without stopping and which is hard enough to make you breathe heavier and your heart beat faster)?

    1 ☐ Less than 1 time per week
    2 ☐ 1 or 2 times per week
    3 ☐ At least 3 times per week

37. If you ride a motorcycle or all-terrain vehicle (ATV), what percent of the time do you wear a helmet?

1 ☐ 75% to 100%
2 ☐ 25% to 74%
3 ☐ Less than 25%
4 ☐ Does not apply to me

38. Do you eat some food every day that is high in fiber, such as whole grain bread, cereal, fresh fruits or vegetables?

1 ☐ Yes   2 ☐ No

39. Do you eat foods every day that are high in cholesterol or fat, such as fatty meat, cheese, fried foods, or eggs?

1 ☐ Yes   2 ☐ No

40. In general, how satisifed are you with your life?

1 ☐ Mostly satisfied
2 ☐ Partly satisfied
3 ☐ Not satisfied

41. Have you suffered a personal loss or misfortune in the past year that had a serious impact on your life? (For example, a job loss, disability, separation, jail term, or the death of someone close to you.)

1 ☐ Yes, 1 serious loss or misfortune
2 ☐ Yes, 2 or more
3 ☐ No

42a. Race

1 ☐ Aleutian, Alaska native, Eskimo, American Indian
2 ☐ Asian
3 ☐ Black
4 ☐ Pacific Islander
5 ☐ White
6 ☐ Other
7 ☐ Don't know

42b. Are you of Hispanic origin, such as Mexican-American, Puerto Rican, or Cuban?

1 ☐ Yes   2 ☐ No

43. What is the highest grade you completed in school?

1 ☐ Grade school or less
2 ☐ Some high school
3 ☐ High school graduate
4 ☐ Some college
5 ☐ College graduate
6 ☐ Post graduate or professional degree

Name _____

Address _____

City _____ State _____ Zip _____

From The Healthier People Network, Inc., 1992, Altanta, GA.

13-4 2000 Federal Health Information Centers and Clearinghouses

The federal government operates many clearinghouses and information centers that focus on specific topics and whose services include distributing publications, providing referrals, and answering inquiries. Many offer toll-free numbers. Unless otherwise stated, numbers can be reached within the continental United States, Monday through Friday, during normal business hours, eastern time. The clearinghouses are listed below by keyword. This document is available from the Internet at www.health.gov/NHIC/Pubs/.

To order printed copies of this publication or to obtain this publication on disk (pdf, html, rtf), contact the ODPHP Communication Support Center, P.O. Box 37366, Washington, DC 20013-7366; fax (301) 468-7394. Inclusion of an information source in this publication does not imply endorsement by the U.S. Department of Health and Human Services. This information is in the public domain. Duplication is encouraged.

National ADOPTION Information
  Clearinghouse (NAIC)
330 C St., SW.
Washington, DC 20447
(888) 251-0075
(703) 352-3488
(703) 385-3206 (Fax)
naic@calib.com (E-mail)
http://www.calib.com/naic
Provides professionals and the general public with easily accessible information on all aspects of adoption, including infant and intercountry adoption and the adoption of children with special needs. NAIC maintains an adoption literature database, a database of adoption experts, listings of adoption agencies, crisis pregnancy centers, and other adoption-related services, as well as excerpts of state and federal laws on adoption. Ultimately,

NAIC's goal is to strengthen adoptive family life. NAIC does not place children for adoption or provide counseling; it does, however, make referrals for such services. NAIC is funded by the Children's Bureau, Administration for Children and Families, and U.S. Department of Health and Human Services.

National ADOPTION Center
1500 Walnut St., Suite 701
Philadelphia, PA 19102
(800) 862-3678
(215) 735-9988
(215) 735-9410 (Fax)
nac@adopt.org (E-mail)
http://www.adopt.org/adopt
Mission is to expand adoption opportunities throughout the United States for children with special needs and those from minority cultures. Offers information and referral services. Provides publications on special needs adoption, single parent adoption, open adoption, and searching for birth parents.

National AGING Information Center
U.S. Administration on Aging
330 Independence Ave., SW
Washington, DC 20201
(202) 619-7501
(202) 401-7620 (Fax)
naic@aoa.gov (E-mail)
http://www.aoa.gov/naic
A service of the U.S. Administration on Aging (AoA). Serves as a central source for a wide variety of program and policy-related materials, demographic information, and other statistical data on health, economic, and social status of older people who live in the United States. Responds to any public inquiry about federal

programs and policies for the elderly, especially those supported under the Older American Act. Maintains a 3,800 bibliographic database of research and demonstration reports and documents, develops and maintains a publications list for AoA, and distributes fact sheets on aging topics for caregivers and older adults. Develops topic- and issue-based Web link pages as a series called *Aging Internet Information Notes.*

National Institute on AGING Information Center
P.O. Box 8057
Gaithersburg, MD 20898-8057
(800) 222-2225
(301) 496-1752
(800) 222-4225 (TTY)
(301) 589-3014 (Fax)
niainfo@jbs1.com (E-mail)
http://www.nih.gov/nia
Provides publications on health topics of interest to older adults, doctors, nurses, social activities directors, health educators, and the public.

U.S. Department of AGRICULTURE
    Extension Service
See the listing in the government section of your telephone book for your local extension office. Provides information on health, nutrition, fitness, and family well-being.

CDC National Prevention Information Network
    (CDC NPIN) (HIV/AIDS, STDs, TB)
P.O. Box 6003
Rockville, MD 20849-6003
(800) 458-5231
(800) 243-7012 (TTY)
(888) 282-7681 (Fax)
info@cdcnpin.org (E-mail)
http://www.cdcnpin.org
Sponsored by the Centers for Disease Control and Prevention (CDC), the CDC National Prevention Information Network (NPIN) is the U.S. reference, referral, and distribution service for information on HIV/AIDS, sexually transmitted diseases (STDs) and tuberculosis (TB). NPIN services are designed to facilitate the sharing of information and resources among people working in HIV, STD, and TB prevention, treatment, and support services. Bilingual staff are available to speak with callers, and all calls are confidential.

National Clearinghouse for ALCOHOL
    and DRUG Information
P.O. Box 2345
Rockville, MD 20847-2345
(800) 729-6686
(301) 468-2600
(800) 487-4889 (TTY/TDD)
(301) 230-2867 (TTY/TDD)
(301) 468-6433 (Fax)
info@health.org (E-mail)
http://www.health.org
Sponsored by the Center for Substance Abuse Prevention, Substance Abuse and Mental Health Services Administration. Gathers and disseminates information on alcohol and other drug-related subjects, including tobacco. Services include subject searches, provision of statistics and other information, and publications distribution. Operates the Regional Alcohol and Drug Awareness Resource Network, a nationwide linkage of alcohol and other drug information centers. Maintains a library open to the public, 8:00 a.m. to 6:00 p.m., Monday through Friday. 800 number offers 24-hour voicemail service.

National Institute of ALLERGY
    and INFECTIOUS DISEASES
Office of Communications Building 31,
    Room 7A-50 31
Center Drive, MSC 2520
Bethesda, MD 20892-2520
(301) 496-5717
(301) 402-0120 (Fax)
niaidoc@flash.niaid.nih.gov (E-mail)
http://www.niaid.nih.gov
Distributes publications and provides reference and referral services to the public, health professionals, and researchers on HIV/AIDS; allergy and asthma; and bacterial, fungal, immunologic, viral, and parasitic diseases. Provides information on diseases such as malaria, hepatitis, Lyme disease, tuberculosis, and sexually transmitted diseases.

National Center for Complementary and
    ALTERNATIVE MEDICINE (NCCAM)
    Information Clearinghouse
P.O. Box 8218
Silver Spring, MD 20907-8218
(888) 644-6226 (Voice and TTY/TDY)
(800) 531-1794 (Fax-back)
(301) 495-4957 (Fax)

nccamc@altmedinfo.org;
   nccam-info@nccam.nih.gov (E-mails)
http://www.nccam.nih.gov
Develops and disseminates fact sheets, information packages, and publications to enhance public understanding about complementary and alternative medicine research supported by the National Institutes of Health (NIH). NCCAM public information is currently free of charge; however, due to printing and duplication costs, only a limited number of copies can be requested. Information specialists can answer inquiries in English or Spanish. After normal business hours, callers have the option of receiving fact sheets and other information by fax.

ALZHEIMER'S DISEASE Education and Referral
   Center (ADEAR)
P.O. Box 8250
Silver Spring, MD 20907-8250
(800) 438-4380
(301) 495-3311
(301) 495-3334 (Fax)
adear@alzheimers.org (E-mail)
http://www.alzheimers.org/
Sponsored by the National Institute on Aging. Provides information and publications on Alzheimer's disease to health and service professionals, patients and their families, caregivers, and the public.

National Institute of ARTHRITIS and
   Musculoskeletal and Skin Diseases
   Information Clearinghouse
1 AMS Circle
Bethesda, MD 20892-3675
(877) 22-NIAMS
(301) 495-4484
(301) 565-2966 (TTY)
(301) 718-6366 (Fax)
niamsinfo@mail.nih.gov (E-mail)
http://www.nih.gov/niams
Designed to help patients and health professionals identify educational materials concerning arthritis and musculoskeletal and skin diseases. Distributes publications and maintains a file on the Combined Health Information Database (CHID) that indexes publications and audiovisuals. Personal information requests from patients are referred to appropriate organizations for additional information.

National Library Service for the BLIND
   and Physically Handicapped
Library of Congress
1291 Taylor St., NW
Washington, DC 20542
(800) 424-8567
(202) 707-5100
(202) 707-0744 (TDD)
(202) 707-0712 (Fax)
nls@loc.gov (E-mail)
http://lcweb.loc.gov/nls
A network of 57 regional and 81 subregional libraries that is administered by the National Library Service for the Blind and Physically Handicapped, Library of Congress. Provides free library service to anyone who is unable to read or use standard printed materials because of visual or physical disabilities. Delivers recorded and Braille books and magazines to eligible readers. Specially designed phonographs and cassette players are available for loan. A list of participating libraries is available in print and online.

U.S. Coast Guard Office of BOATING SAFETY
2100 Second St., SW., Room 3100
Washington, DC 20593-0001
(800) 368-5647
(202) 267-1077
(800) 689-0816 (TTY)
(703) 313-5910 (BBS)
boatweb@mail.rmit.com (E-mail)
http://www.uscgboating.org/
Provides safety information to recreational boaters; assists the public in finding boating education classes; answers technical questions; and distributes literature on boating safety, federal laws, and the prevention of recreational boating casualties.

CANCER Information Service
Office of Cancer Communications
National Cancer Institute
31 Center Dr., Room 10A31
Bethesda, MD 20892-2580
(800) 4-CANCER
(800) 332-8615 (TTY)
(800) 624-2511 (Fax back)
(301) 435-3848
(301) 402-5874 (Fax)
http://www.cancernet.nci.nih.gov
Provides information about cancer and cancer-related resources to patients, the public, and

health professionals. Inquiries are handled by trained information specialists. Spanish-speaking staff members are available. Distributes free publications from the National Cancer Institute. Operates 9 a.m. to 4:30 p.m.

National Clearinghouse on CHILD ABUSE
  and Neglect Information
330 C St., SW
Washington, DC 20447
(800) 394-3366
(703) 385-7565
(703) 385-3206 (Fax)
nccanch@calib.com (E-mail)
http://www.calib.com/nccanch
Serves as a national resource for the acquisition and dissemination of child abuse and neglect and child welfare materials and distributes a free publications catalog upon request. Maintains bibliographic databases of documents, audiovisuals, and national organizations. Services include searches of databases and annotated bibliographies on frequently requested topics.

National CHILD CARE Information Center
243 Church St., NW, 2nd Floor
Vienna, VA 22180
(800) 616-2242
(800) 516-2242 (TTY)
(800) 716-2242 (Fax)
info@nccic.org (E-mail)
http://nccic.org
A project of the Child Care Bureau, Administration for Children and Families, U.S. Department of Health and Human Services. A national resource that links information and people to complement, enhance, and promote the child care delivery system, working to ensure that all children and families have access to high-quality comprehensive services.

NIH CONSENSUS Program Information Center
Office of Medical Applications of Research
P.O. Box 2577
Kensington, MD 20891
(888) 644-2667
(301) 593-9485 (Fax)
http://consensus.nih.gov
A service of the Office of Medical Applications of Research, National Institutes of Health. Provides up-to-date information on biomedical technologies to all health care providers. Offers a 24-hour

voice mail service to order consensus statements produced by nonfederal panels of experts that evaluate scientific information on biomedical technologies. Information specialists available between 8:30 a.m. and 5 p.m. (eastern). Consensus statements can also be ordered by mail, fax, and electronic bulletin board.

U.S. Federal CONSUMER INFORMATION
  Center
Pueblo, CO 81009
(719) 948-4000 (Orders)
catalog.pueblo@gsa.gov (E-mail)
http://www.pueblo.gsa.gov
Helps federal agencies develop, promote, and distribute consumer information to the public through the Consumer Information Catalog and Web site. The catalog, available in print and online, lists over 200 free and low cost federal consumer publications on topics such as product recalls, health, energy conservation, money management, and nutrition. Also offers the Consumer Action Handbook in print and online and the Lista Publicaciones Federales en Español Para El Consumidor.

National Institute on DEAFNESS and Other
  Communication Disorders Information
  Clearinghouse
1 Communication Ave.
Bethesda, MD 20892-3456
(800) 241-1044
(800) 241-1055 (TTY)
(301) 907-8830 (Fax)
nidcdinfo@nidcd.nih.gov (E-mail)
http://www.nidcd.nih.gov
Collects and disseminates information on hearing, balance, smell, taste, voice, speech, and language for health professionals, patients, people in industry, and the public. Maintains a database of references to brochures, books, articles, fact sheets, organizations, and educational materials, which is a subfile of the Combined Health Information Database (CHID). Develops publications, including directories, fact sheets, brochures, information packets, and newsletters.

National DIABETES Information Clearinghouse
1 Information Way
Bethesda, MD 20892-3560
(800) 860-8747

(301) 654-3327
(301) 907-8906 (Fax)
ndic@info.niddk.nih.gov (E-mail)
http://www.niddk.nih.gov/health/diabetes/
    diabetes.htm
The National Diabetes Information Clearing-house (NDIC) is an information and referral service of the National Institute of Diabetes and Digestive and Kidney Diseases, one of the National Institutes of Health. The clearinghouse responds to written, telephone, and e-mail inquiries; develops and distributes publications about diabetes; and provides referrals to diabetes organizations, including support groups. The NDIC maintains a database of patient and professional education materials from which literature searches are generated.

National DIGESTIVE DISEASES Information
    Clearinghouse
2 Information Way
Bethesda, MD 20892-3570
(800) 891-8389
(301) 654-3810
(301) 907-8906 (Fax)
nddic@info.niddk.nih.gov (E-mail)
http://www.niddk.nih.gov/health/digest/nddic.htm
The National Digestive Diseases Information Clearinghouse (NDDIC) is an information and referral service of the National Institute of Diabetes and Digestive and Kidney Diseases, one of the National Institutes of Health. A central information resource on the prevention and management of digestive diseases, the clearinghouse responds to written inquiries, develops and distributes publications about digestive diseases, and provides referrals to digestive disease organizations, including support groups. The NDDIC maintains a database of patient and professional education materials from which literature searches are generated.

National Information Center for Children
    and Youth With DISABILITIES
P.O. Box 1492
Washington, DC 20013-1492
(800) 695-0285 (Voice/TTY)
(202) 884-8200 (Voice/TTY)
(202) 884-8441 (Fax)
nichcy@aed.org (E-mail)
http://www.nichcy.org

Sponsored by the U.S. Department of Education. Assists individuals by providing information in English and Spanish on disabilities and disability-related issues, with a special focus on children and youths with disabilities (birth to age 22). Services include responses to questions, referrals, and technical assistance to parents, educators, caregivers, and advocates. Develops and distributes fact sheets on disability and general information on parent support groups and public advocacy. All information and services are provided free of charge.

OSERS/Communications and Media Support
    Services (DISABILITIES, REHABILITATION)
Office of Special Education and Rehabilitative
    Services (OSERS)
U.S. Department of Education
Switzer Building, Room 3132
330 C Street SW
Washington, DC 20202-2524
(202) 205-8241
(202) 205-4208 (TTY)
(202) 401-2608 (Fax)
http://www.ed.gov/offices/OSERS/
Responds to inquiries on a wide range of topics, especially in the areas of federal funding, legislation, and programs benefiting people with disabling conditions. Provides referrals.

National Center for Chronic DISEASE
    PREVENTION and Health Promotion
    (NCCDPHP)
Technical Information and Editorial Services
Branch Centers for Disease Control and Prevention
4770 Buford Hwy., MS K13
Atlanta, GA 30341-3724
(770) 488-5080
(770) 488-5969 (Fax)
ccdinfo@cdc.gov (E-mail)
http://www.cdc.gov/nccdphp/nccdhome.htm
Provides information and referrals to the public and to professionals. Gathers information on chronic disease prevention and health promotion. Develops the following bibliographic databases focusing on health promotion program information: Health Promotion and Education, Cancer Prevention and Control, Comprehensive School Health with an AIDS school health component, Prenatal Smoking Cessation, and Epilepsy Education and Prevention Activities. Produces bibliographies on topics of interest in chronic

disease prevention and health promotion. The NCCDPHP Information Center collections include approximately 400 periodical subscriptions, 4,000 books, and 400 reference books. Visitors may use the collection by appointment. Produces the Chronic Disease Prevention (CDP) File CD-ROM, which includes the above databases and the CDP Directory, a listing of key contacts in public health.

DRUG POLICY Information Clearinghouse
2277 Research Blvd., Mailstop 2B
Rockville, MD 20850
(800) 666-3332
(301) 519-5212 (Fax)
ondcp@ncjrs.org (E-mail)
http://www.whitehousedrugpolicy.gov/about/
   clearinghouse.html
Supports the White House Office of National Drug Control Policy, National Criminal Justice Reference Service. Staffed by subject matter specialists and serves as a resource for statistics, research data, and referrals useful for developing and implementing drug policy. Disseminates publications; writes and produces documents on drug-related topics; coordinates with federal, state, and local agencies to identify data resources; and maintains a reading room offering a broad range of policy-related materials.

Educational Resources Information Center
   (ERIC) Clearinghouse on Teaching and
   Teacher EDUCATION
1307 New York Ave., NW, Suite 300
Washington, DC 20005
(800) 822-9229
(202) 293-2450
(202) 457-8095 (Fax)
query@aacte.org (E-mail)
http://www.ericsp.org
Sponsored by the U.S. Department of Education. Acquires, evaluates, abstracts, and indexes literature on the preparation and development of education personnel and on selected aspects of health and physical education, recreation, and dance. Publishes monographs, trends and issues papers, ERIC Digests, and ERIC Recent Resources (annotated bibliographies from the ERIC database). Performs computer searches of the ERIC database and sponsors workshops on searching the ERIC database.

U.S. ENVIRONMENTAL PROTECTION Agency
Information Resources Center
1200 Pennsylvania Ave., NW
Washington, DC 20460
(202) 260-5922
(202) 260-5153 (Fax)
library-hq@epamail.epa.gov (E-mail)
http://www.epa.gov
Offers general information about the agency and nontechnical publications on various environmental topics, such as air quality, pesticides, radon, indoor air, drinking water, water quality, and Superfund. Refers inquiries for technical information to the appropriate regional or program office. The public may visit the center between the hours of 8 a.m. and 5 p.m., Monday through Friday, except federal holidays.

National Clearinghouse on FAMILIES
   AND YOUTH
P.O. Box 13505
Silver Spring, MD 20911-3505
(301) 608-8098
(301) 608-8721 (Fax)
info@ncfy.com (E-mail)
http://www.ncfy.com
Links those interested in youth issues with the resources they need to better serve young people, families, and communities. Offers services that can assist in locating answers to questions or in making valuable contacts with other programs.

FEDERAL INFORMATION Center (FIC)
   Program—National Contact Center
P.O. Box 600
Cumberland, MD 21501-0600
(800) 688-9889
(800) 326-2996 (TTY)
http://www.info.gov
Provides information about the federal government's agencies, programs, and services. Information specialists use an automated database, printed reference materials, and other resources to provide answers to inquiries or accurate referrals. Callers who speak Spanish will be assisted. A descriptive brochure on the FIC program is available free from Department 584B at the Consumer Information Center (see listing in this publication). 9 a.m. to 8 p.m. eastern, Monday through Friday, except federal holidays.

FOOD AND DRUG Administration
Office of Consumer Affairs
5600 Fishers Lane
Rockville, MD 20857
(888) INFO-FDA
(301) 443-9767 (Fax)
webmail@oc.fda.gov (E-mail)
http://www.fda.gov.
Responds to consumer requests for information and publications on foods, drugs, cosmetics, medical devices, radiation-emitting products, and veterinary products. 10 a.m. to 4 p.m.

FOOD AND NUTRITION Information Center (FNIC)
National Agricultural Library/FNIC
U.S. Department of Agriculture Agricultural Research Service
10301 Baltimore Ave., Room 304
Beltsville, MD 20705-2351
(301) 504-5719
(301) 504-6856 (TTY)
(301) 504-6409 (Fax)
fnic@nal.usda.gov (E-mail)
http://www.nal.usda.gov/fnic/
One of several information centers located at the National Agricultural Library, part of the U.S. Department of Agriculture's Agricultural Research Service. Provides information on food, human nutrition, and food safety. Resource lists, databases, and many other food- and nutrition related links available on FNIC Web site. Collection includes books, manuals, journal articles, and audiovisual materials. Eligible patrons may borrow directly; others may borrow through interlibrary loan. Hours: 8:30 a.m. to 4:30 p.m., Monday through Friday.

Agency for HEALTHCARE Research and Quality Clearinghouse
P.O. Box 8547
Silver Spring, MD 20907-8547
(800) 358-9295
(410) 381-3150 (outside the United States)
(410) 290-3841 (Fax)
info@ahrq.gov (E-mail)
http://www.ahrq.gov
Distributes lay and scientific publications produced by the agency, including clinical practice guidelines on a variety of topics, reports from the National Medical Expenditure Survey, and health care technology assessment reports.

National HEALTH INFORMATION Center
P.O. Box 1133
Washington, DC 20013-1133
(800) 336-4797
(301) 565-4167
(301) 984-4256 (Fax)
info@nhic.org (E-mail)
http://www.health.gov/nhic
Helps the public and health professionals locate health information through identification of health information resources, an information and referral system, and publications. Uses a database containing descriptions of health-related organizations to refer inquirers to the most appropriate resources. Does not diagnose medical conditions or give medical advice. Prepares and distributes publications and directories on health promotion and disease prevention topics. 9 a.m. to 5:30 p.m.

National Information Center on HEALTH SERVICES RESEARCH and Health Care Technology (NICHSR)
National Library of Medicine
8600 Rockville Pike Building 38A, Room 4S-410, Mail Stop 20
Bethesda, MD 20894
(301) 496-0176
(301) 402-3193 (Fax)
nichsr@nlm.nih.gov (E-mail)
http://www.nlm.nih.gov/nichsr/nichsr.html
The 1993 NIH Revitalization Act created a National Information Center on Health Services Research and Health Care Technology (NICHSR) at the National Library of Medicine. The center works closely with the Agency for Healthcare Research and Quality (AHRQ), formerly the Agency for Health Care Policy and Research (AHCPR), to improve the dissemination of the results of health services research, with special emphasis on the growing body of evidence reports and technology assessments, which provide organizations with comprehensive, science-based information on common, costly medical conditions and new health care technologies.

National Center for HEALTH STATISTICS
Data Dissemination Branch
6525 Belcrest Rd., Room 1064
Hyattsville, MD 20782
(301) 458-4636

nchsquery@cdc.gov (E-mail)
http://www.cdc.gov/nchs
The Data Dissemination Branch of the National Center for Health Statistics answers requests for catalogs of publications and electronic data products; disseminates single copies of publications, such as Advance Data reports; provides information for publications and electronic products sold through the Government Printing Office and National Technical Information Service; adds addresses to the mailing list for new publications; and provides statistical data collected by the National Center for Health Statistics.

National HEART, LUNG, and BLOOD Institute
    (NHLBI) Information Center
P.O. Box 30105
Bethesda, MD 20824-0105
(301) 592-8573
(301) 592-8563 (Fax)
NHLBIinfo@rover.nhlbi.nih.gov (E-mail)
http://www.nhlbi.nih.gov
NHLBI serves as a source of information and materials on risk factors for cardiovascular disease. Services include dissemination of public education materials, programmatic and scientific information for health professionals, and materials on worksite health, as well as responses to information requests. Materials on cardiovascular health are available to consumers and professionals.

National HIGHWAY TRAFFIC SAFETY
    Administration
U.S. Department of Transportation
400 Seventh St., SW
Washington, DC 20590
(800) 424-9393 (Hotline)
(202) 366-0123 (Hotline)
(800) 424-9153 (TTY)
(202) 366-5962 (Fax)
http://www.nhtsa.dot.gov/
Provides information and referral on the effectiveness of occupant protection, such as safety belt use, child safety seats, and automobile recalls. Gives referrals to other government agencies for consumer questions on warranties, service, automobile safety regulations, and reporting safety problems. Works with private organizations to promote safety programs. Provides technical and financial assistance to state and local governments and awards grants for highway safety. 8 a.m. to 10 p.m.

National Resource Center on HOMELESSNESS
    and Mental Illness
345 Delaware Ave.
Delmar, NY 12054
(800) 444-7415
(518) 439-7415
(518) 439-7612 (Fax)
pra@prainc.com (E-mail)
http://www.prainc.com/nrc

HOUSING and URBAN DEVELOPEMENT
    (HUD)
P.O. Box 6091
Rockville, MD 20849
(800) 245-2691
(800) 483-2209 (TDD)
(301) 519-5767 (Fax)
huduser@aspensys.com (E-mail)
http://www.huduser.org
Disseminates publications for the U.S. Department of Housing and Urban Development's Office of Policy Development and Research. Offers database searches on housing research. Provides reports on housing safety, housing for elderly and handicapped persons, and lead-based paint.

INDOOR AIR Quality Information
    Clearinghouse
P.O. Box 37133
Washington, DC 20013-7133
(800) 438-4318
(703) 356-4020
(703) 356-5386 (Fax)
iaqinfo@aol.com (E-mail)
http://www.epa.gov/iaq/
Information specialists provide information, referrals, and publications on indoor air quality. Information is provided about pollutants and sources, health effects, control methods, commercial building operations and maintenance, standards and guidelines, and federal legislation.

National INJURY Information
    Clearinghouse
U.S. Consumer Product Safety Commission
Washington, DC 20207
(301) 504-0424
(301) 504-0124 (Fax)
clearinghouse@cpsc.gov (E-mail)
http://www.cpsc.gov/about/clrnghse.html

Sponsored by the U.S. Consumer Product Safety Commission (CPSC). The clearinghouse collects and disseminates information on the causes and prevention of death, injury, and illness associated with consumer products. Compiles data obtained from accident reports, consumer complaints, death certificates, news clips, and the National Electronic Injury Surveillance System operated by the CPSC. Publications include statistical analyses of data and hazard and accident patterns.

National KIDNEY AND UROLOGIC Diseases
   Information Clearinghouse
3 Information Way
Bethesda, MD 20892-3580
(800) 891-5390 (Toll free)
(301) 654-4415
(301) 907-8906 (Fax)
nkudic@info.niddk.nih.gov (E-mail)
http://www.niddk.nih.gov/health/kidney/
   nkudic.htm
The National Kidney and Urologic Diseases Information Clearinghouse (NKUDIC) is an information and referral service of the National Institute of Diabetes and Digestive and Kidney Diseases, one of the National Institutes of Health. The clearinghouse responds to written inquiries, e-mail, and telephone requests; develops and distributes publications about kidney and urologic diseases; and provides referrals to kidney and urologic disease organizations, including support groups. The NKUDIC maintains a database of patient and professional education materials from which literature searches are generated.

National LEAD Information Center
8601 Georgia Ave., Suite 503
Silver Spring, MD 20910
(800) 424-LEAD (Clearinghouse)
(800) 526-5456 (TDD)
(301) 585-7976 (Fax)
hotline.lead@epamail.epa.gov (E-mail)
http://www.epa.gov/lead/nlic.htm
Sponsored by the Environmental Protection Agency. Responds to inquiries regarding lead and lead poisoning. Provides information on lead poisoning and children, lead-based paint, a list of local and state contacts who can help, and other lead-related questions.

National Center for Education in MATERNAL
   AND CHILD HEALTH Clearinghouse
Suite 701
2000 15th St.
North Arlington, VA 22201-2617
(703) 524-7802
(703) 524-9335 (Fax)
info@ncemch.org (E-mail)
http://www.ncech.org
Sponsored by the Maternal and Child Health Bureau, Health Resources and Services Administration. Provides information to health professionals and the public, develops educational and reference materials, and provides technical assistance in program development. Subjects covered are women's health, including pregnancy and childbirth; infant, child, and adolescent health; nutrition; children with special health needs; injury and violence prevention; and maternal and child health programs and services. Materials include professional literature, curricula, patient education materials, audiovisuals, and information about organizations and programs. Participates in the Combined Health Information Database (CHID) and National Library of Medicine's DIRLINE. Provides online databases: MCHLine, Organizations Database, MCH Projects Database, and Title V Information System. Appointments preferred for onsite visits.

National MATERNAL AND CHILD HEALTH
   Clearinghouse
2070 Chain Bridge Rd., Suite 450
Vienna, VA 22182-2536
(888) 434-4MCH
(703) 356-1964
(703) 821-2098 (Fax)
nmchc@circlesolutions.com (E-mail)
http://www.nmchc.org
Sponsored by the Maternal and Child Health Bureau, Health Resources and Services Administration. Centralized source of materials and information in the areas of human genetics and maternal and child health. Distributes publications and provides referrals.

National Institute of MENTAL HEALTH (NIMH)
Information Resources and Inquires Branch
6001 Executive Blvd., Room 8184
MSC 9663
Bethesda, MD 20892-9663

(301) 443-4513
(301) 443-8431 (TTY)
(301) 443-5158 (MENTAL HEALTH FAX4U—
Fax Information System)
(888) 8ANXIETY (publications on anxiety
disorders)
(800) 421-4211 (publications on depression)
nimhinfo@nih.gov (E-mail)
http://www.nimh.nih.gov
The National Institute of Mental Health (NIMH),
a component of the National Institutes of Health,
conducts and supports research that seeks to
understand, treat, and prevent mental illness. The
institute's public inquiries line is staffed with
trained information specialists who respond to
information requests from the lay public, clinicians, and the scientific community with a variety
of publications. These include printed materials
on such subjects as basic behavioral research,
neuroscience of mental health, rural mental
health, children's mental disorders, schizophrenia,
depression, bipolar disorder, attention deficit
hyperactivity disorder, Alzheimer's disease, panic
disorder, obsessive-compulsive disorder, posttraumatic stress disorder, and other anxiety
disorders. Information and publications on
NIMH-sponsored educational programs on
depressive and anxiety disorders, their symptoms,
and their treatments are also available. A list of
NIMH publications, including several in Spanish,
is available upon request. Information on NIMH-
sponsored meetings, workshops, and symposia is
available on the institute's website.

Office of MINORITY HEALTH
Resource Center
5515 Security Lane, Suite 101
Rockville, MD 20852
(800) 444-6472
(301) 230-7874
(301) 230-7199 (TDD)
(301) 230-7198 (Fax)
LMosby@omhrc.gov; info@omhrc.gov
(E-mails)
http://www.omhrc.gov/
Responds to information requests from health
professionals and consumers on minority health
issues and locates sources of technical assistance.
Provides referrals to relevant organizations and
distributes materials. Spanish-speaking operators
are available.

Clearinghouse for OCCUPATIONAL SAFETY
AND HEALTH INFORMATION
4676 Columbia Pkwy.
Cincinnati, OH 45226-1998
(800) 356-4674
(513) 533-8328
(513) 533-8573 (Fax)
(888) 232-3299 (Fax-on-demand)
pubstaff@cdc.gov (E-mail)
http://www.cdc.gov/niosh
Provides technical information support for the
National Institute for Occupational Safety and
Health (NIOSH) research programs and disseminates information to others on request. Services
include reference and referral, and information
about NIOSH studies. Distributes a publications
list of NIOSH materials. Maintains an automated
database covering the field of occupational safety
and health.

National ORAL HEALTH Information
Clearinghouse
1 NOHIC Way
Bethesda, MD 20892-3500
(301) 402-7364
(301) 907-8830 (Fax)
nohic@nidcr.nih.gov (E-mail)
http://www.nohic.nidcr.nih.gov
A service of the National Institute of Dental and
Craniofacial Research. Focuses on the oral health
concerns of special care patients, including people
with genetic disorders or systemic diseases that
compromise oral health, people whose medical
treatment causes oral problems, and people with
mental or physical disabilities that make good
oral hygiene practices and dental care difficult.
Develops and distributes information and educational materials on special care topics, maintains a
bibliographic database on oral health information
and materials, and provides information services
with trained staff to respond to specific interests
and questions.

NIH OSTEOPOROSIS and Related Bone
Diseases—National Resource Center
1232 22 St., NW
Washington, DC 20037-1292
(800) 624-BONE
(202) 223-0344
(202) 466-4315 (TTY)
(202) 293-2356 (Fax)

orbdnrc@nof.org (E-mail)
http://www.osteo.org/
Sponsored by the National Institute of Arthritis and Musculoskeletal and Skin Disease, National Institute of Child Health and Human Development, National Institute of Dental and Craniofacial Research, National Institute of Environmental Health Sciences, NIH Office of Research on Women's Health, HHS Office on Women's Health, and National Institute on Aging. Provides resources and information to patients, health professionals, and the public on metabolic bone diseases such as osteoporosis, Paget's disease of the bone, osteogenesis imperfecta, and primary hyperparathyroidism. Specific populations include the elderly, men, women, and adolescents.

President's Council on PHYSICAL FITNESS
    and Sports
Hubert H. Humphrey Building, Room 738-H
200 Independence Ave., SW
Washington, DC 20201
(202) 690-9000
(202) 690-5211 (Fax)
http://www.fitness.gov
Conducts a public service advertising program, prepares educational materials, and works to promote the development of physical fitness leadership, facilities, and programs. Helps schools, clubs, recreation agencies, employers, and federal agencies design and implement programs. Offers a variety of testing, recognition, and incentive programs for individuals, institutions, and organizations. Materials on exercise and physical fitness for all ages are available.

POLICY Information Center (PIC)
Office of the Assistant Secretary for Planning
    and Evaluation
U.S. Department of Health and Human Services
Hubert H. Humphrey Building, Room 438F
200 Independence Ave., SW
Washington, DC 20201
(202) 690-6445
pic@osaspe.dhhs.gov (E-mail)
http://aspe.dhhs.gov/pic/
A centralized repository of evaluations, short-term evaluative research reports, and program inspections/audits relevant to the department's operations, programs, and policies. It includes relevant reports from the General Accounting Office,

Congressional Budget Office, and the Institute of Medicine and the National Research Council's Committee on National Statistics, both part of the National Academy of Sciences. Reports are also available from the Departments of Agriculture, Labor, and Education, as well as the private sector. Final reports and executive summaries are available for review at the facility, or final reports may be purchased from the National Technical Information Service. In addition, the PIC online database of evaluation abstracts is accessible through USDHHS home page, http://www.hhs.gov. The database includes over 6,000 project descriptions of both in-process and completed studies. *PIC Highlights,* a quarterly publication, features articles of recently completed studies.

Office of POPULATION AFFAIRS (OPA)
    Clearinghouse
P.O. Box 30686
Bethesda, MD 20824-0686
(301) 654-6190
(301) 215-7731 (Fax)
opa@osophs.dhhs.gov (E-mail)
http://opa.osophs.dhhs.gov/clearinghouse.html
Sponsored by the Office of Population Affairs. Provides information and distributes publications to health professionals and the public in the areas of family planning, adolescent pregnancy, and adoption. Makes referrals to other information centers in related subject areas.

National Clearinghouse for PRIMARY CARE
    Information
2070 Chain Bridge Rd., Suite 450
Vienna, VA 22182
(703) 821-8955 ext. 248
(703) 821-2098 (Fax)
http://www.bphc.hrsa.dhhs.gov
Sponsored by the Bureau of Primary Health Care (BPHC), Health Resources and Services Administration. Provides information services to support the planning, development, and delivery of ambulatory health care to urban and rural areas that have shortages of medical personnel and services. A primary role of the clearinghouse is to identify, obtain, and disseminate information to community and migrant health centers. Distributes publications focusing on ambulatory care, financial management, primary health care, and health services administration of special

interest to professionals working in primary care centers funded by BPHC. Materials are available on health education, governing boards, financial management, administrative management, and clinical care. Bilingual medical phrase books, a directory of federally funded health centers, and an annotated bibliography are available also.

U.S. Consumer PRODUCT SAFETY
   Commission Hotline (CPSC)
Washington, DC 20207
(800) 638-2772 (Toll free hotline)
info@cpsc.gov (E-mail)
http://cpsc.gov/
Maintains the National Injury Information Clearinghouse, conducts investigations of alleged unsafe or defective products, and establishes product safety standards. Assists consumers in evaluating the comparative safety of products and conducts education programs to increase consumer awareness. Operates the National Electronic Injury Surveillance System, which monitors a statistical sample of hospital emergency rooms for injuries associated with consumer products. Maintains a free hotline to provide information about recalls and to receive reports on unsafe products and product-related injuries. Publications describe hazards associated with electrical products and children's toys. Spanish-speaking operator available through the toll-free number listed.

National REHABILITATION
   Information Center
1010 Wayne Ave.,
800 Silver Spring, MD 20910
(800) 346-2742
(301) 562-2400
(301) 595-5626 (TTY)
(301) 562-2401 (Fax)
naricinfo@kra.com (E-mail)
http://www.naric.com
The National Rehabilitation Information Center (NARIC) is a library and information center on disability and rehabilitation. Funded by the National Institute on Disability and Rehabilitation Research, NARIC collects and disseminates the results of federally funded research projects. The collection, which also includes books, journal articles, and audiovisuals, grows at a rate of about 300 documents per month.

RURAL Information Center Health Service
   (RICHS)
National Agricultural Library
10301 Baltimore Ave., Room 304
Beltsville, MD 20705-2351
(800) 633-7701
(301) 504-5547
(301) 504-6856 (TDD)
(301) 504-5181 (Fax)
ric@nal.usda.gov (E-mail)
http://www.nal.usda.gov/ric/richs
Disseminates information on a variety of rural health issues including health professions, health care financing, special populations, and the delivery of health care services. Provides information, referrals, publications, and brief complimentary literature searches to professionals and the public. Posts rural health information on the Internet. RICHS is funded by the Federal Office of Rural Health Policy, the Department of Health and Human Services and is part of the United States Department of Agriculture Rural Information Center, which provides information on rural issues such as economic development and community well-being.

National Center on SLEEP DISORDERS Research
2 Rockledge Center, Suite 10038
6701 Rockledge Dr., MSC 7920
Bethesda, MD 20892-7920
(301) 435-0199
(301) 480-3451 (Fax)
ncsdr@nih.gov (E-mail)
http://www.nhlbi.nih.gov/health/public/sleep
Promotes basic, clinical, and applied research on sleep and sleep disorders by strengthening existing sleep research programs, training new investigators, and creating new programs aimed at addressing important gaps and opportunities in sleep and sleep disorders.

Office on SMOKING and Health
Centers for Disease Control and Prevention
National Center for Chronic Disease Prevention
   and Health Promotion
Mail Stop K-50,
4770 Buford Hwy. NE
Atlanta, GA 30341-3724
(800) CDC-1311
(770) 488-5705
(770) 488-5939 (Fax)

tobaccoinfo@cdc.gov (E-mail)
http://www.cdc.gov/tobacco
Develops and distributes the annual Surgeon General's Report on Smoking and Health, coordinates a national public information and education program on tobacco use and health, and coordinates tobacco education and research efforts within the Department of Health and Human Services and throughout both federal and state governments. Maintains the Smoking and Health database, consisting of approximately 60,000 records available on CD-ROM (CDP File) through the Government Printing Office (Superintendent of Documents, Government Printing Office, Washington, DC 20402). Provides information on smoking cessation, environmental tobacco smoke/passive smoking, pregnancy/infants, professional/technical information, and a publications list upon request.

National SUDDEN INFANT DEATH
    SYNDROME Resource Center
2070 Chain Bridge Rd., Suite 450
Vienna, VA 22182
(866) 866-7437 (Toll free)
(703) 821-8955
(703) 821-2098 (Fax)
sids@circsolutions.com (E-mail)
http://www.sidscenter.org
Sponsored by the Maternal and Child Health Bureau, Health Resources and Services Administration. Provides information and educational materials on sudden infant death syndrome (SIDS), apnea, and other related topics. Responds to information requests from parents, professionals, and the public. Maintains a library/database of public awareness and medical research materials on SIDS and related topics and conducts customized searches of this database and Medline in response to users' requests. Maintains and updates mailing lists of state programs, groups, and individuals concerned with SIDS. Also develops fact sheets, catalogs, and bibliographies on topics of special interest to the SIDS community.

National TECHNICAL INFORMATION
    Service
U.S. Department of Commerce
5285 Port Royal Rd.
Springfield, VA 22161
(800) 553-6847
(703) 605-6900 (Fax)

info@ntis.gov (E-mail)
http://www.ntis.gov/
Sells more than 9,000 federally produced audiovisual programs. Provides catalogs at no cost. Several catalogs cover health-related topics, including alcohol and other drug abuse, emergency fire services, industrial safety, and occupational health.

National WOMEN'S HEALTH Information Center
8850 Arlington Blvd., Suite 300
Fairfax, VA 22310
(800) 994-9662
(888) 220-5446 (TDD)
4woman@soza.com (E-mail)
http://www.4woman.gov
NWHIC is a health information and federal publication referral service that provides a gateway to women's health information from other government agencies, public and private organizations, and consumer and health care professional groups.

National YOUTH VIOLENCE PREVENTION
    Resource Center (NYVPRC)
P.O. Box 6003
Rockville, MD 20849-6003
(866) 723-3968
(800) 243-7012 (TTY)
(301) 562-1001 (Fax)
NYVP@safeyouth.org (E-mail)
http://www.safeyouth.org
NYVPRC is a central source of information on prevention and intervention programs, publications, research, and statistics on violence committed by and against children and teens. The resource center is a collaboration between the Centers for Disease Control and Prevention and other federal agencies.

FEDERAL HEALTH INFORMATION CENTERS AND CLEARINGHOUSES

Agency for Healthcare Research and Quality
    Clearinghouse
(800) 358-9295
(410) 381-3150 (outside the United States)
(410) 290-3841(Fax)
info@ahrq.gov (E-mail)
http://www.ahrq.gov

Alzheimer's Disease Education and Referral
    Center
(800) 438-4380
(301) 495-3311

(301) 495-3334 (Fax)
adear@alzheimers.org (E-mail)
http://www.alzheimers.org/

Cancer Information Service
(800) 4-CANCER
(800) 332-8615 (TTY)
(800) 624-2511 (Fax back)
(301) 435-3848; (301) 402-5874 (Fax)
http://www.cancernet.nci.nih.gov

Centers for Disease Control National Prevention
  Information Network
(800) 458-5231
(800) 243-7012 (TTY)
(888) 282-7681 (Fax)
info@cdcnpin.org (E-mail)
http://www.cdcnpin.org

Clearinghouse for Occupational Safety
  and Health Information—National
  Institute for Occupational Safety and
  Health
(800) 356-4674
(513) 533-8328
(513) 533-8573 (Fax)
(888) 232-3299 (Fax-on-demand)
pubstaff@cdc.gov (E-mail)
http://www.cdc.gov/niosh

Drug Policy Information Clearinghouse
(800) 666-3332
(301) 519-5212 (Fax)
ondcp@ncjrs.org (E-mail)
http://www.whitehousedrugpolicy.gov/about/
  clearinghouse.html

Educational Resources Information Center
  Clearinghouse on Teaching and Teacher
  Education
(800) 822-9229
(202) 293-2450
(202) 457-8095 (Fax)
query@aacte.org (E-mail)
http://www.ericsp.org

Federal Information Center Program—
  National Contact Center
(800) 688-9889
(800) 326-2996 (TTY)
http://www.info.gov

Food and Drug Administration
(888) INFO-FDA
(301) 443-9767 (Fax)
webmail@oc.fda.gov (E-mail)
http://www.fda.gov.

Food and Nutrition Information Center
(301) 504-5719
(301) 504-6856 (TTY)
(301) 504-6409 (Fax)
fnic@nal.usda.gov (E-mail)
http://www.nal.usda.gov/fnic/

Housing and Urban Development
(800) 245-2691
(800) 483-2209 (TDD)
(301) 519-5767 (Fax)
huduser@aspensys.com (E-mail)
http://www.huduser.org

Indoor Air Quality Information Clearinghouse
(800) 438-4318
(703) 356-4020
(703) 356-5386 (Fax)
iaqinfo@aol.com (E-mail)
http://www.epa.gov/iaq/

National Adoption Center
(800) 862-3678
(215) 735-9988
(215) 735-9410 (Fax)
nac@adopt.org (E-mail)
http://www.adopt.org/adopt

National Adoption Information Clearinghouse
(888) 251-0075
(703) 352-3488
(703) 385-3206 (Fax)
naic@calib.com (E-mail)
http://www.calib.com/naic

National Aging Information Center—U.S.
  Administration on Aging
(202) 619-7501
(202) 401-7620 (Fax)
naic@aoa.gov (E-mail)
http://www.aoa.gov/naic

National Agricultural Library
(800) 633-7701
(301) 504-5547

(301) 504-6856 (TDD)
(301) 504-5181 (Fax)
ric@nal.usda.gov (E-mail)
http://www.nal.usda.gov/ric/richs

National Center for Chronic Disease Prevention
and Health Promotion
(770) 488-5080
(770) 488-5969 (Fax)
ccdinfo@cdc.gov (E-mail)
http://www.cdc.gov/nccdphp/nccdhome.htm

National Center for Complementary and
Alternative Medicine Information
Clearinghouse
(888) 644-6226 (Voice and TTY/TDY)
(800) 531-1794 (Fax-back)
(301) 495-4957 (Fax)
nccamc@altmedinfo.org;
nccam-info@nccam.nih.gov (E-mails)
http://www.nccam.nih.gov

National Center for Education in Maternal
and Child Health
(703) 524-7802
(703) 524-9335 (Fax)
info@ncemch.org (E-mail)
http://www.ncemch.org

National Center for Health Statistics
(301) 458-4636
nchsquery@cdc.gov (E-mail)
http://www.cdc.gov/nchs

National Center on Sleep Disorders Research
(301) 435-0199
(301) 480-3451 (Fax)
ncsdr@nih.gov (E-mail)
http://www.nhlbi.nih.gov/health/public/sleep

National Child Care Information Center
(800) 616-2242
(800) 516-2242 (TTY)
(800) 716-2242 (Fax)
info@nccic.org (E-mail)
http://nccic.org

National Clearinghouse for Alcohol and Drug
Information
(800) 729-6686
(301) 468-2600

(800) 487-4889 (TTY/TDD)
(301) 230-2867 (TTY/TDD)
(301) 468-6433 (Fax)
info@health.org (E-mail)
http://www.health.org

National Clearinghouse for Primary Care
Information
(703) 821-8955 ext. 248
(703) 821-2098 (Fax)
http://www.bphc.hrsa.dhhs.gov

National Clearinghouse on Child Abuse
and Neglect Information
(800) 394-3366
(703) 385-7565
(703) 385-3206 (Fax)
nccanch@calib.com (E-mail)
http://www.calib.com/nccanch

National Clearinghouse on Families
and Youth
(301) 608-8098
(301) 608-8721 (Fax)
info@ncfy.com (E-mail)
http://www.ncfy.com

National Diabetes Information
Clearinghouse
(800) 860-8747
(301) 654-3327
(301) 907-8906 (Fax)
ndic@info.niddk.nih.gov (E-mail)
http://www.niddk.nih.gov/health/diabetes/
diabetes.htm

National Digestive Diseases Information
Clearinghouse
(800) 891-8389
(301) 654-3810
(301) 907-8906 (Fax)
nddic@info.niddk.nih.gov (E-mail)
http://www.niddk.nih.gov/health/digest/
nddic.htm

National Health Information Center
(800) 336-4797
(301) 565-4167
(301) 984-4256 (Fax)
info@nhic.org (E-mail)
http://www.health.gov/nhic/

National Heart, Lung, and Blood Institute
Information Center
(301) 592-8573
(301) 592-8563 (Fax)
nhlbIinfo@rover.nhlbi.nih.gov (E-mail)
http://www.nhlbi.nih.gov

National Highway Traffic Safety Administration
(800) 424-9393 (Hotline)
(202) 366-0123 (Hotline)
(800) 424-9153 (TTY)
(202) 366-5962 (Fax)
http://www.nhtsa.dot.gov/

National Information Center for Children
and Youth With Disabilities
(800) 695-0285 (Voice/TTY)
(202) 884-8200 (Voice/TTY)
(202) 884-8441 (Fax)
nichcy@aed.org (E-mail)
http://www.nichcy.org

National Information Center on Health Services
Research and Health Care Technology
(301) 496-0176
(301) 402-3193 (Fax)
nichsr@nlm.nih.gov (E-mail)
http://www.nlm.nih.gov/nichsr/nichsr.html

National Injury Information Clearinghouse
(301) 504-0424
(301) 504-0124 (Fax)
clearinghouse@cpsc.gov (E-mail)
http://www.cpsc.gov/about/clrnghse.html

National Institute of Allergy and Infectious
Diseases, Office of Communications
(301) 496-5717
(301) 402-0120 (Fax)
niaidoc@flash.niaid.nih.gov (E-mail)
http://www.niaid.nih.gov

National Institute of Arthritis and
Musculoskeletal and Skin Diseases
Information Clearinghouse
(877) 22-NIAMS
(301) 495-4484
(301) 565-2966 (TTY)
(301) 718-6366 (Fax)
niamsinfo@mail.nih.gov (E-mail)
http://www.nih.gov/niams

National Institute of Mental Health
(301) 443-4513
(301) 443-8431 (TTY)
(301) 443-5158 (MENTAL HEALTH FAX4U—
Fax Information System)
(888) 8ANXIETY (publications on anxiety
disorders)
(800) 421-4211 (publications on depression)
nimhinfo@nih.gov (E-mail)
http://www.nimh.nih.gov

National Institute on Aging Information
Center
(800) 222-2225
(301) 496-1752
(800) 222-4225 (TTY)
(301) 589-3014 (Fax)
niainfo@jbs1.com (E-mail)
http://www.nih.gov/nia

National Institute on Deafness and Other
Communication Disorders Information
Clearinghouse
(800) 241-1044
(800) 241-1055 (TTY)
(301) 907-8830 (Fax)
nidcdinfo@nidcd.nih.gov (E-mail)
http://www.nidcd.nih.gov

National Kidney and Urologic Diseases
Information Clearinghouse
(800) 891-5390 (Toll free)
(301) 654-4415
(301) 907-8906 (Fax)
nkudic@info.niddk.nih.gov (E-mail)
http://www.niddk.nih.gov/health/kidney/
nkudic.htm

National Lead Information Center
(800) 424-LEAD (Clearinghouse)
(800) 526-5456 (TDD)
(301) 585-7976 (Fax)
hotline.lead@epamail.epa.gov (E-mail)
http://www.epa.gov/lead/nlic.htm

National Library Service for the Blind
and Physically Handicapped
(800) 424-8567
(202) 707-5100
(202) 707-0744 (TDD)
(202) 707-0712 (Fax)

nls@loc.gov (E-mail)
http://lcweb.loc.gov/nls

National Maternal and Child Health
  Clearinghouse
(888) 434-4MCH
(703) 356-1964
(703) 821-2098 (Fax)
nmchc@circlesolutions.com (E-mail)
http://www.nmchc.org

National Oral Health Information
  Clearinghouse
(301) 402-7364
(301) 907-8830 (Fax)
nohic@nidcr.nih.gov (E-mail)
http://www.nohic.nidcr.nih.gov

National Rehabilitation Information Center
(800) 346-2742
(301) 562-2400
(301) 595-5626 (TTY)
(301) 562-2401 (Fax)
naricinfo@kra.com (E-mail)
http://www.naric.com

National Resource Center on Homelessness
  and Mental Illness
(800) 444-7415
(518) 439-7415
(518) 439-7612 (Fax)
pra@prainc.com (E-mail)
http://www.prainc.com/nrc

National Sudden Infant Death Syndrome
  Resource Center
(866) 866-7437 (Toll free)
(703) 821-8955
(703) 821-2098 (Fax)
sids@circsolutions.com (E-mail)
http://www.sidscenter.org

National Technical Information Service
(800) 553-6847
(703) 605-6900 (Fax)
info@ntis.gov (E-mail)
http://www.ntis.gov/

National Women's Health Information Center
(800) 994-9662
(888) 220-5446 (TDD)

4woman@soza.com (E-mail)
http://www.4woman.gov

National Youth Violence Prevention
  Resource Center
(866) 723-3968
(800) 243-7012 (TTY)
(301) 562-1001 (Fax)
NYVP@safeyouth.org (E-mail)
http://www.safeyouth.org

NIH Consensus Program Information Center
(888) 644-2667
(301) 593-9485 (Fax)
http://consensus.nih.gov

NIH Osteoporosis and Related Bone Diseases—
  National Resource Center
(800) 624-BONE
(202) 223-0344
(202) 466-4315 (TTY)
(202) 293-2356 (Fax)
orbdnrc@nof.org (E-mail)
http://www.osteo.org/

Office of Minority Health Resource Center
(800) 444-6472
(301) 230-7874
(301) 230-7199 (TDD)
(301) 230-7198 (Fax)
LMosby@omhrc.gov; info@omhrc.gov
  (E-mails)
http://www.omhrc.gov/

Office of Population Affairs Clearinghouse
(301) 654-6190
(301) 215-7731 (Fax)
opa@osophs.dhhs.gov (E-mail)
http://opa.osophs.dhhs.gov/clearinghouse.html

Office on Smoking and Health
(800) CDC-1311
(770) 488-5705
(770) 488-5939 (Fax)
tobaccoinfo@cdc.gov (E-mail)
http://www.cdc.gov/tobacco

OSERS/Communications and Media Support
  Services (Disabilities, Rehabilitation)
(202) 205-8241
(202) 205-4208 (TTY)

(202) 401-2608 (Fax)
http://www.ed.gov/offices/OSERS/

Policy Information Center
(202) 690-6445
pic@osaspe.dhhs.gov (E-mail)
http://aspe.dhhs.gov/pic/

President's Council on Physical Fitness and Sports
(202) 690-9000
(202) 690-5211 (Fax)
http://www.fitness.gov

Rural Information Center Health Service
(800) 633-7701
(301) 504-5547
(301) 504-6856 (TDD)
(301) 504-5181 (Fax)
ric@nal.usda.gov (E-mail)
http://www.nal.usda.gov/ric/richs

U.S. Coast Guard Office of Boating Safety
(800) 368-5647
(202) 267-1077
(800) 689-0816 (TTY)

(703) 313-5910 (BBS)
boatweb@mail.rmit.com (E-mail)
http://www.uscgboating.org/

U.S. Consumer Product Safety Commission
  Hotline
(800) 638-2772 (Toll free hotline)
info@cpsc.gov (E-mail)
http://cpsc.gov/

U.S. Department of Agriculture Extension Service
See the listings in the government section of telephone book for your local extension office.

U.S. Environmental Protection Agency
  Information Resources Center
(202) 260-5922
(202) 260-5153 (Fax)
library-hq@epamail.epa.gov (E-mail)
http://www.epa.gov

U.S. Federal Consumer Information Center
(719) 948-4000 (Orders)
catalog.pueblo@gsa.gov (E-mail)
http://www.pueblo.gsa.gov

14 Management Concepts and Principles and Their Applications

The occupational health manager must be thoroughly familiar with the organization's purpose, goals, and structures that support the organization's mission, understanding of organizational culture, and dynamics as described in Chapter 9. In addition, knowledge and skills about concepts related to leadership, quality improvement and cost management, and the importance of change in a dynamic environment are essential. This chapter will focus on a discussion of concepts and skills important to effective managerial guidance.

DEFINITIONS

The terms *management* and *leadership* are often considered synonymous and used interchangeably; however, these concepts are different. Leadership is a broader concept than management and is not bound by organizational structures. It involves the process of influencing the behavior of people in their willing efforts toward goal setting and achievement (Hitt, 1993; Tomey, 2000). Management has been defined by numerous authors; however, a discrete yet targeted and encompassing definition is offered by Hersey and Blanchard (1993), who define management as working with and through individuals and groups to accomplish organizational goals.

To accomplish the goals of the organization, the occupational health manager must apply management and leadership skills to facilitate the work of the staff efficiently and effectively. The manager needs to be aware of various managerial and leadership theories and styles, including her or his own, and how this style affects the relationship with and performance of those being managed. For the most part, the occupational health manager will be managing and working with knowledge workers who usually require a great deal of autonomy in carrying out the responsibilities of their jobs. Colleagueship and collaboration are essential ingredients in the management experience.

MANAGEMENT THEORIES

Various management theories describe the relationship and impact of management and leadership styles on the motivation and productivity of workers/staff. Contrary to early management theories that emphasized autocratic leadership and rules and regulations, human relations management focuses on encouraging and empowering workers to develop their potential and enhancing worker efforts to meet their needs for recognition and accomplishment (Beaulieu et al., 1997; Renmick-Breisch, 1998; Douglas, 1996; Tappen, 2001). The occupational health manager will find that understanding and applying principles related to these theories will help in discovering strategies to stimulate worker motivation and creativity. Several theories will be briefly described; however, reference to a good leadership and management text is suggested for a fuller discussion.

MASLOW'S HIERARCHY OF NEEDS

Maslow developed the hierarchy of needs theory in which he classifies a human needs structure into five categories: physiological/survival, safety and security, belongingness/social, self-esteem, and self-actualization (Maslow, 1954). The essence of the theory is that lower level needs (e.g., eating, shelter) must be met before moving on to higher level needs (e.g., recognition, achievement). Although many types of needs or motivators are apparent in the work setting, the occupational health manager needs to recognize that people are different and what satisfies one person may not satisfy another. For example, one employee may have a need for social affiliation; another, good pay and work hours; and yet another, work performance recognition. Depending on one's circumstances, motivators will change; that is, recognition and achievement are likely to be valued by most employees at different points in time. The occupational health manager should be attuned to recognizing these needs.

HERZBERG'S TWO FACTOR THEORY

Herzberg's Two Factor or Motivation-Hygiene Theory was based on interview research conducted with 200 engineers and accountants regarding job situations they found satisfying or dissatisfying. The research indicated that workers are most satisfied with job factors associated with what he called *motivators,* including achievement, recognition, advancement, responsibility, growth potential, and the work itself. Factors that produced dissatisfaction are termed *hygiene* factors and are associated with supervision, policy, work status, work conditions, interpersonal relationships, and job security. Job dissatisfaction leads to increased absenteeism, turnover, and reduced productivity resulting in excessive recruitment, orientation, and job development, which are costly and time consuming. Herzberg believed

Maslow's Needs Heirarchy	Herzberg's Factors	
Personal Growth	Motivators	Work Itself Achievement
Esteem		Advancement Recognition
Belongingness	Hygiene Factors	Interpersonal and Supervisory Relationships
Safety		Technical Supervision Working Conditions Company Policy/Administration
Physiological		Salary

Figure 14-1 Comparison of Maslow's and Herzberg's theories related to human needs and rewards.

that these more personal and environmentally-related hygiene factors do not necessarily motivate but can lower job performance. Although some controversy (based on the research methodology) surrounds this theory, human relations conditions identified as satisfiers and dissatisfiers comparably reflect Maslow's work. A comparison is shown in Figure 14-1.

McGREGOR'S THEORY X AND THEORY Y

McGregor's Theory X and Theory Y (Table 14-1), which describes a philosophy of human nature as applied to managerial relationships, shares some of the same concepts as Maslow's hierarchy of needs and Herzberg's Motivation-Hygiene theory. The basic assumptions underlying Theory X management are that the manager places strong emphasis on the attainment of organizational goals and that workers must be fully directed, controlled, coerced, and punished into performing their jobs. This type of manager assumes that workers inherently dislike their jobs and avoid responsibility and new challenges. Theory X managers will do the thinking and planning for the workers and closely supervise them.

Theory Y managers emphasize the goals of the individual within the context of achieving organizational goals. These managers believe that workers have the self-direction and control skills necessary to meet work performance objectives and enjoy personal achievement and task accomplishment. The Theory Y manager believes that under good working conditions people seek responsibility and are creative and innovative. This manager encourages worker participation in goal setting, delegates authority, supports and enhances job expansion, and uses positive motivations such as praise and recognition to encourage goal attainment.

TASK/RELATIONSHIP THEORY

Hersey and Blanchard (1993) extended the earlier (1960s) work of Blake and Mouton in examining task/productivity and relationship behavior with maturity levels of workers (Table 14-2). Hersey and Blanchard assert that the most effective leadership is dependent on the maturity of the workers. Groups with below average maturity function best under leaders with high task-low relationship orientations, whereas groups with average maturity function best under leaders with high task-high relationship or low task-high relationship. Employees' attitudes toward management are an important factor to consider with respect to their perception of the manager's role. Some employees perceive an authoritarian, highly structured role as desirable; some prefer strong

---

TABLE 14-1   List of Assumptions About Human Nature That Underlie McGregor's Theory X and Theory Y

THEORY X	THEORY Y
1. Work is inherently distasteful to most people.	1. Work is as natural as play if the conditions are favorable.
2. Most people are not ambitious, have little desire for responsibility, and prefer to be directed.	2. Self-control is often indispensable in achieving organizational goals.
3. Most people have little capacity for creativity in solving organizational problems.	3. The capacity for creativity in solving organizational problems is widely distributed in the population.
4. Motivation occurs only at the physiological and safety levels.	4. Motivation occurs at the social, esteem, and self-actualization levels, as well as at the physiological and safety/security levels.
5. Most people must be closely controlled and often coerced to achieve organizational objectives.	5. People can be self-directed and creative at work if properly motivated.

TABLE 14-2	Leadership Styles Appropriate for Varying Maturity Levels of Workers	
MATURITY LEVEL	**APPROPRIATE STYLE**	
M1 Low Maturity Unable and unwilling or insecure	**S1** Telling High task and low relationship behavior	
M2 Low to Moderate Maturity Unable but willing or confident	**S2** Selling High task and high relationship behavior	
M3 Moderate to High Maturity Able but unwilling or insecure	**S3** Participating High relationship and low task behavior	
M4 High Maturity Able/competent and willing/ confident	**S4** Delegating Low relationship and low task behavior	

From *Management of Organizational Behavior*, (6th ed.), by P. Hersey and K. Blanchard, Englewood Cliffs, NJ: Prentice Hall. 1993.

interaction with the manager in decision making and control; others prefer to work autonomously. Individual differences require that the occupational health manager be adaptive.

Traditional management theory is based on McGregor's Theory X, Maslow's primary physiological and safety needs, and Herzberg's hygiene needs. Contemporary management is based on McGregor's Theory Y, Maslow's higher level needs, and Herzberg's motivators. Employee participation in goal direction and planning and empowerment of workers to assume more deci-

sion making responsibility are considered major factors in management philosophy and have been shown to contribute to worker satisfaction.

This overview of management/leadership theories demonstrates a trend toward increased emphasis on human needs and commitment through participation within the context of the organization rather than an emphasis on efficiency in the absence of human relations, recognition, and personal goal fulfillment. The occupational health manager is encouraged to explore these theories and styles, analyze her or his management style within the context of the organization, and determine the most effective management approach that fits the situation, personal style, and objectives. By studying the management process, management and leadership theories, and motivational enhancers, the occupational health manager can gain an increased understanding of effective strategies in working with others in order to accomplish both organizational and personal goals. This is achieved through implementation of defined skills, effective decision making, and managerial functions designed to effectively utilize the skills and talents of all employees. Soliciting input from many sectors about decisions affecting the organization will be a key component in this effort (Fallon, 2001).

MANAGERIAL SKILLS

In a classic article Katz (1955) identifies the following three management skill levels as important to the managerial role:

1. *Technical skills* emphasize the use of knowledge, methods, processes, procedures, techniques, and equipment necessary for the performance of specific tasks and activities.
2. *Interpersonal skills* utilize knowledge about human behavior and interpersonal processes, including an understanding of motivational and leadership concepts and effective communication techniques.
3. *Conceptual skills* are concerned with the ability to understand organizational complexities and dynamics, analyze internal/external trends that affect the organization, and develop and conceptualize ideas that provide a visionary direction for the organization as a whole.

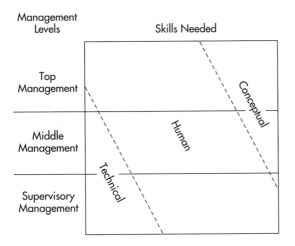

Figure 14-2   Managerial skill mix at various orga-
nizational levels. *(From* Management of Organizational
Behavior: Utilizing Human Resources *(6th ed., pp. 8, 195), Paul
Hersey/Kenneth H. Blanchard, 1993, Englewood Cliffs, NJ:
Prentice-Hall.*

Managers need all three skills to fulfill their role
requirements, but the relative importance and
degree of use of each skill depends on the situation and the manager's position in the authority
hierarchy of the organization.

As illustrated in Figure 14-2, the manager's
skill mix is dependent on the role and level at
which she or he functions in the organization. As
a person advances in the management/organiza-
tional structure, less technical and more conceptual skills are needed (Yukl, 1989). However, top
level executives need to have an understanding
of how these skills interrelate. The occupational
and environmental health nurse may be in the
role of manager of the occupational health unit,
manager of occupational health services, or
regional or corporate nurse or health director.
Managerial skills should be developed to reflect
the level and scope of responsibilities attached to
the position.

Technical skills are particularly important at
the supervisory level in order to train, develop,
and direct workers regarding specialized activities and evaluate their performance. Supervisory
level managers are mainly responsible for
implementing policy and maintaining the work-
flow within the organizational structure.

Interpersonal skills are key for middle managers whose roles are primarily focused on furthering organizational goals and developing

plans to implement policies established at higher
levels. Although this requires some skill in visioning and technical competence, good communication and motivational skills are essential to empower workers to assume increased responsibility
for accomplishing the work goals and objectives.

Conceptual skills, the major responsibility of
top executives, are essential to move the organization forward. This is accomplished through
promoting effective strategic planning, policy
formulation, and program development; recognizing the influence and impact of the external
environment; and understanding interrelationships and intrarelationships among and within
the organizational units. To effectively lead the
organization, input must be actively sought from
all levels in the organization.

Of course, the type, size, and structure of
organizations need to be considered with respect to
managerial skill levels. For example, in organizations where decision making is highly decentral-
ized, technical skills are less important for top level
executives, whereas in smaller organizations that
operate with highly centralized decision making
authority, top level executives may exercise more
intense technical skill abilities. Although middle
managers may be placed in the position to deal
with human relations problems and situations,
interpersonal or human relations skills fall within
the domain of all levels of managers. Organizations
are social systems that require both individual productivity and teamwork to achieve organizational
goals. The occupational health unit manager must
possess the ability to relate to people, communicate
clearly, manage conflict, and promote productivity
through motivation, which is central to human
resource management.

DECISION MAKING

To function effectively, the manager needs to be
skilled in continuously making effective decisions,
which requires familiarity with the decision
making process. As described by Tomey (2000),
decision making is a dynamic, deliberate, cognitive
process consisting of sequential steps that allow for
more rational and accurate problem solving and
action. One decision ultimately affects other
decisions. Steps in the decision making process are
illustrated in Figure 14-3, and a brief discussion of
this process within the context of occupational
health follows.

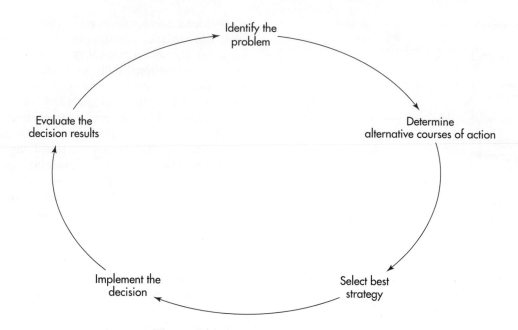

Figure 14-3 Decision making process.

1. *Identify the problem.* The first step in the decision making process is defining the problem and factors that cause this problem. The occupational health manager needs to be able to recognize the problem and gather as much data as needed to fully identify and analyze the problem. For example, if disagreements arise over who is responsible for and has authority over something at work, the real problem may be an inadequate job description or ill-defined task delineation. Once the real problem is identified, possible solutions can be explored.

2. *Determine alternative courses of action.* Usually there are a number of ways to solve a problem. Some solutions may be quick and economical but less effective than others; some may be more effective but may take longer to resolve the problem and may be more costly. The occupational health manager should first determine if a policy exists to handle the situation. If no policy exists, the manager should determine alternative courses of action by using various sources such as experience, benchmarking, literature, consultants, and staff members. Creative ideas are likely to emerge from these sources. The greater the number of

alternatives identified, the higher the probability of problem resolution.

3. *Select the most desirable alternative.* The pros and cons of each alternative should be considered and measured against the current method of handling the problem or situation in order to determine which proposed strategy is potentially the most effective. Resources and constraints such as manpower, human relations, finances, facilities, and equipment must be evaluated to determine potential pitfalls that might be avoided if they can be managed up front. Eagerness to reach a decision may lead to premature solutions, and considering only a few alternatives in haste blocks good decisions. Avoidance of the real problem, lack of clear problem definition, insufficient data, and early statements of attitude by a status figure also interfere with reaching effective solutions as do mixing of idea generation and idea evaluation, decisions made by large groups and lack of staff commitment because the superior who makes the decision does not implement it (Tomey, 2000). The alternative selected should yield the best results within a cost-efficient framework. One alternative is not always clearly

superior to another. Multiple factors should be considered in selecting a strategy, including worker acceptance, morale, time, and risk of failure.

4. *Implement the decision.* A decision made must be put into action, otherwise it is wasted effort. Ideally, coworkers have been involved in the decision making process so that implementation of the decision will not create undue antagonism. Often situations that require change will arouse uncomfortableness, so the manager will need to communicate with staff regarding the best approaches to decision implementation. Involvement of staff will help to increase ownership and decrease resistance.

5. *Evaluate the decision results.* The final step is to evaluate the decision outcome. The manager should allow some time to pass in order for the decision to be integrated. There may be resistance to the decision; however, if the decision was made thoughtfully, management should adhere to its commitment to the decision. If the decision is ultimately unworkable, alternative strategies may need to be invoked.

The occupational health manager can improve the decision making process through the use of tools and techniques such as brainstorming, nominal group process, decision trees, PERT (program evaluation and review techniques) models, Delphi methods, forecasting, critical path analyses, and simulated computer applications and analyses. The manager may make independent decisions or involve the group responsible for decision implementation, depending on the manager's knowledge and expertise relative to the area under consideration, degree of commitment from the group, time constraints, and impact and importance of the decision.

MANAGERIAL FUNCTIONS

The managerial process engages six major functions: planning, financial management, organizing, staffing, directing, and evaluating. The planning function is the most important and provides the framework for all other functions. Although these functions are described sepa-

rately, they are interrelated. As an effective manager, the occupational and environmental health nurse possesses skills in all areas (Tappen, 2001; Tomey, 2000).

PLANNING

Planning, the first managerial function, is critical to the management process. Planning requires conceptual thinking. There are two major types of planning, strategic or long-range planning and operational or short-term planning, the results of which set the stage for effective strategic and operational functioning (Martin, 1998).

The manager engaged in strategic planning asks, Where is the organization going and how will it get there? Strategic planning is used to determine the direction of and resources needed for the organization and assigns responsibilities for strategic management; the goals that come from strategic planning are more generic and less specific than those from operational planning. Strategic planning generally extends 3 to 5 years into the future and begins with an analysis of both the internal strengths and weaknesses of the organization and the external influences that present opportunities and threats to the organization; this analysis is commonly referred to as a *SWOT analysis* (Figure 14-4). This grid can be used to identify the organization's internal strengths and weaknesses, which may include such areas as qualifications and personnel expertise, quality of services, and budgetary resources; opportunities may include new programs and initiatives, improved technology, and new facilities, whereas threats may be new regulations, decreased service satisfaction, and inadequate personnel. After an analysis is done, leaders and managers must define a vision that is clear and feasible and encompasses the values and beliefs of the organization (see Chapter 9), write a mission statement, and specify long-term goals and objectives, including strategies and a timetable to accomplish the objectives. Priorities are determined and resources needed for implementation are identified along with evaluation criteria.

Vision and Mission

The vision is an image of the company or unit that depicts the preferred future, and the mission defines the organization's expectation or purpose for being. The mission of the organization

SWOT Analysis	
Strengths	**Weaknesses**
Opportunities	**Threats**

Figure 14-4   SWOT analysis.

Box 14-1   Examples of Vision and Mission Statements

VISION STATEMENT

The following values guide the Occupational Health Service Center:

• Quality
• Fairness
• Innovation
• Prevention

MISSION STATEMENT

The mission of the Occupational Health Services Center is to deliver comprehensive health care services to promote physical and mental health; to prevent occupational and nonoccupational disease, injury, and disability; and to provide quality-driven cost-effective health services.

---

influences the goals and objectives. Carrying this through the organization to departmental units allows for support of and consistency with the overall organizational vision and mission. Box 14-1 provides an example of a vision statement and a mission statement for an occupational health department.

Goals and Objectives

When planning for occupational health programs and services, the occupational health manager should identify and/or review the overall organizational mission and goals and objectives and determine where in this structure the occupational health unit fits. The occupational health manager should be familiar with the organization's history, structure, value system, and culture, particularly with respect to health care, existing occupational health and safety programs, leadership/management styles, trends in illness/injury, health care costs, professional attitudes, role behaviors, communication lines and patterns, and productivity measures (Hersey & Blanchard, 1993). Although it may seem evident, the occupational health manager must clarify the purpose of the occupational health service or program or both. For example, does the occupational health service exist to reduce work-related risk, improve overall worker health, or reduce health care costs or for a combination of these reasons or for other reasons?

In congruence with the organization's mission and goals occupational health unit goals and objectives should be established to achieve the unit's purpose. Goals are broad statements central to the whole management process, and the planning process explicitly defines the goals. Objectives are specific statements set to achieve the goals and are measurable, realistic, and time-oriented. Goals and objectives may address, for example, existing programs and services or use of resources or innovations and should be prioritized in order of importance. Personnel involved in setting goals and objectives should be familiar with the needs of the organizational unit. For example, while the board of directors and top level administrators usually set organizational goals and objectives, the corporate occupational health director or occupational health manager sets the goals and objectives for the occupational health service in collaboration with other staff members. Goals and objectives should be reviewed periodically to assess progress toward achievement or need for modification or both. Examples of occupational health goals and programmatic objectives are shown in Box 14-2.

Management by Objectives (MBO), first introduced by Peter Drucker in the 1950s, is a tool and philosophy used for both planning and evaluation functions and is aimed at improving worker motivation and productivity (Drucker, 1982). MBO is widely used by U.S. business and in the health care sector. The purpose of MBO is to help workers and managers collaborate and negotiate mutually acceptable goals and performance objectives that can be both unit/program-oriented or individually worker-focused and are results-oriented and measurable. MBO helps broaden participation in day-to-day decision making and focuses on work outcomes. In MBO the manager does not set goals and objectives for the employee; rather, the manager acts as a mentor, collaborator, or coach for the employee. Goal setting is a deliberate act wherein the employee analyzes strengths and weaknesses, reviews the work plan, and establishes measurable objectives. In developing objectives, the employee should review job duties and existing responsibilities, outline proposed or expansion initiatives, and discuss with the manager key areas needing accomplishment.

After the major job responsibilities are identified, expected levels of accomplishment are

---

Box 14-2 **Examples of Occupational Health Goals and Objectives for 2004**

GOAL: IMPROVE THE HEALTH OF PREGNANT WORKING MOTHERS

Objectives

- Provide a series of prenatal education classes stressing the importance of prenatal care and healthy habits (two times during the year).
- Develop communication mechanisms with personal health care providers for appropriate prenatal care monitoring and facilitation of prenatal care.
- Reduce the proportion of pregnant women who smoke (by 80%) through smoking cessation programs.

GOAL: IMPROVE HEALTHY LIFESTYLE HABITS IN THE WORKFORCE

Objectives

- Provide two health promotion programs targeted to meet the health needs of the workforce.
- Reduce the proportion of workers who smoke by 50%.
- Increase the proportion of workers who exercise regularly by 40%.

---

determined. Criteria for expected levels of accomplishment should be results-oriented, established before the fact, time bound, realistic and attainable, measurable and verifiable, written, and agreed on by both the manager and the staff associate employee. Common errors to avoid when developing objectives are writing too many objectives or overly complex objectives, having too high or too low of standards, using too long or too short of a time period, and having imbalanced emphasis, objectives that are not measurable, or objectives for which the cost of measurement is too high.

After objectives, responsibilities, and the achieved expectations are completed, evaluation criteria, against which measurements can be made, must be established. The employee should meet with the manager to establish priorities and develop plans for the accomplishment of the objectives. The manager will determine whether the objectives are compatible with the overall goals of the organization. The manager and the employee should hold periodic reviews to check the employee's progress and make adjustments. An annual review should be held to compare the actual results with the expected levels of accomplishment and to set the objectives for the next period (Tomey, 2000).

MBO fosters employee growth, strengthens employee identification with organizational goals, promotes self-direction, and builds self-esteem. The process allows for feedback and an option to modify objectives and thus provides a more fair evaluation of employee performance (Gillies, 1994; Marquis and Huston, 1998).

Business Proposals/Plans

In the current health care and business environment the occupational health manager is challenged with developing new or expanding existing health programs and services. This is part of the manager's planning function. The formal business plan or proposal is the vehicle often used to acquire resources and gain approval for program implementation (Jarrett, 1989). The plan is a written document that specifies concisely, but in sufficient detail, what the proposed venture or program is and the expectations to be achieved from its implementation. The nurse executive must always keep in mind that she or he will be competing with other departments for scarce funding and should produce evidence of the potential cost-effectiveness of the proposed services, such as how the program will improve employee health and reduce health insurance premiums, workers' compensation claims, or absenteeism. The business plan serves as a guide for efficient project operation and management, an information source, and a document that will facilitate decision making, motivation, and the measurement of performance (Vestal, 1989).

The specific elements, format, and length of a business plan or proposal are not universal, and

---

> ### Box 14-3   Typical Elements of a Business Proposal or Plan
>
> Title page
> Project/executive summary
> Table of contents
> Introduction
> Project description
> Rationale/identification of need
> Alternative approaches
> Operational plan (implementation plan)
> Marketing plan
> Financial plan
> Evaluation plan
> Appendices

the occupational and environmental health nurse should be familiar with the organizational expectations. However, a basic set of components that should be considered for inclusion in any plan or proposal (Box 14-3) is described here.

Title page

The title page should include the title of the proposed project, the author or project leader, the organizational unit, the date of submission, and the anticipated date of project implementation.

Project/executive summary

The project/executive summary section should provide a clear, brief overview of the entire project. This component is often considered the most critical piece of the plan since many reviewers will read only this initial summary and financial plan (to determine if there is any interest in the project proposal). The essence of the project must be condensed into 1 or 2 pages that clearly state the project's purpose and value in relation to the organization's mission and goals, the need or rationale for the project, and the financial implications that include a brief summary of the initial or start-up costs and expected return on investment.

Table of contents

The table of contents should provide an easy reference guide to the major components of the document so that the reader can quickly access specific components as desired.

Introduction

The introduction describes the organization, its goals and objectives, and supporting infrastructure.

Project description

The purpose of the project description is to clearly describe the exact purpose of the project. In addition, goals and objectives, expected outcomes, the project's fit with the overall goals of the organization, the impact of the project on the company's image, timetables, and flowcharts should be presented succinctly and in a logical order.

Rationale/identification of need

The rationale/identification of need provides the justification for the project or program and includes evidence to support the need. For example, if a program for cholesterol and/or high blood pressure screening and monitoring is proposed, supporting evidence might include epidemiologic data such as demographic, risk factor, and morbidity and mortality indicators compared with known population parameters, health insurance claims data, and absenteeism trends for cardiovascular-related illnesses. In addition, the nurse can review a sample of health charts or actively sample the workforce via questionnaires to determine if relative risk factors exist and then provide these data in aggregate form.

Alternative approaches

Alternative approaches to addressing the problem should be discussed. This will provide the reviewer with information that shows that the problem and alternative solutions have been carefully explored. Cost-benefit data for varying alternatives should also be presented. If alternative propositions are of roughly equal cost, the occupational health nurse should state why one alternative is recommended over another. For example, if the proposed project is to offer a fitness and exercise program, alternative strategies might include offering exercise classes on-site, which might entail hiring a fitness instructor or creating or renovating space. In addition, factors associated with employee release time versus off-work time should be considered. Another option could be to contract with a fitness center to have employees utilize the center through a limited voucher system. Each alternative should be described along with anticipated benefits and estimated costs.

Operational plan

The operational plan should be tied to the objectives and is intended to describe how the plan will be carried out. The exact content, of course, will reflect how the objectives will be implemented in terms of human and physical facilities/material resource needs. Information regarding organizational management/charts, personnel to be hired along with targeted activities or responsibilities, plans for training, and how the program or project will be organized to produce the desired outcome should be presented. The physical facilities/materials should be described in terms of new or existing space needs, including renovation or remodeling, capital expenditures for equipment or furniture and maintenance, and consumable supplies and materials. If a contractual arrangement is proposed, it should also be thoroughly described with respect to the operational procedure. Résumés for key personnel and proposed job descriptions can be included in the document appendix.

Marketing plan

The marketing plan should describe how the program or project will be marketed to the target group, including a promotional schedule or calendar, media selection, and advertising plans and materials. Costs for marketing materials need to be included in the financial or budget plan.

Financial plan

The financial plan or budget should address all costs that are associated with the project and are tied to meeting the goals and objectives; these costs include operating and capital expenditures. In the operating budget personnel costs should include compensation and benefits, training, travel, and any other related expenditures such as professional dues or insurance. If consultant services are expected, these will also need to be accounted for in the financial plan. Nonpersonnel items can be categorized and include space (e.g., rent, lease), small supplies, communications (e.g., telephone, postage, computer), and promotional and project materials (e.g., brochures, handouts, videos, refreshments, data analysis). A capital budget should be developed for large expenditures, such as construction or remodeling of physical facilities and high cost equipment such as a Reflotron. Often a budget is prepared for the start-up first-year costs plus the second- and third-year estimated budgets (which might include additional or replacement inventory). Standardized organizational budget forms should be utilized.

Evaluation plan

The evaluation plan should spell out in detail how to measure the outcomes of the project, which should reflect the original objectives. A plan for evaluating anticipated costs of achieving the objectives should be included. For example, measuring programmatic costs of identifying individuals with high blood pressure and referring them for treatment versus the costs of potential cardiovascular morbidity and mortality could be specified. A plan for data analysis and a written report should be included.

Appendices

The appendices should include all supporting documents related to the plan such as charts, job descriptions (Appendix 14-1), and résumés.

Writing business plans or proposals is a process the occupational health nurse will increasingly use in planning and providing for health care programs to the workforce. If not already acquired, the occupational health nurse will need to develop skills to formulate a persuasive business plan utilizing the appropriate organizational format. The occupational health manager can use the business plan as a tool to obtain the resources necessary to achieve the goals and objectives of the occupational health department.

FINANCIAL MANAGEMENT

Financial management involves fiscal planning, identification and allocation of resources, analysis of expenditures, and creative budgetary negotiations. Budgeting is a financial control system defined as a tool for planning, monitoring, and controlling costs (Douglas, 1996). The fiscal manager coordinates fiscal planning, plans and justifies the budget, organizes, implements the budget process, and determines resource requirements within the budget's OR organization's constraints. The fiscal manager also coordinates expenses and budget control, documents needs to other administrative levels, organizes needed resources, explains budgeting to others, and evaluates technology (Huber, 1996; Marquis and Huston, 1996).

A budget is a quantitative plan, the primary purpose of which is to ensure the most effective use of scarce resources over a period of time. The budget is tied to the formal organizational plan set forth to meet the goals and objectives established in the planning process. Participation in the budget from individuals at all levels in the organization is more likely to produce a realistic budget. The presumption is that individuals who are operationally responsible for meeting a part of the overall budget are allowed to help determine budget allocations and have some control over expenditures and outcomes (Finkler, 2000).

Preparation of the budget requires the manager to think and plan ahead, anticipate costs, and monitor and control expenditures. There are many types of budgets (e.g., operating, program, performance, capital, strategic); however, the operating budget and the capital expense budget are probably the ones most familiar to the occupational health manager. Numerous computer programs are available for organizing and preparing budget spread sheets. Through monitoring the budget, deviations from the budget line can be detected and corrective actions taken quickly.

The operating budget is specified for a period of time—generally annually—and is designed to plan for the daily operation of the cost center, a functional unit (in this case the occupational health unit) within the organization that generates costs. The budget projects salary and nonsalary expenditures.

In developing the operating budget, the occupational health manager will need to know historical budget data, unit goals and objectives reflecting projected needs and growth, and quantifiable indicators of resource consumption (e.g., numbers and types of personnel, pieces of equipment, supplies) necessary to accomplish the goals and objectives identified in the program plan.

A review of historical data can help the occupational health manager understand how resources were previously used (Bozman & Childres, 1991), if allocations and expenditures were cost-effective, if unexpected deviations occurred, and if performance objectives were met (Finkler, 2000). All goals and objectives are closely tied to the budget so that

resource allocation is appropriate for conducting the work needed to achieve programmatic/unit goals. Here, the occupational health manager will want to plan for such areas as inflationary costs, new or expanded services or programs (e.g., health screening, surveillance activities), new or updated technology systems, advanced health/medical therapeutics and technologies, and the cost/impact of regulatory mandates.

Armed with historical data, a unit/program plan, and expense data, the occupational health manager can prepare an operating budget. The actual preparation of the operational budget translates goals and objectives into numbers. Although terms or categorical labels may vary from organization to organization, typical cost or line item categories to include in the budget are personnel salaries, benefits, insurance, rent, materials/supplies, equipment, communication, professional/staff development costs, membership fees, travel, and consultants. Examples of items usually considered within the line item categories are shown in Box 14-4. However, it is important to note that line item categories will vary from organization to organization, and the occupational health manager will need to be skilled in budget preparation specific to the organization.

Preparation of the budget should begin several months in advance of the (fiscal or calendar) year of expenditure, at the time the unit/program plan is developed. During the annual planning process, goals and objectives and related budgetary costs are established and readied for approval by top management.

As previously mentioned, projected costs to operate the occupational health unit will in part be derived from historical usage levels. The occupational health manager should review all line item expenditures from the previous year to determine the cost-effectiveness in meeting goals and objectives. The review should indicate if resources were adequate to operate the occupational health unit. If not, adjustments should be factored in to meet actual needs for the next budget period. Inflationary costs, anticipated bonuses, and costs associated with proposed, expanded, or new mandated programs should be incorporated. This might include projected costs for mammography screening for female employees and/or spouses or family members of male employees, expansion of occupational health

Box 14-4 Examples of Line Items Included in an Occupational Health Unit Budget

PERSONNEL

Full-time staff
Part-time staff
Fringe benefits for each individual (e.g., health insurance, pension, vacation/-sick pay)
Taxes
Contract personnel
Substitute personnel
Overtime pay
Shiftwork differential
Merit/bonus supplements

MATERIALS/SUPPLIES

Office supplies (e.g., forms, paper, pens)
Health care supplies
Pharmaceuticals
Health education materials
Photocopying

EQUIPMENT

Desks/chairs
File cabinets
Photocopying machine
Laboratory items/instruments
Equipment rental/maintenance/repair

COMMUNICATION

Telephone
Postage/overnight mail
Fax machine
Print materials (e.g., brochures)
Computer

PROFESSIONAL/STAFF DEVELOPMENT

Conferences/seminar fees
Professional dues
Journals
Certifications

SPECIAL PROGRAMS/PROJECTS

Health promotion activities
Research

TRAVEL

Conferences/seminars and related business trips
Site or other satellite visits

CONSULTANT

In-house site services
External fees (preparatory work, reports)
Travel/lodging

---

services for 24-hour coverage, or start-up costs associated with implementation of a new satellite occupational health service. For example, projected personnel expenditures should include all mixes and quantities (full-time, part-time, contractual) of personnel needed by shift. An example of an occupational health service cost center budget spreadsheet is shown in Figure 14-5.

Capital expenditures are generally related to long-term planning. Capital expenditures include physical changes such as replacement or expansion of the plant, major equipment, and inventories. These items are usually major investments and reduce the flexibility in budgeting because it takes a long time to recover the costs. For example, purchase of an audiometric booth or other types of high cost equipment will fall into this category. The chief executive officer usually establishes the ceiling for capital expenses. Under this budget the occupational health manager must establish priorities if requests exceed availability of funds.

The next step in the budgeting process is obtaining formal approval from top management. The occupational health manager must justify the budget in terms of growth related to projected goals and objectives, outline the rationale for program initiation or expansion, and emphasize the contribution the occupational health service makes in health care cost reduction. This can be carried out by providing data relative to trends in work-related illness and injury, workers' compensation costs, insurance claims, and lost work time and disability management.

Once the budget is operationalized, the occupational health manager is responsible for the ongoing monitoring and controlling of actual expenditures. Regular computerized budget statements or spreadsheets should be utilized that specify each line item actually budgeted, current expenditures, any variance (amount spent over or under budget), and the balance available. This scrutiny should be done at least monthly to be certain that projected and actual expenditures are

BS32A

Budget System
Budget Worksheet
Fiscal Year 2002/03

Page: 1
Date: 2/01/02
Time: 16:15:53

Rev.
(even dollars)

Cost Center 5600 Health Center

Acct Code	Description	2000/01 Actual	(2001/02) YTD Actual	(2001/02) YTD Bud	2001/02 Est Actual	2001/02 Budget	2002/03 Budget	2003/04 Forecast
611110	Salaries: Office							
611210	Sick pay: Office							
611310	Overtime: Office							
616450	Fringe charge: Office							
621111	T & E: Lodging							
621222	T & E: Meals							
621333	T & E: Trans/Tips—No air							
621339	T & E: Air travel							
621444	T & E: Entertainment							
621666	T & E: Other							
621810	T & E: RTP/Greenville							
623110	Employee medical services							
623190	Other employee services							
624240	Dues & registration fees							
625100	Temporary help							
631160	USA forms							
631180	Other printed matter							
632110	Office equipment not capital							
632310	Stationary stock supplies							
632320	Office supplies: O/S purchase							
633110	Chemicals							
633410	Scientific apparatus/supp							
639110	Computer operating supplies							
639120	Subscriptions & pamphlets							
639130	Books							
639220	Photographic supplies							
639244	Other audiovisual							
639250	Reprints, photostat & transl.							
639260	Multilith & offset supplies							
639310	Fin gds inv by IT-med							

Figure 14-5 Example of a budget spreadsheet. *(Courtesy Burroughs-Wellcome Co., Research Triangle Park, NC.)*

Continued

639315	Fin gds inv by IT-diag
639410	Art supplies
639540	Cleaning supplies
639910	Sundry supplies
644110	Electrical supplies
644310	Hardware supplies
653110	Consulting fees
656210	O/S repairs-bldg/mach/equip-ment
656510	O/S maint-comp hrdw & sftw
656610	O/S repairs-office mach
656710	O/S repairs-scientific
659110	O/S laundry service
659910	Other outside services
661110	Telephone & telegraph
683150	Comp hardware-purchases
683180	Computer software
683190	CIS hardware charges
683210	O/S computer charges
684210	Sales tax on purchases
685110	Postage
685910	Sundry freight
689910	Sundry expenses
699107	Travel contingency
699117	Other O/S serv contingency
699134	Sundry supplies contingency
699154	Training & meetings contin-gency
699155	Office supplies contingency
699162	M & R supplies contingency
	Cost center subtotals
662110	Deprec-building & improve
662210	Deprec-machainery & equip-ment
662310	Deprec-computer hardware
662410	Amortz-comp. software
662510	Amortz-land improvements

Below the line totals
Cost center totals

Figure 14-5, cont'd For legend see p. 483.

compatible. If deviations are apparent, problem areas can be identified and minor modifications can then be made to adjust expenditures.

Although the budget process is relatively straightforward, unforeseen problems can occur because organizations are always changing. Examples of unanticipated costs might be associated with new occupational health regulations, staff turnover, budget cuts, or cost overruns. Problems should be analyzed for cause, and solutions should be determined to prevent recurrence as much as possible.

ORGANIZING

Organizing is the third managerial function, wherein the manager organizes the personnel and work to accomplish the plan. While planning is the key to effective management, the organizational structure and infrastructure provide the framework for getting the job done. This involves establishing a formal structure that provides for the coordination of objectives and resources and infrastructure, such as space and equipment, which support good environmental working conditions.

Organizational Concepts

The occupational health manager should be fully familiar with the organizational structure that shows the relationship among people and positions and depicts hierarchical structures that define authority relationships and accountability. This is depicted in an organizational chart or schematic that shows the links among the parts of an organization, areas of responsibility, persons to whom one is accountable, and channels of communication. The visual diagram of a chart is often a more effective means of communicating the organization's structure than is a written description. Vertical charts depict the chief executive at the top, with formal hierarchical lines of authority, often referred to as the chain of command, flowing down (Tappen, 2001; Tomey, 2000). Within this context, line authority represents a chain of command and is a direct line from the manager to the worker that is depicted by a solid line on organizational charts. Line positions are related to the direct achievement of organizational objectives.

In contrast, staff authority supports line authority relationships, and its functions are advisory or service-oriented, such as locating required data and offering counsel on managerial problems. Staff individuals function through influence; they do not have the authority to accept, use, modify, or reject plans. An example of an organizational chart is shown in Figure 14-6.

When a manager communicates with employees, the organizational chart may be used for several purposes, such as outlining administrative authority, defining relationships with other departments and agencies, describing policy and operational levels of the organization, and evaluating strengths and weaknesses of the current structure. The manager can also use the organizational chart to orient new personnel or to present the agency's structural design to others external to the organization.

In addition to the formal organizational structure, informal networks exist that comprise the personal and social relationships not identified on the organizational chart (e.g., individuals who lunch or take breaks together). These networks or structures help employees to meet personal and social needs and to gain recognition. Informal structures have their own modes of communication and are often referred to as the "grapevine" (Hein & Nicholson, 1986). Management should recognize this important structure, its value, and how it operates.

Organizational charts are not used by all managers. Autocratic managers who wish to control and manipulate others may feel that their power would be diminished if employees understood the working environment. Adaptive structures are more difficult to chart because they are more fluid and subject to change. Charts become outdated as changes are made. On charts the informal structure is not diagrammed, the formal structure may be difficult to define, and duties and responsibilities are not described. Charts may foster rigidity in relationships and communications and people may be sensitive about their relative status in the organization and may not want their positions revealed. However, organizational principles can help guide the occupational health manager to clarify relationships and maximize organizational efficiency. These principles are outlined in Box 14-5.

Span of management

The concept of span of management or span of control is important in determining effective

ORGANIZATION

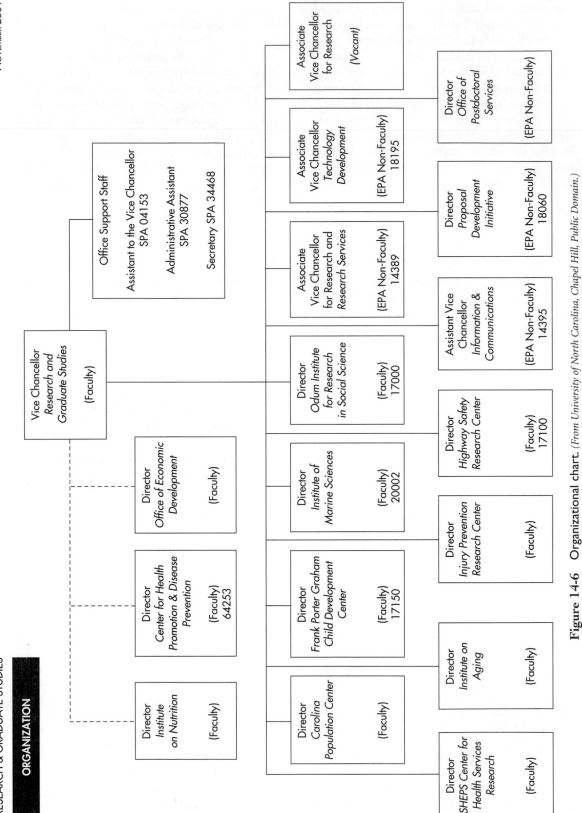

Figure 14-6 Organizational chart. *(From University of North Carolina, Chapel Hill, Public Domain.)*

Box 14-5   Principles for Organizational Efficiency

1. Clear lines of authority
2. Unity of command with each person having only one boss
3. Authority and responsibility relationships clearly defined in writing (reduces role ambiguity)
4. Clear role definition for each worker
5. Delegation of responsibility to the lowest effective level in the organization along with appropriate authority for decision making and goal achievement

---

manager/worker relationships and reflects the scope of coordination of employee activities— that is, the number of workers that can be effectively managed (Tomey, 2000). The span of management will vary within the organization and is influenced by the pace and type of work and the knowledge and skill of the workers. Supervising routine work performance requires less time than supervising innovative work performance because people performing routine work know what is expected of them. However, as the degree of difficulty increases for performing a task satisfactorily, so will the demand on the manager's time and effort (Douglas, 1996). For example, if a new health promotion program such as mammography screening is to be developed, the occupational health manager will need to spend considerable time determining how the program should be organized for implementation, including the training of nurses and other health care personnel with respect to the screening procedures. In addition, as the variability or number of different functions increases, the manager must consider more performance factors and interrelationships, which consumes more time. Interdependent functions of workers require more management time than do independent functions because of the increased need for managerial coordination within and across departments.

The greater the geographical separation of personnel reporting to the occupational health manager, the more limited will be the span of control. Increased emphasis on nonmanagerial responsibilities will also lessen the time the manager has for managing. Supervisors in flat organizational structures have a broader range of management responsibilities than do managers in tall structures, and lower level managers have a broader range of responsibility than do top level managers. In addition, managers of positions where tasks are shared will most likely have a smaller span of control than first-line managers who coordinate employees who do the same task (Gillies, 1994).

Decentralization versus centralization

One characteristic of an organization that influences both productivity and staff morale is the degree of centralization or decentralization of management responsibility. A highly centralized organization is one in which the chief executive officer makes most decisions. Decisions made at the top of an organization must then be filtered down through intermediaries to reach occupational health personnel. Retention of major decision making by top level administrators decreases the need for critical thinking and problem solving by middle and supervisory level personnel and does not increase growth in decision making abilities. Eventually, these workers may become passive and unenthusiastic about their jobs. Usually agencies tend to be more centralized during their early formative years.

Decentralization is the degree to which decision making is diffused throughout the organization. For decentralization to be effective, top managers must adopt a positive attitude toward it, and they need competent personnel to whom they can delegate authority and responsibility. Decentralization of responsibility leads to improvement in worker morale, because it demonstrates a certain degree of trust and confidence in the decision making abilities of others. When middle managers are given the responsibility for managerial decision making, they too may decentralize decision making still further, enabling direct caregivers to help formulate organizational plans, policies, and procedures.

The advantages of decentralization seem to outweigh the disadvantages. When people have a voice in governance, they feel that they are empowered, have more ownership, and are more willing to contribute. This increased motivation provides a feeling of individuality and freedom that in turn encourages creativity and commits the individual to making the system more successful.

Decentralization brings decision making closer to the action. Thus, decisions may be more effective because people who know the situation and have to implement the decision are the ones who make it.

Decentralization develops managers by allowing them to manage and releases top management from the burden of daily administration by freeing them for long-range planning, goal and policy development, and systems integration (Tomey, 2000). On the down side, because decentralization requires more managers and larger staffs, it is more costly.

Delegation

Delegation is the process of assigning work from one organizational level to another (i.e., manager to a subordinate) and should be recognized by the occupational health manager as an opportunity to maximize the utilization of the talents of those to whom the task has been delegated. The manager is responsible for assessing the results of the delegated activity. Learning to live with differences may be difficult for a manager, especially if the manager once performed the tasks now assigned to another worker and finds that the tasks are not performed in the same way (Poulin, 1984).

Assignment of responsibility, delegation of authority, and creation of accountability are the three concepts most often mentioned in relation to the delegation process with which the occupational health manager must be familiar. Responsibility denotes obligation and refers to what must be done to complete a task. Authority is the power to make final decisions and give commands. The person to whom responsibility has been assigned needs authority in sufficient scope to direct delegated duties without frequent consultation with her or his manager. Granting too little authority is a common problem and should be avoided. Although authority is delegated so that responsibilities can be fulfilled, the occupational health manager maintains control over the delegated authority and may recall it at any time.

Accountability refers to an obligation to complete work satisfactorily and to accept the consequences for the outcome. In authority relationships, the occupational health manager is accountable for both her or his and the employee's performance of the task and the selection of the employee to complete it.

Underdelegating occurs often and for numerous reasons (Tomey, 2000). The manager may believe she or he can do the job more quickly than someone else, may resent interruptions to answer questions from those given the task, or may not want to take the time to check what has been done. In addition, the occupational health manager may feel that those to whom the task has been delegated will not keep them adequately informed, or the manager may be unwilling to take risks for fear of being blamed for others' mistakes. If the manager decides to delegate something, she or he must select the appropriate person, communicate the responsibility to that person, grant authority with the responsibility, provide support, monitor the situation, and evaluate the results.

Delegation has the following four "rights":

1. The right task should be within the scope of the person's practice and consistent with the job description.
2. The right person should have the appropriate license or certificate and the demonstrated skill appropriate to the job description and should be able to accept the delegated responsibility.
3. The right communication should be clear, concise, complete, and correct.
4. The right feedback should ask for input, get the person's recommended solution to the problem, and recognize the person's efforts.

Policies and procedures

After a hierarchical structure has been established in the organization, mechanisms are needed to support and maintain it (Fallon, 2001). One such mechanism is the development of policies and procedures aimed at facilitating the work toward achievement of the goals and objectives set forth in the planning process. The occupational health manager must be involved in setting policies and procedures relative to the occupational health unit. Policies are designed to guide workers in their functions and should be comprehensive in scope, stable, fair, unambiguous, and written. Policies are approved and often developed by top management but may originate at any level in the organization (Tomey, 2000). Policies should be consistent with the overall goals of the organization, help solve recurring problems, establish areas of authority, and be accessible and available, usually in a policy manual. Policies should be identified by source, dated, and regularly reviewed, modified, and updated. Elements found in a policy manual will vary depending on the organization and its size but typically include policies related to personnel, medical, leave, and legal issues (e.g., sexual harassment).

Procedures define specific actions, help define steps in the activity being undertaken, and are often departmental in nature rather than organizational. Procedures serve to standardize operations, provide a basis for orientation and staff development, help simplify the work, and increase productivity. Before developing a procedure, the occupational health manager should consider if a procedure is really needed, because goals can be achieved in different ways. However, if procedures are deemed necessary, staff input, if available, should be obtained in the goals' development. Procedures should be dated and written in a consistent format that considers definition, purpose, materials/equipment, steps in the procedure, and documentation. Procedures should be placed in a manual with a table of contents and should be easily accessible. They should be reviewed and updated periodically for accuracy and provided to all staff. Examples of procedures would include chain of custody procedures for urine drug screening, referral and follow-up procedures for employees needing medical evaluation, and procedures for conducting a walk-through.

Position/job description

The position or job description is derived from a job analysis and is the key organizational tool that provides a written summary of the principal duties and scope of responsibility for a particular position (Simms et al., 1985). Position descriptions are developed by the occupational health manager with input from the staff as appropriate and are used to define the job, assist with recruitment and orientation procedures, and provide criteria elements for performance evaluation. The job position is organized according to a standard format that meets the needs of the organization. However, common elements generally include position title, summary purpose statement of the position describing the overall concept and nature of the position, span of responsibility and accountability, list of duties, and qualifications for the position (e.g., knowledge, skills, education, experience). Duties should be

arranged in a logical order, with the primary duties listed first and stated clearly, specifically, and concisely. Position descriptions should be accurate, realistic, current, and dated; however, they should not be so exact as to discourage innovation and creativity. Examples of job descriptions are shown in Box 14-6 and Appendix 14-1.

STAFFING

The staffing function is very important and involves recruitment and selection of personnel, coordination of work schedules, and personnel development to determine the correct mix and number of workers needed to achieve the organizational goals and the skills needed to carry out the program plans. The acquisition of qualified people in any organization is critical for accomplishing goal-driven strategies and growth of the organization and is achieved through a variety of recruitment strategies and interviewing techniques.

Recruitment

Modes of active recruitment include employee recommendations and word of mouth; advertisements in local newspapers, nursing organization bulletins, and nursing journals; recruitment literature, such as flyers and newsletters; posters; career days; job fairs; contacts with schools' graduating classes; placement services; open houses; nursing conventions; and frequent, low cost, credit-carrying continuing education courses for outsiders, and employees.

Word of mouth can be very effective, but it can also lead to the hiring of friends and relatives of the current workforce; this practice may foster nepotism and violate equal opportunity employment requirements. Prior to recruitment, the manager should review the job description for accuracy and revise the document appropriately.

Résumé

All applicants should submit résumés and references when appropriate. A résumé is a summary of information about a person's education, employment, and professional and personal history. It is typically a prerequisite for an interview, because the employer uses the résumé to determine who will be interviewed. Consequently, the résumé should be carefully developed and updated periodically. Résumés should be printed

Box 14-6 **Example of Job Description for Occupational Health Nurse**

Job Title:	Senior Occupational Health Consultant
Department:	Occupational Health Services
Classification:	Exempt
Job Summary:	Direct, manage, and supervise the occupational health unit and staff. In addition, develop and manage health promotion and safety programs in consultation with other members of the occupational health team and community resources.
Educational Requirements:	Graduate from an accredited school with a Bachelor of Science in nursing and licensed as a registered nurse in North Carolina. Prefer a master's degree in occupational health nursing or public health.
Work Experience:	2 to 3 years nursing experience and an additional 1 to 2 years experience in occupational health
Knowledge, Skills, and Abilities Required:	Must be able to assess, plan, develop, implement, and evaluate health promotion programs. Must possess effective management and leadership techniques and advanced communication and interpersonal relationship skills.

The following described job functions are not meant to be all-inclusive but to reflect the general work description for this job.

Position: Senior Occupational Health Consultant

Description of Work

1. Plan, develop, implement, manage, and evaluate occupational health and health promotion programs.
2. Perform needs assessment of the workplace and employees for the purpose of determining need, interest, and scope of occupational health and health promotion programs.
3. Prepare and deliver written and oral presentations/reports for management regarding occupational health and health monitoring programs.
4. Develop written policies, procedures, goals, objectives, and protocols (to be updated annually) for the occupational health and health promotion program.
5. Plan, develop, and promote the necessary facilities, equipment, supplies, and records system to operate the employee health service.
6. Orient, supervise, and evaluate nursing and/or support staff in the occupational health unit. Assign the staff's work, duties, and schedules and provide in-service education and professional growth opportunities for staff.
7. Prepare an annual budget for an occupational health unit/program.
8. Consult with management and other members of the occupational health team such as industrial hygiene, safety, toxicology, and human resources.

9. Use epidemiological methods to determine the major health and safety needs of a group of workers.
10. Calculate the cost-effectiveness of different types of occupational health services and health safety programs.
11. Conduct and/or supervise on-site health promotion programs including classes, individual counseling sessions, and health screenings.
12. Provide treatment for work- and nonwork-related injuries and illnesses.
13. Assist with or conduct accident and injury investigation of workers.
14. Continuously update knowledge of federal, state, and local laws, regulations, and requirements that are applicable to an occupational health and safety program.
15. Develop a written proposal, including a budget for the program, for occupational health and health promotion programs.
16. Participate in the service delivery, educational programs, and research projects of the occupational health service.
17. Assist with management of the safety committee and programs.
18. Supervise the first responder and emergency teams.
19. Utilize community resources with company support by establishing good work relations and with universities and the community emergency planning committee.

on high-quality paper and printer and should never be handwritten. The contents should be well-arranged, with major and minor headings to facilitate reading. The content should be concise yet complete, but not crowded. Résumés should contain a standard set of information.

Identification

Full name, address, telephone number, and e-mail address should appear at the beginning of the résumé.

Job objective

Including or excluding a job objective is controversial. Some say it limits a person's scope of employment, whereas others argue that the personnel manager should know what position the nurse is seeking. Separate résumés for each job, customizing the job objective, and accenting the characteristics that qualify the nurse for a particular job are appropriate.

Education

In reverse chronological order, a person should list the names and locations of schools attended, dates of attendance, and diplomas or degrees conferred. Continuing education, such as workshops, in-service education, and home study courses, indicates an interest in self-improvement and may be appropriate to list.

Work experience

Previous employment should be listed in reverse chronological order by identifying the name and location of each agency, dates of employment, position title, and responsibilities. New graduates or graduate level students can list their student clinical/internship experiences.

Publications and research

All publications including the title, journal, volume, and publication date should be listed. Any research conducted as an individual or as part of research team also should be listed and should include the title of the project, role in the project, and if funded, funding source and amount. This may include student research.

Awards

Any awards and recognitions received should be listed with date of and reason for the award.

Community service

A list of community service activities including the location of service provided, dates, and responsibilities, should be provided.

Reference letters

Reference letters should be used cautiously when evaluating the applicant because the authors may be unfamiliar with the applicant's current work performance and are seldom critical. More emphasis should be placed on comments by previous employers, coworkers, and colleagues. However, letters from personal references may attest to the applicant's character and integrity, which should be highly valued.

Interviewing

A preemployment interview is a critical function requiring much skill and should be conducted with the most qualified applicants. The purposes of the interview are to obtain and give information and judge the applicant on predetermined criteria specific to that job. The interview should be considered by the occupational health manager as a reciprocal experience, with both parties prepared to ask questions and discuss issues relevant to the position (Wallace & Ventura, 1991). Information from the résumé and references can serve to initiate and facilitate discussion during the interview process.

The interview has definite purposes and should avoid social chitchat, although a brief warm-up period may help put the interviewee at ease. One of the main purposes is to learn about the prospective employee. Therefore it behooves the interviewer to concentrate on listening, provide necessary information, and answer questions from the applicant. Managers should avoid giving clues about what pleases or displeases them, should not be argumentative, and should try to avoid premature judgment.

The interview process should have an introduction, body, and closure. The environment and behavioral aspects related to the interview should be considered. The occupational health manager provides introductory information about the job and any relevant historical data. A preplanned set of questions based on criteria established from the job description should be developed to facilitate the interview process (Tomey, 2000; Wallace & Ventura, 1991).

Certainly information about the applicant's knowledge, skills, ability to work with others, congruence of professional goals with that of the organization, willingness to perform the job responsibilities, and other skill areas specific to the position should be addressed. Open-ended or nondirective questions are probably the most valuable method for information gathering because they allow the applicant to express ideas and encourage self-disclosure. Examples of nondirective questions include, What qualifies you for the job? and How do you relate to your peers? Closed-ended questions are directive and can generally be answered "yes" or "no." Questions such as, Do you think you are qualified for this job? and Did you get along with your peers? are directive.

The funnel technique incorporates both open-ended and closed-ended questions. When using the funnel technique, the interviewer starts with an open-ended question such as, What are your professional goals? This gets objective information and sets a nonthreatening tone. The scope of the discussion is then funneled by asking a self-appraisal question such as, How do you plan to accomplish your goals? This elicits subjective information. The interviewer closes the discussion of a particular subject by asking direct questions to clarify the self-appraisal. A direct question might be, What specific type of job would you like?

A grid of topics to explore and the funnel technique can help the interviewer sequence questions in a logical order and decide what kind of questions to ask. Initially, filling in the topics and potential questions may be helpful. The questions may be modified during the interview.

Problem solving approaches to particular situations can also be explored. The manager should be prepared to answer questions from the applicant about the organizational structure and culture, policies and procedures, working conditions and benefits, and specific questions pertinent to the position under consideration. Interviewing principles shown in Box 14-7 should be observed. Verbal and nonverbal behavior by the manager during the interview can affect the applicant's comfort level. Therefore, the occupational health manager should demonstrate respect for the applicant's ideas, listen carefully, and maintain eye contact. Behavioral characteristics of the applicant also should be observed as to style of relationships and comfort with the interview process. For example, the applicant might be asked to interview with several people in a group format, conduct a formal presentation, or attend a social reception. This will provide an opportunity to witness both formal and informal interactions. At closure the interview discussion should be summarized and clarifications made. The applicant should be told what to expect in terms of a decision. Information obtained during the interview should be verified.

Interviewers can talk about the applicant's qualifications, abilities, experiences, education, and interests; the duties and responsibilities of the job; where the job is located; the travel, equipment,

---

Box 14-7   Interviewing Principles

1. Create and maintain a comfortable environment throughout the interview.
2. Conduct the interview according to a pre-planned outline.
3. Explore the applicant's background and future plans before describing the available position.
4. Encourage the applicant to talk freely by asking nondirective, open-ended questions.
5. Listen actively and talk sparingly while the applicant describes [her or] his background and future plans.
6. Be aware of your own and the applicant's nonverbal communications.
7. When describing the available position, give information about job responsibilities and working environment and withhold opinion about the applicant's ability to fill the position.
8. Identify both positive and negative aspects of the job in detail.
9. In concluding the interview, clarify subsequent steps in the selection procedure.

From *Nursing Management: A Systems Approach,* by D. A. Gillies, 1994, Philadelphia: W. B. Saunders.

and facilities available; and the organization's missions, programs, and achievements. However, the interviewer may not ask about lineage, national origin, race, sex, age, marital status, number or age of children, former addresses, religious affiliations, or handicaps. Although the interviewer may ask about academic and professional education, schools attended, and ability to read, write, and speak a foreign language, the interviewer may not ask about the racial or religious affiliation of the schools, the date of the schooling, or the applicant's native language. One may ask about professional organizations but not all memberships. Inquiry into actual convictions that relate to job performance can be asked, not questions relating to arrests (Tomey, 2000).

After all applicants have been interviewed, strengths and weaknesses can be evaluated. Education and experience can be easily compared; however, other characteristics such as interpersonal skills, social style, creativity, and integrity may be more difficult to measure. Once this is done a selection should be made quickly.

Coordination of work schedules

The manager must coordinate staffing of the occupational health unit to carry out the work of the organization. An important aspect to remember is employee orientation. Once hired, employees must have a planned and deliberate orientation to the organization and the occupational health unit. The orientation includes a history of the organization and a description of its vision, purpose, structure, working hours, holiday time, vacation, sick time, paydays, performance standards and evaluation, labor contracts, grievance procedures, parking facilities, eating facilities, health services, and educational opportunities. That is more information than new employees and experienced nurses can remember. The information should be in a handbook to be referenced during the induction. Both the new employees and experienced nurses in new positions need orientation. The manager introduces the nurse to the new job, agency policies, facilities, and coworkers. Orientation is important, and the manager who does not take the time to assist a new employee is making a serious mistake. Communicating regulations and exactly what is expected of the employee diminishes uncertainty, relieves anxiety, and prevents unnecessary misunderstandings. A person's security usually

increases when someone is considerate enough to help that person adjust to a new situation.

No specific rule exists for determining the number of staff needed in an occupational setting. The number will vary, depending on the needs and relative health of the workforce and industry. Staffing involves identifying the type and amount of services provided and the number and type of staff needed to deliver services. The majority of occupational settings are staffed by one nurse; therefore, some issues to be discussed with regard to staffing nurses will be more applicable to multinurse units and regional or corporate settings. When planning how to staff the occupational health unit, the type of setting, number and demographics of workers, types of hazards, worker and management orientation toward health care, and budgeting constraints will influence the type and number of personnel needed. For example, an assessment of the organization and workforce by the occupational health manager may reveal the need for management of lifestyle change issues or repetitive motion problems. The types of personnel recruited, such as a nurse skilled in health promotion or a physical therapist who may be part-time, full-time, or contractual, should reflect this need.

The occupational health manager will want to plan and coordinate the work schedule and take into consideration the number of staff needed, programs offered (especially if they are seasonal or special programs), vacation schedules, absenteeism, professional education needs, turnover, rotation, shift schedules, and special needs of the staff. In addition, consideration should be given to the need for substitute and/or additional personnel if workload demands increase for special programs. However, in occupational health settings the manager may also be responsible for managing clerical, support (e.g., laboratory), and professional (e.g., physicians and counselors) staff. Utilization of these personnel will also need to be planned for and scheduled.

Personnel development

Personnel or staff development is an important aspect of meeting both employee and employer needs. Personnel development is designed to help employees grow in their jobs, acquire new skills, and assume additional decision making responsibilities. Staff development goes beyond orientation; it is a continuing liberal education of the whole person to develop potential fully. Staff development deals with aesthetic senses and technical and professional education and may include orientation, preceptorships, mentorships, skill checklists, internships, in-service education, courses, conferences, seminars, journal or book clubs, programmed learning, and independent study and refresher courses.

Managers play an important role in the support of staff development and have a responsibility to review the goals for the staff development program and provide a budget for those activities. They participate in needs identification and analyze how education effects change in nursing and occupational health services. In addition, managers must be careful to differentiate staff development needs from administrative needs. If staff nurses know how to do a procedure properly but do not do it because the necessary supplies and equipment are not available, the need is administrative rather than educational. Positive reinforcement through recognition, such as oral praise of the unit or acknowledgment of accomplishments in a newsletter, is useful. Staff development also can be related to retention, pay raises, advancement to other positions, or termination.

DIRECTING

Providing direction is more focused on giving guidance, communicating effectively, and managing and effecting change than on providing overbearing supervision. The amount of direction needed varies with the knowledge, experience, and initiative of individual employees and the group as a whole. Everyone needs some direction, no matter how small. People need to know (1) what is expected of them and (2) how to do it. The knowledgeable staff member will know how to do the assigned task or how to obtain the needed information but still needs information about how the work has been divided among members of the team. The less experienced, less knowledgeable employee will need assistance with the how-to-do-it part of the assignment. This assistance does not necessarily have to come from the occupational health manager; it may be delegated to experienced staff members.

Guidance

When new work or a new initiative needs to be completed, the manager must discuss this with

the appropriate employees to determine who is the best fit for the assignment. In many cases an employee who is challenged by the work will "volunteer" for the task. However, the manager has the final authority to assign the responsibility for work completion. This means having a good understanding of the capabilities of the staff and providing learning opportunities and growth experiences. The occupational health manager will also be called upon to provide technical expertise and guidance as needed. When providing direction for the work, effective communication skills are needed.

Communication

Effective communication techniques are central to the leadership function and must flow freely both vertically and horizontally. Vertical communication follows the chain of command, and employee input into decision making is critical to satisfaction. Although communication about accomplishing the work tasks may be directive at times from the manager, more successful communication can be accomplished when the worker and manager mutually agree on task assignment and strategy implementation (Gardner et al., 1991). The employee must feel free to communicate solicited and unsolicited information to the nurse manager. Communication cannot be taken for granted and requires effort.

Lateral or horizontal communication occurs between departments on the same level and between coworkers and is needed primarily to coordinate activities and clarify roles and responsibilities. This type of communication is crucial when multiple departments or parties collaborate on projects. It is also used when staff/advisory personnel provide technical assistance to supervisors or managers.

Informal communication, or the grapevine, exists in all organizations and is a method whereby workers at all levels transmit information to each other. The grapevine transports information much faster; however, information received may be distorted as it passes from person to person. Grapevine information has no formal lines of accountability. Managers should pay attention to informal communication channels in order to recognize sources of information, correct deviations, and pass on messages. Examples of

TABLE 14-3	Effective Communication: Facilitators and Barriers	
FACILITATORS	**BARRIERS**
Clear ideas/purpose	Lack of clarity or precision
Well-organized message	Faulty reasoning/message poorly expressed
Familiarity with problem	Omitting facts or filtering information
Seeking/understanding other's point of view	Using jargon
Avoiding arguments/giving of advice	Selective screening/perception
Positive verbal/nonverbal expressions	Distrust of sender
Nonjudging atmosphere	Potential for punishment
Appropriate confidentiality	Poor listening
Appropriate repetition	Poor/unsafe working conditions and environment
Allowing for feedback	Resistance to change
Well-written, courteous memos	Lack of authority
Timing	Timing

facilitators and barriers to communication are listed in Table 14-3.

Depending on the type of communication behavior displayed, the occupational health manager may need to utilize special communication skills and techniques to deal with employees who demonstrate difficult communication behaviors—that is, those that are hostile, complaining, unresponsive, negative, or overly agreeable. It is important to avoid battles with hostile or aggressive workers but rather deal with them directly and forthrightly and state a position forcefully but in a friendly manner. If an employee has an outburst, the employee should be given the opportunity to calm down, regain control, and then discuss the problem. For workers who continually complain or shed negative thoughts, the manager must acknowledge the comments but then move on to explore alternatives and engage these workers in problem solving (Tomey, 2000). Reading silent or unresponsive individuals is difficult; however, it is important to try to get their thoughts or opinions by directly asking open-ended questions.

Management of Change

As part of the direction function, the occupational health manager will need to manage change. Change is a dynamic, inevitable phenomenon in life that provides a stimulus for growth. In health care, change provides an opportunity to improve the delivery and management of health care services. Although often initiated or allowed to occur in a random or haphazard fashion, change should be introduced in a planned, organized manner by a person who is knowledgeable about change concepts, processes, and predicted outcomes.

Various theories seek to explain the concept of change (Olsen, 1978; Sullivan & Decker, 1988). For example, conflict theory of social change contends that the basis of most organizational change is due to some form of conflict experienced by individuals in the organization. Change is initiated to eliminate the conflict. Systems theory emphasizes that because of the interdependence and reciprocal relationship of one group to another, a change in one part of the system will result in a change in some other part of the system. Attitudinal change at the individual level is reported to be a function of the degree of internal conflict or disagreement between old and new information. In addition, how one perceives a situation and her or his role in conformity to group pressure is a strong influencing factor.

Lippitt et al. (1958) point out that "as a change agent, the manager identifies the problem and helps others become problem aware; assesses the capacity and motivators of individuals for change; explores alternative change options with the individual or group; assesses resources needed; establishes and maintains a helping relationship; recognizes the phases of the change; and guides the process and techniques for the planned change" (p. 126). The classic process of change is well-described by Bennis et al. (1985) and

Restraining forces	↓	↓	↓	↓	↓
Status quo					
Driving forces	↑	↑	↑	↑	↑

Figure 14-7 Forces of change. *(Concept from "Studies in Group Decisions," by K. Lewin, in D. Cartwright & A. Zander (Eds.), Group Dynamics, 1953, Evanston, IL: Row Peterson.)*

involves three phases: unfreezing, moving, and refreezing. Unfreezing involves problem awareness or dissatisfaction with the status quo and recognition of the need for change. Moving involves working toward change through problem identification, exploring alternatives for problem resolution, developing a clear plan for change, and then implementing the plan. The manager plays a critical role here and should be viewed as a facilitator and approachable expert who is available to help, not demand. The success of the change is positively related to the relationship the change agent has to the targeted individual or group (Kemp, 1986).

Assuming the change is accepted, refreezing is the integration of the change into one's life or performance and stabilization of the change, which probably will require reinforcement or practice or both. However, not all change will be accepted. If the change is rejected, the manager or change agent must determine why this occurred and explore new alternatives and plans for accomplishing the task (Kemp, 1986). After the change has been introduced, the consequences should be evaluated both short-term and long-term to determine the effects of the process and outcome.

Lewin's (1953) description of force-field analysis is a classic, widely known approach to planned change. Lewin states that in any situation a dynamic equilibrium of simultaneously operating driving and restraining forces exists to maintain the status quo (Figure 14-7). To create change, the status quo must be unfrozen, which requires either an increase in driving forces or decrease in restraining forces in the situation (Tomey, 2000). Driving forces might include pressure from the manager, a desire to please the manager, a desire to get ahead or receive recognition, or a desire to improve working conditions. Restraining forces might include pressure to conform to group

Box 14-8 Factors Influencing Resistance to Change

- Vested interests
- Routines and habits
- Risk of error
- Fear of failure
- Conflict with personal goals
- Threats to employees
  - Role
  - Economic/job security
  - Self-esteem
  - Social support
- Excessive work pressure
- Conflict with change agent
- Institutional power structure
- Clique forces of conformity

norms or lack of sufficient resources to accomplish unit goals and objectives.

Resistance to change is normal and comes primarily from those who oppose the change (Box 14-8). Change may represent a threat to the employee's role, job security, or self-esteem, or the employee may simply have a low tolerance for change, or the change may be misperceived as to its benefit or impact. Workers may perceive that the change implies (by management) inadequate work performance on their part. An experienced manager will recognize that individuals who complain the most about the change will actually prove to be less resistant than those who remain silent and refuse to discuss their objectives or those who pretend acceptance but have no intention to modify their behavior (Gillies, 1994). Several strategies can be employed to reduce resistance to change (Box 14-9). Different strategies may be useful in different situations, and multiple approaches may be needed.

EVALUATION

The function of evaluation is a key element in determining overall programmatic effectiveness. Employee evaluation involves setting performance standards and criteria, evaluating performance results, and recommending and taking corrective actions. Programmatic evaluation may be done through quality measurement approaches including quality assurance and quality management techniques.

Box 14-9   Strategies to Reduce Resistance to Change

- Involve participants in the change process.
- Start change process with those most receptive.
- Gradually introduce changes.
- Be sure information Is clear.
- Avoid attempts at coercion.
- Employ consultant collaborator, if needed.
- Identify resisters and try to understand reasons for resistance.
- Involve the resisters with specific tasks to increase ownership.
- Divide the clique.
- Provide avenue for compromises.
- Provide rewards, incentives, and positive reinforcement for changes made.
- Foster trusting relationship.

Evaluation of Employees

As mentioned previously, Management by Objectives (MBO) is a tool for both planning and evaluation. MBO emphasizes achievement of objectives rather than personality traits; therefore, it reflects a results orientation. The performance appraisal is a periodic formal evaluation to determine how well the employee has performed her or his duties during a specified period of time. Based on measurable objectives, professional standards of practice, and performance criteria established in advance by the manager and employee, the occupational health manager can objectively complete the performance evaluation or appraisal. Both the employee and the manager know the standard of performance expected and can discuss modifications that may need to be made. In addition to reviewing and discussing organizational/unit goals and objectives, purposes of the evaluation include the following:

1. Determine job competence;
2. Enhance staff development and motivate personnel toward higher achievement;
3. Discover the employee's aspirations and recognize accomplishments;
4. Improve communications between managers and employees and reach an understanding about the objectives of the job and agency;
5. Improve performance by examining and encouraging better relationships between employees;
6. Aid the manager's coaching and counseling;
7. Determine training and developmental needs of employees;
8. Make inventories of talent within the organization and reassess assignments;
9. Select qualified employees for advancement and salary increases;
10. Identify unsatisfactory employees (Swansburg, 1996; Tappen, 2001).

The underlying philosophy is a belief that people perform best and develop most in an environment of participative management, high performance standards that build on individual strengths, prompt feedback that accentuates the positive, and appropriate rewards. Employees are encouraged to "do their thing" while maintaining individual accountability. The manager is a listener and clarifier who readjusts responsibilities on the basis of individual differences.

Advantages of MBO for the employee are that the standard of evaluation is based on the characteristics of a specific person and job; employees have input and some control over their future and employees know the standard by which they will be judged; employees have knowledge of the manager's goals, priorities, and deadlines and have a greater understanding of where they stand with the manager in relation to relative progress; there is a better basis for evaluation than personality traits; MBO emphasizes the future, which can be changed, instead of the past; and MBO stimulates higher individual performance and morale.

Advantages for the manager include a reservoir of personnel data and performance information for updating personnel files; an indication of personnel development needs within the agency; a basis for promotion and compensation; a relationship with the employee that makes the manager a coach rather than a judge; and better managerial planning and use of the employee.

MBO directs work activities toward organizational goals, facilitates planning, provides standards for control, provides objective appraisal criteria, reduces role conflict and ambiguity, and uses and motivates human resources (Tomey, 2000).

Because judgment is involved in the evaluation process, it is highly subject to influences of prejudices, bias, politics, and other extraneous factors that may affect performance ratings. Common errors that may affect the performance appraisal are shown in Box 14-10.

When evaluating the employee, the manager might consider a checklist that can be used to denote the presence or absence (*yes* or *no*) of a desired characteristic or behavior. However, checklists have limited utility because they do not measure the degree (e.g., average, above average, exceptional) of the characteristic being measured and are generally not suitable for measurement of interpersonal relationships.

Rating scales can provide much more data about a desired behavior or characteristic and can be constructed numerically compared with qualitative terms such as poor to excellent, low to high, or almost never to almost always. Figure 14-8 demonstrates several characteristics measured on a 5-point scale from low to high. Using this type of scale, the occupational health manager is able to evaluate each characteristic independently, a set

or group of characteristics, or all characteristics combined. Numerical scores can be tallied, and the manager can then compare groups or sets of characteristics to help target strengths and limitations.

Other types of evaluation include self-appraisal and peer review. In self-appraisal the employee performs a personal evaluation that is used as a basis for discussion with the manager. Peer review is a process whereby a group of like professionals evaluate the employee's performance. Peer review is usually time consuming and costly; however, it generally provides an extensive and objective appraisal of the employee. The group or committee selected to perform the peer evaluation should be representative of and knowledgeable about the practice specialty. To conduct the peer review, appraisal tools will need to be obtained and/or developed to measure the characteristics being evaluated (e.g., technical competence or organizational, leadership, and interpersonal relations skills) and a process must be established. The committee conducting the review must be oriented to the established process and procedure, which may include a review of the employee's self-evaluation, the manager's performance evaluation of the employee, a determination of the employee's contributions to occupational health nursing, a review of external letters critiquing the employee's work and any other supporting documentation (e.g., project reports, publications), and an interview with the employee. After the review is completed, feedback is given to the employee to provide recognition for exceptional performance and information about areas for further growth and development.

Evaluation conference

Although the occupational health manager's formal evaluation of the employee's performance is usually conducted annually, evaluation should

---

> **Box 14-10   Common Errors in Performance Appraisals**
>
> - Using incomplete or inaccurate information
> - Using ambiguous or irrelevant performance measures
> - Using performance measurements never discussed with the employee
> - Overemphasizing the halo effect (allowing one trait to color all other traits) or the horns effect (being hypercritical of the employee's performance—that is, a task could always be done better)
> - Avoiding sensitive or "touchy" subjects
> - Being influenced by personal preferences such as gender, age, and ethnicity
> - Failing to recognize good performance

Characteristic/Behavior	Low	Below Average	Average	Above Average	High
Works well with others	1	2	3	4	5
Demonstrates initiative	1	2	3	4	5
Demonstrates creativity	1	2	3	4	5
Demonstrates leadership abilities	1	2	3	4	5

Figure 14-8   Example of a characteristic/behavior rating scale.

be a continuous process so that the employee has sufficient feedback to maximize performance. Both the manager and employee should be prepared for the performance evaluation conference with adequate time scheduled. Privacy should be afforded and interruptions and distractions avoided. Seating arrangements should be comfortable and reflect equality or collegiality (e.g., sitting side by side or at the corners of a table). Emphasis should be placed on achievement of specific objectives, special or outstanding accomplishments, and observed performance. The employee should be asked to identify areas that she or he perceives need improvement, if any, because this will enhance joint evaluation efforts and reduce the potential for defensiveness. A collaborative discussion about performance improvement, goal setting, and new initiatives or job responsibilities should be encouraged.

If the manager must point out a need for performance improvement, this should be interspersed with favorable performance indicators to avoid setting up a barrier during the evaluation process. If the employee becomes defensive, the manager should listen and not engage in a battle.

Problem solving and goal setting evaluation approaches facilitate and stimulate employee growth (Dubnicki & Sloan, 1991; Townsend, 1991). Through problem solving, the employee discusses problems and expresses ideas and opinions for solutions while the manager listens, reflects, and summarizes. Goal setting is future-oriented and focuses on results. It encourages the employee to determine how to achieve objectives and also enhances teamwork. Before the evaluation is completed, ways in which the manager can help the employee achieve performance goals should be discussed (e.g., additional or reduced responsibilities, resources, time for special projects or research).

The evaluation should be written addressing achievements, accomplishments, and future goals. If weaknesses or performance deviations are evident, these should be documented with recommendations for improvement stipulated within a defined time frame. For changes to be made, recommendations for improvement should be mutually agreed upon, and the employee should understand the consequences of failure to perform. In some structures performance interventions such as positive rein-forcement (e.g., recognition, verbal praise), counseling, or referral to an Employee Assistance Program may be helpful and needed. The evaluation report should be signed and dated by both the occupational health manager and the employee and placed in the performance file to be used as a basis for promotions, pay increases, and other rewards or for disciplinary or termination action if necessary. A progressive disciplinary action program and grievance procedure should be established and uniformly applied to personnel.

QUALITY MEASUREMENT

QUALITY ASSURANCE

Quality assurance in nursing has been of concern since nursing's beginnings when Florence Nightingale called for the systematic collection and analysis of data and the identification of practice standards (Nightingale, 1860). In contemporary times the impetus for quality assurance programs came about as a result of recognizing the need to improve the quality of health care and at the same time reduce health care costs (Dienemann, 1992). Quality assurance activities also assist the professional in self-regulation and accountability for nursing practice (AAOHN, 1999). A quality assurance program involves a measurable means of achieving professional goals with a positive impact on the quality of service provided. Setting standards and comparing actual performance/practice with those standards through defining criteria against which performance can be measured and initiating change to enhance standards compliance is still recognized as the basic foundation for assuring quality performance (Hardy, & Forrer, 1996). Quality assurance programs reflect two major purposes, evaluation and improvement of care or services. The intent of quality assurance expresses a commitment to take action that results in the assurance of quality nursing care (and services) to the public (Lang, 1976), efficiently and effectively, with a minimum expenditure of resources. It is not intended to be a mechanism for disciplining caregivers or trying to find fault or determine blame.

The general framework for quality assurance mechanisms is based on the classic work of Donabedian (1966). Three major approaches form the basis for evaluative mechanisms in quality assurance: structure, process, and outcome. Structural elements relate to the physical setting and organizational modalities designed to facilitate the work (e.g., facilities, personnel); process elements relate to the actual performance of work or process of nursing care/service (e.g., walkthroughs, recordkeeping, examinations) and decision making processes involved; outcome elements relate to the results achieved from the work performed or nursing interventions or service delivered (e.g., reduced work-related injuries, improved working conditions, service satisfaction). Evaluative elements for each of these approaches are listed in Box 14-11. In addition, as an example of the application of components of the Donabedian framework, Rogers et al. (1993) describe the results of a survey regarding employee satisfaction with health services as a quality indicator mechanism for service improvement.

Various methods for quality assurance have been utilized; the most common of these include quality assurance audits, peer review, and quality circles. Establishment of standards of performance and related measurement criteria are necessary in order to conduct an effective audit. Most often practice and performance standards are developed by professional societies, wherein the standard(s) reflects the values and beliefs of the collective profession as to what constitutes competent practice. However, organizations or groups may sometimes develop specific standards tailored to the institutional demands or may develop specific criteria to meet established standards (AAOHN, 1999).

PRACTICE STANDARDS

Deming (1982) encourages the voluntary establishment of standards, thereby avoiding government regulation and allowing for greater freedom of practice. The American Nurses Association (1998) states that the function of professional associations is to establish the scope of practice and desirable qualifications required for general specialty practice. Further, a profession regulates itself through codes of ethics, standards, accreditation agencies, peer review, and certification processes, allowing for appropriate expansion commensurate with public needs, research findings, and demands from the practice environment.

ANA defines standards as authoritative statements by which the nursing profession describes the responsibilities for which its practitioners are accountable. Consequently, standards reflect the values and priorities of the profession. Standards provide direction for professional nursing practice and a framework for the evaluation of practice. Written in measurable terms, standards also define the nursing profession's accountability to the public and the client outcomes for which nurses are responsible. Standards are broad statements that address the full scope of professional nursing practice (ANA, 1998).

The American Nurses Association first developed standards of nursing practice in 1973. Numerous specialty organizations also have independently established standards for practice but utilized different definitions, formats, or other criteria, thus creating confusion as to the standards' utility. ANA standards have been revised and are considered generic and applicable to all registered nurses engaged in clinical practice, regardless of

---

Box 14-11 Evaluative Elements in Quality Assurance

Structural elements may include the following:

- Physical setting
- Philosophy of health by management, employees, health care professionals
- Organizational mission and structure
- Unit goals and objectives
- Human and financial resources
- Operational resources

Process elements may include the following:

- Management of the operation
- Decision making processes
- Collaboration
- Nursing interventions/monitoring
- Services provided
- Records and reports

Outcome elements may include the following:

- Improved health
- Compliance with treatment regimen
- Reduced morbidity and mortality
- Positive changes in knowledge and attitudes about health
- Satisfaction with service delivery

clinical specialty, practice setting, or educational preparation, and describe a competent level of professional nursing care and professional performance (ANA, 1998).

ANA's *Standards of Clinical Nursing Practice* (1998) are categorized as "Standards of Care" and "Standards of Professional Performance" (Box 14-12). Standards of Care describe a competent level of nursing care as demonstrated by the nursing process, which provides the foundation for clinical decision making, whereas Standards of Professional Performance describe a competent level of behavior in the professional role. All nurses are expected to engage in professional role activities appropriate to their education, position, and practice setting.

Standards developed for specialty practice or advanced clinical practice are further defined and determined by those nursing specialties building on the ANA standards and based upon specific criteria relevant to the practice specialty. *Standards of Occupational and Environmental Health Nursing* established by the American Association of Occupational Health Nurses (1999) are slightly different and can be found in Chapter 19.

Even with the availability of standards, nurses must exercise professional judgment based on education and experience in determining what is appropriate, pertinent, and realistic care at any one time (Dienemann, 1992). Standards should remain stable over time because they reflect the values and beliefs of the profession about the practice. However, criteria should be reviewed and revised to reflect advancements in scientific knowledge and technology and utilization of research findings into practice.

QUALITY ASSURANCE MODELS AND INSTRUMENTS

Various quality assurance models, often used in auditing approaches, have been developed to evaluate health care. Because continuous quality improvement is the recent norm, quality assurance is less in the forefront. However, one model is described here. The Marker Umbrella Model for Quality Management (Figure 14-9) (Marker, 1987) offers another approach to quality assurance. Marker describes this model as reflecting nine interdependent universal activities that constitute professional practice in any practice setting. Although Marker advocates the implementation of all nine areas implemented, all should not be implemented at the same time and priorities for implementation should be established. The nine activities include the following:

1. *Standards development* for professional practice should be directed at structure, process, and outcome. Standards should be validated periodically with mechanisms determined for their implementation.
2. *Credentialing* means validating competency both legally and professionally, including licensure, performance monitoring, certification, and skill-based testing.
3. *Continuing education* is vital to maintaining and updating knowledge and skills to support competent nursing practice, creating new competencies, and correcting deviations from noncompliance with existing standards. Methods to achieve this include providing for attendance at continuing education events for new or mandatory competencies and staff development. Tracking of learning events should be included.

Box 14-12   ANA Standards of Clinical Nursing Practice

STANDARDS OF CARE

• Assessment
• Diagnosis
• Outcome identification
• Planning
• Implementation
• Evaluation

STANDARDS OF PROFESSIONAL PERFORMANCE

• Quality of care
• Performance appraisal
• Education
• Collegiality
• Ethics
• Collaboration
• Research
• Resource utilization

From *Standards of Clinical Nursing Practice,* by American Nurses Association, 1998, Washington, DC: Author.

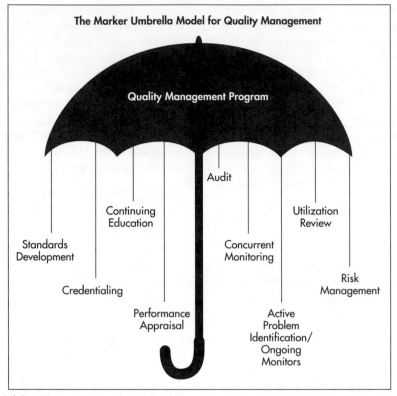

Figure 14-9 Marker Umbrella Model. *(From "The Marker Umbrella Model for Quality Assurance: Monitoring and Evaluating Professional Practice," by C. Marker, 1987,* Journal of Nursing Quality Assurance, *1(3), 52-63.)*

4. *Performance appraisal* is essential to the managerial role and relates to quality assurance with respect to performance matched to standards. This is accomplished through use of an appraisal tool based on the employee's job description; performance standards that define specific expectations relative to a particular position; and monitoring, tracking, and documenting of performance related to nursing care, which are then shared with the employee.

5. *Audit procedures* define a formal process of data collection from a representative sample of individuals or elements to determine compliance with specific care procedures and criteria for meeting standards. Audits should be carried out concurrent with the course of the work to examine structure, process, and outcome criteria. Auditing procedures can include chart reviews, direct observations, and interviews with staff and employee clients.

6. *Concurrent monitoring* may be considered a minireview and usually occurs through a small nonrepresentative sample of observations. Its purpose is to spot-check a specific aspect of care at a designated point by a specific caregiver. Examples of concurrent monitoring activities include observation of physical assessment skills, occupational history taking, medication administration practices, research, and log recording practices.

7. *Active problem identification/ongoing monitoring* involves reporting and documenting problems to identify approaches to improve performance. Report forms, where problems can be logged, and conferences, the results of which are recorded, are valuable data sources for problem identification and monitoring.

8. *Utilization review* involves monitoring and tracking resources for the health unit to determine adequacy and appropriate utilization. This can be done through reviewing budgeting records and workload logs.

9. *Risk management* involves activities designed to prevent loss such as through health hazard evaluations, safety inspections, and periodic health surveillance.

Various tools for quality assurance are available and are often specific to the needs of the nursing specialty. However, quality assurance tools in occupational health nursing are scarce. Examples include an instrument titled "Standards, Interpretation, and Audit Criteria for Performance of Occupational Health Programs" developed by the Department of Environmental Health, Kettering Laboratories, University of Cincinnati, Ohio (AAOHN, 1987); "Assessment Guide for Occupational Health Nursing Practice" (Appendix 14-2) developed by Manchester et al., (1991) based on job descriptions and AAOHN practice standards that use structure and process and outcome criteria for evaluating occupational health programs and services; and a tool titled "Quality Assurance in Occupational Health Nursing" (Appendix 14-3) developed by Jarrett (1987) using the Marker Umbrella Model for Quality Management.

In corporate settings with multiple nurses, these nurses can develop a quality assurance program and utilize it in several different sites. However, establishing quality assurance programs is more difficult in occupational and environmental health nursing settings where nurses often work alone. One alternative is the development of a quality assurance review team by interested peers located within close proximity or by occupational and environmental health nurses representing local AAOHN constituencies. Professional standards for practice from AAOHN can also be used and serve as the basis for specific criteria development.

QUALITY CIRCLES

Quality circles represent another approach to quality assurance wherein a small group of employees (5 to 10) meets generally on a weekly basis to solve problems related to the work (Marks, 1986). The group identifies common problems, and working on one problem at a time, concentrates on the cause or causes of and solutions to the problem. The solution is then presented to management for approval. If the proposal for change or correction is approved, the quality circle implements the action and evaluates its effectiveness.

Once quality assurance programs have been implemented, all staff involved should be given feedback about areas that are positive and areas that need change or correction (Brodbeck, 1992). Reports of favorable findings can serve to enhance and reinforce quality performance. For areas needing modification, strategies such as training, education, skill development, and organization change, need to be determined.

It is important to recognize that quality assurance should be viewed as one mechanism for quality improvement. In many instances quality assurance is linked to risk management in an effort to identify causes of injury and help determine the best resolution to eliminate the problem. In addition, it should be emphasized that improvements in care and service must involve an interdisciplinary approach and commitment from all levels of the organization's structure. Quality health care services will be achieved as the result of positive interactions among professionals and departments working together to build a dynamic mechanism that continuously improves the processes and outcomes of service delivery (Dienemann, 1992).

QUALITY MANAGEMENT

Quality assurance programs should focus on quality work and preventive managing rather than satisfying accrediting bodies or as detecting employees who make errors. Some think that quality assurance activities alone are too restrictive and insufficient for contemporary health care and management needs and that these activities need to be expanded to reflect improvement in client satisfaction based on quality service and management (Tomey, 2000).

Total quality management was first developed in the United States and successfully integrated into the Japanese business structure through the work of Deming, a leading expert in quality improvement (Oberle, 1990). Although the concept of quality management or continuous quality improvement is not foreign to the U.S. business industry, it is a relatively new concept to the health care sector, but one that should be considered seriously as a method to enhance both management and productivity. Quality management incorporates and expands the traditional quality assurance functions while focusing efforts on continuous improvement with a more satisfying outcome. The idea is to do the right thing right the first time, on time, and all the time and to strive always for improvement and client/customer satisfaction (Deming, 1982).

Deming suggests that there must be a shift in management's thinking and managing, which includes changing the philosophy of the organization to value quality, emphasizing empowering the worker to be more productive, and focusing on leadership and team building. Deming outlines a 14-point system encompassing these concepts (Box 14-13) (Walton, 1986).

It is important to note that quality management or improvement focuses on the system, not the employee. According to Deming, 15% of quality improvement focuses on people; the remaining 85% focuses on systems problems (Walton, 1986). Quality improvement can be considered preventive rather than reactive wherein the focus is to anticipate problems so they can be prevented and/or to take corrective action to solve an identified problem in the system to prevent it from occurring again (Widtfeldt, 1992). The focus is on the process of doing the job right to ensure a quality outcome. Thus, time is spent on fixing the system as opposed to fixing broken products. The notion of quality improvement that is prevention-oriented shares the same philosophy as prevention versus cure in health care; that is, it is more cost-effective to prevent an illness than to treat the symptoms and illness.

Another important aspect of quality improvement is customer satisfaction (Casalov, 1991; Ervin, 1992; McLaughlin & Kaluzny, 1990). The occupational and environmental health nurse in the business setting is certainly familiar with total quality management with respect to goods and customer services. This familiarity is or can be carried over into the occupational health unit in terms of satisfaction of employees and other groups or departments who are served by the occupational health unit; satisfaction as demonstrated by staff morale; satisfaction of staff with their own performance; and satisfaction from external groups (e.g., community). For example, Rogers et al. (1993) conducted a satisfaction survey of nearly 500 employees regarding the delivery and perceived quality of occupational health services in a pharmaceutical company. Results indicated high satisfaction with both services delivery indicators (e.g., waiting time) and quality indicators (e.g., provider interaction). One area noted for improvement was the employees' inability to identify specific health care providers. This could potentially have an impact on continuity of care and thus reduce quality. This problem was resolved through the utilization of name tags.

Quality management shifts the focus from the individual to a team with a fundamental concept that if something goes wrong, it's usually not the people but the system that is at fault. Quality management relies on input from employees as a source for change (Hardy & Forrer, 1996). This management philosophy is basically consistent

---

Box 14-13   Deming's Guidepoints for Quality Improvement

1. Create constancy of purpose for improvement in product or service.
2. Adopt the new philosophy related to quality.
3. Cease dependence on inspections.
4. End the practice of awarding business on the price tag alone.
5. Improve constantly and forever the system of production and service.
6. Institute training and retraining on the job.
7. Adopt and institute leadership.
8. Drive out fear.
9. Break down barriers among staff and departments.
10. Eliminate slogans, exhortations, and targets for the workforce.
11. Eliminate quotas for the workforce (including numerical goals).
12. Remove barriers to pride in work performance.
13. Institute a program of education and self-improvement for everyone.
14. Implement the transformation through team effort.

From *Quality, Productivity, and Competitive Position,* by W. E. Deming, 1982, Cambridge, MA: Massachusetts Institute of Technology.

with that of McGregor's Theory Y and Herzberg's motivators.

Laza and Wheaton (1990) emphasize the importance of monitoring the system for improvement. This means that each work process is questioned and evaluated as to its usefulness, efficiency, and effectiveness. For example, Widtfeldt (1992) describes a situation in a Fortune 500 company—whose hypertension screening program had not been evaluated in several years—in which significant numbers of employees walked into the occupational health unit for blood pressure monitoring, thereby disrupting prearranged occupational health unit services. This was both a quality assurance and quality improvement issue. The problem was addressed through reviewing the current Joint National Committee on Detection, Evaluation, and Treatment of High Blood Pressure recommendations for screening high blood pressure and updating the occupational health service program standards and criteria for blood pressure monitoring (quality assurance). By doing this, high-risk individuals could more appropriately be identified and scheduled for blood pressure monitoring and disruption of prearranged occupational health service activities was reduced (quality improvement).

Before initiating a quality management program, the occupational and environmental health nurse must assess the organization, including such elements as customer satisfaction planning, quality assurance, resource utilization, leadership, and teamwork. This is necessary for recognizing the organization's strengths and weaknesses and avoiding potential pitfalls (Arikian, 1991; Johnson & Olesinsi, 1995). Various tools such as flowcharts, Pareto charts, scatter diagrams, and cause and effect diagrams can be useful in analyzing work processes and problem areas.

Rogers (1998) points out that nurses often have more impact on the quality of care than any other member of the health care team; thus, nursing is in a good position to implement quality management. Advantages of quality management include the following:

- Increased quality
- Increased productivity
- Increased savings in time and money
- Increased teamwork
- Increased employee morale
- Employee ownership of the organizational improvement process
- Meeting of accreditation standards
- Decreased rework
- Decreased employee turnover
- Decreased recruitment costs
- Decreased costs

To implement quality management, top administration must commit to the philosophy of continuous improvement in all aspects of work. This will mean not only a change in thinking from the management's perspective but also from the staff. The solution to enhanced quality with cost savings should be embraced.

Occupational and environmental health nurses are often the decision makers with respect to occupational health indicators and unit functioning; thus their expertise is invaluable. More emphasis should be placed on incorporating a team philosophy that utilizes all skills, with less focus on hierarchical occupational nursing decision making.

Summary

The essence of management is to work with others to accomplish organizational goals. To achieve this, the manager must adapt and display management methods that help motivate and support work performance.

While traditional management philosophy has assumed a more authoritarian managerial style, contemporary theory supports participative management with input from employees in the planning, executing, and evaluating of the work and work performance.

It seems appropriate that managerial skills and functions be integrated within a total quality management philosophy with emphasis on continuous improvement. Within this framework all workers share a common bond to not only ensure but improve quality with a reduction in cost. Utilizing contemporary management approaches will also enhance worker self-esteem and ownership of the services and products produced.

References

American Association of Occupational Health Nurses. (1987). *A comprehensive guide for establishing an occupational health nursing service.* Atlanta, GA: Author.

American Association of Occupational Health Nurses. (1999). *Standards of occupational and environmental health nursing*. Atlanta, GA: Author.

American Nurses Association. (1998). *Standards of clinical nursing practice*. Washington, DC: Author.

Arikian, V. (1991). Total quality management. *Journal of Nursing Administration, 21*(6), 46-50.

Beaulieu, R., Shamian, J., Donner, G., & Pringle, D. (1997). Empowerment and commitment of nurses in long-term care. *Nursing Economies, 15*, 32-41.

Bennis, W. G., Benne, K. D., & Chinn, R. (1985). *The planning of change*. New York: Holt, Rinehart, & Winston.

Bozman, A., & Childres, F. (1991). The budgeting process. *AAOHN Update Series, 4*(8), 1-8.

Brodbeck, K. (1992). Professional practice actualized through an integrated shared governance and quality assurance model. *Journal of Nursing Care Quality, 6*(2), 20-31.

Casalov, R. (1991). Total quality management in health care. *Hospital and Health Services Administration, 36*(1), 134-146.

Deming, W. E. (1982). *Quality, productivity and competitive position*. Cambridge, MA: Massachusetts Institute of Technology.

Dienemann, J. (1992). *Continuous quality improvement in nursing*. Washington, DC: American Nurses.

Donabedian, A. (1966). Evaluating the quality of medical care. *Milbank Memorial Fund Quarterly, 44*(3), 166-206.

Douglas, L. (1996). *The effective nurse*. St. Louis, MO: Mosby.

Drucker, P. (1982). *The practice of management*. New York: Harper & Row.

Dubnicki, C., & Sloan, S. (1991). Excellence in nursing and management. *Journal of Nursing Administration, 21*(6), 40-45.

Ervin, D. (1992, January/February). Quality issues in group practice. *MGM Journal*, 25-31.

Fallon, L. F., Jr. (2001). Management theory and applications. *Occupational Medicine: State of the Art Reviews, 16*(3).

Finkler, S. (2000). *Budgeting concepts for managers*. Philadelphia: W. B. Saunders.

Gardner, D., Kelly, K., Johnson, M., McCloskey, J., & Maas, M. (1991). Nursing administration model for administrative practice. *Journal of Nursing Administration, 21*(3), 37-41.

Gillies, D. A. (1994). *Nursing management: A systems approach*. Philadelphia: W. B. Saunders.

Hardy, V. S., & Forrer, J. (1996). A comprehensive quality management approach. *Nurse Manager, 27*, 35-38.

Hein, E., & Nicholson, M. J. (1986). *Contemporary leadership behavior* (2nd ed.). Boston: Little, Brown & Company.

Hersey, P., & Blanchard, K. (1993). *Management of organizational behavior* (6th ed.). Englewood Cliffs, NJ: Prentice Hall.

Hitt, W. D. (1993). The model leader: A fully functioning person. *Leadership & Organizational Development Journal 14*(7), 4-11.

Huber, D. (1996). *Leadership and nursing care management*. Philadelphia: W. B. Saunders.

Jarrett, M. (1989). Writing successful business proposals. *AAOHN Update Series, 3*(21), 1-8.

Jarrett, M. E. (1987). *A questionnaire to identify quality assurance activities in occupational health nursing*. Unpublished manuscript, University of North Carolina at Chapel Hill.

Johnson, J. H., & Olesinsi, N. (1995). Program evaluation, key to success. *JONA, 25*, 53-60.

Katz, R. L. (1955, January/February). Skills of an effective manager. *Harvard Business Review*, 33-42.

Kemp, V. (1986). An overview of change and leadership. In E. Hein & M. J. Nicholson (Eds.), *Contemporary leadership behavior* (2nd ed.). Boston: Little, Brown & Company.

Lang, N. M. (1976). *Issues in quality assurance in nursing: Issues in evaluation research*. Kansas City, MO: American Nurses Association.

Laza, R. W., & Wheaton, P. L. (1990). Recognizing the pit-falls of total quality management. *Public Utilities Fortnightly, 125*, 17-21.

Lewin, K. (1953). Studies in group decisions. In D. Cartwright & A. Zander (Eds.), *Group dynamics*. Evanston, IL: Row Peterson.

Lippitt, R., Watson, J., & Westley, B. (1958). *Dynamics of planned change*. New York: Harcourt Brace.

Manchester, J., Summers, V., Newell, J., Graughan, B., & Spitter, K. (1991). Development of an assessment guide for occupational health nurses. *AAOHN Journal, 39*(1), 7-12.

Marker, C. (1987). The Marker umbrella model for quality assurance: Monitoring and evaluating professional practice. *Journal of Nursing Quality Assurance, 1*(3), 52-63.

Marks, M. (1986, March). The question of quality circles. *Psychology Today, 1*, 36-42.

Marquis, B. L., & Huston, C. J. (1996). *Leadership roles and management functions in nursing, theory and application*. Philadelphia: Lippincott.

Marquis, B. L., & Huston, C. J. (1998). *Management decision making for nurses: 124 case studies*. Philadelphia: Lippincott.

Martin, M. (1998). Achieving the right balance with strategic planning. *Nurse Manager 29*, 30-31.

Maslow, A. H. (1954). *Motivation and personality*. New York: Harper & Row.

McLaughlin, C. P., & Kaluzny, A. D. (1990). Total quality management in health: Making it work. *Health Care Management Review, 15*(3), 7-14.

Nightingale, F. (1860). *Notes on nursing: What it is and what it is not*. New York: Appleton.

Oberle, J. (1990, January). Quality gurus: The men and their message. *Training, 1*, 47-52.

Olsen, M. E. (1978). *The process of social organization.* New York: Holt, Rinehart & Winston.

Poulin, M. (1984). The nurse executive role. *Journal of Nursing Administration, 14*(2), 9-14.

Renmick-Breisch, L. (1998). Motivate! Create a work environment that brings out each nurse's drive to excel. *Nursing Management, 6*(10), 27-29.

Rogers, B. (1998). Occupational health nursing expertise. *AAOHN Journal, 46,* 497-503.

Rogers, B., Winslow, B., & Higgins, S. (1993). Employee satisfaction and occupational health services. *AAOHN Journal, 41,* 58-65.

Sullivan, E., & Decker, D. (1988). *Effective management in nursing.* New York: Addison-Wesley.

Swansburg, R. C. (1996). *Management and leadership for nurse managers,* (2nd ed.). Boston: Jones & Bartlett.

Tappen, R. (2001). *Nursing leadership and management.* Philadelphia: F. A. Davis.

Tomey, A. (2000). *Guide to nursing management.* St. Louis, MO: Mosby.

Townsend, M. (1991). Creating a better work environment. *Journal of Nursing Administration, 21*(1), 11-14.

Vestal, K. W. (1989). Writing a business plan. *Nursing Economics, 6*(3), 121-124.

Wallace, K., & Ventura, M. (1991). Planning the interview for a clinical nurse researcher. *Journal of Nursing Administration, 21*(12), 54-59.

Walton, M. (1986). *The Deming management method.* Putnam, NY: Dodd, Mead.

Widtfeldt, A. (1992). Quality and quality improvement in occupational health nursing. *AAOHN Update Series, 4*(3), 1-8.

Yukl, G. (1989). *Leadership in organizations.* Englewood Cliffs, NJ: Prentice-Hall.

Yuri, H. (1986). Nursing leadership process. In E. Hein & M. J. Nicholson (Eds.), *Contemporary leadership behavior* (2nd ed.). Boston: Little, Brown & Company.

14-1

Job Description for Department Head of Occupational Health Center

JOB DESCRIPTION
U 1300   5/92

Wellcome

INSTRUCTIONS ON HOW TO COMPLETE THIS FORM CAN BE FOUND IN THE SUPERVISOR'S MANUAL

Job Title Health Center Department Head	*Unit* OD	*Dept.* OH&S	*Cost Center* 5600	☐ RTP ☐ GVL ☐ Other
This job description supersedes all previous job descriptions for this position. Management retains the discretion to add to or change the duties at any time.	Compensation Dept. Use Only: Exempt ☐ Grade Code _____ Nonexempt ☐			

JOB SUMMARY

Briefly state the main purpose of and basic responsibilities of the job.

> To plan, develop, and administer the policies and procedures of the RTP Health Centers and manage resources to meet Company needs. To provide health care to RTP and Field Staff employees that is directed toward the promotion, protection, and restoration of worker health within the context of a safe and helpful work environment.

JOB DUTIES AND RESPONSIBILITIES

List in order of importance and/or frequency of occurrence each predominant and significant duty, task, or responsibility. Indicate if the job duty is essential (yes), which means that removing the function would fundamentally alter the job, or not essential (no). For each major job duty list the most important knowledge, skill, or ability (K, S, A) required to accomplish the duty.

JOB DUTIES	ESSENTIAL DUTIES (YES/NO)	REQUIRED K, S, A'S
Assure completion and follow-up of preplacement physical examinations, complying with government regulations, environmental job demands, and physical ability to perform work.	Yes	• Professional interdisciplinary knowledge base including the public health, occupational health, social and behavioral sciences, management and administration and nursing science • Knowledge of EEO standards, handicap laws, ADA, and job demands • Decision making capabilities

JOB DUTIES	ESSENTIAL DUTIES (YES/NO)	REQUIRED K, S, A'S
Manage the Company-sponsored periodic physical exams and medical surveillance programs. Promote employee health and lifestyle changes through individual counseling and referrals to Wellcome Health. Consult with Company physician to gain clarity regarding health related issues. Consult with Safety on environmental and safety concerns.	Yes	• Professional interdisciplinary knowledge base including the public health, occupational health, social and behavioral sciences, management and administration and nursing science • Planning and organizing skills
Verify eligibility of the employee within the sickness and accident/LTD plans. Monitor progress and coordinate community health services for rehabilitation purposes to assist the employee in return to work. Communicate appropriate information to immediate supervisor, Benefits, Human Resources, and Employee Relations.	Yes	• Professional interdisciplinary knowledge base including the public health, occupational health, social and behavioral sciences, management and administration and nursing science • Working knowledge of job demands and ergonomics • Working knowledge of B.W. Co. benefit plan • Working knowledge of community health resources
Manage health services and reimbursement process for Field Staff.	Yes	• Professional interdisciplinary knowledge base including the public health, occupational health, social and behavioral sciences, management and administration and nursing science • Working knowledge of B.W. Co. Flex Formula Insurance • Working knowledge of accounting and budget
Promote, supervise, and perform prompt and effective medical assistance to employees in acute and chronic situations.	Yes	• Professional interdisciplinary knowledge base including the public health, occupational health, social and behavioral sciences, management and administration and nursing science • Working knowledge of job demands • Skill in providing emergency care • Working knowledge of B.W. Co. emergency response plan
Supervise the development and maintenance of accurate, up-to-date medical records and/or reports to track employee health/illness and provide the Company with the needed data, ensuring client confidentiality.	Yes	• Professional knowledge of medical terminology, attention to detail, skill in technical writing • Confidentiality principles

JOB DUTIES	ESSENTIAL DUTIES (YES/NO)	REQUIRED K, S, A'S
Manage Health Center operation and act as a resource and advisor to staff as health care services are rendered to the employee population. Evaluate performance, counsel, and coach as necessary.	Yes	• Professional interdisciplinary knowledge base including the public health, occupational health, social and behavioral sciences, management and administration and nursing science • Leadership skills • Oral and written communication skills • Working knowledge of B.W. Co. policies and procedures
Investigate illness and injury episodes and trends to determine health and safety needs of the employee population. Communicate this information to Safety and/or Wellcome Health Coordinator for program development.	Yes	• Professional interdisciplinary knowledge base including the public health, occupational health, social and behavioral sciences, management and administration and nursing science • Working knowledge of B.W. Co. safety procedures • Working knowledge of Wellcome Health program • Communications skills
Represent the Health Center at B.W. Co. meetings and/or community affairs as requested.	Yes	• Leadership skills • Oral communication skills • Working knowledge of B.W. Co. policies and procedures
Promote the Employee Assistance Program through individual and/or supervisor referrals.	Yes	• Professional knowledge of nursing process • Working knowledge of B.W. Co. policies and procedures • Counseling skills • Oral communication skills
Meets attendance requirements for the job. Other duties as assigned	Yes	Ability to attend work regularly

PROBLEM SOLVING AND DECISION MAKING

In the first column describe three or four of the <u>most important</u> problems that the job incumbent must solve or decisions that must be made to achieve the <u>primary objectives</u> of the job. For each problem, indicate in the second column the checks or controls that exist to help improve the quality or accuracy of the problem-solving/decision-making process. Then, in the third column, estimate the potential impact these problems/decisions can have on the department/unit <u>or</u> Company if handled <u>correctly</u> or <u>incorrectly.</u>

Problem/Decision	Checks/Controls	Potential Impact
Provide medical placement approval for existing or new employees in a job that matches their physical capabilities.	Medical opinions	Job turndowns, additional recruiting costs, lawsuits, increased WC cost and liability
Approval of diagnosis for S&A benefit; judgment of potential long term sequel on and need for LTD benefits.	Medical opinions	Improper use of benefit plan; increased liability to B.W. Co.
Ensure adequate job restrictions to protect B.W. Co. and facilitate employee rehabilitation.	Medical opinions	Increased WC cost and liability; illness/injury to other employees; increased lost work time, low productivity, lawsuits
Interpret and comply with the medical requirements of regulations issued by ADA, OSHA, FDA and other government agencies.	Medical opinions Legal advise	Fines issued by government agencies for failure to comply or improper interpretation; liability of employee lawsuits

CONTACTS WITH OTHERS

List the most significant interactions that the job has within the Company (other than the immediate supervisor and the subordinates) and outside the Company. Under "Purpose of Contacts" indicate the reason why the contacts are made and why they are important to B.W. Co.

Title of Contact	Purpose of Contacts
Managers/Supervisors	To make recommendations to the manager on health-related issues such as job restriction, job assignment, and/or job design.
Safety Department	To communicate potential health/safety hazards in the work place and ask for assistance in investigating.
Human Resources	To recommend the health ability or inability to perform a job as a preemployment applicant or transfer through Operation Opportunity; to recommend job restrictions and/or job reassignment.
Employee Relations	To communicate the health status of employees when requested and advise Employee Relations of the need to drug test based on cause.
Employee Assistance Program	To refer and communicate the counseling needs of individual employees or groups of employees to the designated EAP counselor. Interact with counselor to resolve problems.
Physician's Contract	To ensure provisions of physician's contract are being carried out and monitor the medical services being rendered so that the highest standards of medical practice and services are being offered to B.W. Co. employees.

CREATIVE THOUGHT

What aspects of the position require the highest levels of creative thought (i.e., the conception and formulation of new ideas, techniques, procedures, programs, etc.)?

> Rendering decisions with regard to work area placement and restrictions based on the employee health status and capabilities

WORKING CONDITIONS AND SPECIAL REQUIREMENTS

List any adverse working conditions, exposure to hazardous materials or conditions, travel requirements, requirements for working long hours, at night, weekends, rotating shifts, etc. **ALSO ATTACH A COMPLETED PHYSICAL AND ENVIRONMENTAL JOB DEMANDS FORM, U 294, IF A NORMAL SEDENTARY OFFICE ENVIRONMENT DOES NOT APPLY.**

X   none   see attached   list follows:
────   ──── form U 294   ────

JOB SPECIFICATIONS

Basic Background

Check the <u>minimum</u> education level and list the base level of experience required to successfully perform the job. Include the time length of experience required, if appropriate, as well as the nature of the experience required. If different combinations of education and/or experience could be considered equivalent, check and complete all that apply. Indicate they are alternatives by typing "OR" after each option.

> Education and Experience
> ☒   Four-year college curriculum with a major concentration in nursing.
>   PLUS: Be a registered nurse in the State of North Carolina. Certification in audiometric and pulmonary function testing. Five year's experience in an occupational health nurse setting. Two year's supervisory experience.
> ☒   Other (special certification, licensure, etc., please specify) Certification as an Occupational Health Nurse.

Other Factors to be Considered in Selection Include:

List required KSAs not mentioned under Basic Background, Targeted Selection® Dimensions, and any <u>preferred</u> job related factors.

> • Professional image
> • Experience in health/hygiene counseling; working with variety of patients in outpatient, adult health settings
> • Skills: oral and written communication, integrity, planning and organizing, problem analysis, decision making, leadership, team building
> • Nonsmoker

APPROVALS & DATE	Signature	Date
Immediate Supervisor	_____	_____
Supervisor's Supervisor	_____	_____
Compensation	_____	_____
HR Manager	_____	_____

REQUEST FOR JOB EVALUATION
(To be completed only when submitting the J.D. for Job Evaluation.
Submit to the Compensation Department RTP or Greenville when complete.)

☐ RTP
☐ GVL
☐ Other

Job Title: <u>Health Center Department Head</u> Cost Center: <u>5600</u>
Initiating Supervisor: _____ Department: <u>OH&S</u> Unit: <u>QD</u>
Supervisor's Supervisor: _____ Date of Request: _____

| Please complete checklist | **An incomplete checklist will slow your request for job evaluation.**

1. Please indicate the reason for job evaluation. (Check one)
   ☐ New job
   ☐ Change in existing job responsibility
   ☐ Other (describe) _____

2. ☐ This new job description (JD) makes obsolete the former JD with the
   title _____ in cost center _____.
   -or-
   ☐ N/A

3. ☐ New JD attached

4. ☐ Physical and Environmental Job Demands form, U 294 attached
   -or-
   ☐ N/A. Normal sedentary office environment; no unusual physical and environmental demands involved

5. ☐ Organization chart attached
   -or-
   ☐ Organization chart completed below

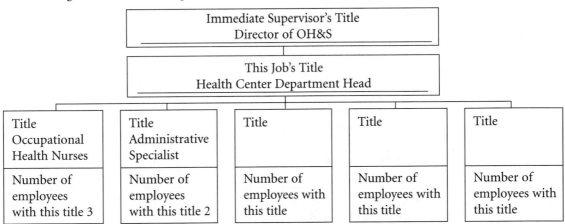

Total number of employees supervised (including employees who report in through the direct reports shown above). __5__

————FOR COMPENSATION DEPARTMENT USE ONLY————

Job Code _____
Job Evaluation by/Date _____
Compensation Department Approval _____

☐ EXEMPT   ☐ NONEXEMPT
Current Grade
Revised Grade

GRADE
TOTAL POINTS

Courtesy of Burroughs–Wellcome.

14-2 Assessment Guide for Occupational Health Nursing Practice

Date:

Evaluator:

Standard	Criteria	Level of Practice					Comments/ Recommendations
		All of the time	Most of the time	Some of the time	Not at all	N/A	
I. FUNCTION The OHN collaborates with management in developing objectives for the employee health service compatible with the company's corporate goals and objectives.	**STRUCTURE** 1. Functions: a. As manager for the health program and policymaker; b. Under the supervision of a qualified occupational health nurse; c. As part of overall management in the development of policies for the health unit.						
	PROCESS 1. Develops philosophy and written goals and objectives for the occupational health program. 2. Conducts periodic reviews of Occupational Health Services to assure goals and objectives being met.						

If not applicable N/A, please explain (i.e., this is not a responsibility of the OHN; this is responsibility of the supervisory nurse, corporate office, physicians, personnel, safety, etc.).

Standard	Criteria	Level of Practice					Comments/ Recommendations
		All of the time	Most of the time	Some of the time	Not at all	N/A	
	3. Keeps informed of legal requirements of occupational health programs and assures compliance with same (i.e., medical surveillance, record keeping, etc.). 4. Communicates findings to other members of management team and makes recommendations for programs and intervention strategies. 5. Conveys cost and benefits of occupational health programs in the workplace to management by: a. Analysis of data; b. Literature documentation.						
	OUTCOME 1. Occupational health programs are developed and implemented to: a. Meet health needs of individual employees; b. Assure optimal health and safety of all employees. 2. Occupational health programs are in compliance with federal and state laws. 3. The OHN is a member of the interdisciplinary team responsible for occupational health and safety.						

If not applicable N/A, please explain (i.e., this is not a responsibility of the OHN; this is responsibility of the supervisory nurse, corporate office, physicians, personnel, safety, etc.).

Standard	Criteria	Level of Practice					Comments/ Recommendations
		All of the time	Most of the time	Some of the time	Not at all	N/A	
II. FUNCTION The OHN administers the employee health service.	**STRUCTURE** 1. The health service is managed by a qualified registered occupational health nurse. 2. The occupational health unit is of adequate size and quality and is suitably located to perform the nursing functions of the occupational health program. 3. The OHN is familiar with the products and processes of the company which affect health.						
	PROCESS 1. Develops and coordinates written policies and procedures with other members of the health team and management. 2. Determines the number and qualifications of nursing and paraprofessional staff that are required for a comprehensive on-site occupational health program. 3. Identifies and supervises the nursing care which can safely be performed by allied health workers. 4. Develops and monitors operating budget. 5. Collects data and prepares reports on the health status of the worker and the existing or potential health hazards in the work environment.						

If not applicable N/A, please explain (i.e., this is not a responsibility of the OHN; this is responsibility of the supervisory nurse, corporate office, physicians, personnel, safety, etc.).

Standard	Criteria	Level of Practice					Comments/ Recommendations
		All of the time	Most of the time	Some of the time	Not at all	N/A	
	6. Provides management with data on trends in health-related statistics in order to inform them of the impact of occupational health program planning and implementation.						
	OUTCOME 1. The occupational health program is comprehensive and an integral part of the workplace. 2. The OHN is responsible for managing the occupational health department.						

If not applicable N/A, please explain (i.e., this is not a responsibility of the OHN; this is responsibility of the supervisory nurse, corporate office, physicians, personnel, safety, etc.).

Standard	Criteria	Level of Practice					Comments/ Recommendations
		All of the time	Most of the time	Some of the time	Not at all	N/A	
III. FUNCTION The OHN defines nursing authority and responsibility based on standards of service and practice established by the nursing profession and collaborates with management in determining the nurses' position in the organization structure.	**STRUCTURE** 1. A written organizational chart is established for the health unit. 2. Written job descriptions are developed and available for all levels of nursing and allied staff. 3. Orientation programs and continuing educational plans are established for all nursing and allied personnel.						
	PROCESS 1. Functions with his/her level of preparation and experience in accordance with state and federal regulations for practice. 2. Attends educational and professional programs and meetings on a regular periodic basis in order to practice and promote state-of-the-art occupational health nursing.						
	OUTCOME 1. Evaluations to measure performance based on completion of activities defined in their job descriptions are conducted on an annual basis by the OHN manager.						

If not applicable N/A, please explain (i.e., this is not a responsibility of the OHN; this is responsibility of the supervisory nurse, corporate office, physicians, personnel, safety, etc.).

Standard	Criteria	Level of Practice					Comments/ Recommendations
		All of the time	Most of the time	Some of the time	Not at all	N/A	
IV. FUNCTION The OHN administers nursing care and develops nursing care procedures and protocols with specific goals and interventions appropriate for employee's needs.	**STRUCTURE** 1. a. There is a written policy and procedure manual for nursing activities. b. A method exists for nursing care procedures and protocols to be communicated to appropriate personnel and health care providers. 2. Recordkeeping and reporting systems are in place which meet legal requirements, ensure continuity of care and confidentiality, and are coordinated with the company's systems. 3. Written, signed, and dated medical directives or protocols are provided and updated at least annually.						
	PROCESS 1. Identifies employee health needs and collaborates with health care providers in establishing nursing care procedures and protocols. 2. Actively participates in: a. Preplacement assessments, periodic and special medical assessments; and b. Determines health risk factors, employee and company needs in relation to job placement.						

If not applicable N/A, please explain (i.e., this is not a responsibility of the OHN; this is responsibility of the supervisory nurse, corporate office, physicians, personnel, safety, etc.).

Standard	Criteria	Level of Practice					Comments/ Recommendations
		All of the time	Most of the time	Some of the time	Not at all	N/A	
	3. Nursing care: a. Is individualized to meet the physical, emotional, social, and cultural needs of employees. b. Ensures optimal opportunities for employees with special needs. c. Is based on measures of prevention and health promotion. 4. Demonstrates professional judgment and skill in patient assessment, nursing care, counseling, and evaluation techniques. 5. Renders professional nursing care and follow-up of occupational and nonoccupational illness and injuries within the scope of the company's Medical Directives and the Nurse Practice Act.						
	OUTCOME 1. Nursing care policies and procedures are recorded and available for review. 2. Nursing care policies and procedures are revised and periodically updated as goals are achieved or changed. 3. Accurate, complete, and concise records of nursing activities are maintained. 4. Records are audited for appropriate treatment and/or referral.						

If not applicable N/A, please explain (i.e., this is not a responsibility of the OHN; this is responsibility of the supervisory nurse, corporate office, physicians, personnel, safety, etc.).

Standard	Criteria	Level of Practice					Comments/ Recommendations
		All of the time	Most of the time	Some of the time	Not at all	N/A	
V. FUNCTION The OHN coordinates responsibilities in the health assessment program and promotes health maintenance and preventions of illness and injury.	**STRUCTURE** 1. The preventive approach to health care, which includes early detection, medical monitoring, health teaching, and counseling with appropriate referral is a primary concern of the occupational health program. 2. Company sponsored health and wellness programs have been established by the OHN to assist employees in improving and maintaining their health. 3. A mechanism exists for the OHN to periodically reevaluate employee health and safety needs.						
	PROCESS 1. Plans, coordinates, implements, and evaluates on-site health education programs. 2. Intervenes appropriately on behalf of individuals and populations at risk of preventable, potential health problems. 3. Intervenes for an employee who evidences an acute illness, injury, or temporary disability condition. 4. Ensure that the employee is informed about his/her current health status. 5. Conducts or collaborates with other team member's regular plant walk-throughs and health tours						

If not applicable N/A, please explain (i.e., this is not a responsibility of the OHN; this is responsibility of the supervisory nurse, corporate office, physicians, personnel, safety, etc.).

Standard	Criteria	Level of Practice					Comments/ Recommendations
		All of the time	Most of the time	Some of the time	Not at all	N/A	
	to assess potential or existing environmental health, and safety hazards. 6. Informs corporate personnel, when appropriate, about adaptations or interventions of the work environment required to meet individual employee health needs. 7. Provides education, support, and motivation in areas of health and safety.						
	OUTCOME 1. Health problems of employees are identified at an early stage. 2. Employees utilize information provided in making decisions and choices about promoting, maintaining, and restoring health, seeking and utilizing appropriate health care personnel and health care resources. 3. Employees demonstrate healthy lifestyle choices, knowledge of health care resources, and an understanding of the means of disease and accident prevention. 4. Employees, including handicapped, chronically and terminally ill, show evidence of participation in the workforce activities to the fullest extent possible in relation to each individual's health status.						

If not applicable N/A, please explain (i.e., this is not a responsibility of the OHN; this is responsibility of the supervisory nurse, corporate office, physicians, personnel, safety, etc.).

Standard	Criteria	Level of Practice					Comments/ Recommendations
		All of the time	Most of the time	Some of the time	Not at all	N/A	
VI. FUNCTION The OHN collaborates with other on-site members of the occupational health team to evaluate the work environment and utilizes outside resources when services are not available within company.	**STRUCTURE** 1. Functions as a member of the interdisciplinary health and safety team and as a resource person to other team members to establish parameters of service. 2. Coordinates the health care of the employees. 3. Is consulted, when appropriate, in selection of personal protection wear. 4. Coordinates and assists in development of safety education program, policies, and procedures.						
	PROCESS 1. Utilizes state, federal, and private agencies and resources for assistance as needed. 2. Provides information to management to assist company in adhering to OSHA regulations, fire codes, SARA, and Hazard Communication, recognizing safety as a priority.						
	OUTCOME 1. The OHN is part of a professional team, the goals of which are to provide a healthy and safe work environment for all employees. 2. The OHN defines his/her role and responsibility in contributing to the provision of a safe and health work environment.						

If not applicable N/A, please explain (i.e., this is not a responsibility of the OHN; this is responsibility of the supervisory nurse, corporate office, physicians, personnel, safety, etc.).

Standard	Criteria	Level of Practice					Comments/ Recommendations
		All of the time	Most of the time	Some of the time	Not at all	N/A	
VII. FUNCTION The OHN establishes and promotes working relationships with appropriate community agencies.	**STRUCTURE** 1. Acts as a member of management team and as a liaison to the community.						
	PROCESS 1. Establishes contact with agencies and services of the community that might be a reciprocal basis for a "good neighbor" policy (i.e., American Red Cross for Blood Drives, CPR, First Aid, Catastrophic Assistance, etc.; American Cancer Society, Police with substance abuse assistance; Fire Department with Right to Know data, etc.) 2. Coordinates employee educational programs with appropriate community agencies.						
	OUTCOME 1. The OHN is an integral part of management team by solidifying good public relations within the community. 2. Community health resources available for support are utilized in accomplishing health service goals and objectives.						

If not applicable N/A, please explain (i.e., this is not a responsibility of the OHN; this is responsibility of the supervisory nurse, corporate office, physicians, personnel, safety, etc.).

From "Development of an Assessment Guide for Occupational Health Nurses," by J. Manchester, V. Summers, J. Newell, B. Graughan, and K. Spitter, 1991, *AAOHN Journal, 39*(1): 7–12.

14-3 Quality Assurance in Occupational Health Nursing

This questionnaire is divided into several small sections, each preceded by directions or comments to assist you in completing the questionnaire.

Standards of practice define and measure nursing accountability and the quality of patient care. The first series of questions addresses professional standards in the occupational health nursing unit where you are currently practicing.

1. Are there written standards of nursing practice for the occupational health nursing unit?

_____ Yes

_____ No

    2. If yes, What is the focus of the standards? (Check those that apply.)

    _____ Characteristics of the physical facilities

    _____ Type, quality, and quantity of equipment and supplies

    _____ Licensure, certification, and formal education

    _____ Staffing requirements

    _____ Continuing education

    _____ Policies and procedures

    _____ Job performance

    _____ Changes in health status of employees expected as a result of nursing care

    _____ Other, please specify: _____

    _____

Continuing education (CE) includes all professional developmental experiences occurring inside and outside the agency you are employed by. The following questions are concerned with the CE activities, with the exception of certification activities, associated with the occupational health nursing unit.

3. Do staff members have the opportunity to attend CE activities (either internal or external) directed at maintaining current competency in existing standards of nursing care?

_____ Yes

_____ No

    If yes, please describe: _____

    _____

    _____

4. Do staff members have the opportunity to attend CE activities that are directed at developing competencies when new standards are implemented?

_____ Yes

_____ No

    If yes, please describe: _____

    _____

    _____

5. Do staff members have the opportunity to attend CE activities that are directed toward correcting identified deficiencies in the knowledge or skills required in the particular practice setting?

_____ Yes

_____ No

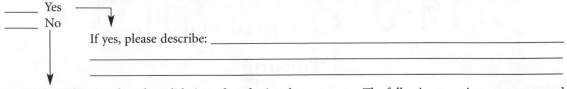

If yes, please describe: _____

_____

_____

Credentialing involves the validation of professional competency. The following questions are concerned with the subject of credentialing in the occupational health nursing unit you are currently practicing in.

6. Are annual licensure validations conducted and documented?

_____ Yes

_____ No

7. Is there periodic certification of staff members for competency in knowledge and skills identified in the unit standards of performance or job description?

_____ Yes

_____ No

If yes, please identify the following that apply:

Certification	How Often
_____ Pulmonary function testing	_____
_____ Hearing conservation	_____
_____ First aid	_____
_____ CPR	_____
_____ Other, please specify: _____	_____
_____	_____
_____	_____

8. Are there approval lists that identify those practitioners certified to practice in high-risk extended nursing roles such as suturing of wounds and prescribing of prescription medications?

_____ Yes

_____ No

_____ Not applicable

Performance appraisals can be utilized to provide staff members with feedback regarding their job performance and compliance to standards. Please answer the following questions dealing with the use of performance appraisals in your practice setting.

9. Is a job performance appraisal instrument used to evaluate your performance?

_____ Yes

_____ No

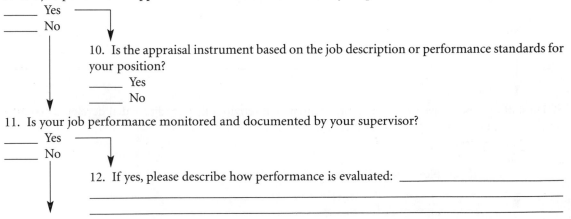

10. Is the appraisal instrument based on the job description or performance standards for your position?

_____ Yes

_____ No

11. Is your job performance monitored and documented by your supervisor?

_____ Yes

_____ No

12. If yes, please describe how performance is evaluated: _____

_____

_____

13. If yes, does your supervisor discuss the results of these monitoring efforts with you on a periodic basis?

_____ Yes

_____ No

If yes, how often? _____

14. If yes, is information on your job performance obtained from these monitoring and review efforts utilized to identify problems and take corrective action?

_____ Yes

_____ No

I would like to gain knowledge of the use of audits in occupational health nursing programs. Please answer the following questions concerning the use of audits in your work setting for questions 15-20.

An audit is defined in the context of this questionnaire as a formal process of data collection from a representative sample.

15. Are audits of nursing practice conducted on site by internal or external reviewers?

_____ Yes (If yes, proceed to question # 16.)

_____ No (If no, proceed to question # 21.)

16. What is the position title of the person responsible for conducting the audits? _____

17. Is there a written schedule that specifies when audits are to be conducted?

_____ Yes

_____ No

If yes, how often? _____

_____

18. Please indicate how audits are utilized to obtain data. (Place a check by those that apply.)

_____ Chart reviews

_____ Direct observation of staff and clients

_____ Staff interviews

_____ Client interviews

_____ Other, please specify: _____

_____

19. Please indicate the purposes for auditing in your unit. (Check those that apply.)

_____ To review compliance to unit standards

_____ To determine how safe and effective a particular aspect of care is

_____ To determine the extent of a problem and which staff members, if any, are responsible

_____ To determine staff satisfaction

_____ To determine client satisfaction

_____ To evaluate staff documentation

_____ Other, please specify, _____

_____

20. On the average, about how many audits are conducted each year? (Please check one.)

_____ 1-2

_____ 3-5

_____ 6-10

_____ 10-20

_____ more than 20

Risk management is concerned with the prevention of loss of human resources. The following questions have been included in order to obtain information on any risk management activities utilized in your occupational health nursing unit.

21. Does a preventive maintenance program exist in the unit to identify, take corrective action, and document safety hazards?
_____ Yes
_____ No

22. Are there standards, policies, and/or procedures that focus on infection control?
_____ Yes
_____ No

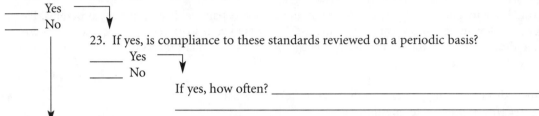

      23. If yes, is compliance to these standards reviewed on a periodic basis?
      _____ Yes
      _____ No

          If yes, how often? _____
          _____

Active problem identification refers to tools utilized by the manager as data sources for tracking events in the unit on a continuous basis. These tools serve a dual purpose in that they identify problems and monitor the results of actions taken to correct problems.

24. Please identify any of the tools listed below that are utilized for this purpose in your work setting. (Check those that apply.)
_____ *Problem identification sheets.* Used by the staff to report complaints and perceived problems in a written manner
_____ *Problem log.* A summarized list of problems identified in the unit, corrective actions (planned or implemented), and evaluations of short- and long-term results of the interventions
_____ *Shift report.* Provides a summation of the shifts' activities and communicates to the manager any problems or events that warrant immediate attention
_____ Other, please specify: _____
_____
_____

_____ None utilized

The next two questions concern the quality assurance activities that review the utilization of resources in the occupational health nursing unit in which you are now practicing.

25. Are unit resources such as staffing, budget monies, equipment, facilities, and supplies monitored and evaluated to determine if they are adequate and are being used in an efficient manner?
_____ Yes
_____ No

      26. If yes, what tools are used to monitor and evaluate resources? (Please check those that apply.)
      _____ *Unit log.* Used to record vital statistics on clients seen in the unit, including any adverse events that occur
      _____ *Unit record.* Used to record information on staff workload, including volume indicators such as number of clients seen per day or number of procedures done per day
      _____ *Budgetary record.* Used to track unit expenditures and compare the current budget status with predetermined budget goals
      _____ Other, please specify: _____
      _____
      _____

For the following question please check those responses that apply.

27. The results of quality assurance activities, if any, are communicated to whom?
_____ There are no quality assurance activities conducted.
_____ Nurses working in the unit
_____ Corporate or supervisor nurse
_____ Medical director or corporate physician
_____ Personnel director/human resources manager
_____ Safety director
_____ General manager
_____Other, please specify: _____
_____

When answering questions #28 and #29, please indicate the extent to which you agree or disagree by circling the appropriate response.

28. Quality assurance programs can assist in the maintenance or improvement of the quality of professional services by occupational health nurses.

| | Strongly | Agree | Uncertain | Disagree | Strongly |
| | Agree | | | | Disagree |

29. A quality assurance program should be an integral part of all occupational health nursing units.

| | Strongly | Agree | Uncertain | Disagree | Strongly |
| | Agree | | | | Disagree |

I would appreciate some information on the participants in this study and their practice settings. Please complete the following questions.

30. What is the total number of years you have practiced as a professional nurse? (Check one.)
_____ Less than 1 year
_____ 1-5 years
_____ 6-10 years
_____ 11-20 years
_____ More than 20 years

31. What is the total number of years you have practiced in an occupational health/employee health setting? (Check one.)
_____ Less than 1 year
_____ 1-5 years
_____ 6-10 years
_____ 11-20 years
_____ More than 20 years

32. Are you a Certified Occupational Health Nurse (COHN)?
_____ Yes
_____ No

33. What degrees/diplomas do you hold? (Check those that apply.)
_____ Associate Degree in nursing
_____ Hospital School of Nursing Diploma Program
_____ Baccalaureate Degree in Nursing

_____ Baccalaureate Degree other than nursing. Please specify:

_____

_____ Masters in nursing

_____ Masters in field other than nursing. Please specify:

_____

_____ Doctorate in nursing

_____ Doctorate in field other than nursing. Please specify:

_____

_____ Other, please specify: _____

_____

34. How many hours per week do you work on the average? (Check one.)
_____ 20 or fewer
_____ 21-39 hours
_____ 40 or more hours

35. Who is your immediate supervisor? (Check one.)
_____ Corporate or supervisor nurse
_____ Medical director or corporate physician
_____ Personnel director/human relations manager
_____ Safety director
_____ General manager
_____ Other, please specify: _____

36. Which of the following best describes your current position? (Check one.)
_____ Staff or general duty nurse
_____ Supervisor nurse or manager
_____ Corporate nurse
_____ Nurse consultant
_____ Nurse educator
_____ Other, please describe: _____

37. How many registered nurses, including yourself, staff the occupational health nursing unit? (Please check one.)
_____ 1
_____ 2-4
_____ 5-10
_____ More than 10

38. If known, please identify your employer's Standard Industrial Classification: _____ If not known, please describe the major product or services of the agency: _____

_____

39. Approximately how many people are employed at the facility? (Please check one.)
_____ fewer than 250
_____ 250-499
_____ 500-999
_____ 1000-1999
_____ 2000-3999
_____ 4000 or more

Thank you for participating in this study.

From "A Questionnaire to Identify Quality Assurance Activities in Occupational Health Nursing," by M. E. Jarrett, 1987, unpublished manuscript, University of North Carolina at Chapel Hill.

15 Legal Responsibility in Occupational and Environmental Health Nursing Practice

Over the past several decades many changes in nursing have resulted in an expanded definition of and expanded practice in nursing. This expansion has led to more comprehensive and explicit standards of practice and competencies, increased the independent functioning of nurses in making diagnoses and providing treatments, and broadened the legal scope of nursing practice. In addition, occupational and environmental health nurses have unique responsibilities related to legislative authority and regulations specific to worker health and safety. Thus, the occupational and environmental health nurse must be familiar with the Occupational Safety and Health Act (1970), recordkeeping requirements and record access, and various legislative mandates that govern occupational health and safety. Although it is impossible to address all statutes and regulations affecting occupational safety and health in this chapter, the following will be addressed: the Occupational Safety and Health Act (1970); major standards and legislative acts that have important implications for occupational and environmental health and nursing practice, including the Hazard Communication Standard, Bloodborne Pathogen Standard, Needlestick Safety and Prevention Act, Recordkeeping Rule, Americans With Disabilities Act, Family and Medical Leave Act, and Workers' Compensation Systems; and the legal responsibilities within the practice framework. The occupational and environmental health nurse must know about new legislation and any changes, modifications, or addenda to any statute or regulation effecting occupational health and safety.

OCCUPATIONAL SAFETY AND HEALTH ACT

All workers are entitled to a safe and healthful work environment. In the last 30 years several public laws and major acts of legislation (Table 15-1) have been enacted to promote and protect worker health and safety. However, the most comprehensive occupational safety and health federal legislation to be enacted is the Occupational Safety and Health Act of 1970 (OSH Act) (Public Law 91-596, 91st Congress, S.2193), signed into law by President Richard M. Nixon on December 29, 1970. The purpose of the OSH Act is "to assure so far as possible every working man and woman in the nation safe and healthful working conditions and to preserve our human resources," (OSH Act, 1970, p. 1). Comprehensive provisions to achieve this goal are embodied in the Act and presented in Appendix 15-1.

The Occupational Safety and Health Act established three separate bodies to administer the major requirements of the Act, including the Occupational Safety and Health Administration (OSHA), the National Institute for Occupational Safety and Health (NIOSH), and the Occupational Safety and Health Review Commission (OSHRC). OSHA, administered by the assistant secretary for labor, was created within the U.S. Department of Labor to carry out regulatory functions prescribed within the purpose of the OSH Act. To accomplish this, the agency focuses on the following three objectives:

TABLE 15-1 Major Federal Occupational and Environmental Health Legislation

DATE	LEGISLATION—RESPONSIBLE AGENCY	PURPOSE
1936	Walsh-Healy Act	Authorizes the federal government to establish occupational safety and health standards for businesses engaged in federal contracts
1969	Federal Coal Mine and Safety Act (amended, 1977)—USDOL	Regulates mine health and safety through mandatory standards governing mine inspections, training, medical monitoring, and control of toxic exposures in the mines
1970	Clean Air Act (amended)—EPA	Regulates air quality through promulgation of standards to control emissions of hazardous air pollutants
1970	Consumer Product Safety Act—CPSC	Requires consumer product manufacturers, distributors, and retailers to notify the CPSC if a product is unsafe or contains a defect that could create a substantial product hazard
1970	Occupational Safety and Health Act—USDOL, OSHA	Requires employers to provide safe and healthful working conditions for all employees
1972	Noise Control Act—EPA	Regulates the identification and control of major noise sources
1972	Clean Water Act—EPA	Regulates pollutant discharge to surface water. Pollution sources are required to meet stringent waste treatment requirements through technology-based standards; industries that discharge wastes to public treatment plants are required to install the best available treatment for toxic pollutant removal and may not discharge wastes that will interfere with or pass through public treatment works and cause them to violate their permits
1972	Federal Insecticide, Fungicide, and Rodenticide Act—EPA	Amended earlier legislation regulating the manufacture, distribution, and use of pesticides
1973	Rehabilitation Act—EEOC	Provides for civil rights of people with respect to discrimination against any employee or candidate for employment on the grounds of physical or mental disability for any position for which the applicant is otherwise qualified
1974	Safe Drinking Water Act—EPA	Regulates water quality through setting of standards to control contaminants that may have an adverse impact on human health (both public drinking water and well water)
1976	Toxic Substances Control Act—EPA	Regulates the production and use of potentially harmful chemicals using a premanufacturing notification (PMN) and standard-setting

CPSC, Consumer Protection and Safety Commission; *EEOC,* Equal Employment Opportunity Commission; *EPA,* U.S. Environmental Protection Agency; *OSHA,* Occupational Safety and Health Administration; *USDOL,* U.S. Department of Labor.

TABLE 15-1	Major Federal Occupational and Environmental Health Legislation—cont'd	
1976	Toxic Substances Control Act—EPA—cont'd	procedure; requires EPA to establish an inventory of chemicals manufactured or processed in the United States (excluding those regulated by FIFRA; Food, Drug, and Cosmetic Act; and the Atomic Energy Act) and to require chemical manufacturers, importers, or processors to perform health hazard testing
1976	Resource Conservation and Recovery Act (RCRA)—EPA	Regulates the storage, transport, and disposal of hazardous waste
1980	Comprehensive Environmental Response, Compensation, and Liability Act (CERCLA) or Superfund—EPA	Remediates environmental releases from pre-RCRA hazardous waste disposal through clean-up procedures and enforcement
1983	Hazard Communication Standard—USDOL, OSHA	Requires chemical manufacturers and importers to evaluate chemicals produced or imported with respect to health hazards and communicate information to employers, employees, and other appropriate parties; employers must develop, implement and maintain a written hazard communication program including labeling, MSDSs, training and recordkeeping
1986	Emergency Planning and Community Right to Know Act—EPA	Establishes a program to deal with emergency situations involving hazardous substances at the local level; requires facilities that store or use hazardous substances to notify local authorities and EPA's National Response Center of their existence
1990	Americans With Disabilities Act—EEOC	Mandates that employers may not discriminate against a qualified individual with a disability with regard to job application, hiring, termination, training, compensation/benefits, medical/job evaluations, advancements, or other conditions of work
1991	Occupational Exposure to Bloodborne Pathogens Standard—USDOL, OSHA	Requires employers to develop and implement procedures to prevent and control exposures to blood or other potentially infectious materials
2000	Needle Safety and Prevention Act	Amends Occupational Exposure to Bloodborne Pathogens Standard to require new engineering controls where appropriate, employee input into decision making, and new recordkeeping requirements for sharps and needlestick injuries

FIFRA, Federal Insecticide, Fungicide, and Rodenticide Act; *MSDS,* material safety data sheet.

1. Improve workplace safety and health by reducing injuries, illnesses, and fatalities.
2. Change workplace culture by increasing employer and employee commitment to improved safety and health.
3. Secure public confidence through excellence in developing and delivering OSHA services (USDOL, OSHA, 2000).

NIOSH is a branch of the Centers for Disease Control and Prevention within the U.S. Department of Health and Human Services and, as described later, is the leading federal occupational safety and health research agency. Among other functions, NIOSH also provides funding for occupational safety and health education for occupational health and safety professionals.

The OSHRC is an independent, quasi-judicial review board composed of three members or commissioners appointed by the president (with the advice and consent of the Senate), each for a 6-year term. The commission is separate from OSHA and hears challenges by employers about OSHA citations and proposed fines. If an employer decides to contest the citation, the prescribed time period for abatement, or the proposed penalty, a written Notice of Contest must be filed within 15 working days with the OSHA area director, who then forwards the case to the OSHRC. The case is first assigned by the commission to an administrative law judge who hears the case, much like in a court of law, and upholds, modifies, or disallows the citation. This decision becomes final within 30 days, unless the commission deems it necessary to review the case report. Commission rulings may be appealed to a U.S. Court of Appeals (USDOL, OSHA, 2000). At any stage of the hearing process OSHA may withdraw the citation, the employer may withdraw its notice of contest, or a settlement agreement may be entered into by the two parties to resolve the dispute. More than 90% of all cases disposed of by OSHRC administrative law judges are terminated prior to case hearings by such actions (Blosser, 1992).

Coverage of the OSH Act, as provided through federal OSHA or an OSHA-approved state plan (discussed later), extends to all employers and employees in the 50 states and all territories and jurisdictions under federal authority. Those jurisdictions include the District of Columbia, Puerto Rico, the Virgin Islands, American Samoa, Johnston Island, and the Outer Continental Shelf Lands as defined in the Outer Continental Shelf Lands Act.

The OSH Act defines an employer as any "person engaged in a business affecting commerce who has employees, but does not include the United States or any State or political subdivision of a State" (OSH Act, 1970, p. 2). OSHA coverage includes employers and employees in such varied fields as manufacturing, construction, longshoring, shipbuilding, ship breaking, ship repair, agriculture, law and medicine, charity and disaster relief, organized labor, private education, and religious groups to the extent they employ workers for secular purposes. Those not covered under the OSH Act include self-employed people; people who work on farms where only immediate members of the family are employed; public employees in state and local governments in their roles as employers; and employees, including mine workers, certain truckers and rail workers, and atomic energy workers, whose working situations are regulated by other federal agencies under other federal statutes. However, where a specific federal agency regulation does not cover a particular area, OSHA standards apply. In some instances, where the division of authority between OSHA and another agency has been unclear, OSHA has entered into agreements or memoranda of understanding to clarify the lines of jurisdiction.

Under the OSH Act the heads of federal agencies are responsible for providing safe and healthful working conditions for their employees and are required to comply with OSHA standards consistent with those issued for the private sector (USDOL, OSHA, 2000). In addition, these agency heads are required to record and analyze injury and illness data, provide personnel training to protect employees from on-the-job hazards, and conduct workplace inspections at least annually to ensure compliance with OSHA standards. Although OSHA has the authority to inspect federal workplaces under certain circumstances, it cannot propose monetary penalties against another federal agency for failure to comply with OSHA standards.

States may seek authority to establish their own occupational safety and health programs by submitting a developmental state plan to OSHA for approval. OSHA's approval will be contingent on the state's ability to demonstrate implementation of all program elements within 3 years, including program administration; standard setting; enforcement and appeals procedures; public employee protection; adequate funding for personnel to carry out the program; training, education, and technical assistance programs; and reporting mechanisms (i.e., illness/injury data). After a state receives final OSHA approval—that is, the state is determined to operate at least as effectively as the federal agency OSHA—up to 50% of the program's operating costs may be funded by OSHA. State standards must be identical to or at least as effective as OSHA standards. When OSHA adopts a new standard, states with approved programs also must issue a corresponding rule (USDOL, OSHA 2000).

State plans covering the private sector also must cover state and local government employees. OSHA rules also permit states to develop plans that cover only public sector (state and local government) employees. In these cases private sector employment remains under federal OSHA jurisdiction. To date, 23 states and 2 territories operate complete plans and 2 cover only the public sector; these can be found on the OSHA website. Federal OSHA continues to cover federal employees and certain other employees specifically excluded by a state plan (e.g., maritime workers and people employed on military bases).

States with approved state plans can respond to accidents and workplace complaints and conduct random unannounced general schedule inspections just like federal OSHA. Citations and proposed penalties are issued under state law, and contests are adjudicated by a state review board or other procedure. States may withdraw from OSHA plan agreements, or OSHA may withdraw approval of a state plan. To date, eight states have withdrawn from OSHA agreements, but OSHA has never withdrawn plan approval.

Some debate has surrounded the effectiveness of state plans. Organized labor has contended that state program enforcement efforts are weak, but state plan administrators believe their enforcement efforts surpass those of OSHA. For example, in fiscal 2000 state plan agencies conducted 54,982 inspections and cited employers for 141,465 alleged violations compared with 46,561 federal OSHA inspections and 80,455 violations during the same period (USDOL, OSHA, 2001a).

OSHA may provide consultation to the employer, upon request, to help identify and correct hazards and provide technical assistance, education, and training. Consultation programs are kept separate from the enforcement program, and information obtained from the consultative activities cannot be given to either state or federal OSHA enforcement personnel unless the employer fails to correct a dangerous deficiency or the employer wishes to request an exception from an OSHA general inspection for a period of 1 year. Employer responsibilities under the Occupational Safety and Health Act are listed in Box 15-1.

NATIONAL INSTITUTE FOR OCCUPATIONAL SAFETY AND HEALTH

Included in the OSH Act is a provision that created the National Institute for Occupational Safety and Health (NIOSH), the principal research agency for occupational safety and health in the nation. As previously stated, NIOSH is a unit within the Centers for Disease Control and Prevention in the U.S. Department of Health and Human Services and is authorized to do the following:

- Develop recommendations for OSHA standards;
- Develop information on safe levels of exposure to toxic materials and harmful physical agents and substances;
- Conduct research on new workplace safety and health problems;
- Conduct on-site investigations to determine the toxicity of materials used in workplaces;
- Fund research/training by other agencies or private organizations through grants, contracts, and other arrangements.

NIOSH conducts research on various workplace safety and health problems, provides technical assistance to OSHA, and develops criteria documents for recommendations on standards for OSHA's adoption. While conducting its research, NIOSH may make workplace investigations, gather testimony from employers and employees, and require that employers measure and report employee exposure to potentially hazardous materials. NIOSH has the authority to enter a workplace to conduct an investigation based on probable cause for believing a problem

---

Box 15-1   Employer Responsibilities Under the OSH Act

- Meet general duty responsibility to provide a workplace free from recognized hazards.
- Keep workers informed about OSHA and the safety and health matters with which workers are involved.
- Comply in a reasonable manner with standards, rules, and regulations issued under the OSH Act.
- Make copies of standards available to employees for review upon request.
- Evaluate workplace conditions.
- Minimize or eliminate potential hazards.
- Make sure employees have and use safe, properly maintained tools and equipment (including appropriate personal protective equipment).
- Warn employees of potential hazards.
- Establish or update operating procedures and communicate them to employees.
- Provide medical examinations when required.
- Provide training required by OSHA standards.
- Report within 8 hours any accident that results in a fatality or the hospitalization of three or more employees.
- Keep OSHA-required records of work-related injuries and illnesses, unless otherwise specified.
- Post a copy of the OSHA Log and Summary of Occupational Injuries and Illnesses for the prior year during each year of the time period specified.
- Post, at a prominent location within the workplace, the OSHA poster informing employees of their rights and responsibilities.
- Provide employees, former employees, and their representatives access to the OSHA Log form at a reasonable time and in a reasonable manner.
- Provide access to employee medical records and exposure records as required by law.
- Cooperate with OHSA compliance officers.
- Not discriminate against employees who properly exercise their rights under the OSH Act.
- Post OSHA citations and abatement verification notices at or near the worksite involved.
- Abate cited violations within the prescribed period.

---

exists but does not have authority to issue citations and penalties. NIOSH conducts health hazard evaluations, which also may be requested by an employee or employee representative or as part of a planned research program (29 U.S.C. 669 (a) (b)). NIOSH also may require employers to provide medical examinations and tests to determine the incidence of occupational illness among employees. However, when tests and examinations are performed as part of a research program, the cost must be borne by NIOSH (USDOL, OSHA, 2000).

NIOSH also develops other types of documents, such as Current Intelligence bulletins, to disseminate new information on workplace hazards and maintains and annually revises the NIOSH Registry of Toxic Effects of Chemical Substances. Under the OSH Act, NIOSH is authorized to conduct directly, or by grants/contracts, education programs to provide an adequate supply of qualified occupational and safety personnel and to provide for consultation and the establishment and supervision of programs for the education and training of employers and employees related to occupational health and safety. NIOSH grants support academic programs through established Education and Research Centers across the country (see Appendix 2-1) and through Training Project Grants specific to a single discipline (e.g., industrial hygiene, occupational health nursing, safety, occupational medicine).

STANDARD SETTING

OSHA is the regulatory agency responsible for promulgating legally enforceable standards that employers must meet to be in compliance with the OSH Act. OSHA standards fall into four major categories: General Industry (29 C.F.R.-1910); Construction (29 C.F.R.-1926); Maritime (29 C.F.R.-1915); and Agriculture (29 C.F.R.-1928). (Box 15-2). OSHA has issued hundreds of occupational safety and health standards

---

Box 15-2   Industry Classifications for Standards

GENERAL INDUSTRY STANDARDS

The broadest category of OSHA regulations, general industry standards generally apply to all industries. Specific standards called vertical standards are applicable for certain industry segments (e.g., pulp, paper, and paperboard mills; textiles; telecommunications) and address unique conditions in these workplaces. Standards that cut across industry boundaries and apply to conditions in many different workplaces (e.g., toxic chemicals, hazardous materials, machine guarding, personal protective equipment) are called horizontal standards. Vertical standards take precedence over horizontal standards.

CONSTRUCTION STANDARDS

Construction standards govern safety and health conditions at building sites. Standards for ladders and scaffolding, excavations and trenches, explosives, and other conditions and equipment found in the building trade are included.

MARITIME STANDARDS

Maritime standards apply to workplaces involved in water-borne commerce conducted within the United States. Rules pertain to work at shipyards, operations at maritime terminals, longshoring activities, and gear certification.

AGRICULTURE STANDARDS

Agriculture standards govern safety and health rules for agricultural operations. Rules include standards for roll-over protective structures for tractors, field sanitation rules for farm laborers, and guarding farm equipment.

The construction, maritime, and agricultural standards are considered vertical standards and take precedence over general industry rules that cover similar hazards.

---

covering a wide range of hazards, such as the following:

- Toxic substances
- Harmful physical agents
- Electrical hazards
- Fall hazards
- Hazardous waste
- Infectious diseases
- Fire and explosion hazards
- Dangerous atmospheres
- Machine hazards

These standards require employers to do the following:

- Maintain conditions or adopt practices reasonably necessary and appropriate to protect workers on the job.
- Be familiar with and comply with standards applicable to their establishments.
- Ensure that employees have and use personal protective equipment when required for safety and health.
- Comply with the OSH Act's "general duty clause" where no specific OSHA standards exist.

For example, if an employee is working with a tool or machine that has the potential to harm or injure the worker, the employer must ensure that the equipment meets recognized safety design criteria, has proper guards and lockout features, is adequately maintained, and that the employee has received appropriate training to use the equipment.

OSHA standards are developed and established through a public standard making process that is laborious and cumbersome, often taking several years. However, this process is necessary to ensure that all interested parties can be heard (McNeely, 1992). The conditions for OSHA's standard setting are specified in statutory provisions and include OSHA-initiated procedures or an OSHA response to a petition for rule making from individuals or groups, NIOSH, other governmental entities, public officials, and any other interested party. OSHA then publishes its intentions in the *Federal Register* as an "Advanced Notice of Proposed Rulemaking" to solicit information to be used in drafting a proposal or as a "Notice of Proposed Rulemaking," which sets forth the new rules' requirements and specifies a time period for the public to respond. Interested parties submit written arguments and pertinent evidence, and OSHA schedules a hearing, if requested. Finally, after considering public comments, evidence, and testimony, OSHA publishes the full text of any standard adopted or amended and the date it becomes effective along with an explanation of the standard and the reasons for implementing it or a determination that no standard or amendment needs to be issued. In addition, OSHA must submit its final rules to Congress for review. Congress can disapprove a rule under an expedited procedure established by the 1996 Small Business Regulatory Enforcement Act (SBREFA). Some critics have stated that OSHA's standard setting agenda is too often set as a result of pressure from specific interest groups and that the agency needs to examine its regulatory goals.

After standards have gone through the rule-making process, final standards are published in the *Federal Register* as required by the OSH Act. Although major standards may take 2 years or more to reach the final rule, under certain conditions OSHA has the authority to set emergency temporary standards that may be put into effect immediately until superseded by a permanent standard. The OSH Act authorizes emergency rulemaking if (1) workers are exposed to grave danger from new hazards or from exposure to substances or agents determined to be toxic or physically harmful; and (2) such an emergency standard is necessary to protect employees from such danger. The emergency temporary standard must be published in the *Federal Register,* where it also serves as a proposed permanent standard, subject to the usual standard adoption procedures. A final permanent standard must be issued no later than 6 months after publication of the emergency standard. Employers may seek a variance order from OSHA—that is, formal permission to deviate from the standard's requirements or time frame. Variances are temporary, permanent, or experimental.

An employer can apply for a *temporary variance* when compliance with a standard or regulation cannot be met by its effective date because professional or technical personnel, material, or equipment is not available or because the necessary construction or alteration of facilities cannot be completed in time. A temporary variance may be granted for the period needed to achieve compliance or for 1 year, whichever is shorter; it is renewable twice, each time for 6 months. A *permanent variance* can be applied for when an employer can prove that working conditions, practices, means, methods, operations, or processes at the worksite are as safe and healthful as compliance with the standard. An employer may apply for an *experimental variance* when participating in an effort to demonstrate or validate new job safety and health techniques and if either the secretary of labor or the secretary of health and human services has approved that effort.

Because OSHA standards are not all inclusive, OSHA may utilize the general duty clause of the OSH Act to address hazards not cited by a particular standard. The general duty clause imposes on employers the general obligation of furnishing workplaces that are "free from recognized hazards that are causing or are likely to cause death or serious physical harm," (OSH Act, 1970, p. 5). Sources of information on standards include the *Federal Register,* available in many public and university libraries, the U.S. Department of Labor, and many OSHA publications available online at http://www.osha.gov.

OSHA WORKPLACE INSPECTIONS

Under the OSH Act, OSHA is authorized to enter and inspect without advance notice every establishment covered by the OSH Act, to enforce its standards. In fact, anyone who alerts an employer in advance of an OSHA inspection can receive a criminal fine of up to $1,000 or a 6-month jail term or both. Similarly, states with their own programs also conduct inspections. If an employer refuses to admit an OSHA compliance officer, a search warrant may be obtained with evidence for cause (Marshall v. Barlows, 1978).

Special circumstances exist under which OSHA may give advance notice to the employer. Even then, such notice will be less than 24 hours. These circumstances include the following:

- Imminent danger situations, which require correction as soon as possible
- Inspections that must take place after regular business hours or that require special preparation
- Cases where OSHA must provide advance notice to ensure that the employer and employee representative or other personnel will be present

• Situations in which the OSHA area director determines that advance notice would produce a more thorough or effective inspection

Because of the limited number of OSHA inspectors, not all 6.5 million workplaces can be inspected annually. The most hazardous workplaces are primary inspection sites according to OSHA's inspection priorities, which include imminent danger to employees, fatalities or catastrophes, employee complaints, referrals, programmed or planned inspections directed toward high hazard workplaces or occupations, and follow-up investigations (Box 15-3). A high hazard industry is one whose injury rate is equal to or higher than the lowest average injury rate for the industry as a whole, as determined by the Bureau of Labor Statistics, or one with a history of OSHA citations for serious health infractions (Blosser, 1992). Industries are selected for inspection on the basis of factors such as death, injury, or illness incidence rates and employee exposure to toxic substances (USDOL, OSHA, 2000).

The OSHA inspection process generally consists of four components: the presentation of inspector credentials, the opening conference, the inspection, and the closing conference (USDOL, OSHA, 2000). When a compliance official arrives at the worksite, official credentials from the U.S. Department of Labor should be presented along with a request to meet with the employer representative. In the opening conference the compliance officer does the following:

• Explains why OSHA selected the establishment for inspection

---

Box 15-3 **OSHA Inspection Priorities**

IMMINENT DANGER

Any condition where there is reasonable certainty that a danger exists can be expected to cause death or serious physical harm immediately or before the danger can be eliminated through normal enforcement procedures. Serious physical harm is any type of harm that could cause permanent or prolonged damage to the body or, while not damaging the body on a prolonged basis, could cause such temporary disability as to require inpatient hospital treatment (e.g., simple fractures, concussions, burns, or wounds involving substantial loss of blood and requiring extensive suturing or other healing aids).

FATALITIES AND CATASTROPHES

Any employee deaths or catastrophes resulting in hospitalization of three or more employees. Such situations must be reported to OSHA by the employer within 8 hours. Investigations are made to determine if OSHA standards were violated and to avoid recurrence of similar incidents.

EMPLOYEE COMPLAINTS

Alleged violation of standards or of unsafe or unhealthful working conditions made by an employee. The Act gives each employee the right to request an OSHA inspection when the employee feels he or she is in imminent danger from a hazard or when the employee feels that there is a violation of an OSHA standard that threatens death or serious physical harm. An employee may file an anonymous complaint to the nearest OSHA office by phone, mail, or fax.

REFERRALS

When another agency has requested an inspection due to threat of high hazard situation.

PROGRAMMED HIGH HAZARD INSPECTIONS

Planned inspections aimed at specific high hazard industries, occupations, or health substances. Industries are selected for inspection on the basis of factors such as the death, injury, and illness incidence rates and employee exposure to toxic substances.

FOLLOW-UP INSPECTIONS

Conducted to determine whether previously cited violations have been corrected. Failure to abate alleged violations may result in additional proposed daily penalties while such failure or violation occurs.

From *All About OSHA* (OSHA Publication No. 2056), by U.S. Department of Labor, Occupational Safety and Health Administration, 2000, Washington, DC: Occupational Safety and Health Administration.

- Determines whether an OSHA-funded consultation program is in progress or whether the facility has received an inspection exemption. If either is the case, the compliance officer usually terminates the inspection
- Obtains information about the establishment
- Explains the purpose of the visit, the scope of the inspection, the walkaround procedures the employee representation, the employee interviews, and the closing conference

The employer or designated representative accompanies the compliance officer on the inspection, and an employee representative selected by the employees (or the union) may also be given the opportunity to attend the opening conference and the inspection.

The two primary components of the inspection are a records check and an inspection walkaround. In examining recordkeeping practices, the compliance officer determines whether the employer has done the following:

- Maintained records of deaths, injuries, and illnesses
- Posted a copy of the totals from the last page of the previous year's Log and Summary of Occupational Injuries and Illnesses (OSHA 300) during the appropriate time frame
- Prominently displayed the OSHA workplace poster

The compliance officer also examines records, where required, of employee exposure to toxic substances and harmful physical agents.

TABLE 15-2   Types of Violations Cited by OSHA and Proposed Penalties

VIOLATION	PROPOSED PENALTY
OTHER THAN SERIOUS VIOLATION A violation that has a direct relationship to job safety and health but probably would not cause death or serious physical harm.	Discretionary penalty of up to $7,000 for each violation, which may be adjusted downward depending on employer's good faith.
SERIOUS VIOLATION A violation where there is substantial probability that death or serious physical harm could result [and] that the employer knew, or should have known, of the hazard.	Mandatory penalty of up to $7,000 for each serious violation, which may be adjusted downward depending on the employer's good history of previous violations, gravity of alleged violation, and business size.
WILLFUL VIOLATION A violation that the employer intentionally and knowingly commits with plain indifference to the law. The employer either knows that what he or she is doing constitutes a violation or is aware that a hazardous condition existed and made no reasonable effort to eliminate it.	Penalties of up to $70,000 may be proposed for each willful violation, with a minimum penalty of $5,000 for each violation. The proposed penalty may be adjusted downward depending on the history of previous violations and business size.
If an employer is convicted of a willful violation of a standard that has resulted in the death of an employee, the U.S. Department of Justice may bring criminal charges, with the offense punishable by a court imposed fine or by imprisonment for up to 6 months or both.	A fine of up to $250,000 for an individual or $500,000 for a corporation may be imposed.

TABLE 15-2	Types of Violations Cited by OSHA and Proposed Penalties—cont'd	
REPEAT VIOLATION		
A violation of any standard, regulation, rule, or order where, upon reinspection, a substantially similar violation is found.	A fine of up to $70,000 for each repeated violation may be imposed.	
FAILURE TO ABATE		
A violation wherein a previous violation has not been abated.	A fine of up to $7,000 for each day the violation continues beyond the prescribed abatement date.	
FALSIFYING RECORDS, REPORTS, OR APPLICATIONS	A criminal fine of $10,000 or up to 6 months in jail or both may be imposed.	
POSTING-REQUIREMENT VIOLATIONS	A civil penalty of up to $7,000 may be imposed.	
ASSAULTING A COMPLIANCE OFFICER OR OTHERWISE RESISTING, OPPOSING, INTIMIDATING, OR INTERFERING WITH A COMPLIANCE OFFICER IN THE PERFORMANCE OF HIS OR HER DUTIES	A criminal fine of not more than $5,000 and imprisonment for not more than 3 years may be imposed.	

From *All About OSHA* (OSHA Publication No. 2056), by U.S. Department of Labor, Occupational Safety and Health Administration, 2000, Washington, DC: Occupational Safety and Health Administration.

During an inspection walkaround the compliance officer and the accompanying representatives proceed through the establishment and inspect work areas for potentially hazardous working conditions. Employees may be asked about safety and health practices and education and training opportunities and practices. Any unsafe or unhealthful conditions observed during the walk-through will be pointed out to the employer and possible corrective actions discussed. Depending on the nature of the visit, the occupational and environmental health nurse may or may not be involved. However, any record reviews will likely involve the nurse, and she or he should be prepared for this inspection and any questions the compliance officer may ask regarding the occupational health and safety program and related hazards.

After the inspection walkaround, a closing conference is held and attended by the compliance officer, employer, and employee representative (optional), either jointly or separately. At this time any unsafe/unhealthful conditions observed, any apparent violations for which a citation may be issued, and any methods to abate the violations are discussed. In addition, employer and employee rights are discussed. Proposed penalties are not discussed by the compliance officer, because this is under the jurisdiction of the OSHA area director.

After the inspection and the report are completed, OSHA may issue citations for violations discovered during the inspection process and determine what penalties, if any, will be proposed. Citations must inform the employer and the employees of the regulations and standards alleged to have been violated and the time frame set for abatement. The citation must be posted at or near the location where the violation occurred for 3 days or until the violation is abated, whichever is longer. Categories of violations that may be cited and accompanying proposed penalties are shown in Table 15-2.

An employer has 15 working days to contest a citation; this must be done in writing to the OSHA area director. The citation is then forwarded on to the Occupational Safety and Health Review Commission.

McNeely (1992) points out that OSHA's enforcement capabilities are limited in scope and force due to the insufficient number of personnel available to conduct inspections and because the appeal process allows for citations to be overturned and penalties to be reduced. Only 2% of the nation's workplaces can be inspected in any given year by OSHA (Council on Occupational and Environmental Health, 1988), whose maximum penalties were not increased until 1990. However, OSHA continues to adjust penalties on the basis of the company size, employer's good faith, and history of compliance (Blosser, 1992).

OSHA STANDARDS

Although several standards have been promulgated by OSHA, it is beyond the scope of this chapter to discuss each one. However, two important standards that have broad implications for occupational and environmental health nursing practice will be described as examples; these are the Hazard Communication Standard and the Occupational Exposure to Bloodborne Pathogens Standard along with its recent revision (2001) in accordance with the Needlestick Safety and Prevention Act, which was signed into law on November 6, 2000. In addition, company sample policy/procedure documents (Bloodborne Pathogens Compliance Program and Lockout/ Tagout Procedure) are given in Appendixes 15-2 and 15-3.

Hazard Communication Standard

Hazard communication is designed to prevent work-related illness and injury through communicating information to workers about the hazards and the risks. The importance of designing and detailing a hazard communication program and involving health care professionals in the program planning, implementation, and evaluation cannot be understated. McNeely (1990) states that if the nurse who sees the employee for health care and health education is not collecting and disseminating the information described in the Occupational Safety and Health Administration's Hazard Communication Rule, then employee health problems that arise from work exposures may go undetected at clinic visits. Furthermore, both the employee and the nurse may lack adequate understanding about the use of personal protective equipment or careful work practices to prevent work-related illness and injury.

According to OSHA, about 32 million workers are potentially exposed to one or more chemical hazards that may cause or contribute to many serious health effects, such as cardiovascular, hepatorenal, respiratory, reproductive, and dermatological problems (USDOL, 1998). An estimated 650,000 chemical products already exist, and hundreds of new ones are being introduced annually. This poses a serious problem for exposed workers and their employers. Because of the seriousness of these health and safety problems, OSHA issued its Hazard Communication Standard (29 C.F.R. 1910, Subpart Z, Toxic and Hazardous Substances) on November 23, 1983, which initially applied to "affected employers and employees within the manufacturing sector." The Hazard Communication Standard was amended in 1985 and again in 1986 and was revised in August 1987 to state that the Hazard Communication Standard (HCS) establishes uniform requirements to make sure that the hazards of all chemicals imported into, produced, or used in U.S. workplaces are evaluated and that this hazard information is transmitted to affected employers and exposed employees (USDOL, 1987). This standard applies to general industry, shipyard, marine terminal, longshoring, and construction employment and covers chemical manufacturers, importers, employers, and employees exposed to chemical hazards.

This information is transmitted by means of a comprehensive written hazard communication program, which includes container labeling and other forms of warning, material safety data sheets (MSDSs), and employee training. The rule also incorporates a "downstream flow of information," which means that producers of chemicals have the primary responsibility for generating and disseminating information and transmitting it to their employees (USDOL, OSHA, 1998). In general the flow of information should work like this:

Chemical manufacturers/importers	Determine the hazards of each product.
Chemical manufacturers/importers/distributors	Communicate hazard information and associated protective measures downstream to customers through labels and MSDSs.
Employers	Identify and list hazardous chemicals in their workplaces.
	Obtain MSDSs and labels for each hazardous chemical if not provided by manufacturer, importer, or distributor.
	Develop and implement a written hazard communication program, including chemical identification, MSDSs, and employee training, about the list of chemicals, and label information.
	Communicate hazard information to their employees through labels, MSDSs, and formal training programs.

The HCS does not apply to hazardous waste regulated by the Resource Conservation and Recovery Act and the Environmental Protection Agency; tobacco and wood products; consumer products packaged for consumer use (food, drugs, cosmetics, alcohol); any drug in solid, final form for direct administration to a patient (i.e., tablets, pills); or manufactured articles with a specific shape that does not release or result in a hazardous chemical exposure.

Meyer and Watson (1992) point out that the formal HCS has placed the emphasis on providing the worker with detailed information about each hazardous substance in the workplace. The authors state that this emphasis has fostered an environment where information is gathered on hazardous material more for the sake of HCS compliance rather than an integration of the information as a component of the total health and safety program. The occupational health and safety professional needs to consider all aspects of information collected and develop a hazardous communication and management program that will be purposeful as well as compliant.

Responsibilities of manufacturers and importers

The quality of the hazard communication program depends on the adequacy and accuracy of the assessment of hazards in the workplace. The HCS requires chemical manufacturers and importers to use available scientific evidence concerning chemical hazards to evaluate chemicals they produce or import and to report such information to their employees and to employers who distribute or use their products. The determination of occupational health hazards is complicated by the fact that many of the effects or signs and symptoms occur commonly in nonoccupationally exposed populations, so that effects of exposure are difficult to separate from normally occurring illnesses. Occasionally a substance causes an effect that is rarely seen in the population at large, such as angiosarcomas caused by vinyl chloride exposure, thus making it easier to ascertain that the occupational exposure was the primary causative factor. More often, however, the effects are more common, such as dermatitis. Also, most chemicals have not been adequately tested to determine their health hazard potential, and data do not exist to substantiate effects.

Regardless of the complexities involved in making a hazard determination, the chemical manufacturers and importers and any employers who choose to evaluate hazards—employers are not obligated to evaluate—are responsible for the quality of the hazard evaluation undertaken. Each hazardous chemical must be evaluated for its potential to cause adverse health effects and physical hazards, such as fires or explosions. (The scope of health hazards covered and criteria related to completeness of the evaluation can be found in the appendix to the Hazard Communication Standard.) Chemicals that are listed in one of the following sources (USDOL, OSHA, 1998) are to be considered hazardous in all cases:

- 29 C.F.R. 1910, Subpart Z, Toxic and Hazardous Substances, Occupational Safety and Health Administration (OSHA)
- *Threshold Limit Values for Chemical Substances and Physical Agents in the Work Environment*, American Conference of Governmental Industrial Hygienists (ACGIH)

In addition, chemicals that have been evaluated and found to be a suspected or confirmed carcinogen in the following sources must be reported as such:

- *Annual Report on Carcinogens,* National Toxicology Program (NTP) (see Chapter 7);
- *Monographs,* International Agency for Research on Cancer (IARC)
- OSHA regulations concerning carcinogens (USDOL, OSHA, 1998)

Written hazard communication program

A written hazard communication program ensures that all employers receive the information they need to inform and train their employees properly and to design and implement employee protection programs. A written program also provides necessary hazard information to employees so they can participate in and support the protective measures in place at their workplace. Covered employers must develop, implement, and maintain at the workplace a written hazard communication program that contains provisions for the following:

- Container labeling and other forms of warning
- Collection, availability, maintenance, and updating of material safety data sheets (MSDSs)
- A list of hazardous chemicals in the work areas cross-referenced with the material safety data sheets;
- Employee information and training
- Methods used to inform employees of the hazards of nonroutine tasks (e.g., cleaning vessels) and hazards associated with chemicals in unlabeled pipes
- Methods to ensure that other employers with employees working on-site (e.g., construction employees working on-site) who may be exposed are provided with information regarding hazards, precautionary and protective measures for these employees, and the labeling system used in the workplace

The written program must be available to employees, their designated representatives, the assistant secretary of labor for occupational safety and health, and the director of the National Institute for Occupational Safety and Health (NIOSH). A sample written hazard communication program is shown in Appendix 15-4.

Labels

The chemical manufacturer, importer, or distributor must ensure that each container of hazardous chemicals leaving the workplace is labeled, tagged, or marked with the chemical identity, appropriate hazard warning, and name and address of the manufacturer, importer, or responsible party. In the workplace the employer must ensure that each container (e.g., bag, barrel, bottle, box, can, cylinder, drum, reactor vessel, storage tank) is labeled, tagged, or marked with the identity of the hazard by chemical or common name and includes health and physical hazards. Hazard warnings may be in the form of words, pictures, or symbols that convey the hazard of the chemical(s) in the container. Labels and/or warnings must be legible, in English (plus other languages, if desired), and prominently displayed. Several exemptions for in-plant labeling requirements include the following:

- Employers can post signs or placards that convey the hazard information if a number of stationary containers that have similar contents and hazards are in the same work area.
- Employers can substitute various types of standard operating procedures, process sheets, batch tickets, blend tickets, and similar written materials for container labels on stationary process equipment if they contain the same information and the written materials are readily accessible to employees in the work area.
- Employers are not required to label portable containers into which hazardous chemicals are transferred from labeled containers and that are intended only for the immediate use of the employee who makes the transfer.
- Employers are not required to label pipes or piping systems.

Material safety data sheets

Chemical manufacturers and importers must develop a material safety data sheet (MSDS), the detailed information bulletin, for each hazardous chemical they produce or import and must provide all MSDSs to distributors or employers with the initial shipment and after an MSDS is updated (examples of MSDSs are shown in the Appendixes 7-1 and 7-2). Each MSDS must be in English and include the following information regarding the hazardous chemical(s):

- Specific identity and common name(s) (including designation as singular substance or mixture)
- Physical and chemical characteristics (e.g., vapor pressure, flash point)
- Physical hazards, including the potential for fire, explosion, and reactivity
- Health hazards, including signs and symptoms of exposure, acute and chronic health effects, and related health information
- Primary routes of entry
- Exposure limits (PELs, TLVs)
- Chemical's status as a carcinogen according to NTP, IARC, or OSHA
- Precautionary measures for safe handling and use, including hygiene practices and procedures for equipment maintenance, clean-up, and leaks
- Control measures, work practices, and use of personal protective equipment
- Emergency and first-aid procedures
- Date and preparation of the MSDS
- Identification of the organization responsible for preparing the MSDS (name, address, telephone number)

Copies of required MSDSs for each hazardous chemical in the workplace must be maintained and made readily accessible during each workshift to all employees in that work area. ANSI standard Z400.1—Material Safety Data Sheet Preparation—may be used, or the nonmandatory MSDS form (OSHA 174), a copy of which can be obtained from OSHA field offices, also may be used as a guide. If hazardous chemicals are used for which an MSDS has not been received, the employer must contact the supplier, manufacturer, or importer to obtain the missing MSDS. A record of the contact must be maintained.

While the type of information to be provided was clearly established, the standard left a great deal of leeway regarding the format of MSDSs. In addition, to protect themselves from liability, chemical manufacturers have begun to use generic safety precautions within their MSDSs, resulting in statements such as "use of respiratory protection required" for a wide range of materials regardless of whether the protection is warranted (Meyer & Watson, 1992).

Employee information and training

One of the most important sections of the Hazard Communication Standard is the require-ment that employers provide workers with training on hazardous chemicals in their work area. This training must be given before workers are assigned to do a job involving potential exposure to hazardous chemicals and whenever a new hazard has been introduced. At a minimum, discussion topics must include the following:

- The HCS and its requirements
- The components of the hazard communication program in the employees' workplaces
- The operations in the work areas where hazardous chemicals are present
- The location and availability of the written hazard communication program, including the list of hazardous chemicals and MSDSs (USDOL, OSHA, 1998)

Under the HCS employee training must include the following elements:

- How the hazard communication program is implemented in that workplace, how to read and interpret information on the labels and the MSDS, and how employees can obtain and use the available hazard information
- The hazards that are posed by the chemicals in the work area and may be discussed by individual chemical or by hazard categories such as flammability
- Measures employees can take to protect themselves from the hazards
- Specific procedures, such as engineering controls, work practices, and use of personal protective equipment (PPE), put into effect by the employer to provide protection
- Methods and observations, such as visual appearance or smell, workers can use to detect the presence of a hazardous chemical to which they may be exposed

The occupational and environmental health nurse can play a key role in this aspect of the risk communication program; however, in an interview study of 24 nurses employed by chemical industries, McNeely (1990) reported limited involvement of occupational and environmental health nurses in all aspects of the hazard communication program. Even though the sample size was small ($n = 24$), many of the nurses lacked knowledge about the hazardous substances at the worksites, health effects related to exposure, and control strategies. Only three nurses were involved in the formal training of employees. In addition, more than half the nurses believed that hazard communication was a safety rather than a health issue. Nurses who perceived hazard communication as part of their job were more knowledgeable about chemical exposures. Occupational and environmental health nurses need to be more involved in the hazard communication program, because they have perhaps the greatest opportunity to teach employees about the hazards both in group and individual encounters.

Trade secrets

A provision is made in the HCS to protect trade secrets. A trade secret is something that gives an employer an opportunity to obtain an advantage over competitors who do not know about the trade secret or who do not use it. For example, a trade secret may be a confidential device, pattern, set of information, or chemical make-up. Chemical industry trade secrets are generally formulas or process data or a "specific chemical identity," which is the type of trade secret information referred to in the Hazard Communication Standard. A specific chemical identity includes the chemical name, the Chemical Abstracts Services (CAS) Registry Number, or any other specific information that reveals the precise designation, but it does not include common names. Information regarding specific chemical identity may be withheld as a trade secret, provided that the MSDS contains information concerning the properties and effects of the hazardous chemical. The standard strikes a balance between the need to protect exposed employees and the employer's need to maintain the confidentiality of a bona fide trade secret. This is achieved by providing for limited disclosure to health professionals who are furnishing medical or other occupational health services to employers and exposed employees and their designated representatives under specified conditions of need and confidentiality. When a treating physician or nurse determines that a medical emergency exists, the chemical manufacturer, importer, or employer must immediately disclose the specific chemical identity of the hazardous chemical. A written statement of need and confidentiality agreement may be required after abatement of the emergency.

In nonemergency situations the specific chemical identity must be disclosed to health professionals (physicians, occupational and environmental health nurses, industrial hygienists, toxicologists, or epidemiologists) who provide medical or other occupational health services to exposed employees and to employees or their designated representatives provided that the request for information is in writing. The request must provide a reasonably detailed description of the need for the information that will be used for one or more of the following purposes:

- To assess the hazards of the chemicals to which employees will be exposed
- To conduct or assess sampling of the workplace atmosphere to determine employee exposure levels
- To conduct preassignment or periodic medical surveillance of exposed employees
- To provide medical treatment to exposed employees
- To select or assess appropriate personal protective equipment for exposed employees
- To design or assess engineering controls or other protective measures for exposed employees
- To conduct studies to determine the health effects of exposure

In addition, the health professional, employee, or employee representative must explain why alternative information is insufficient and detail procedures to be used to protect confidentiality of the information. A written confidentiality agreement not to use the information for any other purpose than the health need stated and not to release information under any circumstances, except to OSHA, must be given.

The occupational and environmental health nurse can play a major role in the implementation and monitoring of the Hazard Communication Standard (Soloman, 1986). The occupational and environmental health nurse can coordinate activities with other team members to accomplish the following:

- Assess hazardous workplace exposures;
- Keep employees informed of the nature and effects of hazardous exposures;
- Recognize the signs and symptoms related to potential/actual exposures;
- Develop strategies to contain exposures;
- Communicate hazardous substance recognition and measures to control exposures to all workers;
- Ensure that emergency and disaster preparedness procedures are in place;

- Make available appropriate and effective personal protective equipment, as necessary;
- Involve workers in the hazard communication program.

A hazard communication program checklist is shown in Appendix 15-5. Observation of workers and collection and review of data, including MSDSs with respect to hazardous exposures, will aid in identifying, controlling, and eliminating hazardous substances.

Bloodborne Pathogens Standard

Exposure to bloodborne pathogens, such as the human immunodeficiency virus (HIV) and hepatitis B virus (HBV), has become a cause for serious concern among workers who may be potentially occupationally exposed through contact with blood and other body fluids containing these and other infectious pathogens. Even though the risk for occupational exposure is small, the potential for exposure remains due to the nature of the work. According to Occupational Safety and Health Administration's (OSHA) estimates, more than 5.6 million workers in health care and public safety occupations could be potentially exposed to these viruses (USDOL, OSHA, 1996). These workers include, but are not limited to, physicians, dentists, dental employees, phlebotomists, nurses, morticians, paramedics, medical examiners, laboratory and blood bank technologists and technicians, housekeeping personnel, laundry workers, employees in long-term care facilities, and home care workers. Other workers who may be occupationally exposed to blood or other potentially infectious materials, depending on their work assignments, include research laboratory workers and public safety personnel, such as fire, police, rescue, and correctional officers (USDOL, OSHA, 1996).

Two diseases are of primary concern. Acquired immunodeficiency syndrome (AIDS), caused by HIV, was first recognized in the United States in 1981, and the incidence has since risen dramatically (CDC, 2001). Hepatitis B occurs in the United States at an estimated rate of 300,000 new cases annually; of these, approximately 8,000 to 12,000 occur in health care workers and result in 200 to 300 deaths per year (USDOL, OSHA, 2001b). OSHA recognized the need for a regulation that prescribes safeguards to protect these workers against health hazards from exposure to blood and certain body fluids, including bloodborne pathogens. Thus, on December 6, 1991, the Occupational Safety and Health Administration (OSHA) published the final rule, Occupational Exposure to Bloodborne Pathogens Standard (29 C.F.R. 1910-1030), with the aim to reduce the risk of occupational exposure to bloodborne diseases. The occupational and environmental health nurse needs to be fully familiar with this standard to ensure employee health and safety and assist management in compliance with the regulations (Goldstein & Johnson, 1991; USDOL, OSHA, 1996).

Scope of application

OSHA's Bloodborne Pathogens Standard (BBPS), which became effective March 6, 1992, applies to all private sector employers and federal civilian employers (USDOL, OSHA, 1996) and includes all persons occupationally exposed to blood or other potentially infectious material (Box 15-4). As defined in the BBPS, an occupational exposure is a reasonably anticipated skin, eye, mucous membrane, or parenteral contact with blood or other potentially infectious materials that may result from the performance of an employee's duties. An exposure incident is a specific eye, mouth, other mucous membrane, nonintact skin, or parenteral contact with blood or other potentially infectious materials that results from the performance of an employee's duties.

Exposure control plan

Under the BBPS employers with occupationally exposed employees are required to develop a written exposure control plan (Box 15-5), which must be made accessible to employees and reviewed and updated annually and whenever new tasks or procedures affect occupational exposure. At a minimum the exposure control plan must include (1) the exposure determination, (2) the procedures for evaluating the circumstances surrounding an exposure incident, and (3) the schedule and method for implementing sections of the standard covering the methods of compliance, HIV and HBV research laboratories and production facilities, hepatitis B vaccination and post-exposure followup, communication of hazards to employees, and recordkeeping. The schedule of how and when the provisions of the standard will be implemented may be as simple as

---

Box 15-4 Exposure Indicators: OSHA Bloodborne Pathogen Standard

A. Bloodborne pathogen (a pathogenic micro-organism that is present in human blood and causes disease in humans)
B. Other potentially infectious material
  1. Human body fluids
     a. Semen
     b. Vaginal secretions
     c. Cerebrospinal fluid
     d. Synovial fluid
     e. Saliva (dental procedures)
     f. Pleural fluid
     g. Pericardial fluid
     h. Peritoneal fluid
     i. Amniotic fluid
     j. Body fluids with visible blood
  2. Any unfixed tissue or organ from a human (living or dead)
  3. HIV-containing cell or tissue cultures, organ cultures, and HIV/HBV-containing culture medium or other solutions; blood, organs, or other tissues from experimental animals infected with HIV/HBV

Box 15-5 Written Exposure Control Plan for Bloodborne Pathogens

EXPOSURE DETERMINATION

- List of job classifications with occupational exposure
- List of all tasks and procedures or groups of closely related tasks and procedures in which occupational exposure occurs and that are performed by employees in specified job classifications
- Exposure determined without regard to use of personal protective equipment

SCHEDULE OF PROCEDURE FOR IMPLEMENTING THE STANDARD COVERING

- Methods of compliance
- HIV/HBV research laboratories and production facilities (as appropriate)
- Hepatitis B vaccination and postexposure follow-up
- Communication of hazard to employees
- Recordkeeping

PROCEDURE FOR EVALUATION OF EXPOSURE INCIDENT

- Documentation of the routes of exposure and how exposure occurred
- Identification and documentation of the source individual, unless the employer can establish that identification is infeasible or prohibited by state or local law
- Examination of the source individual's blood with consent as soon as possible to determine HIV and HBV infectivity and documentation of the source's blood test results. If the source individual is known to be infected with either HIV or HBV, testing need not be repeated to determine the known infectivity.
- Provision of the source individual's test results to the exposed employee, and information about applicable disclosure laws and regulations concerning the source identity and infectious status
- Collection of exposed employee's blood, with consent, as soon as feasible after the exposure incident, and testing of the blood for HBV and HIV serological status. If the employee does not give consent for HIV serological testing during the collection of blood for baseline testing, preserve the baseline blood sample for at least 90 days.
- Provision of HIV and HBV serological testing, counseling, and safe and effective postexposure prophylaxis following the current recommendations of the U.S. Public Health Service
- Provision of information about the exposure incident, regulation, and exposed employee's duties, and of medical records to the evaluating health care provider
- Provision to the employee of a copy of the health care professional's written opinion

a calendar with brief notations describing the methods of implementations and an annotated copy of the standard.

Exposure determination

The exposure determination must be based on the definition of occupational exposure *without regard to personal protective clothing and equipment.* The exposure determination is made by reviewing job classifications within the work environment and listing exposures into two groups. The first group includes job classifications, such as operating room scrub nurses, in which all employees have occupational exposure. Where all employees have occupational exposure, it is not necessary to list specific work tasks. The second group includes those classifications in which some employees have occupational exposure. Where only some employees have occupational exposure, specific tasks and procedures causing occupational exposure must be listed. An example would be in a hospital's laundry facility where some workers would be assigned the task of handling contaminated laundry while others would not.

Exposure prevention and control

The BBPS identifies several approaches to preventing and controlling exposure to blood or other potentially infectious materials; these approaches include risk communication, prevention measures, and control strategies that must be observed. The employer is responsible for providing information and training as described in the standard to each occupationally exposed employee when tasks are initially assigned, when new tasks involve occupational exposures, and annually thereafter (taking into consideration the vocabulary, educational level, and literacy of the employee). Training records must be maintained for a minimum of 3 years.

Risk communication

Communicating risk means that each occupationally exposed employee must be given information and training about the following:

- How to obtain a copy of the Bloodborne Pathogens Standard regulatory text and an explanation of its contents
- The epidemiology, transmission, and symptoms of bloodborne diseases

- The exposure control plan and how to obtain a copy
- How to recognize tasks that might result in occupational exposure
- The use and limitations of engineering and work practice controls and personal protective equipment
- Hepatitis B vaccination issues such as safety, benefits, efficacy, methods of administration, and availability
- Who to contact and what to do in an emergency
- How to report an exposure incident and the postexposure evaluation and follow-up
- The use and meaning of warning labels, signs (where applicable), and color-coding
- A question and answer session on any aspect of the training

Vaccine

HIV and HBV are spread through contact with blood and body fluids and may be transmitted through sexual contact, needle sharing, contact with contaminated blood or blood products, and perinatally (USDOL, OSHA, 2001b). Casual contact is not a mode of transmission. While no vaccine is currently available to prevent HIV infection, an HBV vaccine is available and effective in the protection against HBV infection.

The employer must make the hepatitis B vaccine and vaccination series available to all employees who have occupational exposure and provide a postexposure evaluation and follow-up (described later) to all employees who experience an exposure incident. Vaccines, vaccinations, and follow-up evaluations must be provided at no cost to the employee and at a reasonable time and place and performed by or under the supervision of a licensed physician or another licensed health care professional whose scope of practice allows her or him to independently perform activities required by paragraph (f) of the BBPS. Vaccinations, including boosters, must be administered according to current recommendations of the U.S. Public Health Service. Employees who decline the vaccination must sign a declination form (Appendix 15-6); however, the employee may request and obtain the vaccination at a later date and at no cost if she or he continues to be exposed.

According to the BBPS (USDOL, OSHA, 1991), the hepatitis B vaccination series must be offered within 10 working days of initial assignment to all employees with occupational exposure unless documentation is evident that the vaccination is not required or is contraindicated. Documentation should show that (1) the employee has previously received the complete hepatitis B vaccination series, (2) antibody testing reveals that the employee is immune, or (3) medical reasons prevent taking the vaccinations. Prescreening is not required before receiving the hepatitis B vaccination series. The employer must obtain and provide the employee with a copy of the health care profes-

sional's written opinion stating whether a hepatitis B vaccination is indicated for the employee and whether the employee has received such vaccination. An algorithm for hepatitis B vaccination requirements is shown in Figure 15-1 (Barlow & Handelman, 1993; USDOL, OSHA, 1992).

Universal precautions must be observed. This method of infection control requires the employer and employee to assume that *all* human blood and specified human body fluids are infectious for HIV, HBV, and other bloodborne pathogens.

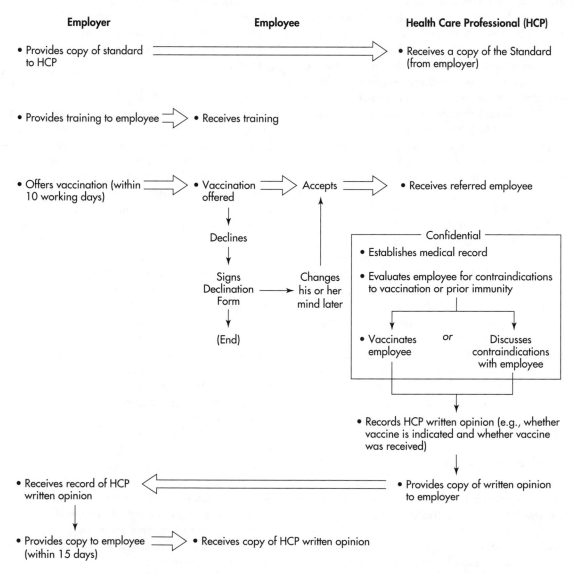

Figure 15-1   Algorithm: Hepatitis B vaccination. *(From "Final Rule: Occupational Exposure to Bloodborne Pathogens—29 C.F.R. part 1910.1030," by U.S. Department of Labor, Occupational Safety and Health Administration, 1991,* Federal Register, *56(235), M004-64182.)*

Where differentiation of types of body fluids is difficult or impossible, *all* body fluids *are* to be considered as *potentially infectious*.

Methods of control

Several types of control strategies are used to eliminate or minimize occupational exposure to bloodborne pathogens; engineering controls and work practice controls are the primary methods used.

Engineering controls are designed to reduce employee exposure in the workplace by either removing or isolating the hazard or isolating the worker from exposure. Self-sheathing needles, puncture-resistant disposal containers for contaminated sharp instruments, resuscitation bags, and ventilation devices are examples of engineering controls. Engineering controls must be examined and maintained or replaced on a scheduled basis.

Appropriate *work practice controls* are designed to alter the manner in which a task is performed and thereby minimize employee exposure. In work areas where reasonable potential for occupational blood and body fluid exposure exists, work practice controls include washing hands immediately after gloves are removed and as soon as possible after skin contact with contaminant; restricting eating, drinking, smoking, application of cosmetics or lip balm, and handling of contact lenses; prohibiting mouth pipetting; preventing the storage of food and/or drink in refrigerators or other locations where blood or other potentially infectious materials are kept; (providing and) requiring the use of handwashing facilities and/or equipment; and routinely checking equipment and decontaminating it prior to servicing and shipping.

Recapping, removing, or bending needles is prohibited unless the employer can demonstrate that no alternative is feasible or that such action is required by a specific medical procedure. When recapping, bending, or removing contaminated needles is required by a medical procedure, this must be done by mechanical means, such as the use of forceps, or a one handed technique. Shearing or breaking contaminated needles is also not permitted. Discarding contaminated sharps/needles into puncture-resistant containers is required, as is affixing appropriate biohazard labels to such sources of hazardous exposure as containers and specimens.

Personal protective equipment is designed to help prevent occupational exposure to infectious materials and must be used if occupational exposure remains after instituting engineering and work practice controls or if those controls are not feasible (USDOL, OSHA, 1996). Protective equipment must not allow blood or other potentially infectious materials to pass through to or reach workers' clothing, skin, or mucous membranes. Such equipment includes, but is not limited to, gloves, gowns, laboratory coats, face shields or masks, and eye protection.

The employer is responsible for providing, maintaining, laundering, disposing, replacing, and assuring the proper use of personal protective equipment and for ensuring that workers have access to it at no cost. Protective equipment should be of the proper size and of the types that take allergic conditions into consideration (USDOL, OSHA, 1996). Precautions for safe handling and use of personal protective equipment, such as appropriate wearing and replacement of damaged or contaminated gloves, gowns, and other equipment and removal and discarding of protective equipment before leaving the work area, are required. Declining to wear or use personal protective equipment is temporarily permitted only under exceptional circumstances (e.g., life threatening situations).

Housekeeping procedures are aimed at keeping the place of employment clean and sanitary and thus reduce the opportunity for exposure to potentially infectious materials. To do this, the employer must develop and implement a cleaning schedule that includes appropriate methods for cleaning and decontaminating all contaminated equipment, surfaces, and waste receptacles; handling and discarding broken glass, contaminated sharps, and regulated waste; and handling and labeling contaminated laundry. Examples include the following:

- Remove and replace protective coverings, such as plastic wrap and aluminum foil when contaminated;
- Use mechanical means, such as tongs, forceps, or a brush and a dust pan, to pick up contaminated broken glassware—never pick up with hands even if gloves are worn;
- Ensure that sharps containers are easily accessible to personnel and located as close as is feasible to the immediate area where sharps are used or can

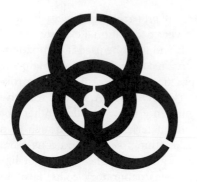

Figure 15-2 Biohazard symbol.

be reasonably anticipated to be found. Sharps containers also must be kept upright throughout use, replaced routinely, closed when moved, and not allowed to overfill;

• Handle contaminated laundry as little as possible and with a minimum of agitation and use appropriate personal protective equipment.

Labels

In order that workers recognize contaminated or potentially infectious material, strict labeling procedures are required. The standard requires that warning labels be attached to containers of regulated waste, to refrigerators and freezers containing blood and other potentially infectious materials, and to other containers used to store, transport, or ship blood or other potentially infectious materials. These labels are *not* required when (1) red bags or red containers are used, (2) containers of blood, blood components, or blood products are labeled as to their contents and have been released for transfusion or other clinical use, and (3) individual containers of blood or other potentially infectious materials are placed in a labeled container during storage, transport, shipment, or disposal (USDOL, OSHA, 1996). The warning label must be fluorescent orange or orange-red, contain the biohazard symbol (Figure 15-2) and the word *BIOHAZARD* in a contrasting color, and be attached to each object by string, wire, adhesive, or another method to prevent loss or unintentional removal of the label.

Postexposure evaluation and follow-up

For all employees who have experienced an exposure incident, a confidential, immediate post-exposure evaluation and follow-up (Figure 15-3) by a health care professional must be provided. This health evaluation should include at a minimum documentation of the exposure route and circumstances; testing (with legal consent) or documentation or both of the source individual's blood as to HIV/HBV status and provision of test results (along with information regarding maintenance of confidentiality and disclosure laws) to the exposed employee; baseline HIV/HBV serologic sampling from the employee with consent (if the employee elects to delay testing, the blood sample must be preserved for 90 days for future testing if desired); counseling; and postexposure prophylaxis as currently recommended by the U.S. Public Health Service.

The employer must provide the health care professional conducting the evaluation a copy of the BBPS, a description of the employee's job duties, all information relevant to the exposure incident and source individual, if known, and the employee's HBV vaccination status and medical history. Within 15 days after evaluation of the exposed employee, the employer must provide the employee with a copy of the health care professional's written opinion. The written opinion is limited to whether the vaccine is indicated and if it has been received. The written opinion for postexposure evaluation must document that the employee has been informed of the results of the medical evaluation and of any medical conditions that resulted from the exposure incident and may require further evaluation or treatment. All other diagnoses must remain confidential and not be included in the written report.

The occupational and environmental health nurse should be involved in counseling exposed employees about the risk of infection, the need for screening, and the methods to prevent transmission of viruses. Because the employee's anxiety level may be heightened, the nurse needs to be aware of the needs of the worker and provide anticipatory guidance. In addition, the nurse can coordinate the education and training program and help develop methods and materials appropriate to the needs and educational levels of the workers.

Recordkeeping

Employers also must preserve and maintain for each employee an accurate record of occupational exposure. This must include the following:

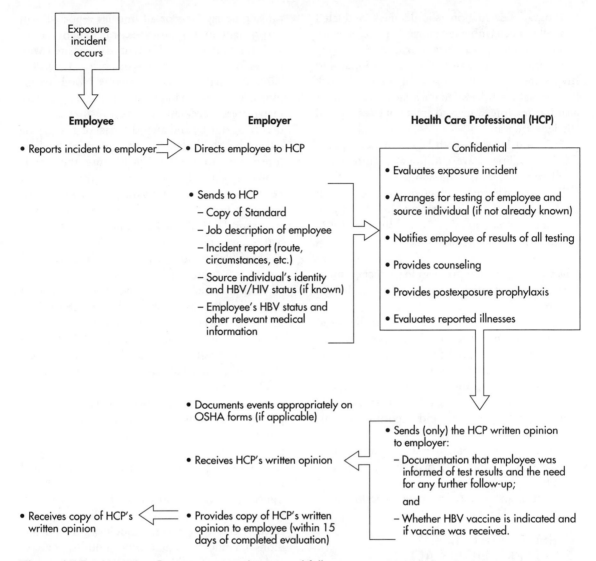

Figure 15-3   Algorithm: Postexposure evaluation and follow-up.   *(Modified from "Final Rule: Occupational Exposure to Bloodborne Pathogens—29 C.F.R. Part 1910.1030," by U.S. Department of Labor, Occupational Safety and Health Administration, 1991,* Federal Register, *56(235), M004-64182.*

- The employee's name and social security number
- The employee's hepatitis B vaccination status, including vaccination dates and any medical records related to the employee's ability to receive vaccinations
- The results of examinations, medical testing, and postexposure evaluation and follow-up procedures
- The health care professional's written opinion
- A copy of the information provided to the health care professional

Medical/health records must be kept confidential and maintained for at least the duration of employment plus 30 years. Maintenance of confidentiality of employee health information is of paramount importance because employees may fear the loss of employment or alienation from coworkers if information is misreported or divulged. The occupational and environmental health nurse will need to devise a policy and procedure for handling health and medical information and records. Accurate training records are kept for 3 years.

Program evaluation should be conducted annually to determine if changes in policies, work practices, education and training, and monitoring procedures are in order. The occupational and environmental health nurse will need to work closely with workers, management, and other health care professionals to create an effective and efficient program.

HIV and HBV research laboratories and production facilities have additional requirements. These can be found in the standard.

The occupational and environmental health nurse can assist management in complying with the standard (Goldstein & Johnson, 1991) through the following methods:

- Developing an effective plan to protect employees from potential exposures to bloodborne pathogens
- Establishing effective control strategies and compliance measures to reduce exposures
- Developing and implementing a vaccination and postexposure follow-up program
- Communicating, through employee training and education programs, information about the nature of the problem and exposure, prevention, and control measures
- Recording information, maintaining and storing records as required, and maintaining confidentiality
- Evaluating and monitoring program performance

NEEDLESTICK SAFETY AND PREVENTION ACT

Epidemiologic evidence has supported the need to develop better protections for the nation's health care workers who are potentially exposed to needlestick injuries resulting in disease (Exposure Prevention Information Network [EPINet], 1999). Evidence suggests that an estimated 800,000 needlestick injuries occur among health care workers each year in the United States, with half of the injuries to nurses. Still, needlestick injuries are seriously underreported, with underreporting rates ranging between 40% and 53% for nurses, between 70% and 95% for physicians, and at 92% for laboratory personnel.

The most common types of devices involved in needlestick injuries are hollow-bore needles,

causing nearly 70% of all injuries reported. Not surprisingly, most injuries occur in patient rooms, with the following five activities associated with the majority of the injuries: disposing of needles, administering injections, drawing blood, recapping needles, and handling trash and dirty linens. Downstream needlestick injuries—that is, those occurring during and after disposal (e.g., carrying out trash, handling dirty linens)—are particularly threatening to the worker because the needle source is generally unknown. The result of any needlestick/sharp injury is the potential for exposure to more than 20 pathogens including HIV, HBV, and HCV. As of December 1998, the CDC had received reports of 54 documented cases and 134 possible cases of occupationally acquired HIV among U.S. health care workers.

Safer needle devices have been shown to reduce needlestick injuries by as much as 86% due to engineering controls with built-in safety features, such as a self-sheathing needle, that are integral to the design. Recessed needles, needleless IV systems, and needle guards are other examples.

Congress was prompted to take action in response to growing concern over bloodborne pathogen exposures from sharps injuries and in response to recent technological developments that increase employee protection. Congress unanimously passed the Needlestick Safety and Prevention Act (Public Law 106-430), which was signed into law on November 6, 2000. This Act requires OSHA to revise the BBPS, broadly categorized into four areas: modification of definitions relating to engineering controls, revision and updating of the Exposure Control Plan, solicitation of employee input, and recordkeeping.

ENGINEERING CONTROLS

The revised standard adds two additional terms to the definition section and alters the definition of one other term. *Sharps With Engineered Sharps Injury Protections* is added and defined as "a nonneedle sharp or a needle device used for withdrawing body fluids, accessing a vein or artery, or administering medications or other fluids, with a built-in safety feature or mechanism that effectively reduces the risk of an exposure incident." This term encompasses a broad array of devices that make injury involving a contaminated sharp less likely and includes, but is not limited to, syringes with a sliding sheath that shields the attached needle after use, needles that retract into a syringe after use, shielded or retracting catheters used to access the bloodstream for intravenous administration of medication or fluids, and intravenous medication delivery systems that administer medication or fluids through a catheter port or connector site using a needle that is housed in a protective covering.

The revised standard also adds the term *Needleless Systems,* which is defined as "a device that does not use needles for the collection of bodily fluids or withdrawal of body fluids after initial venous or arterial access is established; the administration of medication or fluids; or any other procedure involving the potential for occupational exposure to bloodborne pathogens due to percutaneous injuries from contaminated sharps." Examples of needleless systems include, but are not limited to, intravenous medication delivery systems that administer medication or fluids through a catheter port or connector site using a blunt cannula or other nonneedle connection, and jet injection systems that deliver subcutaneous or intramuscular injections of liquid medication through the skin without use of a needle.

The definition of *Engineering Controls* has been modified to include as examples "safer medical devices, such as sharps with engineered sharps injury protections and needleless systems." This change clarifies that safer medical devices are considered to be engineering controls under the standard.

EXPOSURE CONTROL PLAN

The review and update of the Exposure Control Plan is now required to reflect changes in technology that eliminate or reduce exposure to bloodborne pathogens, and to document annually consideration and implementation of appropriate commercially available and effective medical devices designed to eliminate or minimize occupational exposure and improve safety. Thus, the additional provisions require that employers in their written Exposure Control Plans account for innovations in procedure and technological developments that reduce the risk of exposure incidents. This would include, but would not be limited to, newly available medical devices designed to reduce the risk of percutaneous exposure to bloodborne pathogens. Consideration and use of safer medical devices could be documented

in the Exposure Control Plan by describing these devices identified as candidates for adoption, the method or methods used to evaluate devices and the results of evaluations, and the justification for selection decisions. This information must be updated at least annually. The revised Exposure Control Plan requirements make clear that employers must use the safer medical devices as appropriate. If a safer device is not available in the marketplace, the employer is not required to develop any such device.

EMPLOYEE INPUT

In the identification, evaluation, and selection of effective engineering and work practice controls, an employer who is required to establish an Exposure Control Plan must solicit and document input from nonmanagerial employees who are responsible for direct patient care and are potentially exposed to injuries from contaminated sharps. The employer also must document the solicitation in the Exposure Control Plan. No specific procedures for obtaining employee input are prescribed. This provides the employer with flexibility to solicit employee input in any manner appropriate to the circumstances of the workplace. For example, a dental office employing two hygienists may choose to conduct periodic conversations to discuss identification, evaluation, and selection of controls. A large hospital, on the other hand, would likely find that an effective process for soliciting employee input requires the implementation of more formal procedures.

Methods for soliciting employee input may include involvement in informal problem-solving groups; participation in safety audits, worksite inspections, or exposure incident investigations; participation in analysis of exposure incident data or in job or process hazard analysis; participation in the evaluation of devices through pilot testing; and involvement in a safety and health committee.

RECORDKEEPING

The recordkeeping requirements of the standard require that employers maintain a sharps injury log to serve as a tool for identifying high risk areas and evaluating devices. The sharps injury log must contain at a minimum the type and brand of device involved in the incident, the department or work area where the exposure incident occurred, and an explanation of how the incident occurred.

Information in the sharps injury log must be recorded and maintained in a manner that protects the privacy of the injured employee. If data from the log are made available to other parties, any information that directly identifies an employee (e.g., name, address, social security number, payroll number) or information that could reasonably be used to identify a specific employee (e.g., exact age, date of initial employment) must be withheld.

The occupational and environmental health nurse will need to be thoroughly knowledgeable about OSHA laws, regulations, and relevant federal and state laws and collaborate with other departments and disciplines to develop, implement, and evaluate programs that will best protect workers from harm. The occupational and environmental health nurse, working with other health care professionals, can help identify and implement appropriate control strategies and monitor compliance with strategies recommended or required.

RECORDKEEPING AND REPORTING OF OCCUPATIONAL INJURIES AND ILLNESSES

The parts of the OSH Act of 1970 that require covered employers to prepare and maintain records of occupational illnesses and injuries are 29 C.F.R. Part 1904, Recordkeeping and Reporting Occupational Injuries and Illnesses, and Part 1952. The recordkeeping rule has been amended to be effective January 1, 2002. The Bureau of Labor Statistics (BLS) within the U.S. Department of Labor is responsible for administering the recordkeeping system established by the OSH Act. The purposes of keeping records are to permit BLS survey material to be compiled, to help define high hazard industries, and to inform employees of the status of their employer's record.

COVERAGE

Employers of 11 or more employees at any time during the last calendar year must maintain occupational injury/illness records. Exceptions from recordkeeping requirements are size-based and hazard-based. Employers with 10 or fewer employees and several categories of employers are exempt from recordkeeping requirements unless OSHA or BLS informs a specific employer in a notice in writing that they are required to keep records or that they have been selected by the BLS to participate in the Annual Survey of Occupational Injuries and Illnesses. In addition to religious, domestic household, and small employer establishments, exempt categories of employers include those in low hazard retail trade, finance, insurance, real estate, and service industries—Standard Industrial Classification (SIC) 52-89. Table 15-3 provides a listing of partially exempt industries not required to keep OSHA injury and illness records. Exempt employers must comply with OSHA standards, display the OSHA poster, and report to OSHA within 8 hours any workplace incident that results in one or more fatalities or the hospitalization of three or more employees.

FORMS

Where companies employ an occupational and environmental health nurse, OSHA recordkeeping responsibilities are usually managed by the nurse. Thus, the occupational and environmental health nurse must be thoroughly familiar with the regulatory requirements of 29 C.F.R. 1904. The following three forms are used for OSHA recordkeeping:

- OSHA Form 300: Log of Work-Related Injuries and Illnesses (Appendix 15-7A)
- OSHA Form 300A: Summary of Work-Related Injuries and Illnesses (Appendix 15-7B)
- OSHA Form 301: Injury and Illness Incident Report (Appendix 15-7C)

The Log of Work-Related Injuries and Illnesses (Form 300) is used to classify work-related injuries and illnesses and note the extent and severity of each case. When an incident occurs, specific details about what happened and how it happened must be recorded on the log. Employers must keep a log for each establishment or site. The Summary of Work-Related Injuries and Illnesses (Form 300A) shows the totals for the year in each category. At the end of the year the summary is posted in a visible location so that employees are aware of the injuries and illnesses occurring in their workplace. For every injury or illness entered on the log, additional information must be recorded on the Injuries and Illnesses Incident Report (Form 301), which describes how the injury or illness exposure occurred, lists the objects or substances involved, and indicates the nature of the injury or illness and the part(s) of the body af-

TABLE 15-3	Industries Partially Exempt from OSHA Injury and Illness Recordkeeping Requirements		
SIC CODE	**INDUSTRY DESCRIPTION**	**SIC CODE**	**INDUSTRY DESCRIPTION**
525	Hardware stores	729	Miscellaneous personal services
542	Meat and fish markets	731	Advertising services
544	Candy, nut, and confectionary stores	732	Credit reporting and collection services
545	Dairy product stores	733	Mailing, reproduction, and stenographic services
546	Retail bakeries		
549	Miscellaneous food stores	737	Computer and data processing services
551	New and used car dealers	738	Miscellaneous business services
552	Used car dealers	764	Reupholstery and furniture repair
554	Gasoline service stations	78	Motion pictures
557	Motorcycle dealers	791	Dance studios, schools, and halls
56	Apparel and accessory stores	792	Producers, orchestras, entertainers
573	Radio, television, and computer stores	793	Bowling centers
58	Eating and drinking places	801	Offices and clinics of medical doctors
591	Drug stores and proprietary stores	802	Offices and clinics of dentists
592	Liquor stores	803	Offices of osteopathic physicians
594	Miscellaneous shopping goods stores	804	Offices of other health practitioners
599	Retail stores not elsewhere classified	807	Medical and dental laboratories
60	Depository institutions (banks and savings institutions)	809	Health and allied services not elsewhere classified
61	Nondepository institutions (credit institutions)	81	Legal services
		82	Educational services (schools, colleges, universities, and libraries)
62	Security and commodity brokers		
63	Insurance carriers	832	Individual and family services
653	Real estate agents and managers	835	Child day-care services
654	Title abstract offices	839	Social services not elsewhere classified
67	Holding and other investment offices	841	Museums and art galleries
722	Photographic studios, portrait	86	Membership organizations
723	Beauty shops	87	Engineering, accounting, research, management, and related services
724	Barber shops		
725	Shoe repair and shoeshine parlors	899	Services not elsewhere classified
726	Funeral service and crematories		

fected. Substitute equivalent forms are acceptable as long as required information can be detailed and is easily understood.

WORK-RELATEDNESS OF INJURY OR ILLNESS

An injury or illness is considered work-related if an event or exposure in the work environment caused or contributed to the condition or significantly aggravated a preexisting condition.

Work-relatedness is presumed for injuries and illnesses resulting from events or exposures occurring in the workplace, unless an exception specifically applies. Work-related injuries and illnesses that require recording include those that result in death, loss of consciousness, days away from work, restricted work activity or job transfer, or medical treatment beyond first aid.

Any significant work-related injury or illness that is diagnosed by a physician or other licensed health care professional must be recorded, including, cancer, chronic irreversible disease, a fractured or cracked bone, or a punctured eardrum. The following conditions must be recorded when they are work-related:

- Any needlestick injury or cut from a sharp object that is contaminated with another person's blood or other potentially infectious material
- Any case requiring an employee to be medically removed under the requirements of an OSHA health standard
- Tuberculosis infection as evidenced by a positive skin test or diagnosis by a physician or other licensed health care professional after exposure to a known case of active tuberculosis

In the revised recordkeeping rule, two steps are required to determine recordability of a Standard Threshold Shift (STS). The employee must have a confirmed STS in hearing (i.e., case involving an average hearing loss of 10dB or greater in either ear at the 2000 Hz, 3000 Hz, and 4000 Hz frequencies), and the average hearing threshold at the same frequencies in the same ear is greater than or equal to 25dB HL.

Medical treatment includes managing and caring for a patient for the purpose of combating disease or disorder. The following are not considered medical treatments and are NOT recordable:

- Visits to a doctor or health care professional solely for observation or counseling
- Diagnostic procedures, including administering prescription medications that are used solely for diagnostic purposes
- Procedures that can be labeled as first aid as defined in the rules

PRIVACY CASES

Certain restrictions on recording identifying information about an employee now exist in the recordkeeping rule in order to protect the employee's privacy. These are termed *privacy cases*. The following types of injuries or illnesses are to be considered privacy concern cases:

- An injury or illness to an intimate body part or to the reproductive system
- An injury or illness resulting from a sexual assault
- A mental illness
- A case of HIV infection, hepatitis, or tuberculosis

- A needlestick injury or cut from a sharp object that is contaminated with blood or other potentially infectious material (see 29 C.F.R. Part 1904.8 for definition)
- Other illnesses if the employee independently and voluntarily requests that his or her name not be entered on the Log (exception, musculoskeletal disorders [MSDs].

In these situations the employee's name must not be entered on the OSHA 300 Log. Instead, enter *privacy case* in the space normally used for the employee's name. A separate, confidential list of the case numbers and employee names for the establishment's privacy concern cases must be kept updated for Log purposes and to provide information to the government if required. Additional information that may be personally identifiable even though the employee's name has been omitted may also be excluded.

Many specific standards and regulations of the Occupational Safety and Health Administration (OSHA) have additional requirements for the maintenance and retention of records for medical surveillance, exposure monitoring, inspections, and other activities and incidents relevant to occupational safety and health. Reporting of certain information to employees, OSHA, and other governmental agencies is also specified. The occupational and environmental health nurse should also be familiar with these recordkeeping and reporting requirements within these specific standards.

ACCESS TO EXPOSURE AND MEDICAL RECORDS

In 1980 the U.S. Department of Labor issued a standard, Access to Exposure and Medical Records, which was revised in 1988 (USDOL, OSHA, 1993). The purpose of this standard is to ensure the employee or a designated representative access to employee exposure and medical records. Access must be provided within 15 working days of the request. Employee exposure records include environmental monitoring or measurements of a toxic agent, biological monitoring results, material safety data sheets, and any other record that reveals the identity of a harmful or toxic substance (29 C.F.R., Part 1910, 1988). If no exposure records exist, the employer must provide records of other employees with similar job duties. Access to these records does not require written consent of the other employees. The employer must also provide employees and employees' designated representatives access to medical records relevant to the employee.

Employee medical records are those records concerning the health status of the employee and are maintained by health care personnel. These records do not include physical specimens, health insurance claims maintained separately from the record, litigatory records, and separate voluntary employee assistance program records. Prior to employee access to medical records, physicians, on behalf of employers, are encouraged to discuss with employees the contents of their medical records. Access to the medical records of another employee may be provided only with specific written consent of that employee.

The standard provides for special circumstances, such as a terminal illness or psychiatric condition, under which the company physician may deny the employee direct access to record information. However, information must be given to the employee's designated representative with written consent of the employee. This position is difficult to understand and sanctions paternalistic behavior in the standard. In addition, requirements of the Hazard Communication Standard with regard to trade secrets must be observed.

The following requirements regarding retention of exposure and medical records are addressed in the standard:

- Exposure records and data analysis are to be retained for 30 years;
- Medical records are to be retained for the duration of employment plus 30 years;
- Background data for exposure records, such as laboratory reports and work sheets, are to be retained for 1 year;
- Records of employees who have worked for less than 1 year and first-aid records of one-time treatment need not be retained for any specified time period.

The role of the occupational and environmental health nurse in recordkeeping requirements is both a legal and professional obligation. With respect to recordkeeping and disclosure practices, it is necessary to follow the law and document accordingly and at the same time protect the employee's right to privacy (Mistretta, 1990). Legal requirements will dictate the release of occupational injury, illness, and exposure data to specific agencies or individuals. The nurse must have a full understanding of current statutory requirements for recordkeeping procedures and access and should also have a policy in place for protection of employee health records and information disclosure. Only the occupational and environmental health nurse and the physician should have access to the employee's personal health record, and access by other individuals should not be given without the employee's written consent. In addition to the legal requirements, the occupational and environmental health nurse should utilize professional standards and ethical codes as guides to protect employee confidentiality and invasion of privacy. Understanding both the legal and ethical parameters of professional practice will help the nurse in safe and effective recordkeeping practices.

AMERICANS WITH DISABILITIES ACT

In 1990 Congress passed the Americans With Disabilities Act (ADA), which is designed to protect disabled individuals, currently estimated at 43 million, from discrimination. The ADA addresses requirements under five separate titles to end discrimination against people with disabilities (Box 15-6). The employment provisions of Title I of the ADA, Employment, seek to promote independence of disabled individuals through equal employment opportunities. This promotes a human rights appeal rather than compensation appeal to dealing with problems faced by disabled people (Himmelstein et al., 2000). The occupational and environmental health nurse must understand the provisions of the ADA to determine how to best assist the worker and management in implementing these provisions. For example, the occupational and environmental health nurse can help review job descriptions for any physical requirements of a function identified as essential in order to help determine workplace accommodation strategies. In addition, the nurse will want to be actively involved in identifying reasonable accommodations for disabilities, identifying and coordinating outside resources for internal implementation of the ADA, educating employees and management regarding the health and medical implications of the Act, and protecting the confidentiality of the employee's health record (Keim, 1999). The occupational and environmental health nurse must seize the opportunity to participate with management as a member of the business team in defining and coordinating

---

Box 15-6   Americans With Disabilities Act

TITLE I: EMPLOYMENT

Prohibits entities from discriminating against a qualified individual with a disability in all aspects of employment

TITLE II: STATE AND LOCAL GOVERNMENT SERVICES

Prohibits discrimination against individuals with disabilities in providing government services, including public transportation

TITLE III: PUBLIC ACCOMMODATIONS

Requires access to private businesses by individuals with disabilities, thus requiring, where needed,

degrees of alteration, modification, and new construction to the physical structure of the place of business

TITLE IV: TELECOMMUNICATIONS

Requires that telecommunications services in varying forms be made available, to the extent possible, to the hearing impaired

TITLE V: MISCELLANEOUS PROVISIONS

Requires varying provisions for accessibility to recreational and other public areas

---

effective approaches to disability management in the workplace.

COVERAGE

Title I of the ADA states that a "covered entity," which includes private employers, state and local governments, employment agencies, labor unions, and joint labor-management committees (hereinafter referred to as *employer*), cannot discriminate against qualified applicants and employees on the basis of disability. The ADA's requirement applies to all employers with 15 or more employees.

Nondiscrimination

Under the ADA no employer may discriminate against a qualified individual with a disability with regard to job application and testing procedures, hiring assignments and termination, training, compensation, fringe benefits, medical and job evaluations, advancement, or any other term or condition of work (EEOC, 1992). The ADA specifies the following types of actions that may constitute discrimination:

1. Limiting, segregating, or classifying a job applicant or employee in a way that adversely affects employment opportunities for the applicant or employee because of his or her disability
2. Participating in a contractual or other arrangement or relationship that subjects an employer's qualified applicant or employee with a disability to discrimination

3. Denying employment opportunities to a qualified individual because she or he has a relationship or association with a person with a disability
4. Refusing to make reasonable accommodation to the known physical or mental limitations of a qualified applicant or employee with a disability, unless the accommodation would pose an undue hardship on the business
5. Using qualification standards, employment tests, or other selection criteria that screen out or tend to screen out an individual with a disability unless they are job-related and necessary for the business
6. Failing to use employment tests in the most effective manner to measure actual abilities. Tests must accurately reflect the skills, aptitude, or other factors being measured, and not the impaired sensory, manual, or speaking skills of an employee or applicant with a disability (unless those are the skills the test is designed to measure).
7. Discriminating against an individual because she or he has opposed an employment practice of the employer or filed a complaint, or testified, assisted, or participated in an investigation, proceeding, or hearing to enforce provisions of the Act

Disabled Individual

A qualified individual with a disability is defined within the ADA as an individual with a disability who meets the skill, experience, education, and other job-related requirements of a position held or desired, and who, with or without reasonable accommodation, can perform the essential functions of a job. The ADA definition of an individual with a disability is very specific. A person with a disability is an individual who meets one or more of the following criteria:

- Has a physical or mental impairment that substantially limits one or more of his or her major life activities
- Has a record of such an impairment
- Is regarded as having such an impairment

The ADA defines a physical impairment as "any physiological disorder or condition, cosmetic disfigurement, or anatomical loss affecting one or more of the following body systems: neurological, musculoskeletal, special sense organs, respiratory (including speech organs), cardiovascular, reproductive, digestive, genitourinary, hepatic, lymphatic, skin, and endocrine."

The ADA defines a mental impairment as "a (any) mental or psychological disorder, such as mental retardation, organic brain syndrome, emotional or mental illness, and specific learning disabilities."

A person's impairment is determined without regard to any medication or assistive device that she or he may use. Such conditions that would be considered a physical or mental impairment would include orthopedic, visual, speech, or hearing impairments, cerebral palsy, epilepsy, muscular dystrophy, multiple sclerosis, HIV infection, cancer, heart disease, diabetes, drug addiction, and alcoholism. A physical condition that is not the result of a physiological disorder, such as pregnancy, or a predisposition to a certain disease would not be an impairment. Similarly, personality traits such as poor judgment, quick temper, or irresponsible behavior are not themselves impairments.

An impairment is only a disability under the ADA if it substantially limits one or more of the major life activities—that is, the individual must be unable to or have a significantly limited ability to perform an activity compared with an average person in the population (Arruda, 2000a, 2000b; EEOC, 1999, 2000). Factors to consider in making this determination include the nature and severity of the impairment, duration or expected duration, and its permanent or long-term impact (EEOC, 1992). Major life activities include caring for oneself, walking, breathing, performing manual tasks, seeing, hearing, learning, speaking, and working.

An employer may require that an individual not pose a "direct threat" to the health or safety of herself, himself, or others. A health or safety risk can only be considered if it is "a significant risk of substantial harm." Employers cannot deny an employment opportunity merely because of a slightly increased risk. An assessment of "direct threat" must be strictly based on valid medical analyses and/or other objective evidence and not on speculation. This requirement must apply to all applicants and employees, not just to people with disabilities. If an individual appears to pose a direct threat because of a disability, the employer must first try to eliminate or reduce the risk to an acceptable level with reasonable accommodation. If an effective accommodation cannot be found, the employer may refuse to hire an applicant or discharge an employee who poses a direct threat (EEOC, 1992).

ESSENTIAL JOB FUNCTIONS

Essential job functions are those that are fundamental rather than marginal to the job duties. The ADA Title I regulations provide guidance on identifying the essential functions of the job. The first consideration is whether employees in the position actually are required to perform the function. For example, a job announcement or job description for a secretary or receptionist may state that typing is a function of the job, but if the employer has never or seldom required an employee in that position to type, typing could not be considered an essential function (EEOC, 1992).

The next consideration is whether removing that function would fundamentally change the job. According to the ADA regulations, examples of reasons why job functions could be considered essential include the following:

1. The position exists to perform the function;
2. A limited number of other employees are available to perform the function or among whom the function can be distributed;
3. A function is highly specialized, and the person in the position is hired for special expertise or ability to perform the function.

Job Description Questionnaire						
Job Title:						
Department:						
Supervisor:						
1) What Essential (E) Functions do you perform?						
Essential Function	% of time E	Constant E	Frequent E	Occasional E	Is This Function Essential?	Would the Job Change if not done?
2) What Marginal (M) Functions do you perform?						
Marginal Function	% of time M	Constant M	Frequent M	Occasional M	Is This Function Marginal?	Would the Job Change if not done?

3) What education, training, experience, licenses are required for satisfactory performance?

4) What machines or equipment are you responsible for operating?

5) List working conditions such as heat, cold, dust, etc.

6) Do you supervise other emplyees? If YES, give job titles and description of jobs.

7) If you were unable to perform your function, what effect would it have on management?

8) Do you have authority in training others? If YES, describe.

Figure 15-4 Example of job description questionnaire. *(From* Understanding the Americans With Disabilities Act, *by N. Goldenthal, 1993, Beverly, MA: OEM Press.)*

Whether a particular function is essential is a factual determination that must be made on a case-by-case basis. In making this determination, various types of evidence will be considered, including the following:

- The employer's judgment
- The written job descriptions prepared before advertising the position or interviewing applicants for the job
- The amount of time spent performing the function
- The consequences of not performing the function
- The terms of a collective bargaining agreement
- The work experience of those who previously held the job and of those who currently perform similar jobs

Nothing in the ADA prohibits employers from defining physical and other job criteria and tests for a job as long as the criteria and tests are job-related and equally applied (Cross, 1992).

The occupational and environmental health nurse can perform a valuable service in reviewing and collaborating on the identification of requirements of a function stipulated as essential. Kaldor (1992) points out that while recognizing that the job description provides the foundation for any subsequent discussions and decisions around reasonable accommodations, the occupational and environmental health nurse should select a tool or process which facilitates a systematic approach to the job analysis. Data collected in that analysis should include task and process list; essential functions identified; description of how the job is currently done; physical, emotional, intellectual requirements of the essential functions; and comments on what influence the tools, work, and work environment have on the incumbent employee. Once documented, the analysis provides proof of an employer's determination of essential functions for a given position, without regard to a specific applicant. Figure 15-4 is an example of a job description questionnaire with specific reference to essential and marginal functions.

REASONABLE ACCOMMODATION

Reasonable accommodation is a key nondiscrimination requirement of the ADA. Although many disabled individuals can perform jobs without any need for accommodation, many others are excluded from jobs that they are qualified to perform because of unnecessary barriers in the workplace and work environment; these barriers include physical barriers, communication problems, rigid work schedules, and unfounded fears and stereotypes. Under the ADA, when an individual with a disability is qualified to perform the essential functions of a job—except for functions that cannot be performed because of related limitations and existing job barriers—an employer must try to find a reasonable accommodation that would enable this person to perform these functions (Worshop, 1996).

The reasonable accommodation should reduce or eliminate unnecessary barriers between the individual's abilities and the requirements for performing the essential job functions. Reasonable accommodation is any modification or adjustment to a job, an employment practice, or the work environment that makes it possible for an individual with a disability to enjoy an opportunity for equal employment. Legal obligations include the following:

- An employer must provide a reasonable accommodation to the known physical or mental limitations of a qualified applicant or employee with a disability unless she or he can show that the accommodation would impose an undue hardship on the business.
- The obligation to provide a reasonable accommodation applies to all aspects of employment. This duty is ongoing and may arise any time that a person's disability or job changes.
- An employer does not have to make an accommodation for an individual who is not otherwise qualified for a position.
- Generally the individual with a disability is obligated to request a reasonable accommodation.
- A qualified individual with a disability has the right to refuse an accommodation. However, if the individual cannot perform the essential functions of the job without the accommodation, she or he may not be qualified for the job.
- If the cost of an accommodation would impose an undue hardship on the employer, the individual with a disability should be given the option of providing the accommodation or paying that portion of the cost that would constitute the undue hardship.

A reasonable accommodation applies only to accommodations that reduce barriers to employment related to a person's disability; the accommodation need not be the best available as long as it is effective for the purpose, nor is it required primarily for personal use (EEOC, 1992). Some examples of reasonable accommodation include the following:

- Making facilities readily accessible to and usable by an individual with a disability
- Restructuring a job by reallocating or redistributing marginal job functions
- Altering when or how an essential job function is performed
- Providing for part-time or modified work schedules
- Obtaining or modifying equipment or devices
- Modifying examinations, training materials, or policies
- Providing qualified readers and interpreters
- Allowing for reassignment to a vacant position
- Permitting use of accrued paid leave or unpaid leave for necessary treatment
- Providing reserved parking for a person with a mobility impairment
- Allowing an employee to provide equipment or devices that an employer is not required to provide

A good resource to help determine appropriate and useful accommodations is the Job Accommodation Network (JAN) information service from the Department of Labor. The JAN provides worksite accommodation descriptions for several disability-related problems, and these descriptions can be obtained at the websites of various federal agencies (Appendix 15-8). Examples of JAN worksite accommodations for cumulative trauma disorders (Appendix 15-9A) and migraine headaches (Appendix 15-9B) are provided.

The role of the occupational and environmental health nurse can be vital in this process. Critically analyzing the job involved and collaborating with the individual involved is necessary for determining what types of accommodations will help the employee perform the job. The occupational and environmental health nurse can then help select the most appropriate accommodation.

As stipulated, an employer is not required to make a reasonable accommodation if it would impose an undue hardship on the operation of the business—that is, an action requiring "significant difficulty or expense" in relation to the size of the company, resources available, and nature of the operation. Undue hardship is decided on a case-by-case basis. When determining undue hardship, the following factors are considered in the regulations:

1. The nature and cost of the accommodation
2. The overall financial resources of the specific facility where the accommodation is considered and the effect of the accommodation on the expenses and resources of the company facility
3. The overall financial resources of the company, including the total size of the parent company, the number of employees, and the type of company
4. The type of operations of the business, including the business' structure, administrative organization, geographic separateness, and fiscal relationship of the facility to the entire company

It has been suggested that proving undue hardship will be difficult for the employer (EEOC, 1999; Frierson, 1992).

MEDICAL EXAMINATIONS AND INQUIRIES

Another provision of the ADA concerns medical examinations and inquiries (EEOC, 2000). Historically, many employers asked applicants and employees to provide information concerning their physical and/or mental condition. This information often was used to exclude and otherwise discriminate against individuals with disabilities—particularly nonvisible disabilities, such as diabetes, epilepsy, heart disease, cancer, and mental illness—despite their ability to perform the job. The ADA provisions concerning disability-related inquiries and medical examinations reflect the intent of Congress to protect the rights of applicants and employees to be assessed on merit alone while protecting the rights of employers to ensure that individuals in the workplace can efficiently perform the essential functions of their jobs (EEOC, 1992).

Certain restrictions are placed on the employer regarding preplacement examinations and inquiries. "Under the ADA an employer's ability to make disability-related inquiries or require medical examinations is analyzed in three stages: preoffer, postoffer, and employment. At the first stage (prior to an offer of employment) the ADA prohibits all disability-related inquiries and medical examinations, even if they are related to the job . . . The commission explains that a disability-related inquiry is a question (or a series of questions) that is likely to elicit information about a disability" (EEOC, 1999). Disability-related inquiries (which may not be asked about) may include the following (Doe v. Nast & Graf 1994; Executive Order No. 13145, 2000; Griffin v. Steeltek, 1998; Roe v. Cheyenne Mountain Conference Resort, 1997) (note: the EEOC refers to *employee*, but this term also includes applicants):

- Asking an employee whether s/he has (or ever had) a disability or how s/he became disabled, or inquiring about the nature or severity of an employee's disability
- Asking an employee to provide medical documentation regarding his/her disability
- Asking an employee's coworker, family member, doctor, or another person about an employee's disability
- Asking about an employee's genetic information
- Asking about an employee's prior workers' compensation history
- Asking an employee whether s/he currently is taking any prescription drugs or medications, whether s/he has taken any such drugs or medications in the past, or monitoring an employee's taking of such drugs or medications
- Asking an employee a broad question about his/her impairments that is likely to elicit information about a disability (e.g., What impairments do you have?)

Questions that are permitted include the following:

- Asking generally about an employee's well being (e.g., How are you?), asking an employee who looks tired or ill if s/he is feeling okay, asking an employee who is sneezing or coughing whether s/he has a cold or allergies, or asking how an employee is doing following the death of a loved one or the end of a marriage/relationship
- Asking an employee about nondisability-related impairments (e.g., How did you break you leg?)
- Asking an employee whether s/he can perform job functions

- Asking an employee whether s/he has been drinking
- Asking an employee about his/her current illegal use of drugs
- Asking a pregnant employee how she is feeling or when her baby is due
- Asking an employee to provide the name and telephone number of a person to contact in case of medical emergency

"At the second stage (after an applicant is given a conditional job offer, but before she or he starts to work) an employer may make disability-related inquiries and conduct medical examinations, regardless of whether they are related to the job, as long as they are done for all entering employees in the same job category" (42 U.S.C., 1994). For example, an employer may not ask about the applicant's workers' compensation history or about any conditions that might prevent the applicant from doing the job. Applicants may be asked to describe or demonstrate their ability to perform specific job functions. "At the third stage (after employment begins) an employer may make disability-related inquiries and require medical examinations only if they are job-related and consistent with business necessity" (42 U.S.C., 1994).

The ADA requires employers to treat any medical information obtained from a disability-related inquiry or medical examination (including medical information from voluntary health or wellness programs), as well as any medical information voluntarily disclosed by an employee, as a confidential medical record. Employers may share such information only in limited circumstances with supervisor, managers, first aid and safety personnel, and government officials investigating compliance with the ADA.

After making a conditional job offer but before a person starts work, an employer may make unrestricted medical inquiries but may not refuse to hire an individual with a disability based on results of such inquiries unless the reason for rejection is job-related and justified by business necessity (EEOC, 1992). Generally, a disability-related inquiry or medical examination of an employee may be "job-related and consistent with business necessity" when an employer "has reasonable belief , based on objective evidence, that (1) an employee's ability to perform essential job functions will be impaired by a medical condition; or (2) an employee will pose a direct threat due to a medical condition." Disability-related inquiries and medical examinations may follow up on a request for reasonable accommodation when the disability or need for accommodation is not known or obvious. In addition, periodic medical examinations and other monitoring under specific circumstances may be job-related and consistent with business necessity. As previously stated, after employment any medical examination or inquiry required of an employee must be job-related and justified by business necessity. Exceptions are voluntary examinations conducted as part of employee health programs and examinations required by other federal laws. Information about the medical condition or history of the applicant/employee must be collected and maintained on separate forms and in separate medical files and be treated as a confidential medical record. However, exceptions to this include the following:

- Supervisors and managers may be informed regarding necessary restrictions and necessary accommodations;
- First aid and safety personnel may be informed, when appropriate, if the disability might require emergency treatment;
- Government officials investigating compliance with the ADA must be provided relevant information upon request;
- The result of such a physical examination is not used to identify a disability, which is then the basis of withdrawing the offer of employment.

An employer may conduct voluntary medical examinations and inquiries as part of an employee health program (such as medical screening for high blood pressure, weight control, and cancer detection), provided that the following is true:

- Participation in the program is voluntary;
- Information obtained is maintained according to the confidentiality requirements of the ADA;
- This information is not used to discriminate against an employee.

Kaldor (1992) describes the following roles of the occupational and environmental health nurse in this phase of the ADA process:

1. Review existing preplacement examination requirements for compliance;

2. Work with appropriate resources to construct preplacement examinations that accurately test for the essential function-related physical requirements;
3. Coach the consulting physician regarding the ADA prohibition against predictions about future incapacities of an applicant;
4. Protect the confidentiality of these testing results.

Testing for illegal drugs is not considered a medical examination; therefore, employers may continue to conduct drug screening in order to maintain a drug-free workplace (Cross, 1992).

EQUAL EMPLOYMENT OPPORTUNITY COMMISSION

The Equal Employment Opportunity Commission (EEOC) is the federal agency responsible for enforcing the employment requirements of the ADA. An individual must file a complaint of an alleged violation with the EEOC within 180 days of the alleged discriminatory act. If employment discrimination is found, various remedies are available. Several resources that provide assistance in implementing the ADA are listed in the "Resource Directory" section of the *EEOC Technical Assistance Manual.* In addition, several examples of federal agency resources are found in Appendix 15-8. National nongovernmental technical assistance resources (nearly 75) and regional and state locations of federal programs are also listed in the *Technical Assistance Manual.*

FAMILY AND MEDICAL LEAVE ACT

The Family and Medical Leave Act of 1993 (FMLA) was established to afford eligible employees medical leave from work for a certain period of time with a guaranteed right to return to the same or equivalent position with equivalent benefits, compensation, and conditions of employment after the leave has been completed (Danaber, 2001). The Act is intended to balance the demands of the workplace with the needs of families and promote the stability and economic security of families and the national interests in preserving family integrity. The intent of the Act was to accomplish these purposes in a manner that accommodates the legitimate interests of employers and is consistent with the Equal

Protection Clause of the Fourteenth Amendment in minimizing the potential for employment discrimination on the basis of gender while promoting equal employment opportunity for men and women.

The enactment of the FMLA was predicated on two fundamental concerns—the needs of the U.S. workforce and the development of high performance organizations. Increasingly, children and elderly in the United States are dependent upon family members who must spend long hours at work. When a family emergency arises—requiring workers to attend to seriously ill children or parents, to newly born or adopted infants or even to their own serious illness—workers need reassurance that they will not be asked to choose between continuing their employment and meeting their personal and family obligations or tending to vital needs at home.

To be entitled to leave, the employee must have worked for the employer for a total of 12 months and worked at least 1,250 hours during the 12 months immediately before the leave (FMLA, 1993). The law covers employees of private sector organizations and state, local, and federal government agencies.

The FMLA applies to employers with at least 50 employees working within a 75 mile radius and provides up to 12 weeks of unpaid leave during a 12 month period to eligible employees for birth and care of the employee's newborn child; adoption or foster placement of a child with the employee; care of a parent, spouse, or child with a serious health condition; and the employee's inability to work because of a serious health problem. The employee may take leave on an intermittent basis or in the form of a reduced schedule if medically necessary for a serious health condition of the employee, spouse, child, or parent. A married couple working for the same covered employer may be limited to a combined 12 weeks of leave for the birth, foster care placement, or adoption of a child and related care or the care of a parent with a serious health condition.

A serious health consideration means an illness, injury, impairment, or physical or mental condition that involves (1) inpatient care requiring an overnight stay and any related subsequent treatment; (2) any period of incapacity requiring absence of more than 3 workdays and any subsequent treatment or incapacity relating to the same treatment or incapacity relating to the same condi-

tion; (3) any period of incapacity due to pregnancy, or for prenatal care with or without treatment; (4) any period of incapacity or associated treatment due to a chronic serious health condition; (5) any period of incapacity which is permanent or long-term due to a condition for which treatment many not be effective; (6) any period of absence to receive multiple treatments by a health care provider; and (7) a continuing regimen of treatment, including examinations, to determine if a serious health condition exists, and evaluation of the conditions (AAOHN, 1995; FMLA, 1993).

The law requires that the employee provide the employer with reasonable notice of leave; at least 30 days is preferred. However, it is recognized that shorter periods of notice may occur, as with emergency situations. The employer may require medical certification to validate the employee's leave request related to the specific health condition for which the leave is needed. An example of certification by a health care provider is shown in Appendix 15-10. The employer must post a notice specifying information about FMLA. Occupational and environmental health nurses can assist by providing employees with information and by collaborating with human resource personnel to educate employees on their family leave benefits. They might also contribute to the public policy process by documenting the need for family medical leave in smaller workplaces and the impact of employer policies on lower income workers.

WORKERS' COMPENSATION

With the advent of the Industrial Revolution the number and severity of workplace injuries increased, bringing about the need for changes in providing financial and medical support for employees with work-related injuries. Workers' compensation is a legal system through which individuals who sustain physical or mental injuries due to their jobs are compensated for their disabilities and medical costs and some rehabilitation costs, and through which the survivors of workers who are killed receive compensation for lost financial support (Boden, 2000). Excepting federal civilian employees, who are covered by federal laws, primarily the Federal Compensation Act, workers are covered under the various state laws.

The first state workers' compensation law was passed in New York in 1910, but it was later ruled unconstitutional; Wisconsin's 1911 law was the first viable law passed (Howard & Davies, 1985). Currently, each of the 50 states and the District of Columbia has a workers' compensation law, and although the law is specific to each jurisdiction, commonalities exist across statutes. In general, workers' compensation laws provide that in exchange for paying workers' compensation for damages, the employer receives immunity from lawsuits. However, this immunity may not apply under the following circumstances:

- Injuries not covered by workers' compensation
- Injuries sustained by an employee of a noncomplying employer
- Injuries caused by the employer's intentional act
- Injuries sustained while the employer and employee entered into a separate relationship or "dual capacity" independent of their master/servant relationship
- Discharge, demotion, or other punitive action by an employer taken in retaliation for employees' filing workers' compensation claims or otherwise pursuing workers' compensation rights (Nackley, 1987)

WORK-RELATED INJURIES AND DISEASES

To be compensable, occupational injuries and diseases must be work-related. The most common type of workers' compensation claim is the injury that is an unexpected, unintended event (Nackley, 1987). The traditional terms *in the course of* and *arising out of employment* may be used to determine if an injury is work-related and thus compensable. However, because workers' compensation systems are state administered, determinations of similar situations or cases may vary from state to state. Thus, regardless of the terms or language, the determining factor as to whether an injury is compensable should be whether the injury is work-related.

With respect to workers' compensation the definition of occupational disease varies from state to state. However, the obvious application of the definition is one where the illnesses are associated with particular industrial occupations or processes. Virtually any disease that is caused by an industrial trade or process is recognized as an occupational disease. In those jurisdictions in which occupational diseases are distinguished from injuries, coverage is provided by statutes that generally recognize occupational diseases or by statutes that list certain scheduled ailments as recognized occupational diseases associated with certain trades or industrial processes. Sometimes both types of statutes apply.

Some states provide schedules of such diseases; others do not. The schedules of some states may contain only one disease, listed separately from the general accident or injury provision. For example, New York's schedule lists 29 diseases, and Ohio's and North Carolina's list 27 each. The diseases most often occurring on such schedules include the various pneumoconioses, which are associated with exposure to dusts (including coal dust); silicosis from exposure to silica; asbestosis; and radiation illness (Nackley, 1987).

COMPENSATION AND BENEFITS

Awards made to injured workers in workers' compensation systems vary from state to state and are usually designed to compensate the disabled worker or, in the case of the death of an employee, the dependent survivor for economic or wage loss or lost earning capacity. In addition, medical care costs and related expenses, funeral and burial costs, and in most cases, some form of rehabilitation costs are included. Most workers' compensation systems make some effort to compensate injured workers for permanent medical impairment. These awards are usually paid irrespective of any actual or prospective loss of wages and are divided into so-called scheduled awards, usually for loss of limb, eyesight, or hearing or for other defined categories of impairments, disability, or impairment awards.

One reason for establishing these awards was to give injured workers some incentive to return to work; another reason was simply to give the worker some quasi-damage award for the physical impairment endured. The basis of the award is related to the extent of the disability or impairment. Extent of disability is concerned with duration and degree. Duration of disability is concerned with permanent or temporary disability, and degree of disability is concerned with total or partial disability (Table 15-4). As determined by individual state workers' compensation systems, compensation is usually paid weekly and is

TABLE 15-4   Workers' Compensation Disability Awards

DURATION OF DISABILITY	DEGREE OF DISABILITY	
	TOTAL	PARTIAL
Permanent	1. Disability caused by work-related injury or occupational disease that completely removes claimant from substantially remunerative employment (in some jurisdictions) 2. Loss or loss of use of designated part or parts of the body (e.g., loss of both legs, loss of vision of both eyes)	Disability caused by work-related injury or occupational disease that does not remove claimant from substantially remunerative employment but has left the claimant with residual medical impairment expected to be of indefinite duration. (e.g., loss of limb, hearing, or other defined categories of impairment)
Temporary	1. Disability caused by work-related injury or occupational disease that does not appear to be of indefinite duration but keeps the claimant from gainful employment 2. Disability caused by work-related injury or occupational disease that keeps claimant from returning to regular employment. This is the most commonly awarded disability compensation under workers' compensation. It is payable during the acute postinjury phase of disability, while the claimant is in the hospital or recuperating from an injury, and so long as the injury keeps the claimant who has an expectation of returning to the job or to the job market from work. It is intended to compensate a worker for loss of wages during recovery.	Disability caused by work-related injury or occupational disease that does not appear to be of indefinite duration and is not keeping the claimant from gainful employment (e.g., fracture)

From *Workers' Compensations,* by J. V. Nackley, Washington, DC: Bureau of National Affairs. 1987.

calculated as a fraction of the worker's weekly wage at the time of injury or death (e.g., two thirds, three fourths), usually with an upper and lower limit. Compensation payments usually start on the date of the injury and continue until the employee returns to work or as permitted within the defined schedule of the workers' compensation system.

In most U.S. jurisdictions workers' compensation systems are administered by specific agencies, usually referred to as industrial commissions or boards, workers' compensation bureaus, or industrial accident boards. The state agency is almost always given general power over the workers' compensation system. This power includes the authority to investigate claims, collect and disburse funds, employ sufficient staff to perform its statutory duties, and compel employers and insurance carriers to comply with the workers' compensation laws.

As part of the OSH Act, Congress established the National Commission on State Workers' Compensation Laws. The Commission identified the following seven primary obligations of workers' compensation systems:

1. *Compulsory coverage.* Employees could not lose coverage by agreeing to waive their rights to benefits.
2. *No occupational or numerical exemptions to coverage.* All workers, including agricultural and domestic workers, should be covered. All employers, even if they have only one employee, should be covered.
3. *Full coverage of work-related diseases.* Arbitrary barriers to coverage, such as highly restrictive time limits, occupational disease schedules, and exclusion of "ordinary diseases of life," should be eliminated.
4. *Full medical and physical rehabilitation services without arbitrary limits*
5. *Employees' choice of jurisdiction for filing interstate claims*
6. *Adequate weekly cash benefits for temporary total disability, permanent total disability, and fatal cases*
7. *No arbitrary limits on duration or sum of benefits*

Occupational and environmental health nurses are becoming increasingly involved in the management and administration of workplace safety programs, whether through counseling of the injured worker about injury management and worker rights, administration of worker injury claims, or management of the workers' compensation cases. Occupational and environmental health nurses should be thoroughly familiar with the workers' compensation laws and systems in the states in which they practice. Accurate records must be kept, and injuries must be reported and documented promptly so that claims and defenses can be handled effectively.

LEGAL PRACTICE OF NURSING

In the United States each state has a licensure law, generally called the Nurse Practice Act, which defines and regulates the practice of nursing. In most states the law is implemented, interpreted, and enforced by an administrative agency, usually called the Board of Nursing. While nursing licensure laws may differ slightly from state to state, each Nurse Practice Act contains a legal definition of nursing practice that determines the legal scope of nursing practice and provides the legal authority to perform those functions generally defined as nursing (Keener, 1985).

La Bar (1984) states that the definition of nursing practice should be broad to allow for flexibility and utilization of appropriate skills of the professional nurse. In addition, a broader rather than narrower definition can then be interpreted to reflect the expansion of nursing practice as the scope of practice evolves. La Bar collected, reviewed, and analyzed the statutory definitions of nursing practice with respect to certain ANA principles and suggested the following definition of professional nursing practice: the practice of nursing means the performance for compensation of professional services requiring substantial specialized knowledge of the biological, physical, behavioral, psychological, and sociological sciences and nursing theory as the basis for assessment, diagnosis, planning, intervention, and evaluation in the promotion and maintenance of health; the case finding and management of illness, injury, or infirmity; the restoration of optimum function; or the achievement of a dignified death. Nursing practice includes but is not limited to administration, teaching, counseling, supervision, delegation, and evaluation of practice and execution of the medical regimen, including the administration of medications and treatments prescribed by any person authorized by state law to prescribe. Each registered nurse is directly accountable and responsible to the consumer for the quality of nursing care rendered.

Unfortunately, legal boundaries defining the scope of nursing practice are neither clearly delineated between the practice of nursing and the practice of other health professions, nor do they comprehensively and consistently differentiate the expanded role of the nurse from nursing practice in general. However, nursing professional groups and state legislatures seem to be moving toward legal definitions of nursing that adequately reflect specialization and advanced practice (Rogers & Livesey 2000). La Bar (1984) states that the function of the professional association is to upgrade practice, certify individuals in special areas, and establish the scope and qualifications of each practice area.

Each nurse has the responsibility to obtain and be familiar with the nurse practice act that governs nursing practice within the state where she or he practices. In addition, the nurse must know the rules and regulations that further specify nursing functions as set forth by the respective state board of nursing. Keener (1985) lists the following points the nurse should consider when making a determination regarding the legal authority (e.g., nurse practice act) to perform specific nursing functions:

- How does the state nurse practice act define professional nursing? Is it a broad, open-ended statutory definition that authorizes all nursing functions and contains language such as "including but not limited to"? Does it specifically provide for nursing diagnosis and assessment? Does the act contain specific authorization for the expanded scope of nursing practice? Is such practice limited only to certain types of practitioners or specialists with particular credentials?
- Do the Board of Nursing rules and regulations specifically define or limit the scope of nursing practice? Is there a laundry list of functions that nurses are legally permitted to perform? Do the rules and regulations recognize practitioners or specialists? Are specific credentials or certifications required?
- Is there a limitation regarding practicing within the guidelines of medical standing orders and protocols?

If the nurse has questions or needs clarification regarding the statute or regulations or both, the nurse may contact the state nursing board or the state nurses' association to determine what common practices are accepted regarding the use of such protocols and standing orders in the state and whether any statutory, regulatory, or judicial opinions concerning the nurse's legal authority to perform such functions has been issued recently. The nurse should also check other practice acts, such as medicine and pharmacy, where overlapping functions may exist by interpretation, to determine if any statutory prohibitions exist.

The nurse has a duty of care that requires the conforming to a standard of care for protection of the patient or client against unreasonable risk of injury (American Association of Legal Nurse Consultants, 1998). As a professional the nurse must possess and exercise equivalent knowledge and skill levels as a member of the profession in good standing in the same or a similar community; that is, the nurse's conduct will be measured against that of the "reasonably prudent nurse" in a similar situation. Thus, the care that the occupational and environmental health nurse renders to an employee will not be measured against that of a physician. When the nurse's actions or conduct do not meet the required standard, the legal duty of care may be breached, which may be grounds for a case of negligence or malpractice.

Although very few malpractice suits have been filed against occupational and environmental health nurses, the following case is of interest. A nurse cleaned and bandaged a puncture wound sustained by an employee after a piece of metal pierced the employee's forehead. In this particular case, company policy was that employees could only see a physician if the occupational and environmental health nurse made a referral. The nurse continued to treat the reddened area over the next 10 months until it became swollen. By the time the nurse referred the employee to a physician, a basal-cell carcinoma had developed. The nurse and the employer were held liable for damages. The court reasoned that a prudent occupational and environmental health nurse would have explored the wound for potential metal slivers and would have known that failure to heal is a warning sign of cancer. The court also said that the nurse should have referred the employee to a physician much earlier (Cooper v. National Motor Bearing Co., 1955; Wolff, 1984; Yorker, 1989).

Recent case law regarding advanced nursing practice has focused on the practice of two nurses who provided services in a women's health clinic in Missouri. The suit was filed by physicians on the medical licensing board who claimed that the nurses were practicing medicine. As a part of their practice, "the nurses performed a variety of diagnostic and treatment functions, including breast and pelvic examinations, pregnancy testing, Pap smears, gonorrhea cultures, and blood serology; the administration of all kinds of contraceptive methods, including intrauterine devices and oral contraceptives; and the counseling and education of patients." All these functions were performed according to signed physician protocols.

Although lower courts found the nurses guilty of engaging in the practice of medicine, the Missouri Supreme Court unanimously reversed the decision, stating that nurses who could demonstrate appropriate specialized skill, education, and judgment were practicing within the Nurse Practice Act as set forth in the state's statutory definition of nursing. Yorker (1989) emphasizes several important points with respect to this decision. First, the court placed considerable emphasis on the nurses' graduate education. Second, the court was impressed by the overwhelming response of professional groups and private citizens in support of the nurses' expanded role. And third, the court recognized the prevailing trend of independence in nursing practice, even to the point of conceding that the functions of diagnosis and prescription no longer fall within the exclusive territory of the medical doctor.

Rowe (1989) describes an opinion issued by the attorney general of Georgia, which stated that no statutory authority existed for public health nurses to prescribe medications such as birth control pills (for public health clients) by reference to a protocol; therefore, the activity was considered unlawful even though it had been performed by public health nurses by protocol since 1973. The attorney general interpreted Georgia's Nurse Practice Act to authorize (by physicians) only the administration of medications.

Because many medical and nursing functions overlap, nurses need clear statutory authority regarding the use of protocols and the functions that may be delegated by protocols to prevent nurses from being confronted with charges such as practicing medicine without a license (Rowe, 1989). Occupational and environmental health nurses using practice protocols should be aware of the permissible scope of nursing practice in their state and determine that the functions delegated to them by protocol fall within that permissible scope. All protocols requiring delegatory functions should be dated and signed by a physician with defined tasks clearly authorized. The educational preparation a nurse must have to perform tasks should be identified (Wold, 1990). The company policy should distinctly authorize nurses to practice by protocol.

With duties such as recording laboratory results, history taking, physical assessments, screening examinations, and health counseling, the occupational and environmental health nurse must comply with the accepted standard of care generally expected of any nurse when performing such procedures. Of particular importance is keeping accurate records and reporting all observations regarding the client's physical and mental condition, as well as all information given to him or her. However, additional types of recording, such as the delegated keeping of OSHA logs, are specific to occupational and environmental health nursing duties and must conform to the accepted practice therein.

Sometimes the occupational and environmental health nurse may be faced with a dilemma when an ethical decision conflicts with a legal requirement. This may be the case with confidentiality of health information versus disclosure of information when others may be at risk (Rogers, 1988; Yorker, 1989). However, the nurse can utilize ethical codes, frameworks, and standards for practice that will help to guide decisions for safe and effective occupational and environmental health nursing practice (AAOHN, 1999).

Nurse Practice Acts were developed because state governments were concerned with protecting their citizens from unsafe nursing practice. These laws govern all nursing practice within each state, and violation of these laws is a crime. For example, if dispensing medications at the worksite is outside the scope of nursing practice, performance of this function by the occupational and environmental health nurse would be in violation of the law. Little potential for criminal violation in the practice of nursing exists if the nurse is adequately trained and educated and then practices in a reasonable manner.

Summary

The occupational and environmental health nurse is responsible for knowing about federal, state, and local statutes and regulations affecting the occupational health and safety of workers and for implementing appropriate practice strategies to comply with these mandates. The nurse must be thoroughly familiar with the state nurse practice act and recognize the legal parameters for professional nursing practice. As the scope of occupational and environmental health nursing evolves and expands, the nurse will assume greater responsibility in the overall management and delivery of occupational health services. Accountability for legal and professional nursing practice is of paramount importance in ensuring safe and effective health care for all workers.

References

42 U.S.C. §12112(d)(3) (1994a); 29 C.F.R. §1630.14(b) (1998).

42 U.S.C. §12112(d)(4)(A) (1994b); 29 C.F.R. §1630.14(c) (1998).

American Association of Legal Nurse Consultants. (1998). *Legal nurse consulting: Principles and practices.* Washington, DC: CRC Press.

American Association of Occupational Health Nurses. (1995). The Family and Medical Leave Act, advisory. *AAOHN Journal, 7,* insert.

American Association of Occupational Health Nurses. (1999). *Code of Ethics.* Atlanta, GA: Author.

Americans With Disabilities Act of 1990. Pub. L. 101-336, 42 U.S.C.A. 12101 *et seq.* (1991).

Arruda, K. (2000). EEOC's ADA policy guidance: Part I. *AAOHN Journal, 48,* 48-50.

Arruda, K. (2000). EEOC's ADA policy guidance: Part II. *AAOHN Journal, 48,* 197-200.

Barlow, R., & Handelman, E. (1993). OSHA's final blood-borne pathogens standard: Part II. *AAOHN Journal, 41*(1), 8-15.

Blosser, F. (1992). *Occupational safety and health.* Washington, DC: Bureau of National Affairs.

Boden, L. (2000). Workers' compensation. In B. Levy & D. Wegman (Eds.), *Occupational health* (pp. 237-256) Philadelphia: Lippincott Williams & Wilkins.

Centers for Disease Control and Prevention. (2001). http://www.cdc.gov.

Cooper v. National Motor Bearing Co., 288 P. 2d 581 (Cat. 1955).

Council on Occupational and Environmental Health. (1988, Winter). National Association for Public Health Policy: Organizational safety and health legislative agenda, 1989. *Journal of Public Health Policy, 10,* 544-555.

Cross, L. J. (1992). Americans With Disabilities Act: Meeting the requirements. *AAOHN Journal, 40*(6), 284-286.

Danaber, M. (2001). Medical leave under the Family and Medical Leave Act: Understanding the impact of the Act's interpretive guidance. *Journal of Legal Nurse Consulting, 12,* 3-6.

Doe v. Kohn Nast & Graf, P.C., 866 F. Supp. 190, 3 AD Cas. (BNA) 1322 (E.D. Pa. 1994).

EPINet. (1999). *Exposure prevention information network data reports.* Charolettesville, VA: University of Virginia, International Health Care Worker Safety Center.

Equal Employment Opportunity Commission. (1992). *A technical assistance manual on the employment provisions (Title I) of the Americans With Disabilities Act* (EEOC-M-IA). Washington, DC: Author.

Equal Employment Opportunity Commission. *Enforcement guidance: Reasonable accommodation and undue hardship under the Americans With Disabilities Act.* (1999). http://www.eeoc.gov/doc/accommodation.html.

Equal Opportunity Employment Commission. (1999). *Enforcement guidance: Reasonable accommodation and undue hardship under the Americans With Disabilities Act* (20-21, 8 FEP Manual (BNA) 405:7601, 7611). Washington, DC: Author.

Equal Employment Opportunity Commission. *Amending the interpretation: Guidance on Title I of the Americans With Disabilities Act: Final rule,* (2000), http://www.eeoc.gov/regs/-mitigating-final.html.

Exec. Order No. 13145, *To prohibit discrimination in federal employment based on genetic information,* 65 Fed. Reg. 6877 (Feb. 8, 2000).

Family and Medical Leave Act of 1993. Pub. L. 103-3, 29 U. S. C. A. 2601 *et. seq.* (1993).

Frierson, J. (1992). *Employer's guide to the Americans With Disabilities Act.* Washington, DC: Bureau of National Affairs.

Goldstein, L., & Johnson, S. (1991). OSHA Bloodborne Pathogens Standard: Implications for the occupational health nurse. *AAOHN Journal, 39*(4), 182-188.

Griffin v. Steeltek, Inc., 160 F.3d 591, 594, 8 A.D. Cas. (B.N.A.) 1249, 1252 (10th Cir. 1998).

Himmelstein, J., Pransky, G., & Sweet, C. (2000). Ability to work and the evaluation of disability. In B. Levy & D. Wegman (Eds.), *Occupational health* (pp. 257-269) Philadelphia: Lippincott Williams & Wilkins.

Howard, P. H., & Davies, W. (1985). Workers' Compensation: An overview. *AAOHN Update Series, 2*(3), 1-8.

Kaldor, C. S. (1992). The Americans With Disabilities Act: An invitation for occupational health nurse intervention. *AAOHN Update Series, 5*(2), 1-8.

Keener, M. L. (1985). Legal boundaries of nursing practice. *AAOHN Update Series, 2*(1), 1-8.

Keim, K. (1999). Application of the ADA in the workplace: Employment issues. *AAOHN Journal, 47,* 213-216.

La Bar, C. (1984). *Statutory definitions of nursing practice and their conformity to certain ANA principles.* Kansas City, KS: American Nurses Association.

Marshall v. Barlow's, Inc. 436 U.S. 307 54, 55, 114 (1978).

McNeely, E. (1990). An organizational study of hazard communication: The health provider perspective. *AAOHN Journal, 38*(4), 165-173.

McNeely, E. (1992). Tracking the future of OSHA: Regulatory policies into the 90s. *AAOHN Journal, 40*(1), 17-23.

Meyer, A. F., & Watson, D. L. (1992). Hazard communications: A process beyond mere compliance. In *Proceedings of the Occupational Safety and Health Summit* (pp. 49-58). Des Plaines, IL: American Society of Safety Engineers.

Mistretta, E. (1990). Health care records and the law. *AAOHN Journal, 38*(11), 545-547.

Nackley, J. V. (1987). *Workers' compensation.* Washington, DC: Bureau of National Affairs.

Needlestick Safety and Prevention Act, Pub. L. 106-430 (November 6, 2000).

Occupational Safety and Health Act. Pub. L. 91-596, 64 U. S. C. 1590 *et seq.* (1970).

Roe v. Cheyenne Mountain Conference Resort, Inc., 124 F.3d 1221, 7 A.D. Cas. (B.N.A.) 779 (10th Cir. 1997).

Rogers, B. (1988). Ethical dilemmas in occupational health nursing. *AAOHN Journal, 36*(3), 100-105.

Rogers, B., & Livesey, K. (2000). Occupational health nursing practice in health surveillance, screening, and prevention activities. *AAOHN Journal,48*(2), 92-99.

Rowe, B. B. (1989). Expanding the nurse's role to diagnosis and treatment: Understanding the legal significance. *AAOHN Journal, 37*(5), 198-199.

Soloman, C. (1986). Hazard communication and right-to-know. *AAOHN Journal, 34*(6), 264-268.

U.S. Department of Labor, Occupational Safety and Health Administration. (1987). Occupational safety and health standards, subpart Z—Toxic and hazardous substances hazard communication standard, 29CFR part 1910.1200. *Federal Register, 52,* 31877-31892.

U.S. Department of Labor, Occupational Safety and Health Administration. (1991). Final rule: Occupational exposure to bloodborne pathogens—29 C.F.R. Part 1910.1030. *Federal Register, 56*(235), M004-64182.

U.S. Department of Labor, Occupational Safety and Health Administration. (1992). *Enforcement procedures for the occupational exposure to bloodborne pathogens standard—29 C.F.R 1910.1030* (OSHA Instruction CPL 2-2.44C: 1-71). Washington, DC: Office of Health Compliance Assistance.

U.S. Department of Labor, Occupational Safety and Health Administration. (1993). Access to employee exposure and medical records. 29CFR Part 1910-20. *Federal Register, 53,* 38162-38168.

U.S. Department of Labor, Occupational Safety and Health Administration. (1996). *Occupational exposure to bloodborne pathogens* (Publication No. 3127). Washington, DC: Occupational Safety and Health Administration.

U.S. Department of Labor, Occupational Safety and Health Administration. (1998). *Hazard communication guidelines for compliance* (Publication No. 3111, 1991b). Washington, DC: Occupational Safety and Health Administration.

U.S. Department of Labor, Occupational Safety and Health Administration. (2000). *All about OSHA.* (OSHA Publication No. 2056). Washington, DC: Occupational Safety and Health Administration.

U.S. Department of Labor, Occupational Safety and Health Administration. (2001a). *Inspection Report 2001 for Fiscal Year 2000.* Washington, DC: Occupational Safety and Health Administration.

U.S. Department of Labor, Occupational Safety and Health Administration. (2001b). *Occupational exposure to bloodborne pathogens: Needlesticks and other sharps injuries—Final rule.* Washington, DC: U.S. Department of Labor.

Wold, J. L. (1990). Workers' compensation law and the occupational health nurse. *AAOHN Journal, 38*(8), 385-387.

Wolff, M. (1984). Court upholds expanded practice for nurses. *Law, Medicine & Health Care, 12,* 26-29.

Worshop, R. (1996). Implementing the Disabilities Act: Should the scope of the ADA be narrowed? *C Q Researcher, 6,* 1107-1127.

Yorker, B. A. (1984). Scope of practice: Case law. *AAOHN Journal, 37*(2), 80-81.

Yorker, B. A. (1989). Confidentiality—An ethical dilemma. *AAOHN Journal, 36*(8), 346-347.

15-1 Specific Provisions Found in the Occupational Safety and Health Act of 1970

To assure so far as possible every working man and woman in the nation safe and healthful working conditions and to preserve our human resources:

1. By encouraging employers and employees in their efforts to reduce the number of occupational safety and health hazards at their places of employment, and to stimulate employers and employees to institute new and to perfect existing programs for providing safe and healthful working conditions

2. By providing that employers and employees have separate but dependent responsibilities and rights with respect to achieving safe and healthful working conditions

3. By authorizing the secretary of labor to set mandatory occupational safety and health standards applicable to businesses affecting interstate commerce and by creating an Occupational Safety and Health Review Commission for carrying out adjudicatory functions under the Act

4. By building upon advances already made through employer and employee initiative for providing safe and healthful working conditions

5. By providing for research in the field of occupational safety and health, including the psychological factors involved, and by developing innovative methods, techniques, and approaches for dealing with occupational safety and health problems

6. By exploring ways to discover latent diseases, establishing causal connections between diseases and work in environmental conditions, and conducting other research relating to health problems, in recognition of the fact that occupational health standards present problems often different from those involved in occupational safety

7. By providing medical criteria which will ensure insofar as practicable that no employee will suffer diminished health, functional capacity, or life expectancy as a result of his work experience

8. By providing for training programs to increase the number and competence of personnel engaged in the field of occupational safety and health

9. By providing for the development and promulgation of occupational safety and health standards

10. By providing an effective enforcement program, which shall include a prohibition against giving advance notice of any inspection and sanctions for any individual violating this prohibition

11. By encouraging the states to assume the fullest responsibility for the administration and enforcement of their occupational safety and health laws by providing grants to the states to assist in identifying their needs and responsibilities in the area of occupational safety and health, to develop plans in accordance with the provisions of this Act, to improve the administration and enforcement of state occupational safety and health laws, and to conduct experimental and demonstration projects in connection therewith

12. By providing for appropriate reporting procedures with respect to occupational safety and health, which procedures will help achieve the objectives of this Act and accurately describe the nature of the occupational safety and health problem

13. By encouraging joint labor-management efforts to reduce injuries and disease arising out of employment

From *Occupational Safety and Health Act,* Pub. L. 91-596, 64 U. S. C. A. 1590-1620, 1970.

15-2 GoodMark Foods, Inc. Bloodborne Pathogens Compliance Program

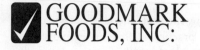

BLOODBORNE PATHOGENS COMPLIANCE PROGRAM

29 CFR 1910.1030

Purpose

To eliminate or minimize exposure to bloodborne pathogens or other potentially infectious materials.

Policy

GoodMark Foods establishes, maintains, and enforces work practices and standard operation procedures to eliminate or minimize contact with blood or other potentially infectious materials.

Definitions

Bloodborne Pathogens. Pathogenic microorganisms that are present in human blood and can cause disease in humans. These pathogens include, but are not limited to, Hepatitis B Virus (HBV) and Human Immunodeficiency Virus (HIV).

Other Potentially Infectious Materials. Includes the following human body fluids: semen, vaginal secretions, cerebrospinal fluid, synovial fluid, pleural fluid, pericardial fluid, peritoneal fluid, amniotic fluid, saliva in dental procedures, and any body fluid that is visibly contaminated with blood.

Occupational Exposure. Actual or potential parenteral, skin, eye, or mucous membrane contact with blood or other potentially infectious materials that may result from the performance of an employee's duties.

Universal Blood and Body Fluid Precautions. According to the concept of universal precautions, all human blood; body components including serum; secretions; tissues; and cerebrospinal, synovial, pleural, peritoneal, pericardial, and amniotic fluids are treated as if they are infectious for HIV, HBV and other bloodborne pathogens.

Regulated Medical Waste. Blood and body fluids in individual containers in volumes greater than 20 ml; microbiological waste, such as laboratory cultures and stocks; and pathological waste such as human tissue, organs, or body parts.

Sharps (Which Are Considered Regulated Medical Waste). Contaminated needles, scalpels, plastic slides and cover slips, broken glass and capillary tubes, ends of dental wires, and other contaminated objects that can penetrate the skin.

Exposure Determination

GoodMark Foods has developed written exposure determinations and maintains a list of all job classifications in which employees have occupational exposure to bloodborne pathogens. All job tasks are classified into one of three categories to facilitate exposure determination:

Category I. Tasks that involve potential for mucous membrane or skin contact with blood, body fluids or tissues or potential for spills or splashes of them.

    Occupational Health Nurse or visiting physician/physician's assistant

Category II. Tasks that involve no exposure to blood, body fluids, or tissues, but employment may require performing unplanned Category I task.

Production Supervisors and Managers

Category III. Tasks that involve no exposure to blood, body fluids, or tissues and Category I tasks are not a condition of employment.

All other employees

Procedure

Preventive Measures

1. Hepatitis B Vaccinations

   Employees who have occupational exposure to bloodborne pathogens are required to take the Hepatitis B Vaccination series. This series is provided to employees at no charge.

   a. The first dose of vaccine is to be made available to employees in Category I within 10 working days of initial assignment. Subsequent doses are to be administered according to current Centers for Disease Control and Prevention recommendations.

   b. The Hepatitis B Vaccine shall be offered to employees in Category II within 24 hours after a cleanup activity occurs as allowed for in the memorandum from the Department of Labor, dated July 6, 1991. Category II employees have the option of taking the Hepatitis B Vaccine Series, at no cost, at any time during their employment.

   c. Employees who decline the Hepatitis B Vaccine are required to sign a Hepatitis B Vaccine Declination Form and have the option of taking the vaccine at a later date if occupational exposures continue.

2. Universal Blood and Body Fluid Precautions

   Universal precautions must be observed. This method of infection control requires the employer and employee to assume that all human blood and specified human body fluids are infectious for HIV, HBV, and other bloodborne pathogens. Where differentiation of types of body fluids is difficult or impossible, all body fluids are to be considered as potentially infectious.

Methods of Control

Engineering and Work Practice Controls

1. Engineering and work practice controls are used as the primary method to eliminate or minimize employee exposure. Where occupational exposure remains after institution of these controls, personal protective equipment will also be used.

2. Handwashing facilities are readily accessible to employees. Additionally, appropriate antiseptic towelettes are provided in each department's first aid kit.

3. There is no potential for "sharps" or contaminated needles at this site, due to the fact that no needles are used.

4. Contaminated instruments are decontaminated with wipes and placed in a labeled, puncture resistant container that is leak proof on the sides and bottom. This container does not require employees to reach into the container where the instruments have been placed.

5. All procedures involving blood or other potentially infectious materials will be performed in such a manner as to minimize splashing, spraying, spattering, and generation of droplets of these substances.

Personal Protective Equipment

1. When there is occupational exposure, appropriate personal protective equipment such as, but not limited to, gloves, gowns, aprons, masks, and eye protection will be provided at no cost to the employee.

2. Appropriate personal protective equipment in appropriate sizes will be available to employees.

3. Use of personal protective equipment by the employees will be monitored and enforced.

4. Hypoallergenic gloves, glove liners, powderless gloves, or other similar alternatives will be readily accessible to those employees who are allergic to the gloves normally provided.

5. Personal protective equipment will be cleaned, laundered, and disposed of at no cost to the employee.

6. Personal protective equipment will be replaced as needed to maintain its effectiveness at no cost to the employee.

7. If blood or other potentially infectious material penetrates a garment, the garment will be removed immediately (or as soon as feasible) and discarded.

8. All personal protective equipment will be removed prior to leaving the work area. When personal protective equipment is removed, it will be placed in an appropriately designated area or container for disposal.

9. Gloves will be worn when it can be reasonably anticipated that the employee may have hand contact with blood, other potentially infectious materials, mucous membranes, and nonintact skin when touching contaminated items or surfaces.

10. Disposable (single use) gloves will be replaced as soon as practical when contaminated or as soon as feasible if they are torn or punctured, and will not be washed or decontaminated or reused.

11. Masks in combination with eye protection devices, such as goggles or glasses with solid side shields, or chin length face shields will be worn whenever splashes, spray, spatter, or droplets of blood or other potentially infectious materials may be generated and eye, nose, or mouth contamination can be reasonable anticipated.

12. Appropriate protective clothing such as, but not limited to, gowns, aprons, lab coats, clinic jackets, or similar outer garments will be worn in occupational exposure situations.

Housekeeping

1. Any contaminated equipment or worksurfaces will be decontaminated immediately after contact with blood or other body fluids using an EPA approved disinfectant such as 1:10 dilutions of bleach, Isolyser, or Red Z.

2. Contaminated disposal items, such as dressings, drapes, etc. that would release blood or body fluids in a liquid or semiliquid state if compressed or items that are caked with dried blood are regulated waste as defined by OSHA. Regulated waste does not require treatment and may be disposed of as general solid waste.

However, while on-site, blood soaked or caked items must be discarded, stored, and transported in closable, leakproof, biohazard labeled containers or disposed of in a container of Isolyzer or Red Z.

Postexposure Procedure

Following a Report of an Exposure Incident

1. An Incident Report, "Employee Exposure to Bloodborne Pathogens," will be obtained from the occupational health nurse or human resources, completed and returned to the supervisor or occupational health nurse before the end of the shift.

2. A confidential medical evaluation and follow-up will be made immediately available to the employee.

3. The occupational health nurse, visiting physician, or human resources will assess the employee's exposure, their Hepatitis B vaccinations, and vaccine response status. This is done by interviewing the employee and reviewing the completed Incident Report Form. The occupational health nurse or human resources manager will confer with the designated physician regarding whether postexposure evaluation and follow-up is needed.

4. If needed, the employee and source patient will be referred to the designated physician for individualized postexposure medical management and treatment of exposed employee(s) on a case-by-case basis, following current communicable disease rules.

5. To ensure that the physician is adequately informed, a copy of the OSHA Bloodborne Pathogens Standard, applicable communicable disease rules, GoodMark Foods, Inc. exposure plan, a description of the specific exposure incident, the infection state of the source, and the vaccination and immunity status of the exposed employee will be sent to the physician at the time of the evaluation.

6. Consult with the designated physician if hepatitis B vaccine is indicated.
7. Completed Incident Report Form should be filed in individual's confidential medical file.
8. Record the circumstances of exposure in the employee's confidential medical file.
9. Obtain copy of the attending physician's written assessment and treatment to be placed in the employee's confidential medical file. The written assessment should include:
   - Whether the hepatitis B vaccine is indicated and if the employee has received the vaccine
   - That the employee was informed of the results of the evaluation
   - That the employee has been told about any medical conditions resulting from exposure to blood or other potentially infectious materials
10. Instruct employee to follow up with physician as directed and discuss treatment and/or concerns with treating physician only.
11. If medical treatment is administered to the exposed employee, record the exposure incident as an injury on the OSHA 300 Log. As of January 1, 2002, such cases will be recorded as a privacy case injury on the OSHA 300 Log.

Training

GoodMark Foods will ensure that all employees with occupational exposure participate in a training program that must be provided at no cost to the employee during working hours.

INCIDENT REPORT: EMPLOYEE EXPOSURE TO BLOODBORNE PATHOGENS

Complete questions 1-9. Give completed report to supervisor, occupational health nurse, or human resources.

1. Employee name: _____ Job title: _____
2. Department: _____ Supervisor: _____
3. Date of exposure: _____ Time of exposure: _____
4. Type of exposure (cut, splash, stick): _____
   Type of fluid: _____ Amount of fluid: _____
   Severity (depth of injury, fluid injected, etc.): _____
   _____

5. Part of the body exposed (mouth, eyes, skin break, etc.): _____
6. Location of exposure (production floor, maintenance, lab, etc.): _____
7. Please describe how and why the exposure occurred (include job duty being performed at time of exposure, extent, and duration of exposure): _____
   _____

8. Personal protective equipment used at time of exposure (gloves, safety glasses, etc.): _____
   _____

9. Date exposure reported: _____ Time exposure reported: _____
   Exposure reported to: _____

THIS SECTION TO BE COMPLETED BY HEALTH CARE PROVIDER/DESIGNATED PERSON

10. Did the employee see a physician regarding the exposure:　　　YES　　　　NO
    If yes, name of physician: _____
    Telephone number: _____
    Physician's instructions:
    _____
    _____

11. Did the employee request to be monitored for HBV, HCV, and HIV antibodies following the exposure:
    YES　　　　NO　　(circle one)
    If no, why not: _____
12. Source of exposure (if known):
    HBV−　　　　HIV+
13. Evaluation/treatment (include condition of skin if applies):
    _____

14. Follow-up of employee (including referrals):
    _____

15. Describe the corrective action taken to prevent recurrence of exposure:
    _____

_____　　　　　_____
　　　Signature　　　　　　　　　　　　　　Date

15-3

GoodMark Foods, Inc. Lock Out/Tag Out Program and Procedures

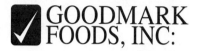
GOODMARK FOODS, INC:

LOCK OUT/TAG OUT POLICY AND PROGRAM

29 CFR 1910.147

(Revised March 2001)

LOCK OUT/TAG OUT PROGRAM AND PROCEDURES

Purpose

To establish the minimum requirements for the lock out/tag out of hazardous energy isolating devices to prevent the unexpected energization or start-up of equipment or release of stored energy.

Scope and Application

These requirements cover the maintenance and/or operation of equipment where the unexpected energization, start-up, or release of stored energy could cause injury to employees. These requirements DO NOT apply to the following:

1. Normal production operations where the employee is not required to remove or bypass guards or safety devices nor to place any part of his/her body into a danger area during the normal operation of the equipment.

Note: The requirements DO apply to individuals who are exposed to electrical hazards as a result of work being done on or near electrical facilities such as panel boxes, electrical disconnects, or electrical equipment.

Definitions

1. *All Employees.* Every employee, regardless of work assignments.
2. *Affected Employees.* Every employee whose job requires him/her to operate equipment or work in an area where lock out/tag out devices are used.
3. *Authorized Employees.* Every employee who has been given the authority, responsibility, and training by his/her manager to implement a lock out/tag out procedure prior to starting maintenance on equipment.
4. *Energy Isolating Device.* A mechanical device that physically prevents the transmission or release of energy. Examples are:
   a. Manually operated electrical circuit breaker
   b. Disconnect switch
   c. Manually operated switch
   d. Slide gate
   e. Slip blind
   f. Line value
   g. Block

Note: Electrical energy isolating devices must simultaneously disconnect all underground supply conductors (e.g., push buttons, selector switches, and other control circuit devices).

5. *Energy Source.* Any source of electrical, mechanical, hydraulic, pneumatic, chemical, thermal, or other energy sources. Examples are:
   a. Energized electrical parts
   b. Hydraulic or pneumatic pressure
   c. Pressurized pipes
   d. Compressed or extended springs
   e. Pressure below atmospheric (vacuum systems)
   f. Flywheels
   g. Batteries
   h. Capacitors
   i. Thermal energy (i.e., residual heat, low temperature)
   j. Residual chemicals causing thermal or pressure buildups
   k. Gravity
   l. Static electricity
6. *Equipment.* A term used in this document to denote tools, appliances, machines, etc. that utilize or produce energy.
7. *Lock Out.* The placement of a lock on an energy-isolating device in accordance with an established procedure to ensure that the energy-isolating device cannot be operated until the lock and tag are removed.
8. *Maintenance.* A term used in this document to denote workplace activities such as constructing, installing, setting up, adjusting, inspecting, modifying, maintaining, and servicing equipment. These activities include cleaning, lubricating, or unjamming equipment and making adjusting or tool changes where employees may be exposed to unexpected energization or start-up of equipment or release of stored energy.
9. *Tag Out.* The placement of a "DANGER—DO NOT OPERATE" tag on an energy isolating device in accordance with an established procedure to indicate that the energy isolating device must not be operated until the tag is removed.

GENERAL REQUIREMENTS

Energy Control Program

The energy control program consists of a lock out/tag out procedure and employee training to ensure that the hazardous energy sources are isolated and rendered inoperative before an employee performs maintenance on equipment where the unexpected energization, start-up, or release of stored energy could cause injury.

Lock Out/Tag Out

1. Energy isolating devices capable of being locked out shall be locked out and tagged according to the lock out/tag out procedure.
2. Energy isolating devices incapable of being locked out shall be tagged out according to the lock out/tag out procedure.
3. Whenever equipment is installed, relocated, or undergoes major modification, renovation, or repair, energy isolating devices capable of being locked out shall be installed.

Full Employee Protection

1. A tag out device alone shall never be used on an energy-isolating device that is capable of being locked out.
2. When a tag out device alone is used because an energy isolating device is incapable of being locked out, additional safety measures shall be taken to reduce the likelihood of inadvertent energization (e.g., removing an isolating circuit element, blocking of a controlling switch, removing a valve handle, opening an extra disconnecting device, etc.).

Energy Control (Lock Out/Tag Out) Procedure

1. A procedure shall be developed, initiated, and utilized for the lock out/tag out of potentially hazardous energies during maintenance of each type of equipment.

   Exception: In certain limited situations, because of the simplicity of a particular piece of equipment and the lock out measures to be used, a documented procedure may not be required when all of the following elements exist:
   a. The equipment has no potential for stored or residual energy.
   b. The equipment has a single, readily identified and isolated energy source.
   c. The isolation and lock out of that energy source will completely de-energize and deactivate the equipment.
   d. The equipment is isolated from that energy source and locked out during maintenance.
   e. A single lockout device will achieve a locked out condition.
   f. The lock out device is under the exclusive control of the AUTHORIZED EMPLOYEE performing the maintenance.
   g. The maintenance does not create hazards for other employees.
   h. There have been no previous incidents involving the unexpected activation or reenergization of the equipment during maintenance.
2. The procedure shall clearly and distinctly outline the scope, purpose, authorization, rules, techniques to be applied, and the measures to enforce compliance. The procedure shall include the following:
   a. A specific statement about the intended use of the procedure
   b. Specific steps for shutting down, isolating, blocking, and securing equipment to control hazardous energy sources
   c. Specific steps for the placement, removal, and transfer of lock out/tag out devices and the responsibility for them
   d. Specific requirements for testing equipment to determine and verify the effectiveness of lock out/tag out devices and other energy control measures
   e. Specialized training, testing, and certifying program for all authorized employees

Protective Materials and Hardware

1. Locks, tags, chains, wedges, key blocks, adapter pins, self-locking fasteners, or other hardware shall be provided for isolating, securing, or blocking equipment energy sources.
2. Locks and tag out devices shall be singularly identified, shall be the only devices used for controlling energy, and shall not be used for other purposes. Lock out/tag out devices shall meet the following requirements:
   a. Lock out/tag out devices shall be capable of withstanding the environment to which they are exposed for the maximum period of time that exposure is expected. Tag out devices shall withstand exposure to weather conditions and wet or damp locations without deteriorating or becoming illegible.
   b. Locks and tag out devices shall be standardized in color, shape, and size. Tag out device print and format shall be standardized.
   c. Lock out devices shall be substantial enough to prevent removal without the use of excessive force or unusual techniques. Tag out devices, including their means of attachment, shall be substantial enough to prevent inadvertent or accidental removal. The attachment means shall be a self-locking, nonreusable nylon cable tie.
   d. Tag out devices shall indicate the name of the authorized employee applying the energy isolation device as well as the equipment name or number being isolated and a brief description of the maintenance being performed.
3. Tag out devices shall warn against hazardous conditions if the equipment is energized and shall include the legend "DANGER—DO NOT OPERATE."

Periodic Inspection

1. The Lock Out/Tag Out Periodic Inspection Form shall be used by managers to conduct periodic inspections of the lock out/tag out procedure, at least annually, to ensure the procedures and the requirements of this standard are being followed. An AUTHORIZED EMPLOYEE other than the employee using the procedure being inspected shall conduct the inspection. Inspection results shall be used to correct any deviations or inadequacies observed. The inspection shall include a review of responsibilities with each AUTHORIZED EMPLOYEE. If tag out only is used for energy control, the inspection shall also include a review of responsibilities with each AFFECTED EMPLOYEE.

2. Periodic inspection shall be certified. The certification shall identify the equipment on which the lock out/tag out procedure was being used, the inspection date the employees included in the inspection, and the name of the person conducting the inspection.

TRAINING AND COMMUNICATION

1. Training shall be provided by managers to ensure that the purpose and function of the energy control program are understood and the employees have the knowledge and skills required for the safe application, usage, and removal of energy controls. Training shall include the following:
   a. ALL EMPLOYEES shall be instructed on the significance of lock out/tag out procedures and the purpose and function lock out/tag out devices. They shall also be instructed to never disturb, bypass, defeat, tamper with, ignore, or attempt to operate any devices or start up any equipment which has a "DANGER—DO NOT OPERATE" tag affixed to it. The "DANGER—DO NOT OPERATE" tag shall only be removed by the AUTHORIZED EMPLOYEE who attached it.
   b. AFFECTED EMPLOYEES shall be instructed on the purpose and use of lock out/tag out procedures.
   c. AUTHORIZED EMPLOYEES shall be instructed on the standard and procedure, how to recognize hazardous energies, and the type and magnitude of the energy available, on the methods and means necessary for energy isolation and control, and on conducting periodic inspections.

2. AUTHORIZED and AFFECTED EMPLOYEES shall also be trained in the following limitations of tags used without lock out devices:
   a. Tags are essentially warning devices and do not provide the physical restraint that is provided by a lock.
   b. Tags shall only be removed by the AUTHORIZED EMPLOYEES who attached them. They shall never be bypassed, ignored, or otherwise defeated.
   c. Tags shall be legible and understandable by all employees who are or may be in the area.
   d. Tags and their attachment means shall be made of materials that will withstand the environmental conditions encountered in the workplace.
   e. Tags may evoke a false sense of security, and their meaning needs to be understood.
   f. Tags shall be securely attached to energy isolating devices so that they cannot be inadvertently or accidentally detached.

3. Retraining shall be provided for AUTHORIZED and AFFECTED EMPLOYEES whenever there is a change in their job assignment, a change in the equipment or process that presents a new hazard, a change in the lock out/tag out procedure, whenever a periodic inspection with that employee occurs, [whenever a] near miss or injury reveals there are deviations from or inadequacies in the employees' use of the procedure, or at least annually. Retraining shall reestablish employee proficiency and introduce new or revised control methods and procedures, as necessary.

4. Training records shall certify that the employee's training has been accomplished and is being kept up to date. The certification shall contain the employee's name, training date(s), and the highest level of training module conducted for each employee (ALL, AFFECTED, or AUTHORIZED).

PROCEDURE FOR APPLYING LOCK OUT/TAG OUT

Implementation of the lock out/tag out procedure shall be performed only by an AUTHORIZED EMPLOYEE. Each lock out/tag out procedure shall cover the following elements and actions and shall be implemented in the following sequence:

1. Notification of Employees
   The AUTHORIZED EMPLOYEE shall notify all AFFECTED EMPLOYEES when lock out/tag out devices are applied or removed.
2. Preparation for Shutdown
   Before equipment is shut down, the AUTHORIZED EMPLOYEE shall know the magnitude, source, and hazards of and the method or means to control each type of hazardous energy.
3. Machine or Equipment Shutdown
   Operating equipment shall be shut down using the normal stopping procedure to avoid any additional or increased hazard.
4. Machine or Equipment Isolation
   Energy isolating devices shall be located and operated such that the equipment is isolated from every energy source.
5. Lock Out/Tag Out Application
   a. A lock out/tag out device shall be affixed to each energy isolating device by the AUTHORIZED EMPLOYEE.
   b. The lock out device shall be affixed in a manner that will hold the energy isolating device in a "safe" or "off" position.
   c. A tag out device shall be affixed in a manner that will clearly indicate the operation or movement of the energy isolating device from the safe or off position is prohibited. When the tag cannot be affixed directly to the energy isolating device, the tag shall be located as close as safely possible to the device, in a position that will be immediately obvious to anyone attempting to operate the device. The tag out device must be completely filled out with the AUTHORIZED EMPLOYEE's name, the equipment name and/or number, as well as a brief description of the maintenance being performed.
6. Stored Energy
   All potentially hazardous stored or residual energy shall be relieved, disconnected, restrained, or otherwise rendered safe. If there is a possibility of reaccumulation of stored energy to a hazardous level, verification of isolation shall be continued until the maintenance is completed or until the possibility of such accumulation no longer exists.
7. Verification of Isolation
   Prior to starting work on equipment that has been locked out and/or tagged out, the AUTHORIZED EMPLOYEE shall verify that isolation and de-energization of the equipment has been accomplished.
   a. After locks and tags have been applied to equipment, verification must be done to ensure that all the energy sources are disconnected and that the equipment is inoperative. Appropriate test equipment must be used to verify that the circuits and equipment are de-energized.
   b. All equipment controls such as push buttons, selector switches, and electrical interlocks must be tested to ensure that equipment cannot be restarted. When equipment is shut down, the off button should be engaged so the equipment will not restart automatically when energized.

Release From Lock Out/Tag Out

Before the lock out/tag out device is removed and energy is restored to the equipment, actions shall be taken to ensure the following:
1. Equipment
   The work area shall be inspected by the AUTHORIZED EMPLOYEE to ensure that nonessential items have been removed and that the equipment components are operationally intact.
2. Employees
   AFFECTED EMPLOYEES shall be notified by the AUTHORIZED EMPLOYEE that the lock out/tag out device is being removed and the work area shall be checked to ensure that all employees have been safely positioned or removed.

3. Lock Out/Tag Out Device Removal

Each lock out/tag out device shall be removed from each energy-isolating device by the employee who applied it. If the employee who applied the lock out/tag out device is not available to remove it, the device may be removed only the employee's manager who shall

a. Verify that the employee who applied the lock out/tag out device is not on the site.

b. Make all reasonable efforts to contact the employee to inform him/her that the lock out/tag out device must be removed.

c. Verify that it is safe to remove the lock out/tag out device and restore the energy to the equipment.

d. Ensure that the employee knows that his/her lock out/tag out device was removed before he/she resumes work at the site. (See accompanying "Lock Out Removal Notice.")

ADDITIONAL REQUIREMENTS

Exceptional Conditions

Exceptional conditions may require equipment to be worked on without being locked out or tagged out. Troubleshooting equipment in an energized state presents a high degree of potential safety hazard and must be performed only by authorized personnel experienced in the functions, operations, and safety hazards of that particular piece of equipment. Due to the nature of troubleshooting work (tracing and identifying faults), it is necessary to allow certain personnel to perform work while the equipment remains energized.

1. Only personnel trained to perform the needed functions are permitted to operate under this procedure.

2. The area supervisor shall barricade the equipment in such a fashion as to maintain operations and protect personnel.

3. Prior to troubleshooting, the area supervisor shall transfer ownership when applicable.

4. IF THE EQUIPMENT MUST BE OPERATED FOR TROUBLESHOOTING PURPOSES, NO ADJUSTMENT OR ALTERATIONS WHICH MAY EXPOSE THE PERSON TO AN INJURY SHALL BE MADE WITHOUT LOCKING OUT THE EQUIPMENT. SPECIFICALLY, REPAIR OR REPLACEMENT OF COMPONENTS REQUIRES A LOCK OUT.

5. All mechanical guards should be in place when equipment is operated. Any guards that must be removed for observation purposes during troubleshooting must be included in the area troubleshooting procedures.

6. Any necessary lock out/tag out devices shall be applied by the person performing the actual repair only.

7. When troubleshooting/repair is complete, the troubleshooter will replace all guards and transfer ownership back when applicable.

When a lock out/tag out device must be temporarily removed from the energy-isolating device and the equipment energized to test, position, or debug the equipment or a component thereof, the following sequence shall be followed:

1. Clear the equipment of tools and materials.

2. Remove employees from the equipment area.

3. Remove the lock out/tag out device.

4. Energize the equipment and proceed with testing, positioning, or debugging.

5. De-energize all systems and reapply energy control measures before continuing maintenance.

Outside Personnel (Contractors, etc.)

These requirements apply to all personnel. Contractors' lock out/tag out devices may vary. However, the same level of control shall be provided by the contractors' isolation devices. Before maintenance work is started, the manager of the area shall ensure that his/her AFFECTED EMPLOYEES and the contractors' employees understand GoodMark Foods' lock out/tag out procedures.

Group Lock Out/Tag Out

When maintenance is performed by more than one AUTHORIZED EMPLOYEE, the lock out/tag out procedures used shall afford a level of protection equivalent to that provided by the implementing of a personal lock out/tag out device. The lock out/tag out procedure used shall comply with the following specific requirements:

1. Primary responsibility for implementation of the procedure shall be assigned to one lead employee who shall attach a group lock out device to each energy isolating device.
2. The lead employee shall ascertain the exposure status of each of the other employees in his/her department.
3. When more than one department is involved in the maintenance activity, one lead employee shall be designated to coordinate the overall activity and ensure continuity of protection.
4. Each employee shall affix his/her personal lock out device to each group lock out when he/she begins work and shall remove each device when he/she stops working on the equipment.

Shift or Personnel Changes

Specific procedures shall be utilized during shift or personnel changes to ensure the continuity of lock out/tag out protection, including provisions for the orderly transfer of lock out/tag out devices between outgoing and incoming employees, to minimize exposure to hazards from unexpected energization or start-up of equipment or release of stored energy. While work is in progress, equipment on which work is being performed must be locked out continuously. When a change in personnel on the job occurs, any incoming employees must lock the equipment before work has begun. The first employee may now remove his lock. Arrangements must be made to keep the equipment locked by individuals involved in the work. The rule of one person, one lock, one key must be followed at all times.

Contractor Work

Contractor work is covered by this document. Any electrical work requires lock out if the circuits involved are capable of being energized. Once cables or other circuit elements are connected at the source, lock out must take place while work continues. Contractors are not permitted to work unless they have been trained in this procedure. The coordinator will arrange for this training.

The coordinator will lock out equipment when a contractor is not present to control the energy sources. When one contractor completes his part of a job and will not be expected to return, the coordinator will control the energy sources during the absence of a contractor. A contractor must not leave a job site unless the lock out is transferred to another contractor, to the coordinator or a check-out lock and sign-off tag are attached.

For service interruptions, the equipment must be locked and tagged by the operating employee or engineer and then turned over to the coordinator and contractor. Two locks would be used in this situation. For example, if the coordinator does not know how to lock out equipment, a knowledgeable plant employee would lock out the equipment and then turn that equipment over to the coordinator and contractor.

Other Hazards

Materials having toxic, caustic, or asphyxiant properties can present serious hazards beyond the scope of this standard. Additional guidelines may have to be met to ensure a safe working environment. Consult with your supervisor prior to starting work.

LOCK OUT/TAG OUT TRAINING

OSHA Standard 29 CFR 1910.147, The Control of Hazardous Energy (Lock Out/Tag Out), took effect in 1989.

The standard affects the servicing and maintenance of equipment where the unexpected energization, start-up, or release of hazardous energy could cause injury. It imposes requirements which must be followed by ALL EMPLOYEES.

ALL EMPLOYEES, regardless of their work assignment, must be trained in the significance of lock out/tag out procedures and on the purpose and function of lock out/tag out devices. The attached training module for ALL EMPLOYEES may be used for this training requirement.

Employees that operate equipment or who work in an area where lock out/tag out devices are used are classified by OSHA as AFFECTED EMPLOYEES. Because of the added exposure, AFFECTED EMPLOYEES require training on the lock out/tag out procedure in addition to the training for ALL EMPLOYEES. The attached training module for AFFECTED EMPLOYEE and the LOCK OUT/TAG OUT PROCEDURE should be used for this training requirement.

Employees that you authorize to maintain or service equipment must receive the same training as ALL EMPLOYEES and AFFECTED EMPLOYEES. In addition, they must understand the standard and be trained to implement lock out/tag out procedures and conduct periodic inspections. They must also be given the knowledge and skills to recognize, isolate, and control hazardous energies and to safely apply, use, and remove energy controls. Finally, they must be trained in the limitations of tags used without lock out devices. The attached information is provided to assist you in developing your AUTHORIZED EMPLOYEE training module.

Please retain the training module for your required retraining and for training new or reassigned employees. Retraining is required for AFFECTED and AUTHORIZED EMPLOYEES whenever there is a change in their job assignment, a change in the equipment or process that presents a new hazard, a change in the lock out/tag out procedure, or whenever a periodic inspection, near miss, or injury reveals there are deviations from or inadequacies in the employees' use of the procedure. Retraining shall reestablish employee proficiency and introduce new or revised control methods and procedures, as necessary.

Training records shall certify that employees' training has been accomplished and is being kept up to date. The certification shall contain the employee's name, the training date(s) and the highest level of training module conducted for each employee (ALL, AFFECTED, or AUTHORIZED).

The standard affects the servicing and maintenance of equipment where the unexpected energization, start-up, or release of hazardous energy could cause injury. It does not apply, however, to cord and plug connected equipment (e.g. PC's, terminals, etc.).

ALL EMPLOYEES, regardless of their work assignment, must understand the significance of lock out/tag out procedures and the purpose and function of lock out/tag out devices.

A Lock Out/Tag Out Procedure must be implemented and followed to ensure all potentially hazardous energy sources are disabled, isolated, and locked out or tagged out before maintenance or service is performed on equipment. Employees must not implement a lock out/tag out procedure unless they are trained and authorized to do so by their manager.

LOCK OUT/TAG OUT TRAINING MODULE FOR ALL EMPLOYEES

Lock out devices consist of locks, chains, blocks, etc., which are used to disable potentially hazardous energies. They must be accompanied by a tag out device to indicate the identity of the person applying the lock out device and to warn against the hazardous conditions if the equipment were to be energized.

A tag with the legend "DANGER—DO NOT OPERATE" and a lock are the only lock out/tag out devices approved for use. They shall not be used for any other purpose.

Locks and tags will be most commonly used in manufacturing and laboratory areas. However, a lock and tag or a tag alone could be attached to a circuit breaker on a panel or to a light switch in an office area.

Employees must never disturb, bypass, defeat, tamper with, ignore, or attempt to operate any devices or start up any equipment which has a "DANGER—DO NOT OPERATE" tag affixed to it. The "DANGER—DO NOT OPERATE" tag shall only be removed by the AUTHORIZED EMPLOYEE who attached it.

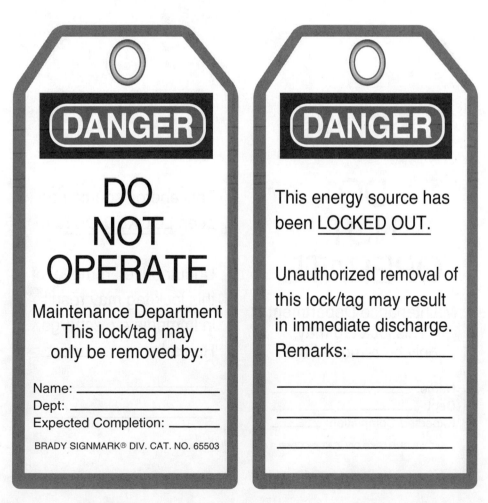

| Front | Back |

LOCK OUT/TAG OUT TRAINING MODULE FOR AFFECTED EMPLOYEES

The site safety standard defines an AFFECTED EMPLOYEE as an employee whose job requires him/her to operate equipment in an area where maintenance is performed on equipment.

AFFECTED EMPLOYEES must understand the information contained in the training module for ALL EMPLOYEES. They must also understand the purpose and use of lock out/tag out procedures.

It is vital to the safety of employees performing maintenance and service on equipment that AFFECTED EMPLOYEES understand the significance of lock out/tag out devices and procedures.

Tag out devices used alone may evoke a false sense of security. Therefore, their meaning must be understood. Tag out devices are essentially warning devices and do not provide the physical restraint that is provided by a lock. Tag out devices shall only be removed by the AUTHORIZED EMPLOYEE who attached them.

Periodic inspection of lock out/tag out procedures will be conducted at least annually to ensure that the procedures and the standard are being followed. This inspection will include a review with all AFFECTED EMPLOYEES regarding their responsibilities under the lock out/tag out procedure when a tag out is used alone.

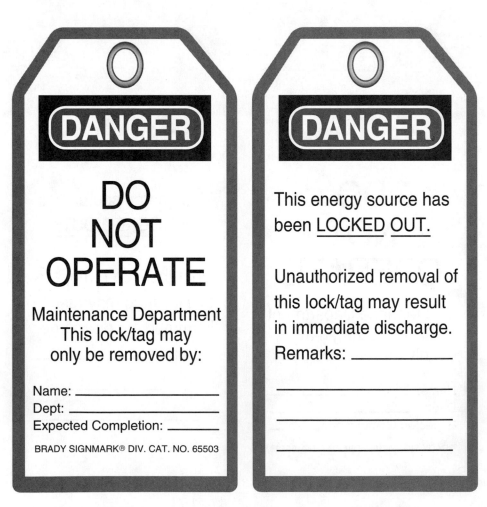

Front   **Back**

LOCK OUT/TAG OUT INFORMATION FOR DEVELOPING TRAINING MODULE FOR AUTHORIZED EMPLOYEES

The OSHA safety standard defines an AUTHORIZED EMPLOYEE as an employee who has been given the authority, responsibility, and training by his/her manager to implement a lock out/tag out procedure prior to starting with maintenance on equipment. Because AUTHORIZED EMPLOYEES are charged with this responsibility, it is important that they receive training in recognizing and understanding all potentially hazardous energy sources that they might be exposed to during their work assignments.

Your AUTHORIZED EMPLOYEES must also be trained in the use of adequate methods and means to isolate and control hazardous energy sources. They must be able to safely apply, use, and remove lock out/tag out devices. They need extensive training in the lock out/tag out procedure, its limitations, and its proper use. They must also be able to conduct periodic inspections of lock out/tag out procedures.

OSHA requires that lock and tags be singularly identified, and they are only devices used for controlling energy and not used for any other purpose. Locks and tags must be standardized in color, shape, or size. Tags must be standardized in print and format. A lock and tag should be obtained for each AUTHORIZED EMPLOYEE. A quantity of unassigned department locks, tags, and multiple locking devices should be obtained to cover the lock out of multiple energy sources.

Managers of employees authorized to implement lock out/tag out procedures must ensure that periodic inspections are conducted at least annually to ensure that the procedures and the standard are being followed by the AUTHORIZED EMPLOYEES. This inspection shall also include a review with all AFFECTED EMPLOYEES regarding their responsibilities when a tag out procedure is being inspected.

LOCK OUT/TAG OUT PERIODIC INSPECTION FORM

Tool/ID # _____   Equipment Name _____

Date of Inspection _____   Authorized Inspector's Name _____

Names of Authorized and Affected Employees Inspected _____

_____

_____

Removal of Equipment From Service			(Circle correct answer)

1. Were all affected employees notified that the machine or equipment was going to be locked out/tagged out? **YES   NO   N/A**

2. Were all the hazardous energy sources and the associated energy isolating devices correctly identified and located? **YES   NO**

3. Was the equipment shutdown performed correctly? **YES   NO**

4. Were the energy isolating devices operating so that the equipment was isolated from all hazardous energy sources? **YES   NO**

5. Were lock out/tag out devices placed on all the energy isolating devices? **YES   NO**

6. Were approved lock out/tag out devices used and listed in the procedure? **YES   NO**

7. Were all potentially hazardous stored energies relieved, restrained, or otherwise rendered safe? **YES   NO   N/A**

8. Was the isolation of hazardous energy sources verified to be affected by testing with appropriate instrumentation and by operating the normal equipment controls after ensuring that no personnel were exposed? **YES   NO**

9. Were the equipment controls returned to the neutral or off position after verifying that the equipment would not start up or cycle? **YES   NO**

10. Were the additional procedures dealing with shift or personnel changes, group lock out/tag out, and testing/positioning of equipment followed? **YES   NO   N/A**

11. Were unique lock out/tag out requirements for this equipment written in the procedure and followed? **YES   NO   N/A**

Release from Lock Out/Tag Out

12. Was the work area checked to ensure that all tools were removed, all shields were properly reinstalled, all interlocks were restored, and that the area was clear of hazards and personnel before the equipment was reenergized? **YES   NO**

13. Were all affected employees notified that the equipment was going to be returned to service? **YES   NO   N/A**

14. Were the lock out/tag out devices removed by the authorized employees who attached them? **YES   NO**

15. Were the energy isolating devices operated to restore energy
     to the equipment?   YES   NO

General Requirements

16. Does the lock out/tag out procedure provide adequate
    employee protection?   YES   NO

17. Did the authorized employees correctly explain their responsibilities
    under the lock out/tag out procedure being inspected?   YES   NO

18. Did the affected employees correctly explain their responsibilities
    under the lock out/tag out procedure being inspected?   YES   NO

NOTE: All "NO" responses require corrective action with dates for completion. Use the space below to specify.

COMMENTS: _____

_____

_____

_____

_____

_____

_____

_____

I certify the completing of this inspection.

Manager's Signature _____ Date _____ Dept. _____

NOTE: Department manager shall retain the completed inspection forms for audit purposes.

SAFETY TAGS

Use of Tags

1. "DANGER—DO NOT OPERATE" Tag
   a. Used to prevent accidental operation or to discontinue the operation of equipment or systems which would create unsafe conditions or damage property. The tag is used in accordance with lock out/tag out procedures.
   b. Used with a lock or other positive locking device.
   c. May be removed only by the person who applied it or the immediate manager in accordance with procedures.
2. "WARNING" Tag
   a. Attached to all new, relocated, or modified equipment and facilities.
   NOTE: The equipment/facility will not be utilized until the installation is complete and all designated personnel have inspected and approved or a caution tag is affixed.
   b. Attached by any of the following: using manager, facilities coordinator, facilities maintenance, equipment maintenance, project engineer, safety engineer, industrial or equipment engineer.
   c. Removed only after all required inspections are complete.
   d. The completed tag must be retained in the using or responsible department. A copy of the completed tag must be placed in the project file by the coordinator or engineer.

LOCK OUT REMOVAL NOTICE

Date/Time: _____

To: _____

    (Name of Employee whose lock is removed)

From: _____

    (Name of Manager removing lock)

1. SAFETY LOCK AND "DO NOT OPERATE" TAGS WERE REMOVED BY ME FROM THE FOL-
   LOWING EQUIPMENT:

   _____

   _____

2. LOCATION:

   _____

   _____

3. FOR THE FOLLOWING REASONS:

   _____

   _____

   _____

_____

(Signature of Manager removing lock)

Distribution (one copy to each):

_____Employee received before next work shift

_____Safety

_____Department Manager removing lock

_____Posted at job side where work was in progress

_____Posted where lock out was removed

CONTROL OF HAZARDOUS ENERGY SOURCE
(LOCK OUT/TAG OUT)
29 CFR 1910.147

Department: _____   Date: _____
Presented by: _____   Method: _____

I, as an employee of GoodMark Foods, Inc., attended the annual training and information program for employees who must use the Lock Out/Tag Out procedure. The program included all pertinent information as mandated in the federal regulations.

Attendees

Print Name   Signature

_____   _____
_____   _____
_____   _____
_____   _____
_____   _____
_____   _____
_____   _____
_____   _____
_____   _____
_____   _____
_____   _____

15-4 Sample Hazard Communication Program

INTRODUCTION

The Hazard Communication Standard requires you to develop a written hazard communication program. The following is a sample hazard communication program that you may use as a guide in developing your program.

OUR HAZARD COMMUNICATION PROGRAM

General Company Policy

The purpose of this notice is to inform you that our company is complying with the OSHA Hazard Communication Standard, Title 29 Code of Federal Regulations 1910.1200, by compiling a hazardous chemicals list, using MSDSs, ensuring that containers are labeled, and providing you with training.

This program applies to all work operations in our company where you may be exposed to hazardous chemicals under normal working conditions or during an emergency situation.

The safety and health manager, Robert Jones, is the program coordinator, acting as the representative of the plant manager, who has overall responsibility for the program. Mr. Jones will review and update the program, as necessary. Copies of the written program may be obtained from Mr. Jones in Room SD-10.

Under this program you will be informed of the contents of the Hazard Communication Standard, the hazardous properties of chemicals with which you work, the safe handling procedures, and the measures to take to protect yourselves from these chemicals. You will also be informed of the hazards associated with nonroutine tasks, such as the cleaning of reactor vessels, and the hazards associated with chemicals in unlabeled pipes.

List of Hazardous Chemicals

The safety and health manager will make a list of all hazardous chemicals and related work practices used in the facility and will update the list as necessary. Our list of chemicals identifies all of the chemicals used in our 10 work process areas.

A separate list is available for each work area and is posted there. Each list also identifies the corresponding MSDS for each chemical. A master list of these chemicals will be maintained by and is available from Mr. Jones' office, Room SD-10.

Material Safety Data Sheets (MSDSs)

MSDSs provide you with specific information on the chemicals you use. The safety and health manager will maintain a binder in his office with an MSDS on every substance on the list of hazardous chemicals. The plant manager, Jeff O'Brien, will ensure that each work site maintains MSDSs for the hazardous chemicals in each work area. MSDSs will be made readily available to you at your work stations during your shifts.

The safety and health manager is responsible for acquiring and updating MSDSs. He will contact the chemical manufacturer or vendor if additional research is necessary or if an MSDS has not been supplied with an initial shipment. All new procurements for the company must be cleared by the safety and health manager. A master list of MSDSs is available from Mr. Jones in Room SD-10.

Labels and Other Forms of Warning

The safety and health manager will ensure that all hazardous chemicals in the plant are properly labeled and updated as necessary. Labels should list at least the chemical identity, appropriate hazard warnings, and the name and address of the manufacturer, importer, or other responsible party. Mr. Jones will refer to the corresponding MSDS to assist you in verifying label information. Containers that are shipped from the plant will be checked by the supervisor of shipping and receiving to make sure all containers are property labeled.

If a number of stationary containers within a work area have similar contents and hazards, signs will be posted on them to convey hazard information. On stationary process equipment regular process sheets, batch tickets, blend tickets, and similar written materials will be substituted for container labels when these documents contain the same information as labels. These written materials will be made readily available to you during your work shift.

If you transfer chemicals from a labeled container to a portable container that is intended only for your immediate use, no labels are required on the portable container. Pipes or piping systems will not be labeled, but their contents will be described in training sessions.

Nonroutine Tasks

When you are required to perform hazardous nonroutine tasks (e.g., cleaning tanks, entering confined spaces), a special training session will be conducted to inform you of the hazardous chemicals to which you might be exposed and the precautions you must take to reduce or avoid exposure.

Training

Everyone who works with or is potentially exposed to hazardous chemicals will receive initial training on the Hazard Communication Standard and the safe use of those hazardous chemicals. The safety and health manager will conduct these training sessions. A program that uses both audiovisual materials and classroom-type training has been prepared for this purpose. Whenever a new hazard is introduced, additional training will be provided. Regular safety meetings will also be used to review the information presented in the initial training. Foremen and other supervisors will be extensively trained regarding hazards and appropriate protective measures so they will be available to answer questions from employees and provide daily monitoring of safe work practices.

The training program will emphasize these items:

- A summary of the standard and this company's written program
- The chemical and physical properties of hazardous materials (e.g., flash point, vapor pressure, reactivity) and methods that can be used to detect the presence or release of chemicals (including chemicals in unlabeled pipes)
- The physical hazards of the chemicals in your work area (e.g., potential for fire, explosion)
- The health hazards, including signs and symptoms of exposure to the chemicals in the work area and any medical condition known to be aggravated by exposure to these chemicals
- Procedures to protect against chemical hazards (e.g., required personal protective equipment and its proper use and maintenance, work practices or methods to ensure appropriate use and handling of chemicals, and procedures for emergency response)
- Work procedures to follow to ensure protection when cleaning hazardous chemical spills and leaks
- The location of the MSDSs, how to read and interpret the information on labels and MSDSs, and how employees may obtain additional hazard information.

The safety and health manager or his/her designee will review the employee training program and advise the plant manager on training or retraining needs. Retraining is required when the hazard changes or when a new hazard is introduced into the workplace. It will be company policy to provide training regularly in safety meetings to ensure the effectiveness of the program. As part of the assessment of the training program, the safety and health manager will obtain input from employees regarding the training they have received and their suggestions for improvement.

Contractor Employers

The safety and health manager upon notification by the responsible supervisor, will advise outside contractors in person of any chemical hazards that may be encountered in the normal course of their work on the premises, the labeling system in use, the protective measures to be taken, and the safe handling procedures to be used. In addition, Mr. Jones will notify these individuals of the location and availability of MSDSs. Each contractor bringing chemicals on-site must provide Mr. Jones with the appropriate hazard information for these substances, including MSDSs, labels, and precautionary measures to be taken when working with or around these chemicals.

Additional Information

All employees or their designated representatives can obtain further information on this written program, the hazard communication standard, applicable MSDSs, and chemical information lists at the safety and health office, Room SD-10.

From *Hazard Communication Compliance Guidelines: OSHA 3111*, by Occupational Safety and Health Administration, 1998, Washington, DC: Author.

APPENDIX 15-5 Hazard Communication

Hazard Communication Checklist

___ 1. Has a list of all hazardous chemicals in the workplace been prepared?

___ 2. Does the company have a method for updating the hazardous chemical list?

___ 3. Has the company obtained or developed a material safety data sheet for each hazardous chemical used?

___ 4. Has a system been developed to ensure that all incoming hazardous chemicals have labels and data sheets?

___ 5. Are procedures in place to ensure labeling for containers of hazardous chemicals?

___ 6. Are employees aware of the requirements of the Hazard Communication Standard and information specific to the workplace?

___ 7. Are employees familiar with the hazards of the chemicals in their workplace?

___ 8. Have employees been informed of the hazards associated with performing nonroutine tasks?

___ 9. Do employees understand how to detect the presence or release of hazardous chemicals in their workplace?

___ 10. Are employees trained about proper work practices and personal protective equipment in relation to the hazardous chemicals in their work area?

___ 11. Does the training program provide information on appropriate first aid, emergency procedures, and the likely symptoms of overexposure?

___ 12. Does the training program include an explanation of labels and warnings that are used in each work area?

___ 13. Does the training describe where employees obtain data sheets and how employees use them?

___   14.   Is a system in place to ensure that new employees are trained before beginning work?

___   15.   Is a system in place to identify new hazardous chemicals before they are introduced into a work area?

___   16.   Is a system in place to inform employees of the hazards associated with newly introduced chemicals?

From *Hazard Communication Compliance Guidelines: OSHA 3111,* by Occupational Safety and Health Administration, 1998, Washington, DC: Author.

15-6 Declination of Hepatitis B Vaccination Form

The following statement of declination of hepatitis B vaccination must be signed by an employee who chooses *not to accept* the vaccine. The statement can only be signed by the employee following appropriate training regarding hepatitis B; hepatitis B vaccination; the efficacy, safety, method of administration, and benefits of vaccination; and the provision of the vaccine and vaccination free of charge to the employee. The statement is not a waiver; the employee can request and receive the hepatitis B vaccination at a later date if she or he remains occupationally at risk for hepatitis B.

Declination Statement

    I understand that due to my occupational exposure to blood or other potentially infectious materials I may be at risk of acquiring hepatitis B virus (HBV) infection. I have been given the opportunity to be vaccinated with hepatitis B vaccine, at no charge to myself. However, I decline hepatitis B vaccination at this time. I understand that by declining this vaccine I continue to be at risk of acquiring hepatitis B, a serious disease. If in the future I continue to have occupational exposure to blood or other potentially infectious materials and I want to be vaccinated with hepatitis B vaccine, I can receive the vaccination series at no charge to me.

Employee Signature _____ Date _____

15-7A Log of Work-Related Injuries and Illnesses

OSHA's Form 300
Log of Work-Related Injuries and Illnesses

You must record information about every work-related injury or illness that involves loss of consciousness, restricted work activity or job transfer, days away from work, or medical treatment beyond first aid. You must also record significant work-related injuries and illnesses that are diagnosed by a physician or licensed health care professional. You must also record work-related injuries and illnesses that meet any of the specific recording criteria listed in 29 CFR 1904.8 through 1904.12. Feel free to use two lines for a single case if you need to. You must complete an injury and illness incident report (OSHA Form 301) or equivalent form for each injury or illness recorded on this form. If you're not sure whether a case is recordable, call your local OSHA office for help.

Identify the person				Describe the case	
(A) Case No.	(B) Employee's Name	(C) Job Title (e.g., Welder)	(D) Date of injury or onset of illness (mo./day)	(E) Where the event occurred (e.g., Loading dock north end)	(F) Describe injury or illness, parts of body affected, and object/substance that directly injured or made person ill (e.g., Second degree burns on right forearm from acetylene torch)

Public reporting burden for this collection of information is estimated to average 14 minutes per response, including time to review the instruction, search and gather the data needed, and complete and review the collection of information. Persons are not required to respond to the collection of information unless it displays a currently valid OMB control number. If you have any comments about these estimates or any aspects of this data collection, contact: US Department of Labor, OSHA Office of Statistics, Room N-3644, 200 Constitution Ave., NW, Washington, DC 20210. Do not send the completed forms to this office.

Attention: This form contains information relating to employee health and must be used in a manner that protects the confidentiality of employees to the extent possible while the information is being used for occupational safety and health purposes.

Year _____

U.S. Department of Labor
Occupational Safety and Health Administration

Form approved OMB no. 1218-0176

Establishment name _____

City _____　　State _____

Classify the case

Using these categories, check ONLY the most serious result for each case:

Enter the number of days the injured or ill worker was:

Check the "injury" column or choose one type of illness:

Death	Days away from work	Remained at work		On job transfer or restriction (days)	Away from work (days)	(M) Injury	Skin Disorder	Respiratory Condition	Poisoning	All other illnesses
		Job transfer or restriction	Other recordable cases							
(G)	(H)	(I)	(J)	(K)	(L)	(1)	(2)	(3)	(4)	(5)
Page totals 0	0	0	0	0	0	0	0	0	0	0

Be sure to transfer these totals to the Summary page (Form 300A) before you post it.

Injury (1)　Skin Disorder (2)　Respiratory Condition (3)　Poisoning (4)　All other illnesses (5)

Page　1 of 1

From *U.S. Department of Labor, Occupational Safety and Health Administration,* http://www.osha-slc.gov/recordkeeping/ OSHArecordkeepingforms.pdf.

15-7B Summary of Work-Related Injuries and Illnesses

OSHA's Form 300A
Summary of Work-Related Injuries and Illnesses

All establishments covered by Part 1904 must complete this Summary page, even if no injuries or illnesses occurred during the year. Remember to review the Log to verify that the entries are complete.

Using the Log, count the individual entries you made for each category. Then write the totals below, making sure you've added the entries from every page of the log. If you had no cases, write "0."

Employees, former employees, and their representatives have the right to review the OSHA Form 300 in its entirety. They also have limited access to the OSHA Form 301 or its equivalent. See 29 CFR 1904.35, in OSHA's Recordkeeping rule, for further details on the access provisions for these forms.

Number of Cases

Total number of deaths	Total number of cases with days away from work	Total number of cases with job transfer or restriction	Total number of other recordable cases
0	0	0	0
(G)	(H)	(I)	(J)

Number of Days

Total number of days of job transfer or restriction	Total number of days away from work
0	0
(K)	(L)

Injury and Illness Types

Total number of...
(M)

(1) Injury	0	(4) Poisoning	0
(2) Skin Disorder	0	(5) All other illnesses	0
(3) Respiratory Condition	0		

Post this Summary page from February 1 to April 30 of the year following the year covered by the form.

Public reporting burden for this collection of information is estimated to average 50 minutes per response, including time to review the instruction, search and gather the data needed, and complete and review the collection of information. Persons are not required to respond to the collection of information unless it displays a currently valid OMB control number. If you have any comments about these estimates or any aspects of this data collection, contact: US Department of Labor, OSHA Office of Statistics, Room N-3644, 200 Constitution Ave., NW, Washington, DC 20210. Do not send the completed forms to this office.

Year_____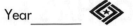

U.S. Department of Labor
Occupational Safety and Health Administration

Form approved OMB no. 1218-0176

Establishment information

Your establishment name _____

Street _____

City _____ State _____ Zip _____

Industry description (e.g., Manufacture of motor truck trailers)

_____

Standard Industrial Classification (SIC), if known (e.g., SIC 3715)

_____ _____ _____ _____

Employment information

Annual average number of employees   _____

Total hours worked by all employees last year   _____

Sign here

Knowingly falsifying this document may result in a fine.

I certify that I have examined this document and that to the best of my knowledge the entries are true, accurate, and complete.

_____   _____
Company executive   Title

_____   _____
Phone   Date

From *U.S. Department of Labor, Occupational Safety and Health Administration,* http://www.osha-slc.gov/recordkeeping/ OSHArecordkeepingforms.pdf.

15-7C Injury and Illness Incident Report

OSHA's Form 301
Injuries and Illnesses Incident Report

This *Injury and Illness Incident Report* is one of the first forms you must fill out when a recordable work-related injury or illness has occurred. Together with the *Log of Work-Related Injuries and Illnesses* and the accompanying *Summary*, these forms help the employer and OSHA develop a picture of the extent and severity of work-related incidents.

Within 7 calendar days after you receive information that a recordable work-related injury or illness has occurred, you must fill out this form or an equivalent. Some state workers' compensation, insurance, or other reports may be acceptable substitutes. To be considered an equivalent form, any substitute must contain all the information asked for on this form.

According to Public Law 91-596 and 29 CFR 1904, OSHA's recordkeeping rule, you must keep this form on file for 5 years following the year to which it pertains.

If you need additional copies of this form, you may photocopy and use as many as you need.

Completed by _____

Title _____

Phone _____ Date _____

Information about the employee

1) Full Name _____

2) Street _____

City _____ State ____ Zip _____

3) Date of birth _____

4) Date hired _____

5) ☐ Male
   ☐ Female

Information about the physician or other health care professional

6) Name of physician or other health care professional
_____
_____

7) If treatment was given away from the worksite, where was it given?

Facility _____

Street _____

City _____ State ____ Zip _____

8) Was employee treated in an emergency room?
   ☐ Yes
   ☐ No

9) Was employee hospitalized overnight as an in-patient?
   ☐ Yes
   ☐ No

Public reporting burden for this collection of information is estimated to average 22 minutes per response, including time for reviewing the collection of information. Persons are not required to respond to the collection of information unless it displays a

> **Attention:** This form contains information relating to employee health and must be used in a manner that protects the confidentiality of employees to the extent possible while the information is being used for occupational safety and health purposes.

U.S. Department of Labor

Occupational Safety and Health Administration

Form approved OMB no. 1218-0176

Information about the case

10)   Case number from the Log   _____ *(Transfer the case number from the Log after you record the case.)*

11)   Date of injury or illness   _____

12)   Time employee began work   _____   AM/PM

13)   Time of event   _____   AM/PM ☐ Check if time cannot be determined

14)   **What was the employee doing just before the incident occurred?** Describe the activity, as well as the tools, equipment, or material the employee was using. Be specific. Examples: "climbing a ladder while carrying roofing materials"; "spraying chlorine from hand sprayer"; "daily computer key-entry."

15)   **What happened?** Tell us how the injury occurred. Examples: "When ladder slipped on wet floor, worker fell 20 feet"; "Worker was spayed with chlorine when gasket broke during replacement"; "Worker developed soreness in wrist over time."

16)   **What was the injury or illness?** Tell us the part of the body that was affected and how it was affected; be more specific than "hurt," "pain," or "sore." Examples: "strained back"; "chemical burn, hand"; "carpal tunnel syndrome."

17)   **What object or substance directly harmed the employee?** Examples: "concrete floor," "chlorine," "radial arm saw." If this question does not apply to the incident, leave it blank.

18)   **If the employee died, when did death occur?** Date of death

current valid OMB control number. If you have any comments about this estimate or any other aspects of this data collection, including suggestions for reducing this burden, contact: US Department of Labor, OSHA Office of Statistics, Room N-3644, 200 Constitution Ave., NW, Washington, DC 20210. Do not send the completed forms to this office.

From *U.S. Department of Labor, Occupational Safety and Health Administration,* http://www.osha-slc.gov/recordkeeping/ OSHArecordkeepingforms.pdf.

15-8 Examples of Federal Agency Resources for Assistance with the Americans With Disabilities Act

American Foundation for the Blind
11 Penn Plaza, Suite 300
New York, NY 10001
Tel: (212) 502-7600
Fax: (212) 502-7777
http://www.afb.org/

American Speech-Language-Hearing Association
10801 Rockville Pike
Rockville, MD 20852
Consumer Help (800) 638-8255 (TDY)
http://www.asha.org/

Association on Higher Education and Disability
(AHEAD)
University of Massachusetts, Boston
100 Morrissey Blvd.
Boston, MA 02125-3393
Tel: (617) 287-3880
Fax: (617) 287-3881
TTY: (617) 287-3882
http://www.ahead.org/

Association for Retarded Citizens of the United
States (ARC)
1010 Wayne Ave., Suite 650
Silver Spring, MD 20910
Tel: (301) 565-3842
Fax: (301) 565-3843
http://thearc.org/

Centers for Independent Living Program
D.C. Center for Independent Living
1400 Florida Ave. NE, Suite 3
Washington, DC 20002
Tel: (202) 388-0033
Fax: (202) 398-3018
TTY: (202) 388-0033

Clearinghouse on Disability Information
Office of Special Education and Rehabilitation
Services
U.S. Department of Education
Switzer Bldg., Room 3132
Washington, DC 20202-2524
(202) 732-1241 or (202) 732-1723
(Voice/TDD)

Developmental Disability Councils
Administration on Developmental
Disabilities
U.S. Department of Health and Human
Services
200 Independence Avenue, SW
Washington, DC 20201
Tel: (202) 619-0257
Toll Free: (877) 696-6775
http://www.hhs.gov/

Disability Online
Disability Employment and Initiatives Unit
Department of Labor/Employment and Training
Administration
200 Constitution Ave., NW
Washington, DC 20210
Tel: (202) 693-3730
Fax: (202) 693-3818
http://wdsc.doleta.gov/disability/

Education and Assistance
Program for Farmers with Disabilities
USDA Extension Service, U.S. Department of
Agriculture
Washington, DC 20250-0900
(202) 720-3377
www.reeusda.gov

Federal Communications Commission
445 12th St., SW
Washington, DC 20554
Tel: (888) 225-5322
TTY: (888) 835-5322
Fax: (202) 418-0232
http://www.fcc.gov/

Information Access Project
National Federation of the Blind
1800 Johnson St.
Baltimore, MD 21230
(410) 659-9314
http://www.nfb.org/

Job Training Partnership Act (JTPA)
  PROGRAMS
Office of Job Training Programs
Employment and Training Administration
U.S. Department of Labor
200 Constitution Ave., NW, Room N-4709
Washington, DC 20210
(202) 535-0580

National Council on Independent Living
1916 Wilson Blvd., Suite 209
Arlington, VA 22201
Tel: (703) 525-3406
TTY: (703) 525-4153
Fax: (703) 525-3409
http://www.ncil.org/

National Council on Disability
1331 F St., NW, Suite 850
Washington, DC 20004
Tel: (202) 272-2004
FAX: (202) 272-2022
TTY: (202) 272-2074
http://www.ncd.gov/index.html

National Center for Medical Rehabilitation
  Research (NCMRR)
National Institute of Child Health and Human
  Development
Bldg. 31, Room 2A32, MSC 2425
31 Center Dr.,
Bethesda, MD 20892-2425
Tel: (800) 370-2943
http://www.nichd.nih.gov/

National Rehabilitation Hospital
102 Irving St., NW
Washington, DC 20010
Tel: (202) 877-6316
TDD: (202) 877-6194
http://www.nrhrehab.org/

Office of Disability Employment Policy (ODEP)
1331 F St., NW, Suite 300
Washington DC 20004
Tel: (202) 376-6200
Fax: (202) 376-6219
TTD: (202) 376-6205
http://www.dol.gov/dol/odep/

U.S. Department of Justice
Civil Rights Division
Office on the Americans with Disabilities Act
P.O. Box 66118
Washington, DC 20035-6118
Tel: (800) 514-0301
TTY: (800) 514-0383
http://www.usdoj.gov/

U.S. Department of Labor
Office of Disability Employment Policy
Job Accommodation Network
P.O. Box 6080
Morgantown, WV 26506-6080
Tel: (800) 526-7234 or (800) 232-9675
Fax: (304) 293-5407
http://www.jan.wvu.edu/

U.S. Equal Employment Opportunity
  Commission
1801 L St., NW
Washington, DC 20507
Tel: (800) 669-4000
TDD: (800) 669-6820
http://www.eeoc.gov/index.html

15-9A Accommodating People With Cumulative Trauma Disorders

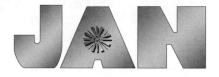

JOB ACCOMMODATION NETWORK

A Service of the U.S. Department of Labor
Office of Disability Employment Policy
Job Accommodation Network
West Virginia University
P.O. Box 6080
Morgantown, WV 26506-6080
(800) 526-7234 in the United States (Voice or TTY)
http://www.jan.wvu.edu

PREFACE

Accommodating People With Cumulative Trauma Disorders

Cumulative trauma disorders (CTDs) account for more than 50% of all occupational illnesses in the United States. According to the Bureau of Labor Statistics (BLS), the most common repetitive task associated with CTDs is placing, grasping, or moving objects other than tools (i.e., scanning groceries). Other work activities, such as typing or key entry, and repetitive use of tools also produce large numbers of CTDs. In 1997 the BLS reported 276,000 CTDs. This statistic coupled with the requirements of the Americans with Disabilities Act (ADA) show why knowing about workplace accommodations for people with CTDs is important. When considering accommodations for people with CTDs, the accommodation process must be conducted on a case-by-case basis. Symptoms caused by CTDs vary from person to person.

When determining effective accommodations, the person's individual abilities and limitations should be considered and problematic job tasks must be identified. Therefore, the person with the CTD should be involved in the accommodation process. Not all people with CTDs will need accommodations to perform their jobs, and many others may need only a few accommodations. For those who need accommodation, the following pages provide basic information about common limitations, symptoms, useful questions to consider, and accommodation possibilities.

The following is only a sample of possibilities to consider; numerous other solutions and considerations may exist. In addition to accommodation ideas, the following material includes information regarding some of the products available to accommodate people with CTDs. The information represents a sample of the possible products and vendors available. Numerous other products and vendors may exist. Also included in this publication is a list of resources for additional information.

This publication was written by Beth A. Loy, Ph.D., a Human Factors Consultant with the Job Accommodation Network. If further information is needed, please call JAN at (800) 526-7234.

CUMULATIVE TRAUMA DISORDERS

The following information regarding CTDs was edited from several sources, including many of the resources listed in the resource section of this publication. The information is not intended to be medical advice. If medical advice is needed, appropriate medical professionals should be consulted.

What are CTDs?

CTDs are disorders that are caused, precipitated, or aggravated by repeated exertions or movements of the body. Continuous use or pressure over an extended period of time results in wear and tear on tendons, muscles, and sensitive nerve tissue. Most common parts of the body affected are the wrists, hands, shoulders, back, neck, and eyes. CTDs are groups of disorders with similar characteristics and may be referred to as repetitive trauma disorders, repetitive strain injuries, overuse syndromes, regional musculoskeletal disorders, and work-related disorders.

Examples of CTDs

Bursitis. Bursitis is inflammation of bursae, which are closed sacs that contain fluid and are located at points of friction in joints. Bursitis can occur in several joints, but the shoulder and knee joints are the most common.

Carpal tunnel syndrome (CTS). CTS is a disorder that causes a prickling or numbness in the hand. It can cause burning pain, decreased hand dexterity, and, in some cases, paralysis. CTS is caused by compression of the median nerve, which runs through a braceletlike bone structure in the wrist, the carpal tunnel, and branches to the thumb and first three fingers. Tendons in the carpal tunnel swell and pinch the nerve.

Cubital tunnel syndrome. Similar to the pain that comes from hitting the funny bone, cubital tunnel syndrome affects the ulnar nerve where it crosses the elbow. The funny bone is actually the ulnar nerve on the inside

of the elbow that runs in a passage called the cubital tunnel.

de Quervain's disease. With de Quervain's disease, pain results from the tendons becoming inflamed on the side of the wrist and forearm just above the thumb.

Epicondylitis. Lateral epicondylitis, sometimes referred to as tennis elbow, can result from excessive activities such as painting with a brush or roller, running a chain saw, and using many types of hand tools continuously. Medial epicondylitis, sometimes referred to as golfer's elbow, can result from activities such as chopping wood with an ax, running a chain saw, and using many types of hand tools continuously.

Guyon's canal syndrome. Similar to carpal tunnel syndrome, Guyon's canal syndrome is a common nerve compression affecting the ulnar nerve as it passes through a tunnel in the wrist called Guyon's canal.

Impingement syndrome. Also known as rotator cuff syndrome, impingement syndrome is a result of the lack of room between the acromion (upper part of shoulder blade bone) and the rotator cuff. Usually the tendons slide easily underneath the acromion as the arm is raised; however, each time the arm is raised, there is a bit of rubbing on the tendons and the bursa between the tendons and the acromion. This rubbing, or pinching action, is called impingement. Continuously working with the arms raised overhead, repeated throwing activities, or other repetitive actions of the arm can result in impingement syndrome.

Myofacial pain syndrome. Also known as temporomandibular joint (TMJ) syndrome, myofacial pain syndrome is a disorder in the joint between the mandible (lower jawbone) and the temporal bone of the skull. Symptoms include blurred vision, sinus problems, and pain in the jaw, head, neck, shoulders, and ears. Treatment ranges from jaw exercises and drug therapy to dental procedures and, in severe cases, surgery.

Radial tunnel syndrome. Radial tunnel syndrome causes aching in the forearm just below the elbow. The symptoms of radial tunnel syndrome can be confused with lateral epicondylitis, tennis elbow.

Tendonitis. Inflammatory condition of a tendon.

Tenosynovitis. Inflammation of the tendon sheaths that may follow trauma, overuse, or inflammatory conditions.

Trigger finger. Trigger finger affects the movement of the tendons as they bend the fingers or thumb toward the palm of the hand. This movement is called flexion.

Thoracic outlet syndrome (TOS). TOS affects the shoulder, arm, and hand.

What Are the Symptoms of CTDs?

The symptoms of CTDs are aching, tenderness, swelling, pain, crackling, tingling, numbness, weakness, loss of joint movement, and decreased coordination in the affected area. The most common body parts affected by CTDs are the fingers, hands, wrists, elbows, arms, shoulders, back, and neck; however, other areas can be affected. Symptoms may appear in any order and at any stage in the development of an injury. A serious injury can develop only weeks after symptoms appear, or it may take years.

How Are CTDs Treated?

Treatments for CTDs vary; exercising alleviates some individuals' symptoms, while other individuals need surgery. The first recommendation is usually to rest the affected area. Vitamin B6 therapy, anti-inflammatory medication, ibuprofen, steroid injections, contrast baths (hot and cold), surgery, and work habit alteration are also treatment options.

What Causes CTDs?

There could be one or several causes of CTDs. The repetition of small, rapid movements; working in a static and/or awkward posture for long periods of time; insufficient recovery time (too few rest breaks); improper workstation setup; forceful movements; excessive grasping; and poor work techniques may contribute. Some associated conditions are broken or dislocated bones, arthritis, thyroid gland imbalance, diabetes, hormonal changes from menopause, and pregnancy. Other risk factors are alcoholism, hemophilia, tumors, acromegaly (increased production of growth hormones), multiple myeloma (cancer of the bone marrow from an uncontrolled growth of plasma cells), and amyloidosis (a group of metabolic disorders where a fibrous protein accumulates in tissues).

QUESTIONS TO CONSIDER WHEN DETERMINING ACCOMMODATIONS

What symptoms or limitations is the individual with a CTD experiencing?

How do these symptoms or limitations affect the person and the person's job performance?

What specific job tasks are problematic as a result of these symptoms and limitations?

What accommodations are available to reduce or eliminate these problems? Are all possible resources being used to determine possible accommodations?

Has the employee with the CTD been consulted regarding possible accommodations?

Once accommodations are in place, would it be useful to meet with the person with a CTD to evaluate the effectiveness of the accommodations and to determine whether additional accommodations are needed?

Do supervisory personnel and employees need training regarding CTDs, other disability areas, or the Americans with Disabilities Act?

ACCOMMODATION CONSIDERATIONS FOR PEOPLE WITH CTDS

(Note: People with CTDs will develop some of these limitations/symptoms but seldom develop all of them. Limitations will vary among individuals. Also note that not all people who have CTDs will need accommodations to perform their jobs and many others may need only a few accommodations. The following is only a sample of the possibilities available. Numerous other accommodation solutions exist as well.)

Fatigue/Weakness

Reduce or eliminate physical exertion and workplace stress.

Schedule periodic rest breaks away from the workstation.

Allow a flexible work schedule and flexible use of leave time.

Allow work from home.

Fine Motor Impairment

Implement ergonomic workstation design.

Provide alternative computer access.

Provide alternative telephone access.

Provide arm supports.

Provide writing and grip aids.

Provide a page turner and a book holder.

Provide a note taker.

Provide ergonomic tools and other adaptations.

Gross Motor Impairment

Modify the worksite to make it accessible.

Provide parking close to the worksite.

Provide an accessible entrance.

Install automatic door openers.

Modify the workstation to make it accessible.

Make sure materials and equipment are within reach range.

Move workstation close to other work areas, office equipment, and break rooms.

Provide carts and lifting devices.

Temperature Sensitivity

Modify worksite temperature.

Modify dress code.

Use fan/air conditioner or heater at the workstation.

Allow flexible scheduling and flexible use of leave time.

Allow work from home during extremely hot or cold weather.

Maintain the ventilation system.

Redirect air conditioning and heating vents.

Provide an office with separate temperature control.

Administrative Considerations

Ergonomics is the science of fitting the job to the worker. When there is a mismatch between the physical requirements of jobs and the physical capacity of workers, work-related CTDs may result. Workers who repeat the same motion throughout their workday, work in an awkward position, use a great deal of force to perform their jobs, and/or repeatedly lift heavy objects are more likely to develop CTDs. Administrative changes can be made to the work environment to decrease the probability of incurring a CTD. Options include [the following]:

Training the employee in ergonomic principles, including proper lifting techniques, adequate maintenance, awkward postures, and correct use of equipment.

Allowing the employee to take rest breaks that include simple, brief exercises such as shoulder shrugs, neck rolls, ankle rotations, leg extensions, overhead stretches, handshakes, and finger spreads. No schedule of rest breaks is universal, but as a general guideline a 1- or 2-minute microbreak every 15 to 20 minutes and a 5 to 10 minute minibreak every hour is recommended. Using an electronic device or other reminder may be helpful to make sure that breaks are taken prior to discomfort.

To reduce stress on eye muscles, an individual should look away from the workstation and refocus on an object at least 25 feet away and blink often.

Varying tasks. An individual should alter positions every 45 minutes (i.e., distribute tasks between right and left hands, alternate between intensive fine motor and gross motor manipulation, and alternate between a sitting and standing position).

Using comfortable hand tools (ergonomic handles), work positions (neutral posture), eliminating sharp edges (cushions), avoiding overgrasping (ergonomic tools), adjusting working heights (adjustable tables and desks), eliminating carrying (using carts), and tool configurations (tool balancers/positioners) to minimize vibration, limit strains, and diminish pinch grip.

Resting feet on the floor or a footrest with knees bent at right angles and thighs parallel to the floor. The lower back should be supported by the chair backrest, and elbows should be bent at right angles, with forearms parallel to the floor. Wrists should be straight, and the head should be looking forward and tilted downward.

Adjusting the chair properly with the backrest giving firm support on the lower back and the front edge of the seat rounded in the back of the thighs.

Placing the keyboard and mouse at a comfortable location (at the same height) and as close together as possible. Elbows should be at the sides, forearms parallel to the floor, and wrists straight.

Properly adjusting monitor. The center of the screen should be eye level and directly in front of the user. The monitor should be at the proper viewing distance, typically 1.5 to 2 feet from the eyes.

EXAMPLE ACCOMMODATIONS FOR PEOPLE WITH CTDS

A journalist with bilateral carpal tunnel syndrome was limited to 2 hours of typing and writing per day. His employer purchased a digital tape recorder, writing aids, and an alternative keyboard; installed speech recognition software; allowed him to take breaks throughout the day; and provided him with office equipment to rearrange his workstation.

An assembly line worker with bursitis in his knee was limited in his ability to stand. His employer gave him a stand/lean stool, provided him with antifatigue matting, and purchased vibration dampening shoe inserts.

A sales clerk with cubital tunnel syndrome lost the ability to move her right hand. The individual needed to use the computer to create reports. Her employer purchased a left-handed keyboard, foot mouse, forearm supports, an articulating keyboard and mouse tray, and an ergonomic chair.

A construction worker with de Quervain's disease had severe inflammation of the wrist and forearm after prolonged use of handtools. The employer provided him with lightweight and pneumatic tools, antivibration tool wraps and gloves, and tool balancers/positioners for stationary work.

A switch board operator with myofacial pain syndrome (TMJ) was having difficulty using the phone and taking messages. The employer gave her a headset, speech recognition software, an adjustable telephone holder, writing aids, and an angled writing surface.

A truck driver with thoracic outlet syndrome was having difficulty driving for long periods of time and unloading bags at his delivery destination. The employer installed a small crane in the back of the trailer and provided him a lightweight aluminum hand truck to help him unload materials. The employer also provided the employee and a steering wheel spinner knob to eliminate prolonged grasping of the steering wheel and an antivibration seat to cut down on fatigue.

A clerical worker who stamped paperwork for several hours a day was limited in pinching and gripping due to carpal tunnel syndrome. The individual was accommodated with adapted stamp handles. Antivibration wrap was placed around the stamp handles. In addition, tennis balls were cut and placed over the wrapped handles to eliminate fine motor pinching and gripping.

A maintenance worker with rotator cuff syndrome was having difficulty reaching cleaning areas and moving cleaning supplies. The employer replaced his tools with long-handled, pneumatic, and lightweight tools. The employer also provided him with an electric cart.

PRODUCTS

There are numerous products that can be used to accommodate people with CTDs. The following pages provide examples of a few of those products. For some products a list of vendors has also been provided. The vendor information came from the Job Accommodation Network's database of products but is not an exhaustive list.

Although all the vendor information was verified in August 1999, products and vendors change quickly, so you may need to check the information again to make sure it is current.
Products include:

Alternative computer input devices
Ergonomic office equipment
Filing accommodations
Independent living aids
Page turners and book holders
Sit/stand workstations
Speech recognition software
Telephones
Tool modifications
Writing and grip aids

RESOURCES

This is a noninclusive list.

Job Accommodation Network
A Service of U.S. Department of Labor Office of
    Disability Employment Policy
West Virginia University
P.O. Box 6080
Morgantown, WV 26506-6080
(800) 526-7234 and (800) ADA-WORK (V/TTY)
(304) 293-7186 (Local Line, V/TTY)
http://www.jan.wvu.edu

Office of Disability Employment Policy
1331 F St. NW
Washington, DC 20004-1107
(202) 376-6200 (Voice)
(202) 376-6205 (TT)
http://www.dol.gov/dol/odep/

Association for Repetitive Motion Syndromes
(ARMS)
P.O. Box 471973
Aurora, CO 80047-1973
(303) 369-0803
http://www.certifiedpst.com/arms
ARMS is a national clearinghouse that provides support and information to at-risk and injured workers, their employers, workers' compensation professionals, the press, and the public at large regarding preventive, therapeutic, medical, and legal aspects of repetitive motion syndromes.

American Industrial Hygiene
Association (AIHA)
2700 Prosperity Ave., Suite 250
Fairfax, VA 22031
(703) 849-8888
http://www.aiha.org
Founded in 1939, AIHA is an organization of more than 12,000 professional members dedicated to the anticipation, recognition, evaluation, and control of environmental factors arising in or from the workplace that may result in injury, illness, or impairment or affect the well-being of workers and members of the community.

American National Standards Institute (ANSI)
1430 Broadway
New York, NY 10018
(212) 642-4900
http://web.ansi.org
ANSI has served in its capacity as administrator and coordinator of the U.S. private-sector voluntary standardization system for 80 years. ANSI promotes voluntary consensus standards.

American Society of Safety Engineers (ASSE)
1800 E. Oakton St.
Des Plaines, IL 60018
(847) 699-2929
http://www.asse.org
ASSE's mission is to foster the technical, scientific, managerial, and ethical knowledge, skills, and competency of safety, health, and environmental professionals.

Canadian Centre for Occupational Health and
Safety (CCOHS)
250 Main St. E.

Hamilton, Ontario, Canada L8N 1H6
(800) 668-4284
http://www.ccohs.ca
CCOHS is Canada's national center for occupational health and safety information.

CTD Resource Network (CTDRN)
2013 Princeton Ct.,
Los Banos, CA 93635
(209) 827-0801
http://www.ctdrn.org
CTDRN was created to bring together existing, online educational publications and provide a vehicle to more assist individuals with cumulative trauma disorders.

Human Factors and Ergonomics Society (HFES)
P.O. Box 1369
Santa Monica, CA 90406
(310) 394-1811
http://hfes.org
HFES's mission is to promote the discovery and exchange of knowledge concerning the characteristics of human beings that are applicable to the design of systems and devices of all kinds.

National Institute for Occupational Safety and
Health (NIOSH)
4676 Columbia Parkway
Cincinnati, OH 45226-1998
(800) 35-NIOSH or (513) 533-8326
http://www.cdc.gov/niosh/homepage.html
NIOSH is part of the Centers for Disease Control and Prevention (CDC) and is the only federal institute responsible for conducting research and making recommendations for the prevention of work-related illnesses and injuries.

National Safety Council
1121 Spring Lake Dr.
Itasca, IL 60143-3201
(630) 285-1121
http://www.nsc.org
The mission of the National Safety Council is "to educate and influence society to adopt safety, health, and environmental policies, practices, and procedures that prevent and mitigate human suffering and economic losses arising from preventable causes."

Occupational Safety and Health Administration (OSHA)

U.S. Department of Labor, Public Affairs Office—Room 3647

200 Constitution Ave, Washington, DC 20210

(202) 693-1999

http://www.osha.gov

OSHA establishes protective standards, enforces those standards, and reaches out to employers and employees through technical assistance and consultation programs.

Rehabilitation Engineering Society of North America (RESNA)

1700 North Moore St., Suite 1540

Arlington, VA 22209-1903

(703) 524-6686

http://www.resna.org

RESNA's purpose is to promote and support the development, dissemination, integration, and utilization of knowledge in rehabilitation engineering and to assure that these efforts result in the highest quality of care and service delivery for all citizens.

15-9B Worksite Accommodation Ideas for Individuals Who Have Migraine Headaches

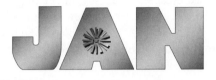

JOB ACCOMMODATION NETWORK
A Service of the U.S. Department of Labor
Office of Disability Employment Policy
Job Accommodation Network
West Virginia University
P.O. Box 6080
Morgantown, WV 26506-6080
(800) 526-7234 in the United States (Voice or TTY)
http://www.jan.wvu.edu
This document was prepared by Mayda LaRosse, MA, Human Factors Consultant for the Job
Accommodation Network

PREFACE

Migraine Headaches

To more than 10 million Americans, migraine headaches can be both physically and psychologically disabling. It affects more women than men (3:1), and the peak years are 35-45 years; but it can affect any age group of people.

Most common types

Classic migraine. Includes a visual aura (a warning sign), usually described as broken zigzag lines, blind spots, flashing lights or double vision—this is usually followed by a headache about 10-30 minutes later. Other symptoms might include speech difficulty, weakness of an arm or leg, tingling of the face or hands, and confusion. The pain from this type of headache is described as intense, throbbing, or pounding and is felt in the temple, ear, jaw around the eye or in the forehead. An attack usually lasts 1 to 2 days.

Common migraine. Most common type in the general population, doesn't have an aura, though some people might experience a mental fuzziness, mood changes, fatigue, or unusual retention of fluid prior to headache. During the headache phase the individual might experience nausea, vomiting, diarrhea, and increased urination.

Both of these types of headaches can strike as often as several times a week or as rarely as every few years. Some individuals might experience them during certain specific times, such as some women may have one prior to menstrual periods, or some individuals might experience these headaches on weekends after a stressful workweek. Some individuals experience sensitivity to light and sound and difficulty with odors.

Cause

There doesn't seem to be a clear cause of migraines. Some scientists believe that a key element is blood flow changes in the brain. Constriction then dilation and inflammation of blood vessels that go to the person's scalp and brain might be the cause of the migraine headaches.

Triggers to a migraine headache might be tension, menstruation, fatigue, use of contraceptives, consumption of alcohol, diet, missing or delaying a meal (which would cause low blood sugar), bright lights, sunlight, fluorescent lights, TV and movie viewing, excessive noise, alteration of sleep-wake cycle.

Treatment

Apply a cold cloth or ice pack to the side of the headache.
Biofeedback training
Stress reduction
Regular exercise (prior to headache) can reduce the frequency and severity of the migraines.
Avoid certain foods that might trigger the headaches, such as cheese, chocolate, nuts, yogurts and lima beans.

Drug therapy

Once the headache occurs [the following can help]: aspirins, aspirin-caffeine combinations such as Midrin, Fiorinal or Fioricet, ergotamine, sumatriptan, dihydroergotamine (DHE).

Preventative treatments

Beta-blockers (such as propranolol, nadolol and atenolol) [and] antidepressants have been found to be helpful for some individuals, as . . . [have] some calcium channel blockers (used to treat hypertension and heart disease) and anticonvulsants medication.

QUESTIONS TO CONSIDER WHEN DETERMINING ACCOMMODATION IDEAS

Issues Related to the Individual

What are the individual's job duties?
What job duties are problematic?
Exactly what does the person have trouble doing within the problematic area? (Be specific.)

Examples of pinpointing:

Absence?

Misses deadlines?
Difficulty concentrating?
How can this be compensated? (This is where an accommodation(s) will be considered.)

General Issues Related to the Worksite

What is the physical layout of the workplace?
What specific equipment is utilized in the work setting?
What kind of lighting is used and what is the noise level in the workplace?
Is the workplace visually distracting, auditorially distracting?
How can the physical environment of the workplace be changed so that the worker will be able to perform his/her job duties?
Can the job duties be restructured so that the worker can perform the duties that are easier for him/her?
What assistive devices or other products could be used that will help the individual perform his/her duties?

WORKSITE ACCOMMODATION IDEAS SPECIFIC FOR PERSONS WITH MIGRAINE HEADACHES

The following are only some accommodation ideas for individuals with migraine headaches. As mentioned before, accommodation solutions should be considered on a case-by-case basis. There may be other accommodation options other than what are listed here. An individual might need none, one, or more accommodations to help him/her be successful in the workplace. As the ADA states, if the accommodation causes an undue hardship to the employer, then it would not be considered reasonable.

Reduce visual and auditory distractions.
Use partitions to block distractions.
Move work area to a more quiet area.
Use environmental sound machines (white noise machines) to mask any noise/sounds that still passes partitions.
Use computer glare screens.
Eliminate fluorescent lighting and replace with full spectrum lighting.
Modif[y] attendance policy and [permit] flexible schedule options to allow the worker to adjust to daily changes.
Use sick/vacation leave without penalty to performance evaluation.

Allow work from home as an option when the job would enable this to be a successful option.

[Provide] proper ventilation system in the work environment and possible use of air purification devices if necessary.

SAMPLE WORKSITE ACCOMMODATION IDEAS FOR INDIVIDUALS WITH MIGRAINE HEADACHES *(taken from actual cases reported to the Job Accommodation Network)*

A systems analyst in a state office has migraine headaches. The office was set up in cubicle format with overhead florescent lighting. The accommodation was to move the person into his or her own office and to use task lighting as oppose to overhead lights. The worker is also sensitive to noise. The office was located next to a noisy garage area, so environmental sound machines were considered to block out some of the background noise that could periodically be a problem.

A laborer for a utility company has migraine headaches in part as a result of the weight of the safety eye wear worn on the job. As the person already wore a hard hat, a visor was added to the hard hat to provide the same protection the glasses had given.

A receptionist for a large company has migraine headaches. A flexible schedule was considered as the accommodation as the worker needed to take off an average of one day a month.

A package operator has migraines and had difficulty with shift rotations. She was reassigned to a daytime position that was temporarily vacant. Later, the person used FMLA to find new medication to help the migraine headaches. The person is currently doing fine in her position working rotating shifts.

A registered nurse with migraine headaches had problems doing her work, including patient care. [Her] employer provided her with time off when needed (once or twice a year).

A production operator with migraine headaches had problems with attendance. [The] employer allowed [the] person to take off approximately 1 day per month.

A consultant was not able to work whenever she had a migraine headache. [The] employee used FMLA during the times that she couldn't make it to work.

A trainer was unable to focus during a migraine headache. [The] employer provided paid leave for these times (1 day per month).

GENERAL RESOURCES FOR MIGRAINE HEADACHES

Job Accommodation Network
A Service of the U.S. Department of Labor's Office of Disability Employment Policy
West Virginia University
P.O. Box 6080
Morgantown, WV 26506-6080
(800) 526-7234 (Voice and TTY)
(304) 293-7186 (Local Line)
(304) 293-5407 (Fax)
http://www.jan.wvu.edu/

U.S. Department of Labor's Office of Disability Employment Policy
1331 F St., NW, Suite 300
Washington, DC 20004-1107
(202) 376-6200 (Voice)
(202) 376-6205 (TDD)
(202) 376-6219 (Fax)
http://www.dol.gov/dol/odep/

American Academy of Neurology
1080 Montreal Ave.
St. Paul, MN 55116
(651) 695-1940 (Phone)
http://www.aan.com

American Council for Headache Education (ACHE)
19 Mantua Rd.
Mt. Royal, NJ 08061
(856) 423-0258 (Phone)
(856) 423-0082 (Fax)
http://www.achenet.org/

Australian Brain Foundation
National/Victoria Branch
746 Burke Rd. Camberwell
Victoria, Australia 3124
1 800 677 579 (Toll Free)
03 9882 2203 (Phone)
03 9882 5737 (Fax)
http://www.brainfunction.org.au/

Migraine Action Association (formerly the
British Migraine Association)
178a High Road
Byfleet, West Blyfeet, Surrey, KT14 7ED
01932 352468 (Phone)
01932 351257 (Fax)
http://www.migraine.org.uk/

Irish Migraine Association
Carmichael House
4 North Brunswick Street
Dublin 7, Ireland
353 01 8724137 (Phone)
353 01 8724157 (Fax)

JAMA (Journal of the American Medical
Association)
http://www.ama-assn.org/special/migraine/
migraine.htm

M.A.G.N.U.M., Inc. (Migraine Awareness Group:
a National Understanding for Migraineurs)
Washington, DC Office
113 South Saint Asaph St., Suite 300
Alexandria, VA 22314
(703) 739-9384 (Phone)
(703) 739-2432 (Fax)
http://www.migraines.org

Migraine Association of Canada
356 Bloor Street East, Suite 1912
Toronto, Ontario M4W 3L4
416-920-4916 (Phone)
416-920-3677 (Fax)
800-663-3557 (To Order Information)
416-920-4917 (24-Hour Information on Line)
http://www.migraine.ca

Migraine Trust
45 Great Ormond Street
London, England WC1N 3HZ
020 7831 4818 (Phone)
020 7831 5174 (Fax)

National Headache Foundation
428 W. St. James Place, 2nd Floor
Chicago, IL 60614-2750
888-NHF-5552 (Phone)
http://www.headaches.org

National Institute of Neurological Disorders and
Stroke
National Institutes of Health
P.O. Box 5801
Bethesda, MD 20892
(800) 352-9424 (Phone)
http://www.ninds.nih.gov/

Neurological Foundation of New Zealand
P.O. Box 110022
Auckland 1030
New Zealand
09 309 7749 (Phone)
09 377 0614 (Fax)

Swiss Migraine Trust Foundation/Migraine
Action
Postfach 4037
4002 Basel, Switzerland
41-61-423 10 80 (Phone)
41-61-423 10 82 (Fax)

There are also newsletters and online computer
resources that can give you more information and
advice about migraine headaches. You can contact
the following places:

Headache newsletter
ACHE (American Council for Headache
Education)
(800) 255-ACHE ext. 2243 (Phone)
http://www.achenet.org

The Excedrin Headache Relief Update newsletter
The Excedrin Headache Resource Center
(800) 580-4455 (Phone)
http://www.excedrin.com

HeadWay newsletter
Glaxo Wellcome Migraine Information Center
(800) 520-8508 (Phone)
http://www.migrainehelp.com/resources.html

15-10

Certification of Health Care Provider (Family and Medical Leave Act of 1993)

Certification of Health Care Provider
(Family and Medical Leave Act of 1993)

U.S. Department of Labor
Employment Standards Administration
Wage and Hour Division

(When completed, this form goes to the employee, ***not to the Department of Labor****.)*	OMB No: 1215-0181 Expires: 06/30/02

1. Employee's Name	2. Patient's Name *(If different from employee)*

3. Page 4 describes what is meant by a **"serious health condition"** under the Family and Medical Leave Act. Does the patient's condition[1] qualify under any of the categories described? If so, please check the applicable category:

(1) _____ (2) _____ (3) _____ (4) _____ (5) _____ (6) _____ or None of the above _____

4. Describe the **medical facts** which support your certification, including a brief statement as to how the medical facts meet the criteria of one of these categories:

5. a. State the approximate **date** the condition commenced, and the probable duration of the condition (and also the probable duration of the patient's present **incapacity**[2] if different):

b. Will it be necessary for the employee to take work only **intermittently or to work on a less than full schedule** as a result of the condition (including for treatment described in Item 6 below)?

If yes, give the probable duration:

c. If the condition is a **chronic condition** (condition #4) or **pregnancy**, state whether the patient is presently incapacitated[2] and the likely duration and frequency of **episodes of incapacity**[2]:

---

[1] Here and elsewhere on this form, the information sought relates **only** to the condition for which the employee is taking FMLA leave.

[2] "Incapacity," for purposes of FMLA, is defined to mean inability to work, attend school, or perform other regular daily activities due to the serious health condition, treatment therefor, or recovery therefrom.

621

6. a. If additional **treatments** will be required for the condition, provide an estimate of the probable number of such treatments.

   If the patient will be absent from work or other daily activities because of **treatment** on an **intermittent** or **part-time** basis, also provide an estimate of the probable number of and interval between such treatments, actual or estimated dates of treatment if known, and period required for recovery if any:

   b. If any of these treatments will be provided by **another provider of health services** (e.g., physical therapist), please state the nature of the treatments:

   c. **If a regimen of continuing treatment** by the patient is required under your supervision, provide a general description of such regimen (e.g., prescription drugs, physical therapy requiring special equipment):

7. a. If medical leave is required for the employee's **absence from work** because of the **employee's own condition** (including absences due to pregnancy or a chronic condition), is the employee **unable to perform work** of any kind?

   b. If able to perform some work, is the employee **unable to perform any one or more of the essential functions of the employee's job** (the employee or the employer should supply you with information about the essential job functions)? If yes, please list the essential functions the employee is unable to perform:

   c. If neither a. nor b. applies, is it necessary for the employee to be **absent from work for treatment**?

8. a. If leave is required to **care for a family member** of the employee with a serious health condition, **does the patient require assistance** for basic medical or personal needs or safety or for transportation?

   b. If no, would the employee's presence to provide **psychological comfort** be beneficial to the patient or assist in the patient's recovery?

   c. If the patient will need care only **intermittently** or on a part-time basis, please indicate the probable **duration** of this need:

_____

_____   _____
Signature of Health Care Provider   Type of Practice

_____   _____
Address   Telephone Number

_____   _____
                                                                                         Date

To be completed by the employee needing family leave to care for a family member.

State the care you will provide and an estimate of the period during which care will be provided, including a schedule if leave is to be taken intermittently or if it will be necessary for you to work less than a full schedule:

_____   _____
Employee Signature   Date

A **"Serious Health Condition"** means an illness, injury impairment, or physical or mental condition that involves one of the following:

1. Hospital Care
   Inpatient care (i.e., an overnight stay) in a hospital, hospice, or residential medical care facility, including any period of incapacity[2] or subsequent treatment in connection with or consequent to such inpatient care.

2. Absence Plus Treatment
   (a) A period of incapacity[2] of **more than three consecutive calendar days** (including any subsequent treatment or period of incapacity[2] relating to the same condition), that also involves:
      (1) **Treatment**[3] **two or more times** by a health care provider, by a nurse or physician's assistant under direct supervision of a health care provider, or by a provider of health care services (e.g., physical therapist) under orders of, or on referral by, a health care provider; or
      (2) **Treatment** by a health care provider on **at least one occasion** which results in a **regimen of continuing treatment**[4] under the supervision of the health care provider.

3. Pregnancy
   Any period of incapacity due to **pregnancy**, or for **prenatal care**.

4. Chronic Conditions Requiring Treatments
   A **chronic condition** which:
      (1) Requires **periodic visits** for treatment by a health care provider, or by a nurse or physician's assistant under direct supervision of a health care provider;
      (2) Continues over an **extended period of time** (including recurring episodes of a single underlying condition); and
      (3) May cause **episodic** rather than a continuing period of incapacity[2] (e.g., asthma, diabetes, epilepsy, etc.).

5. Permanent/Long-Term Conditions Requiring Supervision
   A period of **incapacity**[2] which is **permanent or long-term** due to a condition for which treatment may not be effective. The employee or family member must be **under the continuing supervision of, but need not be receiving active treatment by, a health care provider**. Examples include Alzheimer's, a severe stroke, or the terminal stages of a disease.

6. Multiple Treatments (Nonchronic Conditions)
   Any period of absence to receive **multiple treatments** (including any period of recovery therefrom) by a health care provider or by a provider of health care services under orders of, or on referral by, a health care provider, either for **restorative surgery** after an accident or other injury, **or** for a condition that **would likely result in a period of incapacity**[2] **of more than three consecutive calendar days in the absence of medical intervention or treatment**, such as cancer (chemotherapy, radiation, etc.), severe arthritis (physical therapy), and kidney disease (dialysis).

This optional form may be used by employees to satisfy a mandatory requirement to furnish a medical certification (when requested) from a health care provider, including second or third opinions and recertification (29 CFR 825.306).

Note: Persons are not required to respond to this collection of information unless it displays a currently valid OMB control number.

---

[3] Treatment includes examinations to determine if a serious health condition exists and evaluations of the condition. Treatment does not include routine physical examinations, eye examinations, or dental examinations.

[4] A regimen of continuing treatment includes, for example, a course of prescription medication (e.g., an antibiotic) or therapy requiring special equipment to resolve or alleviate the health condition. A regimen of treatment does not include the taking of over-the-counter medications such as aspirin, antihistamine, or salves; or bed rest, drinking fluids, exercise, and other similar activities that can be initiated without a visit to a health care provider.

Public Burden Statement

We estimate that it will take an average of 10 minutes to complete this collection of information, including the time for reviewing instructions, searching existing data sources, gathering and maintaining the data needed, and completing and reviewing the collection of information. If you have any comments regarding this burden estimate or any other aspect of this collection of information, including suggestions for reducing this burden, send them to the Administrator, Wage and Hourly Division, Department of Labor, Room S-3502, 200 Constitution Avenue, N.W., Washington, D.C. 20210.

DO NOT SEND THE COMPLETED FORM TO THIS OFFICE; IT GOES TO THE EMPLOYEE.

From *U.S. Department of Labor, Employment Standards Administration, Wage and Hour Division,* http://www.dol.gov/dol/esa/public/regs/compliance/whd/fmla/wh380.pdf.

16 Research in Occupational and Environmental Health Nursing

WHY NURSING RESEARCH?

In an applied professional discipline such as occupational and environmental health nursing, research is needed to improve and foster the health and well-being of the worker and the workforce and improve working conditions to support this effort. Coupled with the considerable expansion of the scope of occupational and environmental health nursing practice in the last 25 years, so too has emphasis increased on promoting and conducting occupational and environmental health nursing research and disseminating research findings. The conduct of research is necessary to support and expand the knowledge base that provides the foundation for practice. Research and practice go hand in hand.

Nursing leaders have stressed that nursing care cannot be improved until information-based accountability becomes as much a part of nursing's tradition as humanitarianism (Polit & Hungler, 1999). This means that nurses who incorporate research-based evidence into their practice decisions are being professionally accountable to recipients of care and service.

The professional nurses engaged in research range from those who read the research literature to remain current in their practice to those who actively participate in the development, design, and conduct of research investigations. Increasingly, nurses in practice settings are doing their own research or research in collaboration with other disciplines. This places nurses in a better position to make a contribution to improving practice and advancing nursing knowledge.

This chapter has several purposes. The importance of occupational and environmental health nursing research and the advances made in the field are described, and several examples of the research are discussed. In addition, research preparation and training, the importance of research collaboration, and a brief discussion of the research process will be provided. Although this chapter presents an overview of the research process, the reader, who may have limited knowledge of and familiarity with the research process, is provided only with an appreciation for concepts and procedures involved in the conduct of research. Those interested in becoming more involved in research are encouraged to acquire knowledge and skills to facilitate the experience.

NURSING RESEARCH EVOLUTION AND PREPARATION

Nursing research is concerned with the systematic study and assessment of nursing problems or phenomena, finding ways to improve nursing practice and client care through creative studies, initiating and evaluating change, and taking action to make new knowledge useful in nursing practice. Treece and Treece (1982) have stated that in order to be answerable by research, questions must be conceived that will produce answers through some form of data collection from observation or explanation. In other words, a systematic, carefully designed approach must be used if true and meaningful answers are to be discovered. Research findings are intended to aid nurses in delivering quality health care services and help

627

Box 16-1	**Research Purposes and Relevant Questions**
Describe	• What is the frequency or prevalence of the phenomenon or problem? • What are the characteristics of the phenomenon or problem? • What factors or antecedents are related to the phenomenon or problem?
Explain	• What are the measurable associations between phenomena or problems? • What factors cause the phenomenon or problem? • Does theory explain the phenomenon or problem?
Predict/Control	• What happens if the phenomenon or problem is altered or changed through intervention ($x{\rightarrow}y$)? • Can the occurrence of the phenomenon or problem be controlled or prevented?

document nursing's unique role in the health care system. The major purposes of nursing research are to answer questions or solve problems relevant to the practice field. Generally, this includes identifying the problem and then designing studies that describe, explain, predict, and control the problem or phenomenon under investigation (Box 16-1).

Nursing research has its roots in the work of Florence Nightingale (1859). Nightingale provided care to soldiers during the Crimean War in 1884 and found hospital barracks infested with fleas and rats, sewers under the buildings, numerous open privies, and a general state of filth (Rogers, 1989b). These conditions led to epidemics of cholera and typhus, resulting in thousands of preventable deaths; these epidemics, not battle wounds, were the main cause of death during the war (Cohen, 1984).

While at Scutari, Nightingale organized the recordkeeping practices, and this resulted in a systematic method for data collection and analysis. She was then able to record deaths and mortality causes with accuracy, which enabled her to present these data in diagrams and statistical tables (Figure 16-1). During the first several months of the war the mortality rate among the soldiers was 60% per year due to disease alone; however, after Nightingale's sanitary reforms were implemented, the mortality rate among the soldiers declined rapidly.

Nightingale demonstrated an organized approach to the collecting and reporting of data—a truly unique contribution to nursing research for that period of time. During that period, little nursing research information was added to the nursing literature after Nightingale's work.

As with all scientific inquiry, research is linked with current issues and problems needing answers. Between 1900 and 1940 most of the nursing research centered on nursing education; of major concerns were adequate preparation and educational standards. Resultant studies, including the Goldmark Report and the Brown study (1948), recommended that advanced nursing education in collegiate settings was essential. In the 1950s and 1960s nurses began to focus their research on the characteristics and functions of the nurse. By the 1970s more funding was made available for doctoral preparation of nurse researchers, and the focus of nursing research changed from examining functions and activities to improving care and practice.

The 1980s was marked by an increase in the numbers of qualified nurse researchers and nursing research studies conducted. Of particular importance was the establishment in 1986 of the National Center for Nursing Research (NCNR) at the National Institutes of Health (NIH), whose purpose was to promote and support research training and research projects related to patient care. In the 1990s the NCNR was promoted to full institute status within NIH and became the National Institute for Nursing Research (NINR) in 1993, with nursing research priorities established. During a 10-year span the budget for NCNR/NINR had increased to $55 million in 1996 from $16 million in 1986. Nursing research has begun to focus more effort on nursing practice and outcomes research designed to evaluate

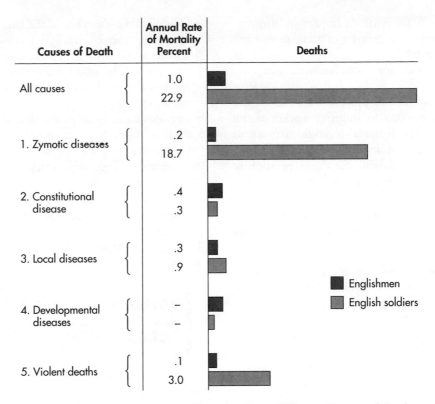

Figure 16-1   Representing the Relative Mortality, From Different Causes, of the Army in the East in Hospital and of the English Male Population, Age 15-45. *(From "Florence Nightingale," by I. B. Cohen, 1984,* Scientific American 25, *128-137.)*

the effectiveness of nursing interventions and health care services.

Research training and education helps the nurse understand and utilize the research process so that scientifically derived solutions to problems can be developed and implemented. Although exposure to, appreciation for, and some application of nursing research occur at the undergraduate level, the graduate level is primarily where nurses become engaged in the knowledge and application of scientific processes and investigations. In general, research roles will vary by preparation and include the following:

- *Associate degree/diploma.* The nurse identifies clinical problems for research; assists in the development of the research and data collection activities; and uses research as a basis for clinical practice.

- *Baccalaureate degree.* The nurse evaluates research for applicability to practice, works with skilled researchers on the development of research projects, uses research to refine and extend the practice, and discusses research findings with colleagues.

- *Master's degree.* The nurse provides clinical expertise related to the research problem, the delivery of care, and the research process and analyzes the practice problems within the context of the scientific process. The nurse also facilitates an environment supportive of nursing research, supports the conduct of research, disseminates research findings, collaborates with other disciplines in scientific investigations, and energizes the integration of research into practice.

- *Doctoral degree.* The nurse develops and conducts independent and collaborative investigations with other scientists and develops methodology for scientific inquiry of phenomena relevant to the practice of occupational and environmental health and safety. In addition, the nurse uses analytical methods and integrates findings to explain and extend scientific knowledge to nursing practice and develops and tests interventions to improve worker health and safety. The nurse also develops fundable proposals and acquires research grant support and provides leadership for the integration of research findings into practice (Rogers, 2001).

The American Nurses Association (1999) states that qualified nursing researchers will do the following:

- Provide leadership for the integration of scientific knowledge with other sources of knowledge for the advancement of practice;
- Conduct investigations to evaluate the contribution of nursing activities to the well-being of clients;
- Develop methods to monitor the quality of the practice of nursing in a clinical setting.

Though many occupational and environmental health nurses may not have had formal academic preparation in nursing research, they are or have opportunities to be involved in research to varying degrees. Agnew and Travers (1990, p. 559) point out that "occupational health nurses have long been involved in research activities but have not always recognized them as such." The authors state that "it often is the nurse who identifies an outbreak of work-related illness, investigates the cause, and initiates the resolution." This underscores the need for being familiar with and understanding the research process and methods and creating opportunities for collaborative relationships with seasoned investigators who can provide primary investigative guidance and serve as mentors, when needed. Collaborative research has several advantages that include, but are not limited to, the following (Rogers, 1988):

- Provides an opportunity, including research mentorship, to develop and expand clinical research skills in the work environment
- Provides an opportunity for the clinician, researcher, and administrator to jointly discuss imperative questions or problems that need solutions

- Combines the expertise of the clinician and the researcher, thereby enhancing clinical integrity and scientific rigor to achieve a mutual benefit and quality, cost-effective health care
- Increases research skills through mutual learning and sharing
- Provides for early dissemination of the research findings from both the research and clinical perspective and allows for a recognition of a valuable partnership, which can lead to new nursing interventions

Those involved in research will find that collaborative efforts stimulate the mind, broaden the learning experience, and lay the foundation for future research opportunities.

ADVANCING OCCUPATIONAL AND ENVIRONMENTAL HEALTH NURSING RESEARCH

A research-based practice is foundational to any professional discipline. Increasingly, research is being conducted by occupational and environmental health nurses to develop and expand knowledge in the field of occupational and environmental health nursing and to test theories and ideas aimed at improving workers' and workplace health and safety. A review of the literature in separate reports by Atkins and Magnuson (1990) and Rogers (1990) shows evidence of advances in occupational and environmental health nursing research. Atkinson and Magnuson reported that from 1984 to 1989 more than 50% of research conducted by occupational and environmental health nurse investigators was concerned with health promotion and interventions to improve healthy lifestyles and stress and coping topics related to worker health. Rogers (1990c) reported that much of the occupational and environmental health nursing research in the early 1980s focused on programmatic activities, role delineation, and scope of practice but that more emphasis was placed on research concerning worker health promotion and protection in the latter part of the decade.

Based on a current review of research-based articles published from 1990 to 1999 in the *AAOHN Journal,* the journal of the professional society the American Association of Occupational Health

Nurses (AAOHN), research related to prevention and health promotion activities and interventions were the most reported ($n = >100$) followed by research related to musculoskeletal problems including back injury ($n = >40$), stress and mental health issues ($n = >35$), and infectious disease issues and interventions ($n = >30$). Other research areas with at least 25 reported publications included occupational and environmental health nursing practice, case management, traumatic injuries, quality assurance and cost-effectiveness of service, and work-related injury and violence studies. Clearly the breadth of occupational and environmental health nursing research has broadened considerably.

Evidence of recognition for occupational and environmental health nursing research was initially established by the AAOHN through the offering of its first research award, the Mary Louise Brown Award in 1983, with this author as the first recipient. Research in occupational and environmental health nursing continued to be emphasized and supported by the profession, and in 1989 a study funded by the AAOHN was conducted to establish occupational and environmental health nursing research priorities (Rogers, 1989a). In 1999 the study was updated, and 12 occupational and environmental health nursing research priorities (Box 16-2) emerged and serve as the stimulus for funding through the

newly created AAOHN Foundation (discussed in Chapter 19). These priorities represent vital areas of importance to improve the health and safety of the U.S. workforce and have been distributed to key agencies and groups (e.g., NIOSH, NINR, NIH) to focus attention on these areas for support in funding opportunities.

Of like importance is the National Occupational Research Agenda (NORA), unveiled by NIOSH and its partners in 1996. NORA provides a framework to guide occupational safety and health research into the next decade (USDHHS, 1996). Approximately 500 individuals and organizations external to NIOSH provided input in the development of NORA, and this effort resulted in 21 occupational safety and research priorities for the nation (Box 16-3). NORA provides a means to target research and funding so that the likelihood of reducing illness/injury can be increased. A high level of agreement exists between the occupational and environmental health nursing research priorities and NORA (Rogers, 2000).

Many of the AAOHN research priorities for occupational and environmental health nursing are being addressed. For example, in the area of health promotion Wilson et al. (1997) conducted a survey study of 200 manufacturing workers and compared health beliefs related to susceptibility, barriers, benefits, severity, self-efficacy, and motivation of participants and nonparticipants in

---

Box 16-2 **Research Priorities in Occupational and Environmental Health Nursing**

1. Effectiveness of primary health care delivery at the worksite.
2. Effectiveness of health promotion nursing intervention strategies.
3. Methods for handling complex ethical issues related to occupational health.
4. Strategies that minimize work-related health outcomes (e.g., respiratory disease).
5. Health effects resulting from chemical exposures in the workplace.
6. Occupational hazards of health care workers (e.g., latex allergy, bloodborne pathogens).
7. Factors that influence workers' rehabilitation and return to work.
8. Effectiveness of ergonomic strategies to reduce worker injury and illness.
9. Effectiveness of case management approaches in occupational illness/injury.
10. Evaluation of critical pathways to effectively improve worker health and safety and enhance maximum recovery and safe return to work.
11. Effects of shiftwork on worker health and safety.
12. Strategies for increasing compliance with or motivating workers to use personal protective equipment.

From "Research Priorities in Occupational Health Nursing," by B. Rogers, J. Agnew, and L. Pompeii, 2000, *AAOHN Journal, 48, 9-16.*

Box 16-3 NORA Priority Research Areas	
DISEASE AND INJURY	Organization of work
Allergic and irritant dermatitis	Special populations at risk
Asthma and chronic obstructive pulmonary disease	
Fertility and pregnancy abnormalities	**RESEARCH TOOLS AND APPROACHES**
Hearing loss	Cancer research methods
Infectious disease	Control technology and personal protective
Low back disorders	equipment
Musculoskeletal disorders of the upper extremities	Exposure assessment methods
Traumatic injuries	Health services research
	Intervention effectiveness research
WORK ENVIRONMENT AND WORKFORCE	Risk assessment methods
Emerging technologies	Social and economic consequences of workplace
Indoor environment	illness and injury
Mixed exposures	Surveillance research methods

From *National Occupational Research Agenda* (Publication No. 96-115), by U.S. Department of Health and Human Services, National Institute for Occupational Safety and Health, 1996, Cincinnati, OH: National Institute for Occupational Safety and Health.

worksite blood pressure and cholesterol screening programs. Significant differences were noted between the groups with respect to likelihood to participate and unpleasantness of the procedure (barrier) and ability to maintain health (self-efficacy).

Helyer et al. (1998) evaluated the effectiveness of a worksite smoking cessation program on 107 military personnel who smoked. Forty-five employees participated in an 8-week program that consisted of lectures, group discussion, and homework built around the concept that smoking is related to psychosocial factors (stress), learned behavior (habit), and addiction to nicotine. Sixty-two employees served as control subjects who did not participate in the program. Of the participants, 26.7% were not smoking 12 months after the program compared with 6.9% of the comparison group. Of the participants who resumed smoking, 64% smoked less than one half the amount they smoked before the program.

Moore (1998) implemented a primary prevention program in the workplace targeted to prevent muscle strains. Physiologic and perception measurements were taken before and after participation in a stretching program developed to improve flexibility through conditioning. A one group pretest/posttest design was used with 60 employees enrolled in a 36-session stretching

program in the workplace. Flexibility was measured by a flexibility profile including the sit and reach test, bilateral body rotation measurements, and shoulder rotation measurements. A statistically significant increase was found in all flexibility measurements at the conclusion of the study for the participants as a total group. The participants' perceptions of their body attractiveness, physical conditioning, and overall self-worth at the program's conclusion, as measured by the Fox Physical Self-Perception Profile, also showed a statistically significant increase. In addition, participants who completed the program had no occurrences of musculosketal injuries during the 2-month period. The results of this study suggest that continued development and implementation of stretching programs in the workplace may benefit employees by increasing flexibility and potentially preventing injuries due to muscle strains. Stretching programs in the workplace also may improve components of employees' perceptions of their physical bodies.

Adams et al. (1995) implemented a health risk appraisal program for 397 employees (with a 47% participation rate) at a university health science center. Data generated on self-reported behaviors indicated that 9% were current smokers, 34% were overweight, and fitness, nutrition, and health practices fell well below recommended levels.

Data generated were used by the nurse practitioner to develop intervention strategies to improve health behaviors.

In the area of primary care Dille (1999) examined the effect of a worksite immunization program implemented at the Hanford nuclear reservation in Washington state. Using a randomized, retrospective case-control survey approach, Dille compared immunized employees (cases) to a group of nonimmunized employees (controls) between the months of October and December 1994 through distribution of a self-administered questionnaire. Bivariate analysis included chi-square tests to study the association between influenza vaccine and rates of influenza-like illness and related complications, rates of employee absenteeism, rates of physician visits, use of prescribed medication, and rates of hospitalization. To assess the economic benefits associated with vaccination, analysis included estimating the direct and indirect costs associated with immunization and influenza-like illnesses, and complications related to influenza-like illnesses.

A total of 1,920 surveys were mailed to nonvaccinated employees, and 960 surveys were mailed to vaccinated employees. As compared with vaccinated employees ($n = 789$ responders), nonvaccinated employees ($n = 931$ responders) reported significantly higher rates of episodes of influenza-like illness (78 per 100 compared with 59 per 100, $p < .01$), influenza related complications (8.0 compared with 5.0, $p < .01$), lost work days (63 per 100 compared with 35 per 100), use of prescription medication (18.6 per 100 compared with 8.7 per 100), and inpatient hospitalization (0.8 per 100 compared with 0.1 per 100). Cost savings were estimated to be $83.84 per person vaccinated. The results of this study suggest this worksite influenza vaccination program produced significant health-related and economic benefit to employee participants and their employers.

Chemical exposures are highly prevalent in selected working populations, thus reflecting one of the AAOHN's research priorities. One of the major issues today is latex exposure. Cohen and Kaufman (2000) studied latex allergy awareness, knowledge, and prevention and control strategies in acute care hospitals. Based on reports from the workers' compensation system and a sentinel health provider network, latex gloves may be one of the most prevalent sources of occupational

skin disorders in Washington state's health care industry. To gather information to understand and address this problem, questionnaires were distributed to 105 acute care hospitals in Washington state. Employee health and infection control specialists were queried on their knowledge about latex allergy, the perceived extent of the problem, and the actions taken to address the problem. With 95 of the hospitals returning completed questionnaires (93% response rate), 30% reported having problems with latex allergies among employees in their facility, with most reporting two or fewer cases. Although adequate knowledge was found about the causes and effects of latex allergies, a lack of knowledge about some areas existed, particularly about the early warning signs of systematic hypersensitivity and the ability of latex protein to adhere to glove powders. More than 60% of all of the hospitals surveyed had made some type of glove alternatives available to affected employees, 4% had designated latex free zones, 4% had cleaned to remove latex dust, and 7% had done nothing to address the issue.

Case management, rehabilitation, and return to work are important areas for occupational and environmental health nursing research and practice, but these areas have not been well-researched. Brines et al. (1999) examined return to work issues from the perspective of injured workers. The investigators surveyed or interviewed 45 workers who had filed a worker's compensation claim from January through September 1995. Workers satisfied with services believed the nurse case manager was able to include them in the plan, whereas workers who were dissatisfied reported feeling unimportant and disrespected in terms of service provision.

Sewitch et al. (2000) reported on the relationships among psychological factors, low back pain, disability, and return to work. The role of psychological factors in recovery from first lifetime low back pain (LBP) was explored in this study. The participants, consecutive clients taken from a physiatry clinic in Montreal, had LBP of less than 3-months' duration, were on sick leave and receiving workers' compensation benefits, and reported the current event as first lifetime LBP. Psychological factors that fluctuate with current events (Psychiatric Symptom Index) and remain stable over time (General Well-Being Scale) were assessed. Outcomes were late return to work (>31 days) and 1-year incidence of compensated recurrence. Lower psychological distress predicted late return to work, and higher well-being, higher aggressiveness, and lower anxiety predicted compensated recurrence. Researchers concluded psychological factors do not impact clients with all types of LBP in the same way. For individuals lacking prior LBP experience, better psychological function increased lengthy work absence. Thus, awareness of the clients' psychological profiles and previous LBP experiences may benefit recovery. For example, in this study younger workers with more years of seniority and less psychological distress were at greater probability of late return to work. Workers with more seniority may be less worried about losing their jobs while on sick leave.

Several studies have been reported in the area of ergonomics. Stoy and Aspen (1999) conducted a study to develop a valid methodology for comparing measured torque repetition data along a ham boning line with symptoms reported in an established clinical database, which included history of cumulative stress disorder symptoms. A musculoskeletal stress measurement system was used to measure torque and repetition data associated with boning hams. Twenty-two surveys were conducted across a representative sample of employees performing this task on three different production lines. Two different knife grips were compared to determine if one method produced lower torque. Data analysis showed an increased rate of reported symptoms by subjects exerting more power as compared to other subjects performing the same task. Operators managed a microbreak in the cycle ranging from 0.88% to 4% of the survey time. Operators not reporting symptoms averaged longer microbreaks than those reporting. The study provided data for structuring a line rotation program for moving people to positions requiring less power.

Cohen-Mansfield et al. (1996) reported the period prevalence and costs of back injuries to nursing staff of long-term care facilities in comparison with nurses employed industry-wide and with other occupations industry-wide. The period prevalence of back injuries to nursing staff in long-term care facilities was highest for nurse aides, followed by liscenced practical nurses (LPNs) and then registered nurses (RNs). Nurses (combined) had a period prevalence of back injuries nearly 1.5 times higher than all employees of long-term care facilities and 6 times higher than all occupations combined industry-wide. Within long-term care facilities nurses sustaining back injuries were younger and had been employed for a shorter period of time than the average for all nurses employed in long-term care facilities. Back injuries accounted for more than half of the indemnity and medical costs of all injuries incurred in nursing homes and industry-wide. The findings highlight the need for better prevention, treatment, and rehabilitation programs. Many back injuries and LBP may be due to a cumulative effect of repeated stress and milder injuries to the back, particularly for nurse aides given the present findings of a markedly higher period prevalence of back injuries compared with other nurses and other long-term care (LTC) employees. Nurse aides are responsible for the majority of the heavy lifting and other "bed and body work." Thus, given their job description, nurse aides will continue to be at high risk for back injuries.

Faucett and Rempel (1996) describe a study related to measuring repetitive strain on the job. The occupational use of video display terminals (VDTs) has been associated with the increasing incidence of upper extremity musculoskeletal disorders, often called cumulative trauma disorders. To guide clinical and policy decisions about the prevention and treatment of these VDT-related disorders, valid and economic measures of total daily VDT use and VDT-related job tasks, such as data entry or editing, will be important. In this study of newspaper reporters and copy editors ($n = 83$), VDT use was measured with employee self-reports and by sampling the work behaviors of a subsample of employees. Behavioral sampling estimated VDT use as a characteristic of the job as opposed to a characteristic of the individual employee performance. Overall, the two techniques of measuring occupational VDT use compared favorably, with the exception that self-reported hours of VDT use tended to exceed the hours of use estimated by behavioral observation for employees who were younger and for those who reported greater job demands. The findings suggest that behavioral sampling is a valid technique for estimating VDT use as a job characteristic.

In the area of reducing work-related adverse health outcomes, Rogers et al. (2000) conducted a comprehensive study of housekeepers in a university setting. This study included survey and in-depth interviews, policy analysis, and walk-throughs of several buildings to identify work-related health hazards and environmental conditions contributing to adverse health outcomes. Several health issues including back injuries, musculoskeletal problems, needlestick injuries, stress, and lack of training, were identified. Strategies are being put in place by university administration to reduce hazards and improve working conditions.

Morris (1999) studied the injury experience of temporary workers in a manufacturing setting. An apparent 2 to 3 times higher injury frequency rate for temporary employees compared with permanent workers was identified in one manufacturing setting. Data were collected using demographic surveys ($N = 20$), three focus group interviews ($n = 13$) with a convenience sample of temporary employees, and four structured interviews with temporary agency owners and managers to explore factors that increase the vulnerability of temporary employees to workplace injuries. Several physical and psychological stressors were identified, such as machine guarding concerns, job insecurity, stress, lack of training, and a perception among the temporary employees that the reporting of work injuries could lead to loss of a temporary work assignment or the opportunity for permanent employment.

In contrast, the agency owners and managers were concerned that reported injuries were not always legitimate. All of them actively used strategies to control their injury experience but faced the challenge of lacking day-to-day control of both the work environment and employee work behaviors. While this preliminary study cannot be generalized to manufacturing worksites, it demonstrates the need for additional research to document the injury experience of temporary employees, identify training needs, and design intervention strategies.

Griest and Bishop (1998) conducted a retrospective study using longitudinal data of audiometric tests to evaluate tinnitus (ringing or other sounds in the ears or head) as a potential early indicator of permanent hearing loss in a population of workers exposed to noise. Data were examined from 91 male employees working in environments with noise levels ranging from 8-hour time-weighted averages of 85 to 101 decibels over a period of 15 years. Results of annual audiometric testing were obtained as part of an ongoing hearing conservation program conducted since 1971 by a steel foundry located in the Portland, Oregon area. Results indicate the prevalence of tinnitus increases more than 2.5 times for workers experiencing maximum threshold shifts greater than or equal to 15 decibels in hearing level (dBHL). Results also provide evidence that reports of tinnitus at the time of annual audiometric testing may be useful in identifying workers at greater risk for developing significant shifts in hearing thresholds.

Another significant occupational and environmental health nursing research priority, hazards to health care workers, is a phenomenon which has been studied by several investigators, mostly within the last 8 to 10 years. Ramsey and Glenn (1996) investigated whether mandatory universal precautions changed nurses' body fluid exposure and reporting rates, hepatitis B vaccination rates, and human immunodeficiency virus (HIV) testing rates. Random cross-sectional surveys of nurses in Tennessee were conducted in 1991 ($n = 145$) before the OSHA Bloodborne Pathogen Standard and in 1993 ($n = 143$) after the standard had been in effect 1.5 years. The questionnaire in both surveys included frequency of body fluid exposures and reporting in the past year, and whether or not the respondent had received the hepatitis B vaccine or had been tested for HIV. The findings indicated that self-reported needlestick injuries decreased by 69%, and other sharps injuries decreased by 81%. Only 4.1% of all exposure incidents reported on this anonymous survey were reported to employee health officials as required, showing no significant difference between 1991 and 1993. Hepatitis B vaccinations significantly increased (61.4% to 82.5%), with a nonsignificant increase in HIV testing (47.2% to 55.6%) from 1991 to 1993. The findings of this study suggest that the universal precautions regulatory mandate has been effective in increasing nurses' compliance to universal precautions.

Sass et al. (1995) conducted a descriptive correlational design study of 178 health care workers (with 45 responding) who were exposed to blood or body fluids or both but did not return for follow-up HIV testing. Depth of exposure as evaluated by the respondent with the health service provider (susceptibility) was a factor in return for follow-up. Further education for those with less invasive exposures was recommended.

Hepatitis B viral infection is a major occupational risk for health care workers; this infection can lead to disability, chronic liver disease, and liver cancer. A health care worker risks a 6% to 30% chance of contracting hepatitis B viral infection after a percutaneous exposure. The duration of immunity after immunization with the hepatitis B vaccine series is unknown.

Funderburke and Spencer (2000) conducted a descriptive study of a convenience sample of 42 health care workers in a large urban hospital to determine hepatitis B immunity in high-risk health care workers 7 years after immunization. The study related immunity to age and site of injection and also described titer results. The study found that 21% of the health care workers had nonreactive titers 7 or more years after immunization. No significant differences existed in the percentages of the reactive participants according to injection site, although intramuscular injection in the deltoid is recommended. No statistically significant relationship was revealed by comparing titer results with age. The low power (.24) shows the need for larger sample sizes, which could be obtained by using multicenter data sites. Future research with national collaboration and standard performance measurement systems could provide crucial information related to hepatitis B immunity in health care workers.

Studies related to cost-containment approaches, evaluation of primary care strategies, and ethics continue to be reported less often than studies on health hazards and health risks to workers. Rogers (1990) has investigated ethical problems facing occupational and environmental health nurses and has identified several recurring issues, such as confidentiality of health information, exposure and right to know issues, and dealing with substance abuse. Conflicts often arise as to how such problems should be managed. Strategies for ethical effectiveness need to be developed.

With the continuing rise of health care costs and increased emphasis on primary health care delivery at the worksite, including family care, strategies to evaluate the effectiveness and efficiency of primary care delivery at the worksite need to be evaluated. Occupational and environmental health nurses must continue to demon-

strate the value of their service by providing positive outcomes for the employee and cost savings for the employer.

These are only a few examples of recent research that were conducted by occupational and environmental health nurse investigators and have an impact on the health of the working population. Knowledge development is needed to measure the effectiveness and impact of interventions that will improve worker health and reduce hazard risk.

CONDUCTING THE RESEARCH

FEASIBILITY

The investigative process involves deliberate steps and activities within a carefully designed framework, or blueprint so to speak. Of clear importance in conducting research is whether the research can be done—that is, is it feasible? The following factors should be considered for the successful completion of the project (Rogers, 1996; Tornquist & Rogers, 1987):

- A research problem of some importance
- Research experience or collaboration with a seasoned researcher for consultation and/or coinvestigation
- A commitment from the researcher to complete the project, because it may take months or years to finish
- Cooperation from management, particularly if the research requires employee time and company involvement
- Adequate time to conduct the study, especially if competing obligations, such as job responsibility, exist
- Accessibility and availability of research subjects
- Sufficient resources, including money, equipment, supplies, and additional personnel if needed, depending on the scope of the project
- Facilities and space in which to conduct the research
- Attention to ethical considerations of the research, including issues related to risk/benefit, potential for harm, informed consent, and maintenance of confidentiality

Consideration of each of these points is important in determining if the research can go forward. Of particular importance is determining funding needs to conduct the research. Appendix 16-1 provides information about potential funding sources. Determining early on the feasibility of conducting the research will save time, money, and energy and help avoid unnecessary frustration.

TERMINOLOGY

Scientific research has specific terminology with which the researcher must be familiar. Basic terms are briefly discussed here.

Concepts are generally abstractions or ideas that are based on observations of certain behaviors or characteristics (e.g., stress, self-esteem, pain, health). A *theory* is a systematic, abstract explanation of some aspect of reality. Concepts are building blocks of theories that are locked together into a coherent system in an effort to explain the world and phenomena around us, including how we live and function in it.

A *variable* is something that varies, such as weight, height, temperature, blood pressure, blood value, and attitude, and takes on different values. For example, the variable *gender* has two values, male and female, whereas, the variable *age* may have values from 0 to more than 100. However, in a research study where all subjects are female, gender would not be a variable (i.e., gender would not vary). Variables that are characteristics of the research subject are such factors as age, health beliefs, or weight and are called *attribute variables.* In the research context, if *relationships* between variables are presumed—that is, one variable affects or influences another variable—those variables are often labeled as independent or dependent. The *independent variable* (IV) is the presumed cause variable, whereas the *dependent variable* (DV), otherwise referred to as the outcome or presumed effect variable, is the variable under investigation. In other words, variability in the dependent variable is presumed to depend on how the independent variable varies. For example, the researcher may investigate the extent to which lung cancer (DV) depends on smoking behavior (IV), the effects of teaching employees about diet and cholesterol (IV) on cholesterol reduction (DV), the use of incentives (IV) to affect employee participation (DV) in health promotion programs, the effect of peer influence (IV) on the use of protective equipment (DV), or the wearing of a certain kind of glove (IV) on reduction of latex allergy (DV). The difference between dependent and independent variables in a research study is usually fairly apparent. The researcher needs to be cautioned, however, not to presume that the independent variable is, in fact, the cause of the dependent variable. Many other factors, such as research design and sampling scheme, which will be discussed later, need to be considered before making conclusions regarding cause and effect. In addition, a variable, such as attitudes about health, can be purely descriptive.

An *operational definition* specifies what the researcher does to make the concept or variable measurable. For example, the variable *weight* will be operationally defined by measuring a subject's weight on scales, after the subject has undressed and has fasted for 10 to 12 hours. If anxiety related to overwork is being measured, then overwork needs to be given a definition, such as working more than 60 hours per week, and anxiety needs to be measured, perhaps through use of a survey instrument, many of which are available. Defining variables operationally allows the researcher to collect data systematically and consistently from all subjects and to communicate exactly what the terms mean.

Other variables of note, *extraneous variables* (or *confounding variables*), may have relevant effects on the dependent variable (other than the independent variable), and the research must take these into account in the design, analysis, and interpretation of the findings. For example, a researcher may be interested in studying whether women who work rotational shiftwork are at higher risk of having low birth weight babies than are women who work regular daytime jobs. Although the key variables of interest are rotational shiftwork (IV) and low birth weight (DV), the researcher will also need to be concerned with the effects of other extraneous variables, such as age, diet, prenatal care, medications, and smoking, all of which can cause low birth weight. Because uncontrolled extraneous variables can lead to erroneous conclusions, the researcher will need to identify these extraneous variables and determine approaches within the design of the study to control for them. For example, control for the variable *smoking* can be accomplished through limiting participation of research subjects to nonsmokers; this eliminates or equalizes the effects of the variable *smoking.* The same would be true of age. The researcher could limit the study participants to those under age 35 or analyze the data relative to age grouping (such as age 20 years or younger, ages 21 to 25 years, 26 to 30 years, and 30 to 35 years).

Data are the pieces of information the investigator collects from the subjects, usually by means of *instruments* or *tools*. Instruments may include questionnaires; rating scales; paper and pencil tests; physiological and biological measurement devices such as thermometers, sphygmomanometers, or blood tests; and a variety of industrial hygiene sampling devices. In quantitative studies the researcher collects quantitative data—that is, information in numeric form. For example, asking about attitudes or perceptions as measured by a scale with a range of 1 through 5 where 1 = *never* and 5 = *almost always* represents quantitative data. The data then are analyzed collectively for the group.

MAJOR STEPS IN A QUANTITATIVE STUDY

The research process is scientifically derived and requires consistency and rigor. The major steps in the quantitative research process (Box 16-4) are briefly described here. In quantitative research the researcher moves from the beginning (asking the question) to the end (arriving at an answer) in a logical sequence or predetermined steps. The research process can be described in five phases: conceptual, design and planning, empirical, analytical, and dissemination (Polit & Hungler, 1999).

Phase 1: Conceptual Phase

This phase requires a strong conceptual or intellectual element, including thinking, reading, conceptualizing, theorizing, reasoning, and insight.

Step 1: Identifying and delimiting the research problem

Selecting the research problem can be the most challenging task of the research process, especially for the beginning investigator. The researcher may have some idea of what she or he is interested in studying but may be unfamiliar with what is known about the subject or concerned with whether the problem is in fact researchable. In addition, the researcher will want to study a problem that is of some significance—that is, address the *So what?* question of whether or not the research idea is important and will contribute to the knowledge base and practice in the discipline, in this case occupational and environmental health nursing.

Sources of research problems

When beginning to identify a research problem for study, there are at least three sources from which ideas can be generated: work experience; trends and patterns in such areas as health, illness, injury, and behavior; and the literature.

Experience. Every work setting has problems, and the researcher may wonder what could improve or alter the situation. For example, what makes some employees use protective equipment while others do not? Is a certain counseling approach more effective in helping employees lower cholesterol levels? Is the use of nursing guidelines or protocols for practice effective in reducing costs? Whatever the problems, curiosity will help generate a research idea.

Trends and patterns. Practitioners can identify research problems from observations of individual cases that form a pattern of occurrence. For example, several workers from the same work area report to the occupational health unit with similar health complaints; the incidence in spontaneous abortions in women workers has increased over a period of time; or violent episodes at work have increased. Trends or

---

Box 16-4 Steps in the Research Process

1. Identify and delimit the research problem.
2. Conduct the literature review.
3. Identify the theoretical or conceptual framework.
4. Formulate the hypothesis.
5. Select the research design.
6. Operationalize the variables.
7. Identify the study population.
8. Develop the sampling plan.
9. Conduct the pilot study.
10. Collect the data.
11. Prepare the data for analysis.
12. Analyze the data.
13. Interpret the results.
14. Communicate the findings.
15. Utilize the information.

patterns that may be occurring lend themselves to investigation.

Literature. Ideas for researchable problems often come from published and unpublished reports. Researchers who publish in various disciplines, including nursing, occupational and environmental health, or related fields, will often suggest problem areas for further research as an extension of their work. Unpublished master's theses or doctoral dissertations also provide fruitful areas for research ideas. Furthermore, questions for study are often stimulated by contradictory results reported by different investigators about the same general area. For example, one researcher may report that work stress is best managed by support groups, but another may report that specific stress reduction techniques are the best approach. Research that further tests these approaches can be useful.

In addition, the AAOHN priorities in occupational and environmental health nursing previously discussed (see Box 16-2) were identified to focus attention on critical areas needing occupational and environmental health nursing research and support for funding (Rogers, 2000). These priorities can be used to generate further thinking and conceptualizing of research areas pertinent to the researcher's interest.

Problem development

The development of a researchable problem requires creativity and thoughtfulness, and the researcher may find herself or himself generating several ideas. The researcher should try not to be critical of these ideas but rather should write down the areas of interest (e.g., ergonomic stressors, job satisfaction among nurses, effective use of personal protective equipment, back injuries in nurses, transmission of communicable diseases, and cost-effectiveness of prenatal care at the worksite) and not worry about the terms or structure used.

After a general topic of interest has been identified, the focus should be narrowed so a researchable problem or question can be developed. Discussing thoughts and ideas with fellow colleagues can help further define or clarify the question. A stem, such as *What types of . . . ?* or *What is the relationship between . . . ?* or *Why do . . . ?*, will need to be added to the topical statement. For example, one might ask, What conditions promote the use of gloves when the potential

for body fluid exposure exists? or What is the relationship between work stress and absenteeism?

Brink and Wood (1988) describe three levels of research and respective types of questions, each based on the amount of knowledge and/or theory about the topic under study. Level I questions are developed when the topic has not been studied, the information is limited, or knowledge gaps exist. Level I questions begin with the *What is/are* stem.

The researcher moves to Level II questions when information on the topic has already been described. Here the researcher focuses on relationships between at least two variables not previously examined together, such as pregnancy outcomes and extended work duty, lifting, or prolonged standing at work. At this level a good foundation for why two variables should be related is based on previous descriptive studies (Rogers, 1990b, 1991). Level II questions may begin with the stem *What is the relationship between . . . ?* and are completed by relating two variables together. At Level III the researcher asks why a relationship exists between the variables, a question that implies that one variable specifically influences the other. A cause and effect relationship is assumed, and the researcher manipulates the independent variable, such as an intervention (e.g., stretching exercise) to predict an outcome. Examples of each level are shown in Box 16-5.

Box 16-5   Examples of Research Questions

LEVEL I
- What is the prevalence of hypercholesterolemia in the worker population?
- What are the characteristics of employees who exercise regularly?

LEVEL II
- Is there a relationship between eating foods prepared at the worksite and hypercholesterolemia in workers?
- What is the relationship between absenteeism and exercise?

LEVEL III
- Why do employees resist or comply with using protective devices?
- Why is there an increase in violence in the workplace?

The research problem normally identifies the key variables (independent and dependent), study subjects, and topic area. Although often stated as a question, the problem may be stated in a declarative form such as: the purpose of this research is to examine the relationship between pregnancy outcome and shift rotation.

Step 2: Conducting the literature review

The literature review involves a comprehensive and systematic examination of available material to help find out more precisely what is known about the topic or area of investigation. Research studies are usually undertaken within the context of an existing knowledge base (Polit & Hungler, 1999). Depending on what the literature reveals, the level of inquiry of the question may change. For example, if the question is, What are the characteristics of employees with back problems? and several research and related articles dealing with that issue are discovered, moving to a second level of inquiry such as, What is the relationship between lifting techniques and back injuries? would be in order. As the topic becomes clearer from the literature review, the question level will also become clearer.

There are several reasons to conduct a literature review. First, determining what is already known about the problem will help avoid unnecessary duplication if the problem has had satisfactory research. Second, reviewing the literature helps to provide a context into which the problem fits; that is, it will help establish links to existing research and build a body of knowledge. And third, the literature review helps identify gaps in research and will then enable the researcher to better define the problem. A study conducted in isolation cannot be clearly evaluated for significance and meaning, whereas a study that links with previous research or theory provides a sense of context and history (Wilson, 1989). The more a researcher's study is linked with other research, the more contribution it is likely to make.

To begin the literature search, the researcher can use manual method print indexes or electronic databases with end user systems, which are quickly becoming the preferred method and are making manual searching obsolete. However, print indexes should not be ignored, because libraries in smaller health care facilities use these sources and some electronic databases do not contain early literature references. Consultation with a librarian may be recommended for more current information sources. The scope of the review should be comprehensive in breadth and depth and should include several types of literature.

Research literature

Research literatue represents the design and results of research investigations and is one of the most important types of information for the review. A review of relevant research literature from nursing and other related disciplines will provide a background for and document progress on a specific topic or problem.

Theoretical and conceptual literature. The information from theoretical and conception literature will provide a theoretical or conceptual context for a research problem. This context or framework will help provide the frame of reference for the research and extend the scope of the researcher's knowledge.

Methodological literature. Methodological literature concerning research similar to the topic area under investigation can be helpful when examining how studies were conducted—that is, what approaches were used, how variables were operationalized or measured, how samples were selected, and how data were analyzed. Understanding how other researchers have conducted similar studies can be helpful. References dealing with statistical tests and instrumentation are also useful.

Clinical literature. Nonresearch, clinical literature provides background information for the topic area and relates experiences with clinical impressions of the problem. However, these sources of literature are of limited value because they provide general information and often are subjective rather than objective in opinion. Nevertheless, they do help broaden the researcher's understanding of the problem.

Sources

Literature references are categorized as either primary or secondary sources. Primary sources are written by the investigator who conducted the study, while secondary sources provide summary descriptions, usually of several research studies, written by someone other than the original researcher. Secondary sources provide useful bibliographic information on primary sources; however, primary sources of the topic area must be read by the researcher to obtain sufficient details about the problem. When the literature is reviewed, written critiques about each article should be put on separate index cards. The researcher will then be able to systematically analyze the literature not only for content but also for flaws, gaps, and methodological weaknesses. For example, if a study has a sample size of five volunteers and the author generalizes its findings to a workforce of 1,000, caution in interpretation should be exercised.

Two electronic bibliographic databases that are particularly useful to nurse researchers are CINAHL (Cumulative Index to Nursing and Allied Health Literature) and MEDLINE (Medical Literature On-line). The CINAHL database covers materials dating from 1982 to the present from more than 950 journals plus relevant books, book chapters, and nursing dissertations covering fields such as cardiopulmonary services, emergency services, health education, respiratory therapy, social sciences, medical records, and laboratory technology. In addition to bibliographic information (i.e., title, author, journal information), the CINAHL database provides abstracts for more than 300 journals.

The MEDLINE database was developed by the U.S. National Library of Medicine and is widely considered the premier source for biblio-graphic information about biomedical literature. MEDLINE covers more than 3,600 journals with more than 8.5 million records and incorporates information from Index Medicus, International Nursing, and other sources in the areas of communication disorders, population biology, and reproductive biology. Table 16-1 displays common electronic databases relevant to nurses in occupational and environmental health. Print-based indexes that are particularly useful to nurses include CINAHL, International Nursing Index, Index Medicus, Hospital Literature Index, and Nursing Studies Index.

After the search is completed, sorting the information into logical categories, such as etiology of the problem, social and demographic characteristics, treatment, and prevention control, will help organize thoughts conceptually.

Step 3: Identifying the theoretical or conceptual context

Theory guides the researcher in understanding not only what happens related to certain phenomena (e.g., stress, pain, or anxiety) but also why these phenomena occur. Theories help link facts and concepts together and represent the researcher's best efforts to explain relationships between variables (e.g., anxiety and pain), predict what will happen (e.g., anxiety increases pain), and ultimately control or change the phenomena of concern (e.g., decrease pain through visualization or medication). The relationship between theory and research is reciprocal; theory guides,

TABLE 16-1	Common Electronic Databases Used in Occupational and Environmental Health
CancerLit	Cancer Literature
CINAHL	Cumulative Index to Nursing and Allied Health Literature
EMBASE	Excerpta Medica
HealthSTAR	Health Service, Technology, Administration and Research
HSDB	Hazardous Substance Database
MEDLINE	Medical Literature On-line
NIOSH TIC	NIOSH Database
PsychINFO	Psychology
RTECS	Registry of Toxic Effects of Chemical Substances
TOXLINE	Toxicology
TOXNET	Toxicology Database

Note: Search homepages of agencies (e.g., OSHA, EPA, NIOSH) for links to other sources of databases.

is amenable to testing, and generates ideas for research, while research from empirical data helps to validate or add to theory.

Not all research is conducted within a theoretical context; many nursing research studies are still at a descriptive point that may later serve as the basis for theory development. Although fitting a problem to a theory enhances its value, scientific meaning, and knowledge building, artificially cramming a problem into a theoretical framework serves no purpose; in other words, there is no point in fabricating a link if one does not exist (Polit & Hungler, 1999). Conceptual models are less well-developed attempts at organizing phenomena, but these models provide the inexperienced researcher with an important step in beginning to establish factual links between variable relationships. An imaginative mind can create a conceptual model that later may be developed into a theory.

Step 4: Formulating the hypothesis

After the problem has been identified, the literature reviewed, all variables conceptualized, and an appropriate theoretical or conceptual framework identified, the researcher will specify researchable questions to be answered and then move to hypotheses to be tested. A research hypothesis is a tentative prediction or explanation of the relationship between two variables. A question often arises as to whether a hypothesis is always necessary or if a research question is sufficient. Descriptive research aimed primarily at describing phenomena generally proceed without hypotheses, and research questions are used to gather data and provide a beginning foundation for later research, which often generates hypotheses. In these cases research questions will serve as the basis for inquiry.

A hypothesis, by setting direction and interconnecting and predicting relationships between two or more variables, requires a theoretical basis and helps extend knowledge about the phenomenon under investigation by testing an idea (Rogers, 2001). Within the framework of previous research or theory, a hypothesis usually flows from a researcher's observations or experiences. A hypothesis must be written clearly and specifically so that variables are identifiable and definable. A hypothesis may be simple or complex. A simple hypothesis predicts the rela-

tionship between one independent variable and one dependent variable, whereas a complex hypothesis predicts the relationship between two or more independent and two or more dependent variables. Examples of hypotheses are provided in Table 16-2.

The testing of a hypothesis is the center of empirical research and must indicate an anticipated relationship between two or more variables. After the hypothesis is developed, it is subjected to empirical testing through the collection, analysis, and interpretation of data. Not all investigations are designed to test a hypothesis but instead may answer questions to provide a foundation for empirical hypothesis testing later.

Phase 2: Design and Planning Phase

In this phase of the research project the researcher decides on the methods and design needed to answer the research question/hypothesis and plans for collection of data. These methodological decisions are critical for the validity of the study, because a flawed design cannot support the study conclusions.

Step 5: Selecting the research design

The research design is the blueprint or plan for conducting the research, and the selection of the research design is guided by the purpose of the research and the questions/hypotheses being posed. There are many types of research designs; however, only commonly used designs will be briefly discussed, for purposes of example. Reference to a good research text will be helpful in determining which type of design is most appropriate to answer the research question(s).

Experimental research

True experimental research is scientific investigation that is characterized by the properties of manipulation, randomization, and control. Manipulation occurs when the investigator does something, often referred to as the treatment or intervention, to the experimental group(s). Randomization involves the random assignment of subjects to experimental or control groups. Random assignment of subjects actually eliminates the systematic bias in the groups and equalizes attributes such as age, education, and marital status that may affect the dependent or outcome variable. The investigator will need to decide on a method to

TABLE 16-2	Examples of Hypotheses		
HYPOTHESIS	**INDEPENDENT VARIABLE**	**DEPENDENT VARIABLE**	**SIMPLE OR COMPLEX**
Women workers are more likely to frequent the occupational health unit than are male workers.	Gender (female versus male)	Occupational health unit visits	Simple
Nurses who randomly rotate shifts are more likely to have a higher number of sick days and decreased job satisfaction than nurses scheduled by block rotation.	Schedule method (random versus block rotation)	Absenteeism Job satisfaction	Complex
A relationship exists between worker age, gender, and work experience and knowledge about use of protective equipment.	Demographic characteristics (age, gender, experience)	Knowledge and use of protective devices	Complex
Younger workers are more likely to have on-the-job accidents than are older workers.	Age	Accidents	Simple

randomly assign subjects to groups; however, the most frequent approaches used are assignment by random number tables or computer-generated numbers.

Control involves managing the experiment through careful manipulation, randomization, and use of at least one control or comparison group. For example, suppose 30 employees with high cholesterol are enrolled in a study to test the effectiveness of two types of nursing interventions in reducing blood cholesterol levels. One intervention involves individual counseling, and the other utilizes individual counseling plus structured group teaching. The investigator will randomly assign (e.g., through use of a random table) 10 subjects to each intervention group and the third group of 10 subjects (control group) will receive the usual but no special treatment. After the intervention is completed, the investigator will then compare all group outcomes—that is, cholesterol levels—to test the effectiveness of the interventions.

Several types of experimental designs can be used, such as pretest-posttest, posttest only, Soloman four-group, and factorial design; however, a discussion of these designs is beyond the scope of this text, and the reader should consult a research text for a detailed discussion.

Quasi-experimental designs are similar to experimental research designs in that they involve manipulation of the independent variable but lack either randomization or a control group. These types of designs are obviously weaker but are useful if the researcher cannot randomly assign subjects to experimental or control groups, as happens when volunteer subjects are used. Several types of quasi-experimental designs are available to the researchers.

Nonexperimental research

Much of the research that is conducted does not involve applying a treatment or intervention (i.e., manipulation of an independent variable) as previously described; the research may be purely descriptive or relational in nature. Because the research is nonexperimental, cause and effect cannot be presumed. Descriptive research is designed to obtain information or facts about certain variables of interest, thereby determining the characteristics of the variables. Descriptive surveys should be conducted when lack of knowledge about a variable or population precludes the use of a theoretical base for the study. Studies of a single variable or characteristic in one population do not mean the variable or characteristic is the same in another population; therefore, further description of a variable in another population would be appropriate for study. In descriptive research no cause and effect relationships exist and no predictions can be made. A survey of employees about their health beliefs or a record review of the types and frequency of health visits to the occupational health unit are examples of descriptive research.

Another example of nonexperimental research is a correlational design in which investigators suspect a relationship between variables (that have already occurred) based on previous research. The purpose of correlational research is to describe relationships among variables rather than to test theory (although the findings may support existing research or theory). The investigator may be uncertain if one variable affects another or vice versa or whether there is any association at all. All variables are measured as they exist, and therefore the independent variable, if known, is not controlled. The study of the relationship between stress and premenstrual symptoms and disability or the examination of the relationship between length of employment or age and accidents would be examples of correlational research.

Other types of nonexperimental research include historical, methodological, or epidemiologic research. Historical research involves examining and analyzing records or data concerning previous events through the use of historical evidence. This research is often undertaken to examine trends relating to past events that may relate to present behaviors or practices. For example, examining the historical roots of occupational and environmental health nursing related to the development and enhancement of independent functioning will help further define

and extend professional occupational and environmental health nursing roles and practice.

Methodological research is aimed at studying the development and validity of research approaches or tools used in research designs. This research is concerned with the internal aspects of research involved with obtaining, organizing, or analyzing data that affect the validity of the research findings. Examples of methodological research include research dealing with development of research instruments, validity and reliability testing of instruments, and studies related to bias in research or to increasing response rates of subjects, such as the timing of telephone calls when telephone interviews are used.

Epidemiologic research is population-based and may use both experimental and nonexperimental types of research designs. However, the two most common types of research, cohort and case-control, are nonexperimental in design. In cohort studies—sometimes referred to as prospective studies—subjects without disease or the health outcome of interest are categorized as with or without exposure and followed forward in time for observation of the occurrence of the disease or problem. For example, in a common type of cohort study groups with the characteristic under investigation, such as workers exposed to a specific chemical (independent variable), are compared with unexposed workers, and then the incidence of disease or adverse health outcome (dependent variable) is statistically measured in both groups over time and compared. Measurement may be through clinical examinations, self-reports of health effects, or standardized test measurements (Gordis, 1999).

Case-control studies, also referred to as retrospective studies, are conducted in the opposite direction; that is, subjects diagnosed with a disease or reporting certain symptoms (cases) are identified and compared with persons without the disease or symptoms (controls). The researcher then goes back in time to determine if a certain exposure or risk occurred. The intent is to identify factors in the past that may account for or contribute to disease/symptom occurrence. For example, if a cluster of cancer cases (dependent variable) occurred in a worker population, this may be investigated by determining through a review of past exposure records what types of specific exposure occurred (e.g., chemical) (independent variable), and then a comparison of exposures can be made with a similar worker population without cancer to determine risk estimates.

Step 6: Operationalizing the variables

After research questions or hypotheses have been stated, variables (previously discussed) need to be defined and measured in the research context; that is, variables need to be operationally defined. The operational definition specifies a concrete definition of how a variable will be measured. Biophysiological measurements, self-report, or observation are common techniques used for the measurement of the variable and collection of data. For example, in a study involving an intervention aimed at blood pressure reduction, the variable *blood pressure* would be easy to define and measure. The operational definition might state that the blood pressures of research subjects would be measured weekly at a specific location, with the employee at rest for 5 minutes, and with a calibrated sphygmomanometer. The measurement of all variables must be consistent for all study subjects.

Many variables measured in nursing research deal with attitudes and behaviors and psychological, social, or health quality concepts that may be less easily operationalized; however, many instruments use such forms of measurement as self-report stress, coping, risk perception, and social support. The researcher needs to develop or choose an instrument that can validly measure the concepts under study. This is both a challenging and complex task.

Issues related to reliability and validity of the instrument must be considered. Reliability of an instrument is the degree of consistency in the measurement of responses of the attribute under study. Types of reliability include (1) stability, which refers to the extent to which the same results are obtained on repeated administrations of the instrument (also referred to as test-retest), (2) internal consistency, wherein all items included measure a certain attribute, not some other tangential attribute, and (3) equivalence, wherein the instrument produces the same (or equivalent) results when administered by two different observers or raters. Validity refers to the degree to which an instrument measures what it is supposed to measure. Types of validity include (1) content validity, which is concerned with the

sampling adequacy of the content area being measured, and (2) criterion-related validity, which focuses on the relationship or correlations between the instrument and an outside criterion (e.g., an instrument to measure self-performance would be validated by manager ratings).

Step 7: Identifying the study population

The term *population* refers to the aggregate of all the subjects. During the planning phase of quantitative studies the researcher identifies the population specifications or characteristics required for study inclusion. For example, a researcher might specify registered nurses who work in home health in the United States. The target population is the total group of interest that meets defined criteria to which the researcher would like to generalize her or his findings. The accessible population is the group from which the sample will actually be drawn. For example, a target population might be all employees who work for General Motors, but the accessible population might be restricted to those in Michigan.

Step 8: Developing the sampling plan

When conducting research, in most cases data are not gathered from an entire population; rather a sample or subset of the population is generally used. Although this is much more practical and cost-effective, the researcher must always be concerned that the sample addresses the characteristics of the population. The process of sampling is intended to enable the researcher to make statements about the larger group based on a smaller group. The principle aim in sampling is to be concerned with how representative the sample is of the larger population. How does one go about doing this? Sampling plans are categorized into two major approaches: probability and nonprobability sampling. Probability sampling involves some form of random selection of subjects from the accessible population so that each subject has the same chance of being selected or included in the sample. Because this sampling procedure is a more rigorous approach, accurate representations of the population in samples is much more likely to occur and generalizability of the findings is increased.

Nonprobability sampling involves selection of subjects in a nonrandom method (e.g., volunteers), and thus there is no way to determine the probability or chance for each subject to be included in the selection. The results, therefore, are usually only representative of and generalized to the sample itself. However, many studies utilize nonprobability sampling. When using nonprobability sampling approaches, caution in interpreting the findings needs to be emphasized. The researcher can choose from among several basic types of probability and nonprobability sampling approaches.

Probability sampling

Simple random sampling. This type of sampling allows each subject to have an equal chance of being selected into the sample. After the population has been defined, subjects or elements are selected, often through a computer-generated sampling frame, or they may be consecutively numbered and, using a table of random numbers, randomly drawn from the population until the desired sample size is obtained.

Systematic sampling. Systematic sampling involves drawing subjects from a listing of names at a specified sampling interval, such as every tenth subject. Procedurally, the desired sample size (n) will need to be known in advance, as well as an estimate of the population size (N). By dividing N by n, the sampling interval is established. For example, if you decided to interview 100 workers (n) from a population of 5,000 workers (N), the sampling interval would be 50 (5,000/100 = 50); that is, every fiftieth employee from the list of 5,000 would be sampled for interviewing, resulting in 100 workers interviewed.

Stratified random sampling. Stratified random sampling is similar to simple random sampling except that the population is first grouped together into strata such as age, gender, and occupation. Subjects are then selected randomly from each stratum in either equal numbers or proportionately, depending on the size or number in each stratum. For example, using gender as the stratifying variable, if the worker population of 1,000 consisted of 70% women and 30% men, drawing a proportionate stratified sample of 100 employees would include 70 women and 30 men.

Cluster sampling. Because obtaining a list of all potential subjects is not always possible or because the cost of doing so is prohibitive (especially in large-scale surveys), cluster or multistage sampling may be employed. Cluster sampling involves successive random sampling of units and elements. It requires that the population be divided into clusters or groups, and clusters are then randomly selected by either simple or stratified methods, after which the subjects themselves are randomly selected from the clusters. For example, suppose a large corporation that employs 80,000 workers has 100 sites nationwide. A random sample of 20 sites might be drawn, which is then followed by random sampling of the desired number of employees within each site.

Nonprobability sampling

Convenience or accidental sampling. Convenience or accidental sampling is used frequently by researchers and obtains subjects who are the most readily available. For example, asking for volunteers or distributing questionnaires to a classroom of students constitutes a sample of convenience. Because of the inherent bias associated with subjects obtained by this type of sampling scheme, convenience sampling has weaknesses; however, it is commonly used because of cost or population access issues.

Quota sampling. Quota sampling is not random but allows for some built-in representation in the sampling plan. The researcher first divides the population into groups or strata, such as gender, and then selects the sample by convenience based on proportions of subjects in each stratum.

Purposive sampling. Purposive sampling is accomplished by the researcher handpicking the subjects for the study based on certain criteria. Here the researcher uses her or his judgment to decide who is representative of the population. Although not usually recommended for obvious reasons of bias, this type of sampling approach is useful when the investigator may want to pretest an instrument with a handpicked sample of workers in order to refine the instrument for later use with the actual research subjects.

Step 9: Conducting the pilot study

In many cases a pilot study is advisable in order to iron out any details or correct previously unforeseen problems with the project. The pilot study will help determine if any modifications need to be made in the design or data collection procedures. For example, the researcher may find out that individuals will not participate in the study because of the types of procedures employed to collect the data (e.g., subjects may be unwilling to have certain invasive tests performed or refuse to answer certain sensitive questions). In addition, the researcher will want to know if participants can understand the directions and questions on survey instruments and, if an interview is conducted, how much time is involved.

The pilot study should mimic as closely as possible the actual study. Subjects selected for the pilot study should possess the same characteristics as subjects who will be selected for the actual study, and data collection procedures should be carried out in the same proposed manner. After pilot data are collected and examined, revisions or modifications should be incorporated to reduce or eliminate anticipated problems.

Phase 3: Empirical Phase

This phase involves the collection of research data and preparation of data for analysis. This data collection phase may be very time consuming, depending on the procedures used and scope of the project.

Step 10: Collecting the data

The actual data collection phase of the project will probably be the most time intensive but also the most fun. This phase should proceed in an orderly, consistent, and systematic way to minimize confusion and bias, which could occur if data were collected haphazardly.

There must be a preestablished plan for collecting the data, and the scope of this plan must be dependent on the research questions or hypotheses and the chosen design. The researcher needs to be concerned about several procedural aspects (depending on the type of design and variables to be measured), including determining measurement instruments (e.g., questionnaires, blood tests, weight scales, and reliability and validity testing), determining measurement approaches (e.g., mailed or telephone surveys, interviews, observations) and settings for data collection (e.g., home, clinic), training data collectors, establishing administrative and clerical procedures (e.g., coding questionnaires, scheduling appointments, mailing surveys, collecting specimens or

responses, follow-up on nonrespondents), and implementing procedures for confidentiality and anonymity, as appropriate, including storing data securely. During this phase the researcher begins to feel that the project is actually real.

Step 11: Preparing the data for analysis

Preliminary steps to prepare the data for analysis are usually necessary. For example, the researcher should look through the questionnaires to determine if they are usable (i.e., not left blank). If data are collected through use of open-ended questions, responses will need to be categorized and assigned a numerical form. For most types of quantitative data, computer analysis will be used. Data may need to be coded—that is, giving verbal data numeric values such as *yes* = 1 and *no* = 2. Coded data will need to be entered into a computer file with an individual record for each subject. Data will then need to be verified, which may entail rechecking the data entered in its entirety. Even after data verification, a few errors are likely to persist from input mistakes. Data cleaning—that is, checking for outliers, strange codes, and consistency checks—will be required to minimize any errors. After the data have been cleaned, a duplicate file copy should be made and stored.

Phase 4: Analytical Phase

This phase involves the interpretation and analysis of raw data in order to present information in the context of meaning to the consumer.

Step 12: Analyzing the data

Data analysis techniques will be derived from the research question(s) (Rogers, 1991), and data analysis should be planned at the time the research questions, hypotheses, and design are formulated. Data are basically analyzed through descriptive and inferential statistics. Descriptive analysis summarizes the data through reporting of the variable frequencies; measures of central tendency such as the mean, median, or mode; and examination of relationships between variables.

For example, if 40 occupational and environmental health nurses took a knowledge test about migraine headaches and the results were a random accounting of test scores as shown in Table 16-3, this would have little meaning. However, when distributed by frequency as

TABLE 16-3 **Point Test Scores for Occupational and Environmental Health Nurses**

50	100	85	90	100	70	80	85	85	90
90	60	85	95	75	85	90	65	85	75
65	70	90	85	75	60	85	80	95	85
75	80	80	90	80	50	90	85	90	80

TABLE 16-4 **Frequency Distribution of Occupational and Environmental Health Nurses' Test Scores**

POINT SCORE	FREQUENCY (F)	PERCENT (%)
50	2	5
60	2	5
65	2	5
70	2	5
75	4	10
80	6	15
85	10	25
90	8	20
95	2	5
100	2	5
	n = 40	100%

Total point score = 3,230
Mean = 80.75
Standard deviation = 11.86

shown in Table 16-4, the distribution of scores with lowest and highest according to the scores, the most common score, and the clustering of scores becomes apparent. For example, the data in Table 16-4 show that most (55%) occupational and environmental health nurses scored at least 85 points on the test and only 15% scored below 70. Ordering the data in such a fashion gives the data both form and meaning and allows for a description of the data. In addition, the mean (x), which is the sum of the scores divided by the number of scores, is the most widely used measure of central tendency and can be determined from the data (x = sum of scores (3230)/number of scores (40) = 80.75).

Inferential analysis almost always involves using more sophisticated statistical measures to test for significance between variables or support or reject hypotheses (Rogers, 1998). The statistical tests to be chosen will depend on the research questions and type of data collected. The analysis should be planned in consultation with a biostatistician up-front when the study is designed.

Step 13: Interpreting the results

The researcher will need to report the results of the statistical analyses with respect to the overall aims of the project, its theoretical underpinnings or conceptualization, specific questions being answered or hypotheses tested, existing body of research knowledge, and limitations of the research methods used.

Being cautious is preferred when reporting conclusions about research findings. The researcher must always remember that even when statistical significance is achieved it does not necessarily reflect a causal relationship, as when the research design is nonexperimental or when tests of significance examined associations between variables rather than for causation. In addition, because statistical tests are based on probability, the possibility that the results are due to chance always exists. The researcher should consider alternative explanations for the findings, particularly within the limits of the research design; if alternatives can be eliminated, the researcher may feel more confident about her or his interpretation of the findings. In addition, caution must be taken in generalizing the findings beyond the sample, particularly when nonprobability sampling has been used.

When the researcher is testing hypotheses, they are either accepted or rejected rather than proved or disproved. Sometimes the results will be statistically nonsignificant; however, the researcher should not reword the hypotheses to obtain statistical inference. Rather, a consideration of alternative theories or explanations should be explored and considered for future research.

In addition, if a particular treatment or intervention was deemed successful, others may want to utilize it in other settings or with other populations. Therefore the researcher will need to be careful about generalizing research findings within the context of the sampling scheme. The researcher also needs to report and interpret the findings within the context of what already is known. This will then affect knowledge development and expansion and identify areas for future research.

Phase 5: Dissemination Phase

When the researcher undertakes a research project, she or he should have a concomitant commitment to disseminating the results. A number of approaches can be used to accomplish this task; however, the primary methods are through writing and speaking.

Step 14: Communicating the findings

The results of research findings are of little use if they are not communicated to others. This can be done through the written word or oral presentation.

Written presentation

Written reports of scientific work allow for information dissemination to a much broader audience and can be in the form of an article, abstract, technical report, thesis, dissertation, or

---

> **Box 16-6**   **Typical Format for Research Article**
>
> 1. Title page
>   a. Title of study
>   b. Authors' names
>   c. Institutional affiliation
> 2. Abstract
>   a. Summary of research purpose, methods, findings
> 3. Sections of the article
>   a. Introduction
>   (1) Statement and significance of the problem
>   (2) Purpose of the study
>   b. Background/literature review
>   c. Conceptual/theoretical framework
>   d. Methods
>   (1) Design, variable definition, sampling, setting, instrumentation
>   (2) Procedures for data collection
>   e. Results
>   (1) Descriptive, inferential
>   (2) Tables, graphs
>   f. Discussion
>   (1) Interpretation of results
>   (2) Limitations, conclusions, implications for nursing and future research
> 4. References
> 5. Figures/models (optional)
>   Appropriate for further clarification of the study/findings

---

book. Because the written report is for someone else; the material should be presented so that it is readable, understandable, and organized; it should emphasize the important points, and avoid jargon or condescension. Research papers are presented in a different format than are clinical articles and generally include the major categories of introduction, background/literature review, theoretical/conceptual framework, methods, results, and discussion (Box 16-6).

If this is the first published paper, the researcher will want to refer to a writing reference, such as Strunk and White's (2000) *Elements of Style*, fourth edition, and the *Publication Manual of the American Psychological Association*, fifth edition (2001). In addition, other published works can be examined for style and format, and colleagues who have previously published might be asked if they would review and critique the manuscript.

Oral presentation

An oral presentation usually occurs at a professional society meeting. Although the research presentation usually follows a format similar to the research article, it will often be presented more concisely and with more attention focused on the results. Organization is important when presenting research. The researcher should state the purpose and major objectives and only briefly mention the supporting literature or provide this information in a handout. The researcher should provide sufficient detail about the study design, measurement instruments, and data collection procedures but not dwell on this aspect of the talk.

Results of the study are the meat of the matter and the bulk of the time should be focused here. The findings should be clearly explained and visual aids used, especially when reporting numerical values and statistical tests. When presenting the findings, their implication with respect to practice must be discussed.

The technical quality of visual aids is important because this will play a large role in conveying the message. The research presentation can be practiced before friendly colleagues to get constructive criticism and adjust the speech where necessary. In the actual presentation the researcher should try to be calm and organized, field questions appropriately, and not panic. The key point is to get the message across.

Step 15: Utilizing the findings

Ideally, the concluding step of a high quality study is to plan for utilization of the findings in practice. Although researchers may not be able to put a utilization action plan in motion, they can lay out strategies or recommendations as to how the study findings can be incorporated into practice. Evaluations can then be made as to the relevance and effectiveness of the strategies in real world situations.

QUALITATIVE RESEARCH

Another approach to research is through the conduct of qualitative studies. Qualitative research has been described as holistic—that is, concerned with humans and their environment in all of their complexities and based on the premise of describing the human experience (Morse & Field, 1995). Qualitative research often involves the researcher trying to comprehend those experiences under study. The focus of investigation is process- rather than structure-oriented, and data analysis techniques are oriented toward description. For example, if the research question is, How do workers feel about the consequence of a hazardous exposure and reproductive toxicity?, the investigator is trying to access perceptions and experiences. Although these data could be obtained through a structured questionnaire, much would probably be lost in the translation.

The design for a qualitative study is often referred to as an emergent design—that is, one that emerges as the researcher reflects about what has been learned based on the inquiry of study informants.

Various approaches can be used to gather information in qualitative studies. For example, ethnography involves the description and interpretation of cultural behavior. The aim is to learn from members of a cultural group their understanding of issues as they define that understanding. Data collection involves extensive field work for months or even years as the researcher actively participates in cultural activities and events to learn more about the culture.

Phenomenology involves trying to understand what the life experiences of people are like. The research focus is what people experience or perceive in regard to some phenomenon and how they interpret it. The main source of data typically is in-depth discussion with several groups (e.g., focus groups) in which the researcher helps the informant describe the lived experience without leading the discussion. Descriptive data are gathered, and in the analysis common themes begin to emerge and an understanding and definition of the phenomenon under study can be determined.

A third type of qualitative research is grounded theory, which has become an important research method for the study of nursing phenomena. Developed in the 1960s, grounded theory is an approach to study the social processes and structures in order to have a better understanding of the social and psychological experiences related to real phenomena. In-depth interviews generally with samples of 25 to 50 informants are the most common data source, but observations and reviews of documents may also be used.

ETHICS IN RESEARCH

Protecting the rights of human subjects involved in the conduct of research is imperative. These rights include the right to self-determination; the right to informed consent; the right to full disclosure; the right to privacy, confidentiality, and anonymity; and the right to protection from harm (AAOHN, 1999a, 1999b; Rogers, 1990b). Self-determination means that people should have control over their own destiny and the freedom to voluntarily choose to participate in a research study without coercion or fear of recrimination. Research subjects should be given full disclosure of information, and deception by withholding of information is unwarranted. Informed consent, usually written, to participate in a study should be obtained when the research involves more than minimal risk (i.e., more than that encountered in everyday living).

Privacy is the right of a person to determine what information will be shared with or disclosed to others. An invasion of privacy occurs when private information, such as that collected through surveys or interviews, is collected under false pretenses. Confidentiality means that information divulged by a research subject will be guarded and not made public or shared with others. Breaches of confidentiality can be quite harmful emotionally and socially for the subject.

Anonymity occurs when the subjects' identities cannot be linked with their responses. Code numbers should be used on questionnaires rather than identifying information, and all data should be analyzed in the aggregate, with pseudonyms used to protect subjects. For example, names of hospitals or companies should not be used; giving general occupational and geographic information, such as an airline industry in the northeast, would be more appropriate.

Research subjects should be protected from harm or discomfort whether it be physical, mental, or emotional. Any research that has the potential for inflicting permanent damage is highly questionable, regardless of the benefits.

In general, great care should be taken to ensure that research subjects' rights are fully protected. Ethics in research is a complex phenomenon when the researcher is engaged in scientific inquiry for the betterment of society. However, the safeguards that exist to protect study subjects are designed to protect the researcher as well and will enable the investigator to develop sensitivity to ethical considerations.

Summary

Occupational and environmental health nursing provides a rich field for the conduct of research focused on improvement of worker health through health promotion and protection strategies that need to be tested. In addition, the use of theories and conceptual models in the development of occupational and environmental health nursing will need to be expanded to enhance the growing body of knowledge. Nurses need to be skilled in the conduct of research through education and the actual doing of the research. Those less skilled should work with a mentor or do collaborative research to gain the experience needed to acquire and maintain scientific rigor. The AAOHN Research Priorities (see Box 16-2) can provide ideas or topics for research; however, the researcher should select a topic that is of interest and is significant to knowledge development. Finally, research findings must be disseminated through publications and presentations and the findings must be utilized in practice because this reflects the ultimate success of research.

The process of doing research is one of rigor and requires thought and attention to concepts, design, and detail. The product, developing more effective approaches to manage employee health care, will clearly add to improving occupational and environmental health services and continue to expand our knowledge base.

References

Adams, J., Mackey, T., Lindenberg, J., & Baden, T. (1995). Primary care at the worksite. *AAOHN Journal*, *43*, 17-22.

Agnew, J., & Travers, P. (1990). Editorial: Occupational health nursing research. *AAOHN Journal, 38*(12), 509.

American Association of Occupational Health Nurses. (1999a). *Code of Ethics.* Atlanta, GA: Author.

American Association of Occupational Health Nurses. (1999b). *Standards of occupational and environmental health nursing practice.* Atlanta, GA: Author.

American Nurses Association. (1999). *Standards of Practice.* Washington, DC: Author.

American Psychological Association. (2001). *Publication Manual of the American Psychological Association* (5th ed.). Washington, DC: Author.

Atkins, J., & Magnuson, N. (1990). Occupational health nursing research, June 1984 to June 1989. *AAOHN Journal, 38*, 560-566.

Brines, J., Salazar, M. K., Graham, K.Y., Pergola, T., & Connon, C. (1999). Injured workers' perceptions of case management services. *AAOHN Journal, 47*, 355-364.

Brink, B., & Wood, M. (1988). *Basic steps in planning nursing research.* Boston: Jones and Bartlett.

Brown, E. L. (1948). *Nursing for the future.* New York: Russell Sage.

Cohen, I. B. (1984). Florence Nightingale. *Scientific American, 250*, 128-137.

Cohen, M. A., & Kaufman, J. D. (2000). Latex sensitivity in Washington state acute care hospitals. *AAOHN Journal, 48*, 297-304.

Cohen-Mansfield, J., Culpepper, W. J., & Carter, P. (1996). Nursing staff back injuries. *AAOHN Journal, 44*, 9-16.

Dille, J. (1999). A worksite influenza immunization program. *AAOHN Journal, 47*, 301-309.

Faucett, J., & Rempel, D. (1996). Musculoskeletal symptoms related to video display terminal use. *AAOHN Journal, 44*, 33-39.

Funderburke, P. L., & Spencer, L. (2000). Hepatitis B immunity in high risk health care workers. *AAOHN Journal, 48*, 325-331.

Gordis, L. (1999). *Principles of epidemiology.* Baltimore, MD: Johns Hopkins University Press.

Griest, S. E., & Bishop, P. M. (1998). Tinnitus as an early indicator of permanent hearing loss. *AAOHN Journal, 46*, 325-29.

Heyler, A. J., Brehm, W. T., Gentry, N. O., & Pittman, T. A. (1998). Effectiveness of a worksite smoking cessation program in the military. *AAOHN Journal, 46*, 238-245.

Moore, M. (1998). A workplace stretching program. *AAOHN Journal, 46*(12), 563-568.

Morris, J. A. (1999). Injury experience of temporary workers in a manufacturing setting. *AAOHN Journal, 47*, 470-78.

Morse, J. M., & Field, P. A. (1995). *Qualitative research methods for health professionals.* Thousand Oaks, CA: Sage.

Nightingale, F. (1859). *Notes on nursing: What it is, and what it is not.* Philadelphia: J. B. Lippincott.

Polit, D., & Hungler, B. (1999). *Nursing research: Principles and methods* (6th ed.). Philadelphia: J. B. Lippincott.

Ramsey, P. W., & Glenn, L. L. (1996). Nurses' body fluid exposure reporting, HIV testing and Hepatitis B vaccination rates. *AAOHN Journal, 44*, 129-137.

Rogers, B. (1989a). Establishing research priorities in occupational health nursing. *AAOHN Journal, 37*, 493-500.

Rogers, B. (1989b). Florence Nightingale and research: The historical link. *AAOHN Journal, 37*(6), 238-9.

Rogers, B. (1990a). Ethics and research. *AAOHN Journal, 38*, 581-585.

Rogers, B. (1990b). The question and rite answer, Part I: Levels of research questions. *AAOHN Journal, 38*, 502-503.

Rogers, B. (1990c). Research in occupational health nursing. *Recent Advances in Nursing, 26*, 137-155.

Rogers, B. (1991). The question and rite answer, Part II: Planning for data analysis. *AAOHN Journal, 39*, 42-44.

Rogers, B. (1996). Researchability and feasibility issues in conducting research. *AAOHN Journal, 44*, 58-59.

Rogers, B. (1998). Descriptive analysis of research data. *AAOHN Journal, 46*(5), 43-44.

Rogers, B. (2000). *Housekeepers' health study.* Unpublished manuscript.

Rogers, B. (2001). Research. In M. Salazar (Ed.), *Core Curriculum for Occupational and Environmental Health Nursing* (2nd ed., pp. 411-423). Philadelphia: W. B. Saunders.

Rogers, B., Agnew, J., & Pompeii, L. (2000). Research priorities in occupational health nursing. *AAOHN Journal, 48*, 9-16.

Sass, J., Bertolone, K., Denton, D., & Logsdon, C. (1995). *AAOHN Journal, 43*, 507-513.

Sewitch, M. J., Rossignol, M., Bellavance, F., Leclaire, R., Esdail, J., Suissa, S., Proulx, R., & Dupuis, M. (2000). First lifetime back pain and physiatry treatment. *AAOHN Journal, 48*, 234-242.

Stoy, D. W., & Aspen, J. (1999). Force as repetition measurement of hamboning: Relationship to musculoskeletal symptoms. *AAOHN Journal, 47*, 254-60.

Strunk, W., & White, E. B. (2000). *The elements of style* (4th ed.). Needleham Heights, MA: Allyn and Bacon.

Tornquist, E., & Rogers, B. (1987). Research proposals: The significance of rite study. *AAOHN Journal, 35*, 190.

Treece, L., & Treece, J. (1982). *Elements of research in nursing.* St. Louis, MO: Mosby.

U.S. Department of Health and Human Services, National Institute for Occupational Safety and Health. (1996). *National Occupational Research Agenda,* (Publication No. 96-115). Cincinnati, OH: National Institute for Occupational Safety and Health.

Wilson, H. (1989). *Research in nursing* (2nd ed.). Redwood City, CA: Addison-Wesley.

Wilson, S., Sisk, R. J., & Baldwin, K. A. (1997). Health beliefs of blue collar workers. *AAOHN Journal, 45*, 254-260.

16-1 Selected Potential Funding Sources Relevant to Occupational and Environmental Health and Occupational and Environmental Health Nursing

ORGANIZATION	APPLICATION DEADLINE
Agency for Health Care Policy and Research Rockville, Md. (301) 443-3091	February 1, June 1, October 1; January 15, May 15, September 15 for small grants
American Association of Occupational Health Nurses Foundation Atlanta, Ga. (770) 455-7757	December 1
American Cancer Society New York, N.Y. (404) 320-3333	April 1, November 1
American Federation on Aging Research New York, N.Y. (212) 570-2090	January 15
American Foundation for AIDS Research Los Angeles, Calif. (213) 857 5900	Two step process: August and December
American Lung Association New York, N.Y. (212) 315-8700	November 1
American Nurses Foundation Washington, DC (202) 789-1800	June 1

Diabetes Research and Education Foundation Bridgewater, N.J. (908) 658-9322	September 30
March of Dimes Foundation White Plains, N.Y. (914) 428-7100	Varies
Metropolitan Life Foundation New York, N.Y. (212) 578-7049	None
Ruth Mott Fund Flint, Mich. (313) 232-3180	March, July, November
National Institute for Nursing Research Bethesda, Md. (301) 496-0526	February 1, June 1, October 1
National Institute for Occupational Safety and Health Atlanta, Ga. (800) 356-4674	February 1, June 1, October 1
National Institutes of Health (Cancer; Eye; Heart, Lung, & Blood; Allergy/Infectious Diseases; Arthritis/Musculo Skeletal/Skin; Child Health; Nursing; Diabetes/Digestive/Kidney; Environmental Health; General Medical; Drug Abuse; Mental Health; Alcohol; Neuro/Communicative Disorders) Bethesda, Md. (301) 496-7441-Inquire for individual Institute	February 1, June 1, October 1
National Library of Medicine Bethesda, Md. (301) 496-6131	February 1, June 1, October 1
National Science Foundation Washington, DC (202) 375-7880	None
PPG Industries Foundation Pittsburgh, Pa. (412) 434-2970	September
Prudential Foundation Newark, N.J. (201) 802-7354	None

Robert Wood Johnson Foundation   None
Princeton, N.J.
(609) 243-5957

Sigma Theta Tau International   March 1
Indianapolis, Ind.
(317) 634-8171

Smokeless Tobacco Research Council   June, December
New York, N.Y.
(212) 697-3485

17 Ethical Perspectives in Occupational and Environmental Health Nursing Practice

Ethical conflict is nothing new in occupational and environmental health nursing practice. Traditional concerns about confidentiality of employee health records, hazardous workplace exposures, issues of informed consent, risks and benefits, and dual duty conflicts are now married with newer concerns of genetic screening (Koh & Jeyaratnam, 1998; Rawbone, 1999), worker literacy and understanding, work organization issues, and untimely return to work.

This chapter provides a discussion of ethical theories and principles and related ethical dilemmas in occupational and environmental health nursing practice. This is followed by a model for ethical decision making that is applied to a case example. How the public views nurses and nursing with regard to ethical behaviors is then discussed.

ETHICAL ISSUES AND PRACTICE

Much attention has been paid to societal ethical issues such as right to life or right to die, organ transplantation, euthanasia, the use of scarce health care resource dollars for expensive technological advances, and health care access. However, ethical issues in occupational health settings have received far less attention in part because these issues are somewhat different in nature and are often subtle and insidious rather than overt (Rogers, 1988). Recent research suggests that occupational health professionals and managers face challenges in an effort to protect and improve worker health (Rogers, 2001) and that these challenges include issues related to

privacy of employee health information, balancing of costs and benefits, truth telling, worker notification and right to know, health screening and surveillance of employees, substance abuse by both employees and health care providers, workplace discrimination, worker and employer compliance with health protection and surveillance, professional competence and unethical/illegal acts (e.g., fraudulent credentials), and whistle-blowing. In addition, understanding language in the face of illiteracy, cultural differences, and diversity presents ethical complexities related to the effective transmission of the information necessary to protect workers from hazardous substance exposures. In corporate environments where the primary mission is to produce a successful product while ensuring corporate survival and profitability, conflicts may be created if health and safety issues compromise the profit goal (Philipp et al., 1997). Issues related to the worker's right to know about exposure to hazardous substances may result in company liability and economic loss. In addition, long-term consequences that affect the worker, family, and community and result from potentially hazardous workplace exposures have yet to be fully explored.

Fry (2000) states that the nurse as a moral agent is concerned with values, choices, priorities, and duties for the good of the individual, the profession, and society. In the face of these concerns what is needed is a more systematic way of approaching ethical issues confronting nursing at all levels, from the clinical provider/client encounter to the level of policy making for the delivery of health and nursing care.

In most occupational health settings the occupational and environmental health nurse bears the primary responsibility for management of the occupational health unit and provision of direct health services. Thus, the nurse has dual responsibility and acts as both an agent of the company and an advocate for the worker. Adherence to professional standards and codes are foundational to the nurse's practice and provide guidance and direction for safe and ethical care. This requires the nurse to always act in the best interest of the client and make informed decisions within the parameters of professional practice to which the nurse is held accountable. Characteristics of a professional are shown in Box 17-1.

Professions develop codes of ethics that indicate collective philosophies about what constitutes professional practice. Ethical principles that help health care professionals to deal effectively with ethical dilemmas are embodied in established professional codes of ethics (Rodham, 1998). Ethics is not law but rather a guide for moral action. These codes provide for an expression of values and beliefs that guides professional practice and ethical obligations and specifies professional responsibility and accountability to the health care consumer and society. Rather than define rules and regulations for conduct, codes are generally intended to create an awareness of ethical considerations and to provide a framework for ethical decision making by the health care professional. The AAOHN *Code of Ethics* and *Interpretive Statements* (AAOHN, 1998) detail seven principle areas for ethical practice and behavior. In addition, the *Code of Ethics* should be recognized as a policy document and shared with management to effect a better understanding of the occupational and environmental health nurse's practice (Rogers, 2001). The guiding *Code of Ethics* from the American Association of Occupational Health Nurses and the *Code of Ethics for Nurses* from the American Nurses Association are shown in Boxes 17-2 and 17-3 respectively.

Box 17-1   Characteristics of a Professional

- Possesses expertise, formal education, or special technical competence
- Has a unique degree of autonomy that entitles her or him to exercise judgment
- Consciously conforms to a cede or standard
- Feels a sense of service to humanity
- Acknowledges a responsibility higher than making a living
- Instills public trust

Box 17-2   *Code of Ethics*: American Association of Occupational Health Nurses

- Occupational and environmental health nurses provide health care in the work environment with regard for human dignity and client rights, unrestricted by considerations of social or economic status, professional status, or the nature of the health status.
- Occupational and environmental health nurses promote collaboration with other health professionals and community health agencies in order to meet the health needs of the workforce.
- Occupational and environmental health nurses strive to safeguard the employees' rights to privacy by protecting confidential information and releasing information only upon written consent of the employee or as required or permitted by law.
- Occupational and environmental health nurses strive to provide quality care and to safeguard clients from unethical and illegal actions.

- Occupational and environmental health nurses, licensed to provide health care services, accept obligations to society as professional and responsible members of the community.
- Occupational and environmental health nurses maintain individual competence in occupational health nursing practice based on scientific knowledge and recognize and accept responsibility for individual judgments and actions while complying with appropriate laws and regulations (local, state, and federal) that impact (sic) the delivery of occupational and environmental health services.
- Occupational and environmental health nurses participate, as appropriate, in activities such as research that contribute to the ongoing development of the profession's body of knowledge while protecting the rights of subjects.

From *Code of Ethics,* by American Association of Occupational Health Nurses, 1998, Atlanta, GA: Author.

ETHICAL THEORIES AND PRINCIPLES

The word *ethics,* derived from the Greek *ethos,* originally meant customs, habitual usages, and conduct of character. The word *morals,* derived from the Latin *moralis,* means customs or habits or beliefs that reflect a standard of right and good. These terms are often used interchangeably to describe acts related to conduct, character, and motives that are described as good, desirable, or right or, conversely, as bad, undesirable, or wrong (Davis & Aroskar, 1983). Socrates, in the Crito dialogue, argued that a person must let reason rather than emotion determine her or his ethical decisions (Jameton, 1984). To accomplish this, individuals must have factual information regarding the situation and keep their minds clear as they deliberate the issue. It is not enough to appeal to what people generally think, since they may be wrong. The answer must be found by informed reasoning that individuals regard as correct and not by what will happen to them as a consequence, or what others will think of them, or how they feel about the situation (Rest & Patterson, 1986).

Although standards or ethical codes and principles provide guidance regarding acts of care, individuals still can face tough ethical dilemmas and choices. A dilemma involves a choice between equally unsatisfactory alternatives and is sometimes thought of as a choice between the lesser of two evils. For example, in a situation where the ethical code guides an individual to maintain confidentiality, that person may decide to break confidentiality to protect the health or lives of others. This example shows that in honoring one ethical principle (i.e., beneficence—in this case, protecting others) another can be violated (i.e., autonomy—in this case, breaching confidence). Hence, although ethical principles can guide decision making, they can never be complete enough to anticipate all possible situations involving moral decisions. Nevertheless, individuals may be faced with conflicting principles and will need to determine which choice brings the most benefit and the least risk. Furthermore, they need to understand that answers to ethical dilemmas will not be arrived at easily or quickly (Aroskar, 1989; Koh & Jeyaratnam, 1998).

The study of ethics falls within the broader domain of philosophy, and ethics is defined as a value or a standard adhered to by an individual,

---

Box 17-3   *Code of Ethics for Nurses:* **American Nurses Association**

1. The nurse, in all professional relationships, practices with compassion and respect for the inherent dignity, worth, and uniqueness of every individual, unrestricted by considerations of social or economic status, personal attributes, or the nature of health problems.

2. The nurse's primary commitment is to the patient, whether an individual, family, group, or community.

3. The nurse promotes, advocates for, and strives to protect the health, safety, and rights of the patient.

4. The nurse is responsible and accountable for individual nursing practice and determines the appropriate delegation of tasks consistent with the nurse's obligation to provide optimum patient care.

5. The nurse owes the same duties to self as to others, including the responsibility to preserve integrity and safety, to maintain competence, and to continue personal and professional growth.

6. The nurse participates in establishing, maintaining, and improving health care environments and conditions of employment conducive to the provision of quality health care and consistent with the values of the profession through individual and collective action.

7. The nurse participates in the advancement of the profession through contributions to practice, education, administration, and knowledge development.

8. The nurse collaborates with other health professionals and the public in promoting community, national, and international efforts to meet health needs.

9. The profession of nursing, as represented by associations and their members, is responsible for articulating nursing values, for maintaining the integrity of the profession and its practice, and for shaping social policy.

From *Code of Ethics for Nurses,* by American Nurses Association, 2001, Washington, DC: Author. http://www.ana.org.

Box 17-4   Major Ethical Theories

TELEOLOGICAL (CONSEQUENTIALIST) THEORY

The rightness or wrongness of an action is determined by the results of that action . . . by its consequences. One ought to do that which is conducive to one's goals. The end justifies the means.

Utilitarianism is the most common teleological theory. It is often thought of as the "greatest happiness" principle, or the greatest good for the greatest number.

John Stuart Mill, philosopher

DEONTOLOGICAL (FORMALIST) THEORY

The rightness or wrongness of an action is based on the nature of the action, or the motives behind the action, but not on the results or consequences of the action. One can determine the rightness of an action based upon principles.

Every individual is worthy of respect and must be honored and revered. It means doing your duty. One deserves respect for one's action only if that action was done for the sake of doing the moral thing (i.e., from a respect for one's moral duty).

Immanuel Kant, philosopher

group, or organization in an attempt to define principles in order to decide which actions are desirable or undesirable (Beauchamp & Childress, 1994; Fry, 2000). Ethical theories and principles guide ethical decision making; thus, familiarity with these tenets is important. Teleological and deontological theories (Box 17-4) are the most widely discussed ethical theories and provide the foundation for application of principles (Beauchamp & Childress, 1994). Decisions about ethical dilemmas in occupational and environmental health nursing can be formulated within these theories and principles.

Teleological theory (utilitarianism or consequentialist theory) focuses on the consequences of an action and gauges the worth of the action by the end or results rather than the means to achieve the end. This theory focuses on providing the greatest good or least harm for the greatest number. Policy formulation based on cost-benefit analysis, wherein the greatest benefit is achieved by the most for the lowest cost, and the provision of health services to those who will benefit the most from the services are examples of utility (Fry, 2000; Rogers, 2002).

Deontological theory (formalist theory) focuses primarily on the action itself and asserts that rightness and wrongness are inherent in the act independent of the consequences of the act.

Box 17-5   Examples of Ethical Issues Facing Occupational and Environmental Health Nurses

AUTONOMY: THE RIGHT TO SELF-DETERMINATION; A FORM OF PERSONAL LIBERTY

Confidentiality
Right to know
Paternalism
Informed consent
Withholding information

BENEFICENCE: ACTIONS THAT CONTRIBUTE TO THE WELFARE OF OTHERS

Screening for potential health hazards
Health promotion activities
Breach of confidentiality (to protect others)
Walk-throughs
Research

NONMALEFICENCE: THE DUTY TO DO NO HARM

High-risk jobs
Second party-induced hazard/substance abuse at work
Incompetent, unethical, illegal practices

JUSTICE: FAIRNESS OR GIVING PEOPLE THEIR DUE

Discrimination
Distribution of benefits and burdens
Cost containment versus quality

For example, deontologists assert that truth telling is always essential and should never be violated for any reason. Utilitarians on the other hand may argue that when truth telling does more harm than good (e.g., telling a psychiatric patient information that may severely jeopardize her or his mental health), the obligation to tell the truth may not need to be honored.

Ethical principles extend from deontological theory, and the most widely observed principles (Box 17-5) are autonomy, nonmaleficence, beneficence, and justice. Autonomy is a form of personal liberty whereby the individual deliberates about and chooses a plan that determines her or his own course of action. Inherent in this principle is the right to self-determination. Adherence to this principle requires that the individual's values and goals be considered in major decisions that affect her or his welfare (Childress, 1990; Mezey, 1994). This rules out paternalism (when one person claims to know what is best for another) in decision making and thereby precludes health professionals or others making decisions for employees without their input and consent.

Autonomy, as characterized by self-determination, relates to issues such as informed consent, confidentiality and right to privacy, right to refuse treatment, right to know about potential workplace health hazards, and worker inclusion in decision making. Potential dilemmas include the use of hazard pay for dangerous jobs; access to/denial of exposure information by employers, which may reinforce knowledge gaps about toxic exposures and their long-term consequences; access to medical records by management personnel, which may result in denial of promotion or loss of job or other forms of punitive or coercive behavior; and maintenance of confidentiality concerning a substance-abusing employee who handles heavy equipment that can harm other workers (Rogers, 1990).

Of significant concern is the use of predictive or genetic screening to identify genetic risk factors in workers. The extent to which people may be considered to be at higher genetic risk depends on both the relevance and interpretation of the test, and ultimately, how that information will be used is of great importance. Who will have access to this information? Will individuals be denied employment or access to selected jobs based on

these data? In this regard, there is much potential to violate the right of autonomy (Rawbone, 1999).

The second principle, nonmaleficence, is often referred to as the "no harm" principle. Foundational to most professional ethical codes, this precept encompasses the concepts of both avoidance of harm and avoidance of risk of harm. For example, an employee with a known hearing loss should not be placed in a job situation that will further compromise hearing, and a pregnant employee should not be exposed to potential or known teratogens that may jeopardize her health or that of her fetus. The performance of preplacement, periodic, and mandatory examinations help identify work-related hazards and help occupational health professionals in their decision making to protect the health of the employee.

Occupational and environmental health nurses are widely recognized as employee advocates as evidenced by their contributions to employee health and welfare. Beneficence, the third ethical principle, requires that health care professionals act in the best interest of the worker. Interventions aimed at health promotion and health protection, such as wellness, screening, and health surveillance programs that benefit the employee through primary and secondary prevention efforts, exemplify this principle. The identification of potential health hazards or employees at increased risk of illness and injury and recommendations for risk reduction represent positive health interventions aimed at worker protection. Examples include the installation of engineering control devices such as needle/sharps containers in patient rooms or clinic areas, the provision of nonlatex gloves when latex is not needed, and the development of a back injury prevention program for workers with back problems or previous injury. Walk-throughs by the occupational and environmental health nurse to identify health and safety hazards and recommend risk reduction programs are also included under the rubric of this principle.

Although screening and health surveillance programs benefit the employee through early detection of potentially serious occupational and nonoccupational disease, care should be taken to observe ethical principles related to screening and to select an appropriate screening test, secure reliable testing procedures and laboratories, and protect individuals' rights (Box 17-6). Mandatory

---

Box 17-6   Prerequisites for Ethical Screening Programs

1. The purpose of the screening must be acceptable ethically.
2. The means used to obtain information must be appropriate to its intended use.
3. High-quality laboratory services must be used.
4. Notification of screening must be given.
5. Individuals screened have a right to be informed of results.
6. Appropriate counseling programs to interpret results and referral options for treatment must be available before and after screening.
7. Confidentiality must be protected.

Effectiveness

		+	−
Efficiency	+	Health improvement Reasonable/low cost (A)	Health decline Reasonable/low cost (C)
	−	Health improvement High cost (B)	Health decline High cost (D)

Figure 17-1   The balance between health care effectiveness and cost efficiency.

---

screening programs and the access and availability of test results demand cautious evaluation to ensure worker autonomy and protect confidentiality and right to privacy. For instance, serious concerns center on whether urine drug screening should be required, how data should be obtained and stored, and the repercussions based on results of unreliable testing procedures.

Increasingly, biomedical tests such as urine drug screening are being used in ways that reveal social and personal information. Although the tests seem simple, test sensitivity and specificity as a result of operator errors, inconsistent laboratory testing, and scientific inaccuracy may be problems. This type of screening may place the employee in the position of proving innocence, may result in unwarranted job loss, has the potential for discriminatory usage, and can be viewed as a method of social control that might offend societal expectations of privacy.

The fourth principle, justice, is directed toward treating employees fairly, equally, and without discrimination. This includes providing equal opportunity for disabled people regarding job availability and promotion, and assuring that individuals will not be discriminated against because of a health condition, such as acquired immunodeficiency syndrome or other chronic diseases, when they are able to perform the job. This concept is embodied in the Americans With Disabilities Act (1990). An employee's history of sexual activity or alcohol consumption and her or his general

health status may be considered risk information with respect to the potential for discrimination (D'Arruda, 2001). Singling out certain individuals or work groups to perform unpleasant or hazardous jobs also would violate this principle.

Issues related to health care costs and benefits cut across all of the ethical principles, as may be the case with many dilemmas (Rogers, 1992). However, embodied in the notion of justice is treating people fairly and equally with respect to health care access, delivery, and quality. It must always be emphasized that cost containment is never a substitute for providing quality health care to all employees. Thus, no employee should receive substandard care, and all employees should have equal care delivery and access options within the scope of their benefits. Yet at the same time the occupational and environmental health nurse manager needs to recognize that when cost becomes an issue, she or he must determine how any given level of effectiveness is to be achieved at the lowest cost—that is, efficiently. Effectiveness and efficiency in health care delivery move together (Rogers, 2002). As shown in Figure 17-1, to maintain a balance in quality health care costs, both effectiveness and efficiency must move in positive directions, indicating the achievement of the goal of health improvement at a reasonable or low cost (Box A). Diversions in the balance are shown in the remaining boxes. Box B depicts an improvement in health but with wasteful use of resources or extremely high cost expenditures. Box C indicates that health goals are not achieved and that limited resources were expended or perhaps adequate funds were unavailable to assist in health improvement. Box D represents not only the failure to provide quality care at extraordinary costs but poor health outcomes as well. From both an ethical and cost containment standpoint, effectiveness and efficiency must be part of the health care professional's practice.

Providing quality health care must be the overriding concern and should not be compromised on the basis of dollars. If cost containment becomes the precedent, in the long run the occupational health professional, the employee, and the company will be dissatisfied, and both effectiveness and efficiency will be compromised. This is not to say that a careful review of all programs should not be conducted with priority determinations made about which programs have the most value in meeting employee health needs. However, in some cases quantity may need to be sacrificed for quality (Rogers, 2002).

Health care practitioners and providers are placed in positions that require moral considerations—that is, questioning what ought to be done in a health situation from an ethical standpoint. Dilemmas are difficult problems that have no easy solutions; however, understanding and utilizing ethical theories and principles will help the occupational and environmental health nurse to arrive at a resolution.

In many instances ethical principles provide health care professionals with a guide to weigh the risks and benefits with respect to individual health and welfare and the development of policies and procedures to safeguard individuals' rights and protect their health. The occupational and environmental health nurse must examine the situation with respect to the guiding principles and ensure that the benefits of the action clearly outweigh the risks.

ETHICAL DECISION MAKING

To resolve ethical problems, the occupational and environmental health nurse needs to recognize and understand both personal and corporate values and know that these values may often compete. Nielsen (1989) points out that the consequences of addressing issues of organizational ethics can be unpleasant: one can be punished or fined; one's career can suffer; or one can be ostracized. Within the context of the corporate environment two approaches to addressing ethical problems in the workplace may be considered:

(1) intervening as an individual to work against others and organizations who perform unethical acts and (2) leading an ethical organizational change by working with others and the organization to promote integrity. Acting individually will probably require some form of whistle-blowing and can entail significant risk, particularly if the company culture demands conformity. Thus, if the individual knows how to lead, the corporate management is reasonable, the degree of risk and severity of risk is understood, and the changes can be made within a reasonable time frame, trying to lead an organizational change may be a more effective and safer approach.

When a person encounters a dilemma, the answer is not clear cut, and often one principle conflicts with another. For example, how long should a substance abuse problem be dealt with if others are at potential risk of harm? Should the burden of a potential toxic exposure, no matter how small, be shared by all or only a few? Should all health care workers be informed of the HIV status of a patient or an employee? Should mandatory testing for HIV be required for all health care workers involved in invasive procedures? Should pregnant workers be allowed to work in hot or cold environments? Ethical problems raise awareness and questions as to how problems can be resolved, what criteria should be used in decision making, and what ethical principles influence the decision to resolve (Fry, 1994).

Notifying workers about exposures to toxic substances is clearly embodied in the 1970 Occupational Safety and Health Act, the 1976 Toxic Substances Control Act, and more recently in the 1983 Hazard Communication Standard, and notification now has been extended to the public by the Community Right to Know provisions of the Superfund Amendment Reauthorization Act (SARA). Underlying the legal requirements of these acts is the ethical imperative of autonomy, wherein workers have the right to participate in decisions to minimize risk and limit exposure through workplace controls. For example, issues related to right to know include short-term and latent effects on personal health, reproductive toxicity, concern about the physical and mental integrity of future offspring, appropriate and scientifically and technically sound test measurements, identification of who should be notified and what constitutes the content, and the

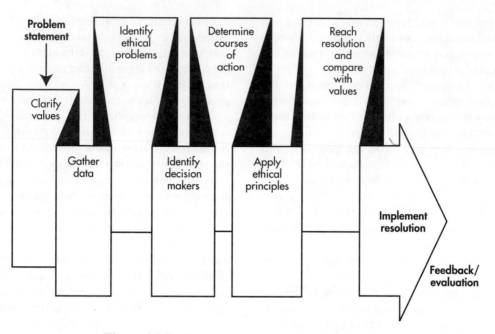

Figure 17-2 Components of ethical decision making.

appropriateness of notification without causing unnecessary fears and anxiety.

To arrive at a rational, deliberate resolution to an ethical problem within the parameters of leading an ethical organizational change, a model for ethical decision making is presented (Figure 17-2) (Rogers, 1991). This framework includes the following steps: (1) statement of the problem, (2) value clarification, (3) data gathering, (4) identification of the ethical problem, (5) identification of the decision makers, (6) determination of courses of action, (7) application of ethical principles, (8) reaching of a resolution, (9) resolution implementation, and (10) feedback or outcome evaluation. A case example is used to illustrate the model from conceptual and applied points of view.

CASE EXAMPLE

A pregnant employee is concerned about exposure to hazardous chemical substances in her work and reports this to the staff occupational and environmental health nurse. The nurse plans an investigation to assess the risk. The worker's supervisor becomes aware of the proposed investigation and reports this activity as unnecessary to the nurse manager, who agrees. The supervisor says that he "knows best" and that this type of investigation will unduly alarm all employees.

Problem Statement

The problem identified should be clearly stated and validated. In this case example the problem identified by the employee is a risk of hazardous exposure. Validation of the problem can be done initially through employee interviews, walk-through observations, and sampling.

Values Clarification

Values clarification enhances understanding and analysis of an individual's personal belief system and the way that a person ideally should act toward others as compared with real actions. In the workplace setting, values clarification should also include recognition of the corporate value system. In this case example the following types of questions should be considered: What constitutes risk and how is it perceived by different parties? Is there an acceptable risk level? Who should have access to information and what should be disclosed? Is there a difference in opinion among health care professionals, employees, management, and peers about the risk? Who, if anyone, will be harmed from the exposure?

Data Gathering

To develop an informed decision, as much information as possible should be collected about the problem and any contributory factors. In this case example, data regarding the type, concentration, and duration of exposure will be helpful. Recent literature as well as Material Safety Data Sheets should be reviewed along with pertinent information obtained from observations and environmental sampling. Determination of high-risk groups, identification and validation of potential and actual adverse health effects, and knowledge of control measures and compliance with recommended safety standards should be evaluated.

Identification of the Ethical Problem

An ethical problem is complex, and the solution will have far-reaching effects on many areas of human concern. It is important to know which ethical principles (autonomy, nonmaleficence, beneficence, and justice) are being compromised or violated in order to determine the associated benefits and risks. In this case example all principles are involved. For example, questions related to this hazardous exposure include the following:

- What are the exposure limits and who should receive exposure notification (autonomy)?
- What level of risk will be allowed and tolerated (nonmaleficence)?
- Is there a causal relationship between exposure and disease or outcome (nonmaleficence)?
- Are protective controls and monitoring systems in place and, if not, why not (beneficence)?
- What are the implications of crude or unreliable monitoring measurements (nonmaleficence, beneficence)?
- Are there select groups at risk of exposure (justice)?

Once these issues are delineated, other types of ethical concerns also can be determined. For example, is it a case of withholding the truth about a hazardous substance or an issue of uninformed voluntary consent? What type of harm will be imposed (i.e., physical or psychological) and who will be affected (i.e., employee, unborn child)? The more clearly one can identify the ethical problem, the more precise the analysis can be.

Identification of the Decision Makers and Involved Parties

All persons involved in the decision making, such as the worker or workers, managers, health care professionals, labor union officials, and family members, if appropriate, and the nature of their involvement should be known (Hardwig, 1990; Rogers, 1991). In this case example the employee, occupational health care professionals, and private physician/obstetrician should be involved in a discussion of the problem. Management should be involved with respect to notification of the exposure, its impact, and work-related recommendations. Other involved parties may include family members, coworkers, or other employee supports such as clergy, as determined by the employee.

Information about worker-manager relationships, control mechanisms, and factors affecting the individual's ability or freedom to make a decision should be obtained. Failure to deal with this component of ethical analysis could lead to the wrong people making the wrong decisions for the wrong reasons. Paternalism in decision making may interfere with the reasoning process and must be avoided.

Determination of Courses of Action

In any given situation there are usually several potential courses of action. The employee and the health care professionals, with consultation from the private physician, should discuss the situation, and recommendations should be communicated to management. The purpose of the proposed actions and related potential or probable consequences of these actions should be explored fully. Sometimes none of the solutions seem desirable, and the employee may need to choose the option that will produce the most good (or least harm). In addition, the issue of feasibility needs to be considered; that is, can a strategy be implemented and what is the cost? For example, alternative strategies determined in this case example might include the following:

- Control of hazardous exposures through engineering redesign of the work station, which will have cost implications
- Use of appropriate protective devices to minimize exposure and the institution of a monitoring and surveillance program that may be less costly
- Institution of administrative controls through job rotation or temporary reassignment at the same pay rate

Research regarding the effectiveness of exposure minimization will be important to consider in the development of alternative courses of action.

The issue of exposure and protection of the unborn fetus, and resultant corporate liability from possible harm, is of concern. How this is handled if the worker believes she should be allowed to continue working in the environment because the financial rewards are greater will be an important consideration if temporary reassignment is recommended and instituted stable pay maintained.

Application of Ethical Principles for Resolution

Herein the ethical principles (autonomy, nonmaleficence, beneficence, justice) should be reexamined: Are the worker's right to know and right to make an informed decision compromised (autonomy)? Is the employee at risk of a potential or known toxic exposure without appropriate disclosure or from withholding of information (nonmaleficence and autonomy)? Are the company and health care professional assuming a position of knowing what is best for the worker (autonomy/paternalism)? All ethical principles should be weighed in terms of benefits and risks. Principles should be applied within the framework of benefit maximization and risk minimization. Once the principles and any violations are applied, resolutions to deal with the problem can be identified.

Reaching of a Resolution

The person deciding the course of action to take must carefully think through the problem, weigh the ethical principles in the balance, and recommend a resolution that is rational, feasible, and defensible. All decision making is hampered by limited capabilities, and a person must select the most beneficial option. One can, of course, be wrong in the choice; however, acting with integrity according to the knowledge possessed and in keeping with one's obligations and values is imperative while in search of a satisfactory outcome.

Resolution Implementation

Once the appropriate resolution is determined, details of the action—that is, what is to be done, by whom, and under what conditions—should be stated and then implemented. In this case

example, costly engineering controls may not be needed if administrative transfer is an effective resolution.

Feedback/Outcome Evaluation

After a resolution is recommended and implemented, feedback about the outcome of the decision should be obtained. Who benefited? What were the costs? Was the resolution acceptable or should another course of action be tried? The problem may have no real solution, but a resolution that is just, reduces harm, and affords some measure of autonomy and beneficence may be acceptable.

Although not common in the occupational health setting, ethics committees, which are used frequently in hospital environments, are helpful in dealing with ethical issues (Blake, 1992). These committees are usually multidisciplinary in composition and thereby bring a variety of expertise for problem delineation and problem solving. Establishment of these types of bodies can help in the overall problem solving and evaluation.

THE PUBLIC'S VIEW OF HONESTY AND ETHICS IN THE PROFESSIONS

The Gallup Organization conducts an annual survey to rate the honesty and ethics of various professions. In the 2001 poll, conducted through telephone interviews of a randomly selected national sample of 1,005 adults, the top three professions rating high or very high in terms of honesty and ethical standards were firefighters (90%), nurses (84%), and the U.S. military (81%) (Figure 17-3).

The Gallup Poll was conducted in November of 2001, which was the first year that U.S. citizens were asked to rate firefighters and members of the military and only the third year that nurses were rated. Nurses came in first in 1999 (the first year the survey included nurses) and in 2000; they were given high ratings by 73% and 79% of respondants in each of the respective years, and supplanted pharmacists, who had come in first every year from 1988 to 1998. Table 17-1 shows the ratings of various professions on the dimensions of honesty and ethics from 1977 to 2001.

This is no real surprise to nurses. Health care given by nurses is of high quality and consistent

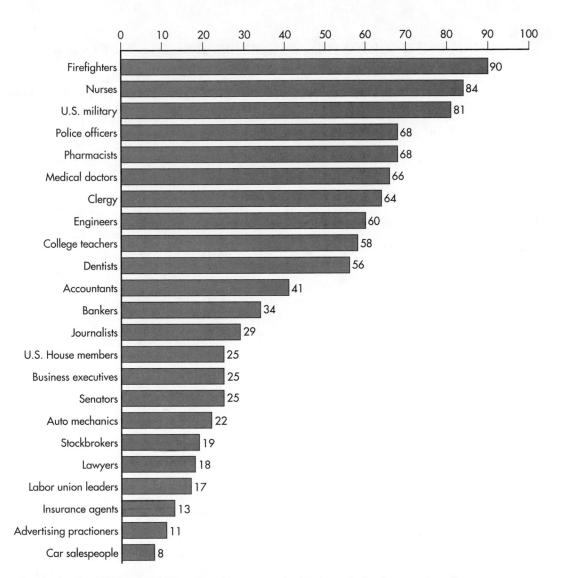

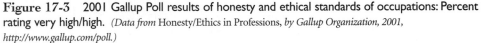

Figure 17-3   2001 Gallup Poll results of honesty and ethical standards of occupations: Percent rating very high/high.   *(Data from* Honesty/Ethics in Professions, *by Gallup Organization, 2001, http://www.gallup.com/poll.)*

with professional codes and standards, which is reflected in the values of caring, advocacy, and accountability. Bishop and Scudder (1996) point out that caring is a way of being with others that assures them of personal concern for their well-being. This way of being fosters trust, mutual concern, and positive attitudes that promote good health.

As an advocate, the nurse speaks for or in support of the best interests of the client, including populations at risk (Rogers, 2002). An advo-

cate has been described as someone who helps a person do what that person cannot do without help but does so in a way that liberates the individual from limitations imposed by his or her disability (Bishop & Scudder, 1996). In addition, this means that the nurse takes appropriate action regarding any instances of incompetent, illegal, or unethical practice by health care professionals or any action on the part of others that places the rights or best interests of the client in jeopardy (ANA, 2001).

TABLE 17-1 Gallup Poll Results of Honesty and Ethical Standards of Occupations, Years 1977-2001: Percentage Rating Very High/High

Year	1977	1981	1983	1985	1988	1990	1991	1992	1993	1994	1995
Firefighters											
Nurses											
U.S. military											
Police officers	37	44	41	47	47	49	43	42	50	46	41
Pharmacists		59	61	65	66	62	60	66	65	62	66
Medical doctors	51	50	52	58	53	52	54	52	51	47	54
Veterinarians											
Clergy	61	63	64	67	60	55	57	54	53	54	56
Grade school teachers											
Engineers	46	48	45	53	48	50	45	48	49	49	53
College teachers	46	45	47	53	54	51	45	50	52	50	52
Dentists		52	51	56	51	52	50	50	50	51	54
Accountants											
Bankers	39	39	38	38	26	32	30	27	28	27	27
Journalists	33	32	28	31	23	30	26	27	26	20	23
U.S. House members	16	15	14	20	16	20	19	11	14	10	10
Business executives	19	19	18	23	16	25	21	18	20	22	19
Senators	19	20	16	23	19	24	19	13	18	12	12
Auto mechanics											
Stockbrokers		21	19	20	13	14	14	13	13	15	16
Lawyers	26	25	24	27	18	22	22	18	16	17	16
Labor union leaders	13	14	12	13	14	15	13	14	14	14	14
Insurance agents	15	11	13	10	10	13	14	9	10	9	11
Advertising practitioners	10	9	9	12	7	12	12	10	8	12	10
Car salespeople	8	6	6	5	6	6	8	5	6	6	5

From *Honesty/Ethics in Professions,* by Gallup Organization. http://www.gallup.com/poll. 2001.

1996	1997	1998	1999	2000	2001
					90
			73	79	84
					81
49	49	49	52	55	68
64	69	64	69	67	68
55	56	57	58	63	66
				63	66
56	59	59	56	60	64
			57	62	
48	49	50	50	56	60
56	55	53	52	59	58
53	54	53	52	58	56
				38	41
26	34	30	30	37	34
23	23	22	24	21	29
14	12	17	11	21	25
17	20	21	23	23	25
15	14	19	17	24	25
			24	22	22
15	18	19	16	19	19
17	15	14	13	17	18
16	15	15	17	17	17
11	12	11	10	10	13
11	12	10	9	10	11
8	8	5	8	7	8

Accountability is related to the client's rights to competent levels of nursing care and specifies that the nurse is responsible for providing health care services consistent with performance standards. The public expects nurses to provide competent care, which reflects a moral sense inherent in competent nursing practice (Bishop & Scudder, 1996). Nurses perform daily many activities and interventions in doing good acts for clients, and the public seems to sense that the nurse is concerned with empowering the client to make appropriate health care choices (Rogers, 2002). Nurses have an ethical interest in doing good for their clients, which includes fostering self-determination and justice.

Summary

Ethical problems in occupational health are pervasive and increasingly complex. Occupational and environmental health nurses, other health care professionals, and corporate managers must understand the ethical challenges encountered, differentiate ethical imperatives, develop approaches to handle these problems, and evaluate the impact of decisions. The nurse as a moral agent is concerned with values, choices, and duties related to the good of individuals and larger societies and with upholding and advancing the standards and codes of the profession. In this role the occupational and environmental health nurse not only brings a special expertise to resolving occupational health dilemmas but also needs to be able to structure the issues so that sound and deliberate decisions are made using a reasoned approach. Knowledge of ethical theories and principles and understanding their application to occupational health problems is essential to the decision making process. The nurse must acquire, enhance, and utilize these skills to provide effective leadership and guidance in the ethics of health care.

References

American Association of Occupational Health Nurses. (1998). *Code of ethics.* Atlanta, GA: Author.

American Nurses Association (2001). *Code of ethics for nurses.* Washington, DC: Author.

Americans With Disabilities Act of 1990. Pub. L. 101-336, 42 U. S. C. A. § *et. seq.* (1991).

Aroskar, M. (1989). Community health nurses: The most significant ethical decision-making problems. *Nursing Clinics of North America, 24,* 967-975.

Beauchamp, T. C., & Childress, J. E. (1994). *Principles of biomedical ethics.* New York: Oxford University Press.

Bishop, A., & Scudder, J. R. (1996). *Nursing ethics.* Boston: Jones and Bartlett.

Blake, D. (1992). The hospital ethics committee. *The Hastings Center Report, 22*(1), 6-12.

Childress, J. (1990). The place of autonomy in bioethics. *The Hastings Center Report, 20*(1), 12-16.

D'Arruda, K. (2001). Legal update—Application of the ADA to contingent workers. *AAOHN Journal, 49,* 323-324.

Davis, A., & Aroskar, M. (1983). Ethical dilemmas and nursing practice. Norwalk, CN: Appleton Century-Crofts.

Fry, S. T. (1994). *Ethics in nursing practice: A guide to ethical decision-making.* Geneva: International Council of Nurses.

Fry, S. T. (2000). Ethics in community-oriented nursing practice. In M. Stanhope and J. Lancaster (Eds.), *Community and public health nursing* (5th ed.), (pp. 116-137). St. Louis, MO: Mosby.

Gallup Organization. *Honesty/ethics in professions.* (2001). http://www.gallup.com/poll.

Hardwig, J. (1990). What about the family? *The Hastings Center Report, 20*(2), 5-10.

Jameton, A. (1984). *Nursing practice—The ethical issues.* Englewood Cliffs, NJ: Prentice-Hall.

Koh, D., & Jeyaratnam, J. (1998). Biomarkers, screening and ethics. *Occupational Medicine, 48,* 27-30.

Mezey, M. (1994). The patient self-determination act: Sources of concern for nurses. *Nursing Outlook 42,* 30.

Nielsen, R. (1989). Changing unethical organizational behavior. *The Academy of Management, 3,* 123-130.

Phillipp, R., Goodman, G., Harling, K., & Beattle, B. (1997). Study of business ethics in occupational medicine. *Occupational and Environmental Medicine, 54,* 351-356.

Rawbone, R. G. (1999). Future impact of genetic screening in occupational and environmental medicine. *Occupational and Environmental Medicine, 56,* 721-724.

Rest, K., & Patterson, W. (1986). Ethics and moral reasoning in occupational health. *Seminars in Occupational Medicine, 1,* 49-51.

Rodham, K. (1998). Manager or medic: The role of the occupational health professional. *Occupational Medicine, 48,* 81-84.

Rogers, B. (1988). Ethical dilemmas in occupational health nursing. *AAOHN Journal, 36,* 100-105.

Rogers, B. (1990). Making the case for ethics in occupational health. *Dangerous Properties of Hazardous Materials, 10,* 2-8.

Rogers, B. (1991). Ethical decision making in occupational settings. NIOSH grant-K 010H0072.

Rogers, B. (1992). Ethics and cost containment. *Continuing Professional Education, 4*(26), 1-8.

Rogers, B. (2001). Why a code of ethics? *AAOHN Journal, 49,* 11-12.

Rogers, B. (in press). Health care costs and quality: A balance. *AAOHN Journal, 50.*

International Occupational Health

As workplaces grow globally, the need to better understand varying practice parameters and occupational and environmental health issues and problems clearly will increase. With diverse populations and cultures in need of occupational health and safety services, occupational and environmental health professionals will need to reach across actual and virtual borders to connect knowledge so it can be applied to achieve the best possible health outcomes for employees (Rogers, 2000). This chapter will describe international occupational health issues along with strategies for occupational health improvement discussed by the World Health Organization, travel health issues and the role of the occupational and environmental health nurse, and ethical challenges related to international occupational health.

GLOBAL OCCUPATIONAL HEALTH

About 2.4 billion (45%) of the worldwide population of 5.4 billion and 58% of the population aged 10 years or older comprise the world's workforce. If informal work and work at home is taken into consideration, the proportion of the working population is even higher. Some 1.8 billion (75%) workers live and work in developing countries and about 600 million (25%) in the industrialized world. Nearly 8 of 10 workers are estimated to be in the developing world (WHO, 1995, 1999).

Work may have either a positive or an adverse effect on the health of the worker. In the most favorable circumstances, work provides the income for meeting the necessities of life and also has a positive impact on social, psychological, and physical health and well-being. At the same time, a high level of occupational health and safety contributes to the achievement of productivity objectives and provides high quality and performance in working life (WHO, 1995).

Although many countries have improved working conditions, the majority of the world's workers still labor where conditions do not meet the minimum standards and guidelines set by the International Labor Organization (ILO) and the World Health Organization (WHO). Workers in all countries are entitled to the basic benefits of federal labor and health and safety laws, including workers' compensation. However, the ILO reports that occupational health and safety laws cover only 10% of the population in developing countries and omit many major hazardous industries and occupations. These omissions include agriculture, fishing, forestry, construction, small scale businesses, and the informational sector (LaDou, 2002). Conditions at work and in the work environment for many occupations and in many countries still involve a distinct and even severe hazard to health that reduces the well-being, working capacity, and even the life span of working individuals (WHO, 1995).

Wide variations in economic and occupational structures, work conditions, quality of work environment, and health status of workers exist in different regions of the world, different countries, and different sectors of economies. Global trade has tripled in the past 20 years, and trade services have grown even faster (LaDou, 2002). Because of the high prevalence of manual and heavy physical work combined with the lack of coverage of general health and social protection, developing and newly industrialized countries have much to do if they are to develop occupational health services. This includes strengthening infrastructures, training human resources, establishing registration systems for occupational injuries and diseases, establishing occupational health institutes, establishing and updating legislation and standards, and performing inspections for compliance with regulations. At the same time, the implementation of new technologies, new demands for productivity and quality, and the need to support work innovation and motivation will lead to new types of work organization, new forms of employment (including self-employment and subcontracting), new work time arrangements, and new management systems (WHO, 1995).

Increasing rates of unemployment are expected because of the increase in productivity as a result of technological development, new divisions of work, high population growth, and economic recession in different regions. In many industrialized countries agricultural and manufacturing processes will become less labor intensive, and the service sector is not likely to absorb all the excess workforce no longer needed by production. International economic organizations and the ILO have emphasized that the only way to respond effectively to such a vast employment challenge is the promotion of small scale businesses and self-employment.

After the year 2000 more rapid aging of the workforce is expected in many developing countries. In some industrialized countries the aging of the workforce and the simultaneous negative or zero growth of the population will lead to an unusually high number of the elderly and an unusually low number of the young living in these countries.

Estimates indicate that 120 million injuries with 200,000 fatalities and 68 million to 150 million cases of occupational disease occur among the global workforce annually (ILO, 2000). In addition to occupational injuries and diseases, workers in developing countries suffer several maladies due to bacterial, viral, and parasitic infections; malnutrition; poor hygiene; and poor sanitation. Such conditions further reduce working capacity and aggravate the effects of occupational hazards.

Mechanical factors and physical and chemical agents are the main problems in manufacturing industries, while pesticides, heavy physical work, organic dusts, biological factors, and accidents are the occupational hazards faced by agricultural workers. Occupational accidents, traditional physical hazards, ergonomic deficiencies, and occupa-

tional diseases are pressing problems in all countries, particularly in overly industrialized countries, and the need for further preventive and control measures is often poorly recognized.

The least developed countries that still employ the majority (up to 80%) of the workforce in agriculture and other types of primary production face occupational health problems that are different from those experienced in the industrialized countries. Heavy physical work, often combined with heat stress, occupational accidents, pesticide poisonings, organic dusts, and biological hazards, will be the main causes of occupational morbidity. In the least developed countries these occupational factors are aggravated by numerous nonoccupational factors such as parasitic and infectious diseases, poor hygiene and sanitation, poor nutrition, general poverty, and illiteracy (Takala, 1999).

Several new problems in occupational health are related to a number of factors that include the following: implementation of new technologies; use of new chemicals and materials; application of new biotechnology; accidents in new production systems; infections such as HIV, hepatitis C, and other new viral and microbial diseases; reemergence of old epidemics such as tuberculosis; growing migration and mobility of people and workers; and new types of organization of work. Numerous ergonomic problems and heavy physical workload are associated with musculoskeletal disorders, causing wide-scale loss of working capacity. The growing performance demands, time pressure, and emotional workload in certain occupations (such as health care) are connected with stress symptoms and adverse health consequences.

In some countries more than half of the workers in certain high risk industries may show clinical signs of occupational disease, which also has an adverse effect on working capacity. According to the WHO (1995), some 200 biological agents, viruses, bacteria, parasites, fungi, molds and organic dusts have been associated with occupational exposures. In the industrialized countries approximately 15% of workers may be at risk of viral or bacterial infection, allergies, and respiratory diseases. In many developing countries the most likely sources of exposure are organic and biological agents. The hepatitis B and hepatitis C viruses and tuberculosis infection (particularly among health care workers), asthma (among people exposed to organic dust), and chronic parasitic diseases (particularly among agricultural and forestry workers) are the most common occupational diseases resulting from such exposures. The growing mobility of people from disease endemic areas to areas of low risk has increased the risk of disease, particularly to health care personnel.

About 100,000 different chemical products are in use in modern work environments, and the number is growing constantly. Exposures are most prevalent in industries processing chemicals and metals, in the manufacture of several consumer goods (such as metal products and plastic boats), in the production of textiles and artificial fibers, and in the construction industry. Chemicals are increasingly used in virtually all types of work, including nonindustrial activities such as hospital and office work, cleaning, cosmetic and beauty services, and numerous other services. The extent of exposure varies widely according to the industry, activity, and country.

Growing attention was paid in the 1980s to the risk from reproductive health hazards of work and workplace exposures (Paul & Frazier, 2000). Some 200 to 300 chemicals known to be mutagenic or carcinogenic tend to have adverse effects on reproduction (including infertility in both genders, spontaneous abortions, fetal death, teratogenesis, fetal cancer, fetotoxicity, or impaired fetal or newborn development) (Frazier & Hage, 1998). Numerous organic solvents and toxic metals are associated with adverse effects on reproductive health. Many biological agents, such as certain bacteria, viruses, and zoonoses-related agents, and heavy physical work are also associated with an increased risk of reproductive disorders. Reproduction hazards caused by ionizing radiation have been well-established, and hazards from nonionizing radiation are under intensive study. Both male and female workers may be affected by occupational hazards, but particular concern is given to the protection of women of reproductive age and during pregnancy. In addition to the conventional preventive actions of occupational health and hygiene services, special arrangements have been made in some countries to remove pregnant women from exposure that may be hazardous to the health of the mother or the fetus.

About 300 to 350 different agents—chemical (e.g., benzene, chromium, nitrosamines, asbestos), physical (e.g., ultraviolet radiation, ionizing radiation) and biological (e.g., aflatoxins, tumor viruses)—have been identified as occupational carcinogens. The most common cancers resulting from occupational carcinogenic exposures are cancers of the lung, bladder, skin, mesothelium, liver, haematopoetic tissue, bone, and soft connective tissue.

About 3,000 allergenic factors are estimated to be in the environment, most of them occurring as occupational exposures. Allergic dermatoses are one of the most prevalent occupational diseases and can lead to incapacity to work and the need to move the worker to another occupation. Occupational asthmas are caused by exposure to certain organic dusts, microorganisms, bacteria, fungi and molds, and organic and inorganic chemicals.

Mechanical factors, unshielded machinery, unsafe structures at the workplace, and dangerous tools are one of the most prevalent environmental hazards in both industrialized and developing countries and affect the health of a high proportion of the workforce. Also, hazards caused by traffic in many countries are starting to reach epidemic dimensions.

Workers may be exposed to physical factors such as noise, vibration, ionizing and nonionizing radiations, and microclimatic conditions, which are known to affect health. Between 10% and 30% of the workforce in industrialized countries and up to 80% in developing and newly industrialized countries are exposed to such physical factors, and in some high risk sectors, such as mining, manufacturing, and construction, all workers may be affected. Noise-induced hearing loss has been found to be one of the most prevalent occupational diseases in both developing and industrialized countries.

Between 10% and 30% of the workforce in industrialized countries and between 50% and 70% in developing countries may be exposed to heavy physical workloads or to nonergonomic working conditions such as lifting and moving of heavy items or repetitive manual tasks. The occupations most heavily exposed to physical workloads are miners, farmers, lumberjacks, fishermen, construction workers, storage workers, and health care personnel (particularly those caring for the elderly). Repetitive tasks and static muscular load are found in many industrial and service occupations. Damage to the cardiorespiratory or musculoskeletal system and traumatic injuries may be the consequence of such an overload of hazardous factors.

Many workers in industrialized counties judge their work to be stressful. Psychological stress caused by time pressure and hectic work has become more prevalent during the past decade. Other work factors that may have adverse psychological effects include heavy responsibility for human or economic concerns, monotonous work, work that requires constant concentration, shift work, work under the threat of violence (e.g., police or prison work), and isolated work. Psychological stress and overload have been associated with sleep disturbances, burn out syndromes, and depression.

In many industrial and service occupations, including health services, irregular working hours and frequent shift work are associated with several physiological and psychosocial problems that affect the health of workers and require exceptional capacity for adaptation. In some countries up to 30% of industrial workers work shifts (WHO, 1995).

The special occupational health problems of working women are recognized in both the developing and industrialized countries. In developing countries, heavy physical work, the double work burden of job and family, less developed working methods, and traditional social roles are the factors that increase the occupational health problems of female workers. In industrialized countries, where women also have the double work burden, lower paid manual jobs are often left to female workers. Also the design of machinery and work tools are often made according to male anthropometry, although female workers use such equipment. Women may also face problems of occupational exposures that are hazardous to reproductive health. In many service occupations, female workers may be exposed to the threat of violence from clients or to sexual harassment from fellow workers. Some studies indicate a higher than average risk of unemployment among low paid female workers, which may also have negative social and health consequences on families. Equal job opportunities for women and men and equal payment for the same job are still rarely seen around the world (WHO, 1995).

The industrialized countries are moving to the so-called postindustrialized stage, which is characterized by a low proportion of employment in agriculture (2.55%), no more than one-third (33.33%) in production industry, and the rest in services. As occupations change, work requires more mental ability, independence, and a high standard of competence and skill. Traditional occupational injuries and diseases will still occur, but they will affect a comparatively small number of high risk groups. Psychological problems at work, including symptoms of stress, will be the most common occupational health problem in the industrialized countries in this decade, as it was in the 1990 decade. Certain new psychosocial problems have been recognized, such as stress from threat of violence among women service workers who work alone and from dealing with work organization concerns.

Occupational health needs are becoming more specific and more complex. Such needs should be taken into consideration in designing training programs for experts. In spite of positive developments in general health services, primary health care and specialized services, a special occupational health service with appropriate support systems, including clinical services for the diagnosis and treatment of occupational diseases, are still needed. The earliest possible prevention and control of preventable hazards would help minimize economic loss at national, company, and individual levels and would have a positive impact on the further development of work, health, productivity, and quality.

New types of employment and new occupational settings are being created as the result of certain types of part-time work, distant work, home work, family industries, work involving traveling, and self-employment. New mechanisms for providing occupational health service for such work environments should be created, and new strategies to provide training, information, and advice for such groups of workers remain to be developed. Continuous monitoring of the possible occupational health effects of such new technologies should be exercised, and care should be taken to introduce scientific criteria for the planning of healthy and safe technologies and work environments.

Preventive strategies aim to eliminate or reduce to acceptable levels the occurrence of hazardous agents and factors in the work environment, preferably at their source of generation/dissemination, if not there then during their path of transmission, and as a last resort through protection of the worker. Information, training, and education of workers and employers on hazards and their prevention (including on emergency response) should also be part of such strategies. To ensure the continued efficiency of preventive measures, environmental monitoring and health surveillance of workers, including biological monitoring whenever appropriate, should be carried out. The importance of anticipatory preventive action, by the selection of the safest and least polluting processes, equipment, and materials, as well as the correct location and ergonomic design of workplaces, cannot be overemphasized.

The most successful economies have demonstrated that workplaces designed according to good principles of occupational health, safety, and ergonomics are also the most sustainable and productive (WHO, 1995). Furthermore, experience from many countries shows that a healthy economy, high quality products or services, and long-term productivity are difficult to achieve in poor working conditions with workers who are exposed to health and safety hazards. The available scientific knowledge and practical experiences of workplaces that have achieved the best results in the development of occupational health indicate the value of several principles. These principles are common denominators in occupational settings that have shown the best results in health, safety, and economic success and include the following:

- Avoidance of hazards (primary prevention) and use of safe technology
- Government responsibility
- Authority and competence to regulate and control working conditions
- Optimization of working conditions
- Integration of production and health and safety activities
- Primary responsibility of the employer or entrepreneur for health and safety at the workplace
- Recognition of employees' own interest in health at work
- Cooperation and collaboration on an equal basis
- Participation, right to know, and ethics
- Continuous follow-up
- Development of good working conditions

The way that work is organized, the management style, and the extent to which the worker can determine or regulate his or her work and participate in decisions about it have been shown in several studies to make a positive impact on health, prevent overload at work, counteract stress, and promote work motivation and productivity. In the midst of rapid change the need to learn new jobs and new skills requires an environment that is conducive to learning and adaptation. Effective management of such changes requires further development of the principles of openness, participation, and informed consent. Many industrialized countries with the strongest traditions in occupational health and safety can show constantly declining trends of occupational accidents and traditional occupational diseases as a result of adopting the principles just listed.

Successful prevention requires multidisciplinary expert competence on the following:

- Knowledge of the mechanism of action of hazardous factors and conditions
- Development and utilization of information on the causal relationship between risk factor and health outcome
- Knowledge of how the causal relationship can be broken
- Resources, tools, and mechanisms for the implementation of preventive measures
- Political, managerial, and target-group support for the preventive program

WHO GLOBAL HEALTH STRATEGY

Occupational health problems are not only problems for the worker, but above all, they are problems of work and the work environment. The work environment is greatly affected by the type of economic activity, occupation, company, size of workplace, and geographic and climatic conditions. The WHO recognizes the seriousness of the health problems of working populations, particularly the underserved in developing countries. Little attention has been given to those in agriculture, small business, construction, and mining. To address the work-related health issues and focus on both promotion and protection of workers worldwide, the WHO has developed the Global Strategy on Occupational Health for All (WHO, 1995; WHO, 1999).

The objective of this strategy was that by the year 2000 the countries where trends in occupational health and safety were already positive should have demonstrated a further improvement of occupational health and safety indicators by showing a reduction of the difference between levels of health and safety of low risk and high risk occupations and businesses. In countries where the present trends were negative, positive development was expected, and legal and other actions, including the development of necessary resources and infrastructures, should have been taken to make such positive trends possible. All countries should have shown a progressive development of OHS, with the ultimate objective of covering all workers with such services irrespective of the sector of the economy, size of company, occupation, mode of employment, or nature of self-employment.

Ten objectives guiding this strategy are mentioned in Chapter 13 and will be briefly discussed here as important to overall occupational health worldwide.

Objective 1: Strengthening of International and National Policies for Health at Work and Development of the Necessary Policy Tools

The priority of occupational health should be elevated on both national and international agendas, and appropriate resources should be provided for strengthening occupational health programs at both levels. Occupational health programs should be considered integral components of socioeconomic development and include the following:

- Updating of legislation and standards
- Definition and, if needed, strengthening of the role of the competent authority
- Emphasis on the primary responsibility of the employer for health and safety at work
- Establishment of mechanisms for tripartite collaboration among government, employers, and trade unions for implementation of national and occupational health programs
- Education and training of experts, employers, and employees
- Development of occupational health services
- Analytical, advisory services, and research
- Development and, if needed, establishment of registration systems of occupational accidents, diseases, and, if possible, exposures

- Action to ensure collaboration between employers and employees at workplace and business level

Objective 2: Development of Healthy Work Environments

In most countries hazardous exposures and factors that have adverse effects on the health of workers are still found in a high number of workplaces. Most hazardous work conditions are in principle preventable, and the primary prevention approach should be the most cost-effective strategy for their elimination and control. International scientific and expert support (WHO) should produce scientifically based guidelines for primary prevention of priority occupational hazards and should generate health-based criteria standards for guidelines for the development of healthy work environments.

Every country should carry out national surveys representative of all workplaces and occupations and examine the occurrence, distribution, and levels of occupational health and safety hazards and thus identify priority problems. Strengthened national actions should be initiated with clear objectives for reduction and prevention of priority hazards at work, such as high risk chemical and physical exposures and unreasonable physical workload or psychological workloads that lead to severe occupational accidents and diseases.

Objective 3: Development of Healthy Work Practices and Promotion of Health at Work

Many occupational hazards can be effectively avoided and controlled through the adoption of appropriate working practices by the worker and through providing him or her with information, tools, work organization, and work aids that enable the performance of work tasks without risk to health. Workers' lifestyles may have a specific or general impact on their occupational health and safety and working capacity. Health education on avoiding the combined effects of harmful lifestyle factors and occupational exposures should be effectively provided. Health promotion that introduces healthy lifestyles and supports the maintenance of such lifestyles with appropriate information, counseling, and education measures should be undertaken and preferably included in OHS programs.

Objective 4: Strengthening of Occupational Health Services

In many developing and newly industrialized countries no more than 5% to 10% of the working population—and in several industrialized countries less than 20% to 50%—have access to competent OHS in spite of the evident needs. Yet, the emerging problems of occupational health call for the development of OHS for all workers in all sectors of the economy and in all businesses, including the self-employed. Disciplines relevant for OHS include occupational medicine and nursing, occupational hygiene, work physiology and physiotherapy, ergonomics, safety, and work psychology. Each country should include in its national occupational health policy and program, objectives and actions for the gradual development of OHS for all workers, starting with those at highest risk and those in underserved groups. The preventive approach should be given the highest priority. Countries are encouraged to provide the support services and other infrastructures needed for development of multidisciplinary OHS. Emphasis should be given to the needs of OHS for the self-employed, agricultural workers, people employed in small businesses, and migrant workers. In most instances such services can be provided by primary health care units specially trained in occupational health.

Objective 5: Establishment of Support Services for Occupational Health

The WHO can give guidance and transmit experience and, if necessary, give advice to countries on why and how to organize the expert services for occupational health. International collaboration between experts providing expert advising services should be encouraged. Governments and authorities responsible for occupational health should ensure the availability of expert services for OHS, including a quality assurance and quality management element.

Objective 6: Development of Occupational Health Standards Based on Scientific Risk Assessment

To ensure minimum levels of health and safety at work, standards that define the safe levels of various exposures and other conditions of work are needed. The WHO should continue its efforts to produce principles and scientific bases for health-based standards concerning the major occupational exposures and other conditions of work, including chemical, physical, biological, and ergonomic factors. International collaboration and international harmonization of standards should be encouraged. Each country should adopt a basic set of standards to be used as criteria for the evaluation of the occupational health and safety aspects of various exposures, including chemical, physical, biological, and ergonomic factors. Where formal standards are not feasible or appropriate (e.g., on psychological factors), guidelines and codes of practices should be prepared. The bodies responsible for occupational health and safety should collaborate with employers' and workers' organizations when standards are being set. Countries should collaborate in the production of a scientific basis for standards.

Objective 7: Development of Human Resources for Occupational Health

Occupational health is a broad activity that utilizes the basic knowledge of several disciplines. Competent occupational health activities require appropriate training in these fields. In collaboration with scientific communities, other international bodies such as ILO and ICOH, and with support from the Network of WHO Collaborating Centers in Occupational Health and relevant professional associations, the WHO should prepare appropriate guidelines for training curricula for the key experts and expert groups in occupational health. Where individual countries are not able to carry out appropriate training programs at a national level, the WHO, through its Network of Collaborating Centers in Occupational Health, should establish training programs for training and education of experts in occupational health. Countries with well-established training capacities in occupational health should be encouraged to provide expert advice and support in the organization of such training programs subregionally or bilaterally.

Each country should include an element of training of sufficient numbers of experts to implement a national program and ensure sufficient personnel resources for OHS. Governments should ensure that the necessary elements of occupational health will be included in the basic training curricula of all who may in the future deal with occupational health issues. Training in occupational health also should be given in connection with vocational training and in training programs for workers, employers, and managers. In all training the need for a multidisciplinary approach in occupational health should be taken into consideration, ensuring involvement of occupational medicine and nursing, occupational hygiene, ergonomics and work physiology, occupational safety, and other relevant fields.

Objective 8: Establishment of Registration and Data Systems, Development of Information Services for Experts, Effective Transmission of Data, and Raising of Public Awareness Through Public Information

Analysis of reliable data, establishment of trends in occupational health, and recognition of priorities at national and local levels are of utmost importance both for the creation of policies and for occupational health practices. At least one well-developed focal point should have sufficient library resources and modem data systems for the country. This focal point should be linked with international information and data networks. Progressive development of national networks is currently needed to provide technically feasible and cost-effective solutions. Development of national data systems should be supported by appropriate training. International data banks on new observations of occupational hazards and outcomes should be established by the Network of WHO Collaborating Centers in Occupational Health. Each country should, through its WHO Collaborating Center, link into the WHO data bank of new occupational hazards and outcomes.

Objective 9: Strengthening of Research

Research is critical to the development of occupational administration and planning, training and education, risk identification, assessment, and practice. Research centers should be established, and the main tasks of such centers are the following:

1. Provide the necessary critical mass of scientific and human resources that can offer expert support to national programs and transfer international knowledge into the country;

2. Provide scientific and advisory support for policy makers and decision makers in the development of occupational health;
3. Support and guide the development of state, local, and company programs in occupational health;
4. Provide research, training, information, and service support for all involved in the development of occupational health.

The national research center should survey the occupational health and safety situation, help develop competence and methodology in occupational health, and respond to national occupational health problems.

Objective 10: Development of Collaboration in Occupational Health and With Other Activities and Services

Occupational health activities have several links with other parallel activities, such as occupational safety, environmental health and protection, primary health care, and specialized hospital-based health care. In certain situations, such as emergency response, occupational health activities are expected to collaborate intensively with several other services, such as rescue groups, fire services, and police. In all such collaborative links the role of occupational health experts is to provide expert knowledge on potential hazards in the work environment and their effects on the health of those exposed to them. The WHO Collaborating Centers in Occupational Health have a central role in the development of occupational health and safety at both national and international levels.

Each country should establish a focal point for WHO occupational health programs. Each country should establish a national body for ensuring multisectoral collaboration in occupational health and for encouraging all relevant bodies, such as other health sectors, the U.S. Department of Labor, environmental health groups, and relevant professional bodies, to participate. Collaboration of occupational health bodies with representatives of the national scientific community and the training and education institutions such as universities should be encouraged. Collaboration should be encouraged with extension and promotion organizations and industrial and trade associations.

Although occupational health and safety has improved, particularly in industrialized countries, occupational health hazards continue to plague all workers, particularly those in developing countries. Because global business is increasing, the occupational and environmental health nurse professional will need to be familiar with and cognizant of occupational health and health needs in other nations. The WHO has identified 10 strategies for occupational health worldwide that can provide guidance in building capacities to deal with occupational health hazards; all occupational health professionals must be familiar with this document.

TRAVEL HEALTH

Because international business travel has grown substantially in the last decade with the increase in the global economy, occupational health professionals must be keenly aware of the health problems and challenges faced by international business travelers. Numerous illnesses and injuries are associated with international business travel, the scope of which is too extensive to be covered here. However, of particular concern are risks related to vector-borne diseases, and risks/diseases related to drink and food (particularly Traveler's Diarrhea), and psychological issues. The role and function of the occupational and environmental health nurse is emphasized.

VECTOR-BORNE RISKS AND DISEASES

Although vaccines or chemoprophylactic drugs are available against internationally prevalent vector-borne diseases such as yellow fever and malaria, none exist for most other mosquito-borne diseases such as dengue, and travelers still should be advised to use repellents and other general protective measures against arthropods. The effectiveness of malaria chemoprophylaxis depends on patterns of resistance and compliance with medication. For many vector-borne diseases, no specific preventatives are available.

According to the CDC (2001), the principal approach to prevention of vector-borne diseases is avoidance. Tick and mite-borne infections characteristically are diseases of place; whenever possible, known foci of disease transmission should be avoided. Many vector-borne infections can be prevented by avoiding rural locations. Certain mosquito-borne arboviral and parasitic infections are transmitted seasonally, and simple changes in itinerary can greatly reduce risk for acquiring certain infections.

Travelers should be advised that exposure to arthropod bites can be minimized by modifying patterns of activity or behavior. Some vector mosquitoes are most active in twilight periods at dawn and dusk or in the evening. Avoidance of outdoor activity during these periods can reduce risk of exposure. Wearing long sleeved, tucked in shirts, long pants, and hats will minimize areas of exposed skin. Repellents such as permethrin-based repellents applied to clothing, shoes, tents, mosquito nets, and other gear will enhance protection. When exposure to ticks or biting insects is a possibility, travelers should be advised to tuck their pants into their socks and to wear boots, not sandals. Permethrin-treated clothing repels and kills ticks, mosquitoes, and other arthropods and retains this effect after repeated laundering. There appears to be little potential for human toxicity from permethrin-treated clothing. The insecticide should be reapplied after every five washings.

CDC (2001) indicates that most authorities recommend repellents containing N,N diethyl-metatoluamide (DEET) as an active ingredient to repel mosquitoes, ticks, and other arthropods when applied to the skin or clothing. Formulations containing less than 35% DEET are recommended because the additional gain in repellent effect with higher concentrations is not significant when weighed against the potential for toxicity. Travelers should be advised to use lower concentrations for children (no more than 10% DEET). Repellents with DEET should be used sparingly on children 2 to 6 years of age and not at all on infants younger than 2 years of age. Travelers should be advised that the possibility of adverse reactions to DEET will be minimized if they take the following precautions:

1. Apply repellent sparingly and only to exposed skin or clothing;
2. Avoid applying high concentration products to the skin;
3. Avoid inhaling or ingesting repellents or getting them in the eyes;
4. Avoid applying repellents to portions of children's hands that are likely to have contact with the eyes or mouth;

5. Avoid using repellents on wounds or irritated skin;
6. Wash repellent-treated skin after coming indoors.

If a reaction to insect repellent is suspected, travelers should wash treated skin and seek medical attention. Bed nets, repellents containing DEET, and permethrin should be purchased before traveling and can be found in hardware, camping, sporting goods, and military surplus stores.

Travelers should be advised that during outdoor activity and at the end of the day, they should inspect themselves and their clothing for ticks. Ticks are detected more easily on light colored or white clothing. Prompt removal of attached ticks can prevent some infections. When accommodations are not adequately screened or air conditioned, bed nets are essential to provide protection and comfort. Bed nets should be tucked under mattresses and can be sprayed with a repellent, such as permethrin. Permethrin will be effective for several months if the bed net is not washed.

RISKS FROM DRINK AND FOOD

Contaminated drink and food are common sources for the introduction of infection into the body (CDC, 2001). Among the more common infections that travelers can acquire from contaminated food and drink are *Escherichia coli* infections, shigellosis or bacillary dysentery, giardiasis, cryptosporidiosis, and hepatitis A. Other less common infectious disease risks for travelers include typhoid fever and other salmonelloses, cholera, infections caused by rotavirus and Norwalklike viruses, and a variety of protozoan and helminthic parasites (other than those that cause giardiasis and cryptosporidiosis). Many of the infectious diseases transmitted in food and water also can be acquired directly through the fecal-oral route.

Water

Water that has been adequately chlorinated, using minimum recommended water treatment standards employed in the United States, will afford significant protection against viral and bacterial water-borne diseases. However, chlorine treatment alone, as used in the routine disinfection of water, might not kill some enteric viruses and

the parasitic organisms that cause giardiasis, amebiasis, and cryptosporidiosis. In areas where chlorinated tap water is not available or where hygiene and sanitation are poor, travelers should be advised that only the following might be safe to drink: (1) beverages, such as tea and coffee, made with boiled water; (2) canned or bottled carbonated beverages, including carbonated bottled water and soft drinks, and (3) beer and wine.

Where water might be contaminated, travelers should be advised that ice also should be considered contaminated and should not be used in beverages. If ice has been in contact with containers used for drinking, travelers should be advised to thoroughly clean the containers, preferably with soap and hot water, after the ice has been discarded. It is safer to drink a beverage directly from the can or bottle than from a questionable container. However, water on the outside of beverage cans or bottles might be contaminated also. Therefore, travelers should be advised to dry wet cans or bottles before they are opened, and to wipe surfaces clean with which the mouth will have direct contact. Where water might be contaminated, travelers should be advised to avoid brushing their teeth with tap water.

Treatment of water

Travelers should be advised of the following methods for treating water to make it safe for drinking and other purposes:

• *Boiling* is by far the most reliable method to make water of uncertain purity safe for drinking. Water should be brought to a vigorous rolling boil for 1 minute and allowed to cool to room temperature; ice should not be added. This procedure will kill bacterial and parasitic causes of diarrhea at all altitudes and viruses at low altitudes. To kill viruses at altitudes above 2,000 meters (6,562 feet), water should be boiled for 3 minutes or chemical disinfection should be used after the water has boiled for 1 minute. Adding a pinch of salt to each quart or pouring the water several times from one clean container to another will improve the taste.
• *Chemical disinfection* with iodine is an alternative method of water treatment when it is not feasible to boil water. However, this method cannot be relied upon to kill *Cryptosporidium* unless the water is allowed to sit for 15 hours

TABLE 18-1	Treatment of Water With Tincture of Iodine	
	DROPS TO BE ADDED PER QUART OR LITER	
TINCTURE OF IODINE	**CLEAR WATER**	**COLD OR CLOUDY WATER**
2%	5	10

before it is drunk. Two well-tested methods for disinfection with iodine are the use of tincture of iodine (Table 18-1) and the use of tetra-glycine hydroperiodide tablets (for example, Globaline, Potable Aqua, or Coughlan's). These tablets are available from pharmacies and sporting goods stores. The manufacturers' instructions should be followed.

• *Chlorine*, in various forms, can also be used for chemical disinfection. However, its germicidal activity varies greatly with the pH, temperature, and organic content of the water to be purified and, therefore, it can produce less consistent levels of disinfection in many types of water.

Chemically treated water is intended for short term use only. If iodine disinfected water is the only water available, it should be used for only a few weeks.

Food

To avoid illness, travelers should be advised to select food with care (CDC, 2001). All raw food is subject to contamination. Particularly in areas where hygiene and sanitation are inadequate, the traveler should be advised to avoid salads, uncooked vegetables, and unpasteurized milk and milk products such as cheese and to eat only food that has been cooked and is still hot or fruit that has been peeled by the traveler personally. Undercooked and raw meat, fish, and shellfish can carry various intestinal pathogens. Cooked food that has been allowed to stand for several hours at ambient temperature can provide a fertile medium for bacterial growth and should be thoroughly reheated before serving.

Consumption of food and beverages obtained from street food vendors has been associated with an increased risk of illness. If the business traveler is accompanied by children, caution should be taken. Some species of fish and shellfish can contain poisonous biotoxins, even when well-cooked. The most common type of biotoxin in fish is ciguatoxin, which is present in many fish, including red snapper, grouper, amberjack, and sea bass, and a wide range of tropical reef fish contain the toxin at unpredictable times. The flesh of the barracuda is the most toxic-laden and should always be avoided. Caution should be taken with all types of fish. Travelers should be advised not to bring perishable seafood with them when they return to the United States from high risk areas. The easiest way to guarantee a safe food source for an infant younger than 6 months of age is to have the infant breast feed. If the infant has already been weaned from the breast, formula prepared from commercial powder and boiled water is the safest and most practical food.

Travelers' Diarrhea

Epidemiology

According to the CDC (2001), Travelers' Diarrhea (TD) is a syndrome characterized by a twofold or greater increase in the frequency of unformed bowel movements. Commonly associated symptoms include abdominal cramps, nausea, bloating, urgency, fever, and malaise. Episodes of TD usually begin abruptly, occur during travel or soon after returning home, and are generally self-limited. The most important determinant of risk is the destination of the traveler. Attack rates of 20% to 50% are commonly reported in both men and women. High risk destinations include most of the developing countries of Latin America, Africa, the Middle East, and Asia. Intermediate risk destinations include most of the southern European countries and a few Caribbean islands. Low risk destinations include Canada, northern Europe, Australia, New Zealand, the United States, and some of the Caribbean islands. TD is slightly more common in young adults than in older people. The reasons for this difference are unclear but could include a lack of acquired immunity, more adventurous travel styles, and different eating habits. Attack rates are similar in men and women. The onset of TD is usually within the first week of travel but can occur at any time during the visit and even after returning home.

TD is acquired through ingestion of fecally contaminated food or water or both. Both cooked and uncooked foods might be sources if they have been improperly handled. Especially risky foods include raw or undercooked meat and seafood and raw fruits and vegetables. Tap water, ice, and unpasteurized milk and dairy products can be associated with increased risk of TD; safe beverages include bottled carbonated beverages (especially flavored beverages), beer, wine, hot coffee or tea, and water boiled and appropriately treated with iodine or chlorine. The place food is prepared appears to be an important variable, with private homes, restaurants, and street vendors listed in order of increasing risk.

TD typically results in four to five loose or watery stools per day. The median duration of diarrhea is 3 to 4 days. Approximately 10% of the cases persist longer than 1 week, approximately 2% longer than 1 month, and less than 1% longer than 3 months. Persistent diarrhea is, thus, quite uncommon and can differ considerably from acute TD with respect to etiology and risk factors. Approximately 15% of ill people experience vomiting, and 2% to 10% have diarrhea accompanied by fever or bloody stools or both. Travelers can experience more than one episode of TD during a single trip. Rarely is TD life threatening.

Etiology

Infectious agents are the primary cause of TD. People traveling from developed countries to developing countries frequently experience a rapid, dramatic change in the type of organisms in their gastrointestinal tract. These new organisms often include potential enteric pathogens. Those who develop diarrhea have ingested an inoculum of virulent organisms sufficiently large to overcome individual defense mechanisms, and this results in symptoms.

Enteric bacterial pathogens

Enterotoxigenic *Escherichia coli, salmonella* organisms, and *shigella* organisms are recognized agents that cause TD in up to 20% of travelers to developing countries.

Viral enteric pathogens: Rotaviruses

Along with the newly acquired bacteria, the traveler can also acquire many viruses (CDC, 2001). For example, as much as 36% of diarrheal illnesses in travelers (median 22%) was associated with rotaviruses in the stools. However, a comparable number of asymptomatic travelers also had rotaviruses, and up to 50% of symptomatic people with rotavirus infections also had nonviral pathogens.

Parasitic enteric pathogens

Although less commonly implicated as the cause of TD than bacteria, enteric protozoa are recognized etiologic agents of TD including *Giardia intestinalis* (0% to 12%), *Entamoeba histolytica* (0% to 5%), *Cryptosporidium parvum* (2% to 5%), and *Cyclospora cayetanensis* (1% to 11%). The likelihood of a parasitic etiology is higher when diarrheal illness is prolonged. *E. histolytica* should be considered when the individual has dysentery or invasive diarrhea (bloody stools).

Prevention

Four possible approaches to prevention of TD include (1) instruction regarding food and beverage consumption, (2) immunization, (3) use of nonantimicrobial medications, and (4) use of prophylactic antimicrobial drugs. Data indicate that meticulous attention to food and beverage consumption, as mentioned previously, can decrease the likelihood of developing TD. Most travelers, however, encounter difficulty in observing the requisite dietary restrictions. No available vaccines and none that are expected to be available in the next 3 years are effective against TD.

Several nonantimicrobial agents have been advocated for prevention of TD. Available controlled studies indicate that prophylactic use of difenoxine, the active metabolite of diphenoxylate (Lomotil), actually increases the incidence of TD, in addition to producing other undesirable side effects. Antiperistaltic agents (for example, Lomotil and Imodium) are not effective in preventing TD. No data support the prophylactic use of activated charcoal. Bismuth subsalicylate, taken as the active ingredient of Pepto Bismol (2 ounces 4 times a day, or 2 tablets 4 times a day), has decreased the incidence of diarrhea by about 60% in several placebo-controlled studies. Side effects include temporary blackening of the tongue and stools, occasional nausea and constipation, and, rarely, tinnitus. Available data are not sufficient to exclude a risk to the traveler from the use of such large doses of bismuth subsalicylate for a period of more than 3 weeks. Bismuth subsalicylate should be avoided by travelers with aspirin allergy, renal insufficiency, and gout and by those who are taking anticoagulants, probenecid, or methotrexate. In travelers already taking aspirin or related salicylates for arthritis, large concurrent doses of bismuth subsalicylate can produce toxic serum concentrations of salicylate. Caution should be used in giving bismuth subsalicylate to children and adolescents with chickenpox or influenza because of a potential risk of Reye's syndrome. Bismuth subsalicylate has not been approved for infants and children younger than 3 years of age. Bismuth subsalicylate appears to be an effective prophylactic agent for TD but is not recommended for prophylaxis of TD for periods of more than 3 weeks. Other agents such as Lomotil and activated charcoal have not proven effective (CDC, 2001).

Controlled data that are available on the prophylactic value of several other nonantimicrobial drugs have shown these agents not to be effective. Because of the uncertain risk involved in the widespread administration of antimicrobial agents, their prophylactic use is not recommended. Although it seems reasonable to use prophylactic antibiotics in certain high risk groups, such as travelers with immunosuppression or immunodeficiency, no data directly support this practice. There is little evidence that other disease entities are worsened sufficiently by an episode of TD to risk the rare undesirable side effects of prophylactic antimicrobial drugs. *Therefore, prophylactic antimicrobial agents are not recommended for travelers* (CDC, 2001). Instead, available data support the recommendation that travelers be instructed in sensible dietary practices as a prophylactic measure. This recommendation is justified by the excellent results of early treatment of TD as outlined in the following section. Some travelers might wish to consult with their physicians and, after the risks and benefits are clearly understood, might elect to use prophylactic antimicrobial agents for travel under special circumstances.

Treatment

Travelers with TD have two major complaints for which they desire relief: abdominal cramps and diarrhea. Many agents have been proposed to control these symptoms, but few have been demonstrated to be effective in rigorous clinical trials.

Nonspecific agents

A variety of "adsorbents" have been used in treating diarrhea. Activated charcoal has been found to be ineffective in the treatment of diarrhea. Kaolin and pectin have been widely used for diarrhea. While the combination appears to give the stools more consistency, it has not been shown to decrease cramps and frequency of stools or to shorten the course of infectious diarrhea. Lactobacillus preparations and yogurt have also been advocated, but no evidence supports use of these treatments for TD. Bismuth subsalicylate preparation has been shown to decrease the frequency of stools and shorten the duration of illness. There is concern about taking large amounts of bismuth and salicylate without supervision, especially for people who might be intolerant of salicylates, have renal insufficiency, or take salicylates for other reasons.

Antimotility agents

Antimotility agents are widely used in treating diarrhea of all types. Natural opiates (paregoric, tincture of opium, and codeine) have long been used to control diarrhea and cramps. Synthetic agents, such as diphenoxylate and loperamide, come in convenient dosage forms and provide prompt symptomatic but temporary relief of uncomplicated TD. However, they should not be used by people with high fever or with blood in the stools. Use of these drugs should be discontinued if symptoms persist beyond 48 hours. Diphenoxylate and loperamide should not be used in infants younger than 2 years of age.

Antimicrobial treatment

Travelers who develop diarrhea with three or more loose stools in an 8-hour period, especially if associated with nausea, vomiting, abdominal cramps, fever, or blood in the stools, might benefit from antimicrobial treatment. The effectiveness of antibiotic therapy will depend on the etiologic agent and its antibiotic sensitivity. The antibiotic regimen most likely to be effective is ciprofloxacin. Other fluroquinolones, such as norfloxacin, ofloxacin, or levofloxacin might be equally as effective. Fewer side effects and less widespread antibiotic resistance has been reported with the fluoroquinolones. Travelers should be advised to consult a physician rather than attempt self-medication if the diarrhea is severe or does not resolve within several days; if blood or mucus (or both) is in the stools; if fever occurs with shaking chills; or if dehydration accompanies persistent diarrhea.

Oral fluids

Most cases of diarrhea are self-limited and require only simple replacement of fluids and salts lost in diarrheal stools. This is best achieved by use of an oral rehydration solution such as World Health Organization oral rehydration salts (ORS) solution (Table 18-2). This solution is appropriate for treating as well as preventing dehydration. Travelers should be advised that ORS packets are available at stores or pharmacies in almost all developing countries.

Precautions for children and pregnant women

Although infants and children do not make up a large proportion of travelers to high risk areas, some children do accompany their families. Teenagers should follow the advice given to adults, with possible adjustments of doses of medication. Physicians should be aware of the risks of tetracyclines for infants and children younger than 8 years of age. Few data are available about the usage of antidiarrheal drugs in infants and children. Drugs should be prescribed with caution for pregnant women and nursing mothers.

Psychosocial issues

Psychosocial issues (i.e., stress, anxiety, culture shock, adjustment) can occur when traveling to or living and working in new physical, cultural, and organizational environments (Rogers & Reilly, 2000). Of particular concern are family and cultural issues, feelings of isolation, and loss of familiar interests. Whenever a business traveler travels, there are always important family concerns to consider. For the short-term traveler, separation from family may create stress and anxiety for both the traveler and family members. For the spouse at home additional responsibilities may increase, leading to feelings of overload, even temporarily. This may be particularly true if the at-home spouse works outside the home and then has to manage the household without help.

For the long-term business traveler, spouse and children may accompany the traveler. Of note is the issue of culture shock for all family members. This means dealing with and learning a new language, becoming familiar with the mores of the community and society, and adapting to new foods, learning environments, and social structures. The spouse may have to deal with a business traveler who may be "on the road" quite a bit in the host country. Children may have issues with schooling and social networks and may exhibit regressive behavior, clinginess, school phobia, and distress.

For the family in general, feelings of isolation may occur, especially for the spouse who may have few social ties or networks. Loss of a job, contact with friends, familiar community events, family medical issues, and church may also be important issues.

ROLE OF THE OCCUPATIONAL AND ENVIRONMENTAL HEALTH NURSE IN TRAVEL HEALTH

Initially, the occupational and environmental health nurse must be involved in developing policies and procedures for a comprehensive travel health program (e.g., destination assessment, health assessment). The nurse will be involved with health and risk factor assessment, immunization management, exposure risks, travel kit preparation, safety/security, predeparture counseling and education, and posttravel evaluation.

The occupational and environmental health nurse begins preparing travelers by assessing their needs prior to departure. Ideally, the traveler should seek health care advice 4 to 6 weeks before traveling. The assessment begins with knowing the countries or regions to be visited, the duration of the trip, and

TABLE 18-2	Composition of World Health Organization Oral Rehydration Solution (ORS) for Diarrheal Illness	
INGREDIENT	**AMOUNT**	
Sodium chloride	3.5 grams per liter	
Potassium chloride	1.5 grams per liter	
Glucose	20.0 grams per liter	
Trisodium citrate*	2.9 grams per liter	

*An earlier formulation that used sodium bicarbonate 2.5 grams per liter had a shorter shelf life but was physiologically equivalent and might still be produced in some countries.

the living accommodations of the traveler. Employees traveling out of the country for an extended period of time or traveling to under-developed countries should do so with a copy of their completed health history, health care provider examination, laboratory work, and a list of regularly taken medications. A physical examination, immunizations, and counseling also may be necessary. Risk factors and immunization status should be reviewed during this assessment (AAOHN, 2001).

The nurse should review all health risks (e.g., chronic diseases, immune status), lifestyle issues and risks, and medications. Employees should pack a supply of useful drugs: aspirin, analgesics, cough mixture, and, if going to an underdeveloped country, a broad-spectrum antibiotic. Travelers should always take their usual medications with them, as well as a physician's letter for customs officials if the quantities are large or the drugs are not approved for use in the final destination (e.g., codeine-based drugs in Asia). It is wise to carry prescription drugs from home even if substitutes are available overseas; for some classes of medication, especially heart and hormone drugs, the bioavailability of the active ingredient (the drug's potency) may differ between manufacturers, and this difference is often enough to cause symptoms due to under-dosage or overdosage (DeJongh & Rey-Herme, 1998). Diabetic patients carrying insulin needles generally have no difficulty at customs checks.

Travelers should be informed about important issues related to medications, especially narcotics and syringes. Narcotics for medical use are regarded by nearly all customs officials as illegal; this also applies to stimulants such as methylphenidate (Ritalin). Even with a letter from the original prescribing physician, the traveler will be fortunate if all that happens is confiscation with a warning. Therefore, as a general rule, it is recommended not to travel with narcotics for any reason (DeJongh & Rey-Herme, 1998).

Immunizations provide protection against a number of diseases, and the traveler should be current on routine immunizations (Thompson et al., 1996). In reviewing immunization, the three Rs of travel immunization—routine, required, and recommended—need to be determined based on country-specific indications and knowledge of current immunizations recommended by the CDC (ISTM, 1999) (Box 18-1).

Routine immunizations are those needed for childhood/adult protection according to current public health recommendations. Required immunizations are those that are legally mandated for the crossing of international borders. Documentation of yellow fever immunization may be required by border health officials from those entering yellow fever endemic zones in Africa and South America or traveling from these areas to nonendemic regions. Although cholera is no longer a required immunization according to international health regulations, occasionally officials at border crossings may require documentation. Meningococcal meningitis vaccine is required by officials in Saudi Arabia for pilgrimage to the Hajj. Proof of diphtheria immunization may be required for travel to the Hajj from the former Soviet Union. Based on a risk assessment of the itinerary, the style of travel, and the traveler's underlying health, the traveler may be advised to obtain selected immunizations for prevention of travel-related infections. The traveler's immunization record should be kept current and reviewed periodically with consideration of destination and length of stay (AAOHN, 2001).

Box 18-1   Routine, Required, and Recommended Immunizations for Travel

ROUTINE IMMUNIZATIONS

- Tetanus/diphtheria
- Polio
- MMR
- Influenza
- Pneumococcal
- Varicella

REQUIRED IMMUNIZATIONS

- Yellow fever
- Meningococcal

RECOMMENDED IMMUNIZATIONS

- Hepatitis A
- Hepatitis B
- Typhoid
- Meningococcal meningitis
- Poliomyelitis
- Rabies
- Japanese encephalitis
- Cholera

From *Introduction to Travel Medicine,* by International Society of Travel Medicine, 1999, Atlanta, GA: Author.

Major exposure risks include the vector-borne and foodborne and waterborne diseases discussed earlier in this chapter. The major cause of morbidity to travelers under the age of 55 is motor vehicle accidents (Rose, 2000). The Association of Safe International Road Travel indicates that death rates from motor vehicle accidents are 20 to 80 times higher in some countries than in the United States (Rose, 2000) (Figure 18-1). Many road accidents involve tourists when drivers lose control due to fatigue or alcohol or are not familiar with roads. Jet lag also places travelers at

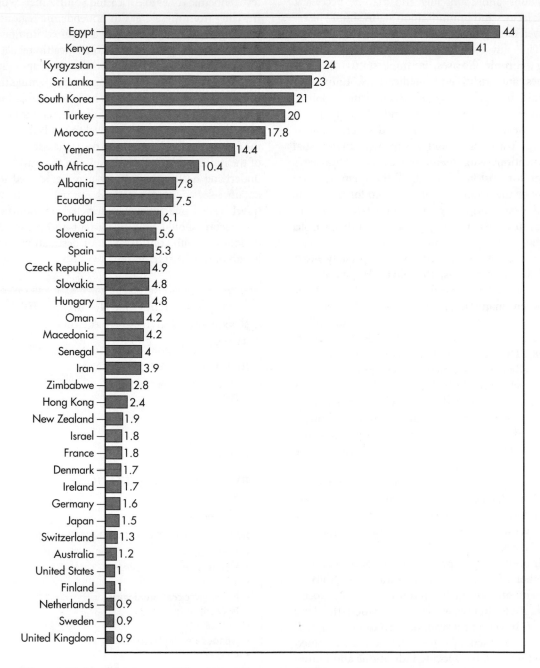

Figure 18-1 Fatalities per 100 vehicle kilometers, 1995. *(From Association for Safe International Road Travel, 1997.)*

risk for injury due to fatigue, irritability, and short attention span. Each year an estimated 750 U.S. citizens die on international roads and at least 25,000 are injured (Rose, 2000).

Business travelers should be provided with a predeparture self-care kit with instructions that include an oral thermometer and instructions on how to take one's temperature; sun screen; first aid supplies, such as topical cleanser, antibiotic ointment, and bandages; over-the-counter remedies for common problems such as headache, musculoskeletal pain, nasal congestion, indigestion, allergy, contact dermatitis, diarrhea, and constipation; select prescription medications and supplies, such as medication for sleep, syringes, and general antibiotics; and dental emergency kits.

Some supplies should be included based on a regional or health risk assessment: antibiotics; antifungal cream; antimalarials; Epi-pens; supplies of regular prescription medications adequate to last the trip; prescriptions for special problems, such as jet lag (short acting benzodiazepine hypnotic, [e.g., Restoril]) or high altitude; and travel-specific and personal hygiene supplies (Saphire, 1996).

Safety and security for travelers is critical. Crime is a potential problem, especially when traveling in large cities. The risk of being kidnapped, hijacked, or taken hostage has greatly increased for business travelers (AAOHN, 2001). Foreign targets are at significant risk and are ideal for those involved in criminal activity. The traveler will want to access the U.S. State Department Website about safety issues and travel warnings related to each country. Box 18-2 identifies safety and security measures travelers should consider.

The occupational and environmental health nurse will want to provide the employee with a general predeparture counseling and education session on a variety of topics, including types of endemic diseases; food and water safety issues; sexually transmitted diseases; health care and delivery options and safety issues at the destination; special precautions for pregnant women, children, and travelers with medical conditions; and psychosocial issues. Many resources are available that both the traveler and the health care professional will find useful (Box 18-3).

Postassignment evaluation should be part of a comprehensive travel health plan for the employee and family, if indicated. A health examination and debriefing can be held with the employee to discuss any problems encountered

---

Box 18-2   Personal Safety and Security Measures for Travelers

- Avoid advertising wealth and foreign status to the extent possible.
- Avoid carrying large amounts of cash if at all possible; use credit cards where possible.
- Travelers checks are even safer but cannot be cashed everywhere one goes, especially outside large cities; U.S. dollars take up less space that most paper currencies and therefore are more easily concealed.
- Consider wearing a concealed money belt when traveling outside urban areas.
- Keep a smaller amount of cash in your wallet or billfold than you actually possess; in the event of robbery you could surrender this and claim it as all you have.
- Women should not carry strap handbags; men should not put their wallet in their hip pocket.
- Do not change money on the black market; the same precautions apply to the supply, sale, and smuggling of antiques, drugs, and any other contraband items.

- Use hotel safes and beware of leaving valuables in your room; if you have to take a sleeper train journey overnight, lock your bag to the carriage rack with a bicycle lock.
- Protect confidential personal and commercial information, including data on personal computer or floppy discs.
- When looking for entertainment, stay with major respectable hotels or those establishments recommended by the senior management of such hotels.
- In many countries, women walking alone are considered easy targets for harassment and crime.
- Street crime—pickpockets, purse-snatchers, and muggers—is rising worldwide.
- Know the nearest fire exit (i.e., stairway) when staying in any hotel or apartment above the first floor and carry a small flashlight to find the exit, as well as a passport (or copy) and money, for emergencies.

From "Travel and Expatriate Medicine," by R. DeJongh and P. Rey-Herme, in J. Herzstein, B. Bunn, and L. Fleming (Eds.), *International Occupational and Environmental Health Medicine* (pp. 211-222), 1998, St. Louis, MO: Mosby.

Box 18-3 Travel Medicine Resources

AMERICAN SOCIETY OF TROPICAL MEDICINE AND HYGIENE (ASTMH)

http://www.astmh.org

Travel and Tropical Medicine Clinic Directory, *American Journal of Tropical Medicine and Hygiene*, overseas opportunities, grants and fellowships, positions, ASTMH Newsletter, clinical tropical medicine and travel medicine online discussion group, annual scientific meeting. Non-profit professional organization.

CENTERS FOR DISEASE CONTROL AND PREVENTION (CDC)

http://www.cdc.gov/travel/travel.html

1 (404) 332-4559 (CDC traveler's health hotline)
1 (888) 232-3299 (CDC FAX information toll-free line)

Public health information on diseases, health conditions, and health hazards worldwide, official requirements and recommendations for overseas travelers with regards to vaccines and malaria, updated frequently. U.S. government agency.

FEDERAL AVIATION ADMINISTRATION (FAA)

http://www.faa.gov

Statements on air travel security.

INTERNATIONAL ASSOCIATION FOR MEDICAL ASSISTANCE FOR TRAVELERS (IAMAT)

http://www.iamat.org/

1 (519) 836-0102

Worldwide Directory of English-Speaking Physicians, World Climate Charts, Malaria Risk Charts, and other travel medicine information

based on WHO information and expert sources. Free information. Nonprofit organization, supported by voluntary donations.

INTERNATIONAL SOCIETY OF TRAVEL MEDICINE (ISTM)

http://www.istm.org

Travel Clinic Directory, *Journal of Travel Medicine*, newsletter, international travel medicine online discussion group, international membership meeting every 2 years. Nonprofit professional organization.

SHORELAND, INC. (PUBLISHERS OF TRAVEL HEALTH ONLINE AND TRAVAX)

http://www.tripprep.com

Health conditions, health requirements, and health recommendations, country by country, plus summary of U.S. State Department advisories, updated frequently. Private publisher of travel health information (TRAVAZ) used by many U.S. and overseas clinics.

U.S. STATE DEPARTMENT

http://www.travel.state.gov

1 (202) 647-5225 (Recorded phone line)
1 (202) 647-3000 (Automated fax line)

Information sheets on countries worldwide and travel warnings.

U.S. EMBASSIES

http://www.usembassy.state.gov

Country-specific information.

WORLD HEALTH ORGANIZATION

http://www.who.int/en/

International travel and health, vaccination requirements, and health advice.

---

during travel, along with recommendations for future travelers. Employee assistance programs should be offered to the employee if needed.

ETHICAL CHALLENGES

Ethical positions should not change in their meaning of honoring the principles of doing what is morally right from an international perspective. Human rights dictate that people should be treated with dignity and respect regardless of their geographic location. This means that exposures in and of themselves are harmful regardless of the country or region of occurrence. However, cul-

tural and religious differences often bring different sets of values.

Goodman (1998) points out that cultural differences underlie many of the most difficult ethical issues faced in international health, issues such as confidentiality, monitoring, and disclosure. Respect for others' cultures is sometimes taken to constitute a license to abandon one's own core values. Similarly, sometimes people suppose that the sociological fact of cultural-ethical diversity entails some form of moral relativism. These are common and understandable views. They are, however, mistaken.

In many circumstances accommodating local values in one's professional practice is acceptable as long as one does not compromise on deeper moral

---

Box 18-4   International Code of Ethics for Occupational Health Professionals:
General Categories of Duties and Responsibilities

1. Aims and advisory role
2. Knowledge and expertise
3. Development of a policy and a program
4. Emphasis on prevention and prompt action
5. Follow-up of remedial actions
6. Safety and health information
7. Commercial secrets
8. Health surveillance
9. Information to the worker
10. Information to the employer
11. Information to a third party about potential dangers
12. Biological monitoring and investigations
13. Health promotion
14. Protection of community and environment
15. Contribution to scientific knowledge
16. Competence, integrity, and impartiality
17. Professional independence
18. Equity, nondiscrimination, and communication
19. Clause on ethics in contracts of employment
20. Records
21. Medical confidentiality
22. Collective health data
23. Relationships with health professionals
24. Combating of abuses
25. Relationships with social partners
26. Promotion of ethics and professional audit

Modified from *International Code of Ethics for Occupational Health Professionals,* by International Commission on Occupational Health, 1997, Geneva, Switzerland: Author.

---

questions. It is one thing to try to accommodate and not disparage folk medical beliefs, for instance, but it might be quite another to neglect a patient who has magical or other false beliefs about illness.

In general, how one deals with issues of practice concern are determined by statutory regulations. However, when ethical issues arise, guidance to addressing these issues is offered by codes of ethics. Many disciplines have their own set of ethical codes. The International Commission on Occupational Health (ICOH) has adopted the *International Code of Ethics for Occupational Health Professionals* (ICOH, 1997), which states that each employer has the responsibility for the health and safety of the workers in his or her employment. Each profession has its responsibilities, which are related to the nature of its duties. When specialists of several professions are working together within a multidisciplinary approach, they should base their action on some common principles of ethics and should understand each others' obligations, responsibilities, and professional standards. Special care should be taken with respect to ethical aspects, in particular when there are conflicting rights, such as the right to the protection of employment and the right to the protection of health or the right to information and the right to confidentiality, as well as individual rights and collective rights.

The ICOH's code of ethics is guided by basic principles of ethics, which include the following (ICOH, 1997):

Occupational health practice *must be performed according to the highest professional standards and ethical principles. Occupational health professionals must serve the health and social well-being of the workers, individually and collectively. They also contribute to environmental and community health.*

The obligations of occupational health professionals *include protecting the life and the health of the worker, respecting human dignity, and promoting the highest ethical principles in occupational health policies and programs. Integrity in professional conduct, impartiality, and protection of the confidentiality of health data and the privacy of workers are part of these obligations.*

Occupational health professionals are experts *who must enjoy full professional independence in the execution of their functions. They must acquire and maintain the competence necessary for their duties and require conditions that allow them to carry out their tasks according to good practice and professional ethics.* (p. 4)

Further, within the Code of Ethics, 26 duties and obligations of occupational health professionals are outlined. Box 18-4 gives the general category of these duties and responsibilities; however, the reader can obtain a full text copy from ICOH (from their website http://www. ICOHSG.org).

Summary

With global connections ever-growing, the world community is becoming more aware and cognizant of health issues worldwide. This is true of the business community and related occupational health issues. Occupational and environmental health nurses have a great opportunity to learn about work-related hazards in global communities and the impact of those hazards on workers. In addition, travel health issues are very important for the worker, company, and occupational health professional, and the occupational and environmental health nurse will have a large role to play in managing these programs. Ethical challenges will need to be explored using ethical codes as a frame of reference for ethical decision making.

References

AAOHN Advisory. (2001). Travel health. *AAOHN Journal, 49,* 320 A.

Centers for Disease Control and Prevention. *Health information for international travel 2001-2002.* (2001). http://www2.ncid.cdc.gov/travel/yb/utils/ybDynamic.asp.

DeJongh, R., & Rey-Herme, P. (1998). Travel and expatriate medicine. In J. A. Herzstein, N. B. Bunn III, and L. E. Fleming, J. M. Harrington, J. Jeraratnam, & I. R. Gardner (Eds.), *International occupational and environmental health medicine* (pp. 211-222). St. Louis, MO: Mosby.

Frazier, L. M., & Hage, M. L. (1998). *Reproductive hazards of the workplace.* New York: John Wiley & Sons.

Goodman, K. N. (1998). Ethical challenges. In J. A. Herzstein, N. B. Bunn III, L. E. Fleming, J. M. Harrington, J. Jeyaratnam, & I. R. Gardner (Eds.), *International Occupational and Environmental Medicine* (pp. 86-96). St. Louis, MO: Mosby.

International Commission on Occupational Health. (1997). *International code of ethics for occupational health professionals.* Geneva, Switzerland: Author.

International Labour Office. (2000). *Encyclopedia on occupational health and safety* (4th ed.). Geneva, Switzerland: Author.

International Society of Travel Medicine. (1999). *Introduction to travel medicine.* Atlanta, GA: Author.

LaDou, J. (2002). Occupational health in industrializing countries. *State of the Art Reviews in Occupational Medicine, 17,* 349-355.

Paul, M., & Frazier, L. (2000). Reproductive disorders. In B. Levy and D. Wegman (Eds.), *Occupational health.* Philadelphia: Lippincott Williams & Wilkins.

Rogers, B. (2000). International perspectives in occupational and environmental health nursing. *AAOHN Journal, 48,* 160.

Rogers, H. L., & Reilly, S. M. (2000). Health problems associated with international business travel. *AAOHN Journal, 48,* 376-384.

Rose, S. R. (2000). *International travel health guide.* Northhampton, MA: Travel Medicine.

Saphire, L. S., & Doran, B. (1996). International travel preparedness. *AAOHN Journal, 44,* 123-127.

Takala, J. (1999). International agency efforts to protect workers and the environment. *International Journal of Occupational and Environmental Health, 5*(1), 30-37.

Thompson, M. C., Holihan, E. H., & MacNeal, B. (1996). Health on the road: Developing a program for international travelers. *AAOHN Journal, 44,* 300-309.

World Health Organization. (1995). *Global strategy on occupational health for all.* Geneva, Switzerland: Author. http://www.who.int/oeh/OCHweb/OCHweb/OSHpages/GlobalStrategy/GlobalStrategy.htm

World Health Organization. (1999). *Fourth network meeting of the collaborating centers in occupational health* (document no. WHO/SDE/OEH/99.8). Geneva, Switzerland: Author.

19

Professionalism in Occupational and Environmental Health Nursing

CHAPTER

Occupational and environmental health nurses are the largest group of occupational health professionals. The traditional role of the occupational and environmental health nurse has expanded substantially in the last two decades beyond emergency care and surveillance, monitoring, and treatment of occupational illness and injury. This expanded role now includes prevention of occupational and nonoccupational illness and injury, health promotion, primary care, risk and case management, research, and administrative functioning. To support the role functions and advance the specialty of occupational and environmental health nursing, professional development, competency enhancement, and growth are essential. This chapter will focus on professional issues relevant to the practice and advancement of the occupational and environmental health nursing specialty. The growth and advancement of expertise in the specialty will be fostered through the monitoring and continued development of professional activities and behaviors that support the profession and the discipline (Chamberline & Lanhorn, 2001).

PROFESSIONAL ASSOCIATION

Professional associations or societies generally exist to improve and advance the profession through standard setting, educational programs, support of research initiatives, and promoting the public's understanding of the body of work in the field. The American Association of Occupational Health Nurses (AAOHN) is the professional association of nurses who practice occupational and environmental health nursing; AAOHN is engaged in the following:

- Promoting professional excellence and opportunities through education and research
- Establishing professional standards of practice and code of ethics
- Influencing legislative, regulatory, and policy issues
- Promoting internal and external communications
- Establishing strategic alliances and partnerships

With regard to the specialty of occupational and environmental health nursing, AAOHN has a responsibility to do the following:

- Define the scope of practice and set standards and competencies for practice;
- Develop standards of professional conduct as described in the AAOHN *Code of Ethics;*
- Promote and provide continuing education;
- Advance the profession by encouraging and supporting research in the discipline;
- Advocate for the practice in business, government, and other sectors;
- Provide up-to-date information through publications such as the *AAOHN Journal* and practice advisories;
- Develop tools and resources in occupational and environmental health that support the practice;
- Develop collaborative relationships and partnerships in the work of promoting and protecting the health of America's workforce.

The occupational and environmental health nurse must be cognizant of the role of the professional association in supporting the work of the nurse, the profession, and the discipline itself.

A variety of resources and guidance materials are available to all occupational and environmental health nurses. Some of these are briefly described in what follows and throughout the text. However, the occupational and environmental health nurse will benefit from supporting and being supported by the professional association.

COMPETENCY ENHANCEMENT IN OCCUPATIONAL AND ENVIRONMENTAL HEALTH NURSING

The professional nurse practices according to the legal scope of practice that is defined in licensure law in each state—generally titled the Nurse Practice Act—and is regulated in each state by an administrative agency, usually termed the Board of Nursing. After being licensed, nurses must maintain and further develop competency in practice. This is done in several ways. Professional societies set forth standards of practice or care that provide authoritative statements about practice responsibilities for which the nurse is accountable. *Standards of Occupational and Environmental Health Nursing* (AAOHN, 1999) provide guidance for professional practice, are criteria-based and measurable, serve as a means to ensure accountability to the public and the profession, and evolve over time to reflect the changing scope of practice and development of new knowledge (Chamberlin & Rogers, 1997). This means that the occupational and environmental health nurse must remain competent in the current and evolving scope of practice as reflected in the standards for practice and, guided by the AAOHN *Code of Ethics* (see Chapter 17), must use ethical judgment in decision making about practice issues.

The AAOHN has identified 11 professional practice standards (Box 19-1) that describe a competent level of performance with regard to the nursing process and professional roles of the occupational and environmental health nurse. The criteria that have been developed for each standard are key measurable indicators of competent practice that permit occupational and environmental health nurses to evaluate their practice relative to the standards. Every occupational and environmental health nurse should have a copy of and review the practice standards and criteria, and these should be utilized to guide and support the nurse's judgment in reaching expected outcomes related to interventions, pro-

grams, and services and to enhance professional development and performance.

The AAOHN has developed the *Core Curriculum in Occupational and Environmental Health Nursing* (AAOHN, 2001). The *Core Curriculum* delineates concepts and principles to support the knowledge base of the specialty practice. References and resources identified in the text assist in attaining and building progressive levels of competence. An underlying assumption is that occupational and environmental health nurses also have the responsibility to be informed about the latest technological developments that enhance service delivery and to develop effective communication skills (AAOHN, 2001). Occupational and environmental health nurses must understand trends and issues that affect practice, organizational dynamics, and, consequently the health and safety of workers. The *Core Curriculum* is designed as a comprehensive resource to assist occupational and environmental health nurses in the theoretical and practical application of this knowledge base and also can be used as a teaching tool.

AAOHN has developed *Competencies and Performance Criteria in Occupational and Environmental Health Nursing* (White et al., 1999), which includes nine competency categories delineated by three levels (competent, proficient, expert) and performance criteria for each stated competency. These competencies and levels are discussed in more detail in Chapter 3, and the competencies can be found in Appendix 3-1. The competencies will assist the nurse (White et al., 1999) by providing information on the following:

- Self-assessment tools
- Curricula for academic and professional education
- Curricula for independent learning
- Accreditation of education programs
- Certification processes
- Occupational and environmental health public policy

The competencies also may be a resource to aid in the following:

- Career planning
- Recruitment of professionals into the specialty
- Planning and evaluation of occupational and environmental health services
- Hiring and job performance evaluation

Box 19-1   **Standards of Occupational and Environmental Health Nursing Practice***

STANDARD I: ASSESSMENT

The occupational and environmental health nurse systematically assesses the health status of the individual client or population and environment.

STANDARD II: DIAGNOSIS

The occupational and environmental health nurse analyzes assessment data to formulate diagnoses.

STANDARD III: OUTCOME IDENTIFICATION

The occupational and environmental health nurse identifies outcomes specific to the client.

STANDARD IV: PLANNING

The occupational and environmental health nurse develops a goal-directed plan of care that is comprehensive and formulates interventions to attain expected outcomes.

STANDARD V: IMPLEMENTATION

The occupational and environmental health nurse implements interventions to attain desired outcomes identified in the plan.

STANDARD VI: EVALUATION

The occupational and environmental health nurse systematically and continuously evaluates responses to interventions and progress toward the achievement of desired outcomes.

STANDARD VII: RESOURCE MANAGEMENT

The occupational and environmental health nurse secures and manages the resources that support an occupational health and safety program.

STANDARD VIII: PROFESSIONAL DEVELOPMENT

The occupational and environmental health nurse assumes accountability for professional development to enhance profession growth and maintain competency.

STANDARD IX: COLLABORATION

The occupational and environmental health nurse collaborates with employees, management, other health care providers, professionals, and community representatives.

STANDARD X: RESEARCH

The occupational and environmental health nurse uses research findings in practice and contributes to the scientific base in occupational and environmental health nursing to improve practice and advance the profession.

STANDARD XI: ETHICS

The occupational and environmental health nurse uses an ethical framework as a guide for decision making in practice.

From *Standards of Occupational and Environmental Health Nursing,* by American Association of Occupational Health Nurses, 1999, Atlanta+, GA: Author.
*Performance measurement criteria can be found in the document, which can be obtained from AAOHN.

- Links with other domestic and international organizations

As an integrated framework, the standards of practice, core curriculum, competencies, and code of ethics provide the basis for scope of practice, knowledge, skill, and legal and ethical practice.

Certification is a process by which a nongovernmental agency or association validates, based on predetermined standards of nursing practice, registered nurse's qualifications, knowledge, and practice in a defined functional or clinical area of nursing (American Board for Occupational Health Nurses, Inc., 2002). The American Board for Occupational Health Nurses, Inc. (ABOHN) is the certification body for occu-

pational health nursing. ABOHN sets the criteria and standards for certification, uses the AAOHN definitions and standards for occupational and environmental health nursing as the practice parameter, and bases the examination content on the practice patterns and parameters for occupational health nursing (AAOHN, 2001). Currently, three certifications are available in occupational health nursing:

1. *COHN.* The Certified Occupational Health Nurse credential is offered to the registered nurse with an associate, diploma, or higher degree or the international equivalent. The focus of the credential is on the nurse's role as clinician, advisor, and coordinator.

2. *COHN-S.* The Certified Occupational Health Nurse Specialist credential is offered to the nurse with a baccalaureate or higher degree and focuses on the nurse's role as educator, manager, clinician, and consultant.
3. *COHN/Case Manager (CM)* or *COHN-S/CM.* The COHN or COHN-S certification is required as a prerequisite for this occupational health case manager credential. Therefore, the roles validated by those credentials form the basis of occupational health nursing case management.

The basic eligibility requirements to sit for the certification examination (in each area) are registered nurse licensure, current occupational health nursing employment and work experience, and a specified number of documented continuing educational contact hours related to occupational health. Depending on the certification desired, other requirements (e.g., a degree) may be needed (ABOHN, 2002). In addition, requirements may change depending on changes such as those to the standards or the scope of practice. ABOHN can provide an application and the most current certification requirements. For continuing competency, the primary responsibility to remain current with the evolving scope of practice and work responsibilities rests with the individual health care professional. The occupational and environmental health nurse has responsibility to do the following (Interprofessional Workgroup on Health Professions Regulation, 1997):

- Practice in accordance with the professional standards of practice;
- Understand their role in the context of the work setting;
- Take action in unsafe practice situations;
- Keep professional responsibility to the client(s) as the highest priority;
- Engage in self-assessment and reflection of competencies (White et al., 1999).

MENTORING

Mentoring is an important component of professional growth and development because it is a process that provides guidance and assistance in the development of skills and abilities. Mentoring differs from formal training because mentors,

through counseling, role modeling, and example setting, work directly with the protégé who learns and acquires needed skill assets (Randolph, 2001).

Role modeling and mentoring are important professional behaviors for occupational and environmental health nurses to develop. Mentoring offers many benefits (Short, 2002). The protégé will develop a network of colleagues and opportunities, which will enhance decision making skills. Protégés also develop increased self-confidence and independence through observing and trying out the practices of the mentor. However, it should be emphasized that the mentor must encourage the protégé to integrate her or his own personality and valued skills into practice. Mentoring also provides the protégé with an opportunity to observe and learn negotiating skills in dealing with management, organizations, and other disciplines and develop effective and positive power bases.

The mentor will benefit from the satisfaction of knowing that the success and careers of others have been promoted. Mentoring also provides the mentor with teaching opportunities and reciprocal learning. Finally, mentoring creates an important growth aspect for the mentor in terms of sharing knowledge, experiences, and ideas and helping to create career enhancement opportunities for others.

ADVANCING THE PROFESSION, PRACTICE, AND DISCIPLINE

As reflected in the *Standards of Occupational and Environmental Health Nursing* (AAOHN, 1999), the nurse is to be held accountable for engaging in professional development to enhance professional growth and competency and for contributions to advance scientific knowledge, which improves practice. This is accomplished through lifelong learning and scientific development of the knowledge base through research. The occupational and environmental health nurse determines lifelong learning needs, based on self-assessment, and initiates a plan to meet these needs through academic and continuing education and independent study (Chamberlin & Lawhorn, 2001). This may mean obtaining additional academic qualifications and certifications needed for job performance or for personal or professional achievement.

As described in Chapter 2, NIOSH-funded Occupational Safety and Health Education and Research Centers are the primary resource for education and training in occupational safety and health for such occupational safety and health practitioners as occupational and environmental health nurses, occupational physicians, industrial hygienists, and safety professionals. These centers provide academic, research, continuing education, and outreach programs. Occupational health nurses can obtain Master's degrees as specialists in the field and as nurse practitioners. Doctoral education may also be pursued to prepare occupational health nursing researchers (Institute of Medicine, 2001). A listing of the Occupational Safety and Health Education and Research Centers is found in Appendix 2-1 in Chapter 2.

Continuing education through attending conferences, workshops, and independent study is essential to both maintain and update knowledge and to acquire certification, recertification, and licensure. The nurse will need to acquire information relevant to the occupational safety and health sciences and related skill areas such as management, research, and leadership.

Advancing scientific knowledge is foundational to any practice discipline. For occupational and environmental health nurses to build a body of knowledge to improve the practice, they must participate in and conduct the research to support this effort. From a practice perspective this means the nurse should actively integrate research findings into practice and help identify researchable practice problems. After problems are identified, nurses skilled to do so conduct the research so answers can be derived and practice theories can be developed and applied. This will add new knowledge or theory to expand the specialty. Often research is conducted through the benefit of grant funding as written by the occupational and environmental health nurse principal investigator and other collaborators. Funding sources vary and include governmental sources and nongovernmental sources, such as the AAOHN Foundation, which funds several research grants, primarily based on AAOHN Research Priorities as identified in Chapter 16, in addition to academic and continuing education and leadership grants. The occupational and environmental health nurse professional disseminates information learned through scholarly publication and presentation at scientific forums so information can be shared with colleagues and practitioners of other disciplines. Theories and research recommendations can then be tested in the field to further develop and refine the body of knowledge in occupational and environmental health nursing.

LEADERSHIP

Professionalism includes providing leadership and acting in a leadership capacity. Leadership is provided in several ways, including but not limited to the following:

- Influencing and developing policy for occupational health and safety programs and initiatives in the work organization
- Influencing governmental legislation and regulation
- Influencing and empowering peers to become involved in occupational health and safety issues
- Participating in leadership activities in the work organization, with the public, and in professional societies
- Engaging in leadership election opportunities in professional societies, voluntary organizations, and government

Leadership also entails creating partnerships with other groups, organizations, and disciplines to advance policy directives in occupational safety and health that support a safe and healthy work environment and workforce. Collaboration must be sought out, nourished, and sustained.

Summary

Professionalism in occupational and environmental health nursing has several facets aimed at ensuring and promoting the professional development of the occupational and environmental health nurse and advancing the profession, the practice, and the science of the discipline. All professional occupational and environmental health nurses are obligated to remain competent in their practice, and many resources exist to support this behavior. Career and professional growth will be a successful outcome.

References

American Association of Occupational Health Nurses. (1999). *Standards of occupational and environmental health nursing.* Atlanta, GA: Author.

American Association of Occupational Health Nurses. (2001). *Core curriculum in occupational and environmental health nursing.* Philadelphia: W. B. Saunders.

American Board for Occupational Health Nurses, Inc. (2002). http://www.abohn.org.

Chamberlin, E., & Lawhorn, E. (2001). Professional issues: Advancing the specialty in the AAOHN.

Chamberlin, E., & Rogers, B. (1997). Credentialing study: An AAOHN report. *AAOHN Journal, 45,* 431-437.

Institute of Medicine. (2000). *Safe work in the 21st century.* Washington, DC: National Academy Press.

Interprofessional Workgroup on Health Professions Regulation. (1997). *Continued competency summit: Assessing the issues, methods, and realities for health care professionals conference.* Chicago: Author.

Randolph, S. F. (2001). Mentoring and training in public health. In L. Rowitz (Ed.), *Public health leadership.* Gaithersburg, MD: Aspen.

Short, J. (2002). Mentoring: Career enhancement for occupational and environmental health nurses. *AAOHN Journal, 50,* 135-141.

White, K., Cox, A., & Williamson, G. (1999). Competencies in occupational and environmental health nursing. *AAOHN Journal, 47,* 552-568.

20 Occupational and Environmental Health Nursing: Tomorrow's Challenges

Occupational and environmental health nursing has evolved and expanded significantly and dramatically into a highly specialized practice recognized globally as a profession and discipline with aims to protect and promote worker health and safety. As occupational and environmental health nurses face the twenty-first century, increased emphasis will be placed on issues related to the following:

- Health promotion and primary health care at the worksite directed at enhancing quality of life and healthy lifestyle changes, reducing preventable death and disability, and wisely containing health care costs
- Impact of work organization
- Ways of dealing with threats of violence, including terrorism at the workplace and in our communities
- Workforce diversity
- Genetics and workplace interaction
- Continued competency development

This chapter will discuss these trends and issues as they affect the work and health of society and nursing's role as providers of a comprehensive multidisciplinary approach in preparation for the future in occupational and environmental health and safety.

HEALTH, HEALTH PROMOTION, AND WORK-RELATED HEALTH CARE DELIVERY

A major issue of concern today in the corporate environment is the control of health care costs, primarily through health insurance coverage. While costly illnesses like heart disease and stroke are declining, they remain leading causes of death. Cancer rates continue to rise, and smoking rates, which have decreased in the nation as a whole, continue to rise among young women. Lung cancer exceeds breast cancer as the leading cause of death in women.

With the percentage of the elderly in the population increasing, illnesses such as hypertension, cancer, cirrhosis of the liver, and diabetes will be more prevalent. Infectious diseases also will affect the workplace not only in terms of worker quality of life and lost work time, but also regarding invasion of privacy, maintenance of confidentiality, potential exposure of the health care worker to viral and bacterial agents, and health care costs. New strategies will need to be developed to address early morbidity and premature mortality and the improvement of positive self-health practices.

Despite steadily decreasing during the last decade, the number of work-related fatalities remains consistently elevated. The risk of injury for younger workers is 5 times greater than for older workers, and this will increase with more younger workers in the workforce. Worldwide, tens of millions of accidents occur every year (an average of 160,000 per day) in industry alone, and each year industrial accidents and illnesses disable millions of workers for the rest of their lives. Traumatic injuries, such as those related to farming and forestry; injuries and illnesses caused by thousands of toxic chemicals, particularly new chemicals whose effects are not immediately obvious; and stress-related diseases remain important challenges in need of investigation.

Nearly 50% of U.S. workers are employed in offices, and this proportion will significantly increase. Musculoskeletal problems related to poorly designed work stations and stress related to human devaluation and increased productivity pressures will increase.

In recent years the delivery of health care has shifted from hospitals to clinics, homes, and the workplace, and this trend is expected to continue. It is evident that alternative health care and preventive programs such as aging programs; corporate health programs; prenatal, family, child and infant care programs at the workplace; and home visiting will become increasingly prevalent. While increased emphasis is placed on the delivery of these preventive and health promotion programs, health monitoring and surveillance will become more important, and physicians and other health care providers will want to be seen as health care managers, placing them in direct competition with the occupational and environmental health nurse.

Self-care or self-help, which often involves participation in health promotion programs, is the preferred choice of health intervention for many, and this particular approach to health care at the worksite is increasing. Some corporations view health promotion programs, such as smoking cessation and improved nutrition programs, as a method to improve their cost savings and increase worker productivity during the initiation and building of corporate wellness efforts. Many, however, still do not see the connection between health and productivity, and as a result, health promotion programs may be fragmented, disjointed, or nonexistent. Increased efforts must be aimed at focusing management and worker thinking to develop and participate in health promotion programs. Integration of health into all aspects of work life that meet individual worker needs based on a health profile will increase the overall quality of life.

Occupational and environmental health nurses will become more involved in environmental health while environmental agents alone, or in conjunction with lifestyle and genetic factors, increasingly cause adverse effects resulting in disease, dysfunction, disability, and death. Issues that need to be addressed include impaired reproductive and developmental health, such as occurs with lead exposure; air pollution and respiratory health; worker exposure to agricultural chemicals; the effects of chemical runoff into soil and drinking water; skin and other cancers associated with sun exposure; and waste management.

The National Institute of Environmental Health Sciences reports that a growing number of studies show that minorities and the poor are disproportionately affected by pollutants (National Institute of Environmental Health Sciences, 1992). By living in residences near industrial worksites or hazardous waste dumps, in smog-filled inner cities, or simply in older houses containing lead paint, some in these population groups face a higher risk just by staying home. In addition, minorities show greater incidences of specific diseases, such as asthma, and are more likely to experience higher chemical and repetitive motion exposures because of their high representations in certain occupations, such as meatpacking and farm work. The need for occupational and environmental health nurses to work in health care employee health centers will increase in order to focus more services on health care workers; these workers make up a special population at significant risk of various occupational health hazards, including ergonomic deficiencies, stress, chemical toxins, and infectious diseases related to contact with blood or body fluids. In addition, few comprehensive health promotion programs are offered in hospital-based settings (Rogers & Haynes, 1991).

New programs will need to be developed to maximize worker health and keep the employee at work. For example, one sixth of all workers are women in childbearing years. The establishment of prenatal programs can be viewed as providing cost saving and health promotion, and the occupational and environmental health nurse can serve as the catalyst to accomplish this goal. Data related to illness and pregnancy, neonatal illness, absenteeism, risk factors, and educational needs of mothers and fathers will need to be collected and analyzed by the occupational and environmental health nurse to determine the need for such programs as nutrition, stress management, and lifestyle risk factors. Programs can be offered on-site, or referrals will need to be made. The nurse will either need to retool to provide prenatal care or education or develop a listing of community resources necessary to meet the needs and the challenges.

Mastroianni (1992) describes the importance of child care arrangements in reducing stress, anxiety, and potential illness in working mothers. The occupational and environmental health nurse will be instrumental in developing postnatal services for mothers who return to work and who may need to find day care accommodations, resolve such conflicts as separation and breast-feeding, and arrange for infant health care, which necessitates off-work time. If on-site day care is not feasible, establishment of a resource book for area day care facilities would be extremely helpful. Other helpful areas include establishing parental support groups, parenting programs, and options for maintaining breastfeeding needs and providing childhood immunizations.

Primary care delivery and health promotion activities will be increased at the worksite not only for workers but for their families. Many health care services provided by nurses and nurse practitioners, such as screening services, monitoring chronic conditions, and worker health assessments, have been demonstrated to be effective, efficient, and of good quality.

The occupational and environmental health nurse will assume increased responsibility for case management services to help determine safe and effective levels of worker physical and mental capacity necessary to perform the job. For example, as case manager the nurse will help coordinate extended health care services to employees with complex illnesses or injuries and work with community agencies to find the most appropriate and cost-effective services (McCloskey et al., 1987). The occupational and environmental health nurse will play a more prominent role in education and training not only for the worker but for management. This will entail developing both general and specific programs to increase awareness, knowledge, and understanding of risk factors and interactive effects associated with health, illness, and injury. Coupled with this, the nurse will be responsible for data analysis regarding the incidence/prevalence of injury and illness, epidemiological trends and patterns, and work practices related to the injury/illness events.

As discussed in Chapter 1, health care costs continue to rise. The occupational and environmental health nurse as the health care manager will be in a position to provide for quality cost-effective care through overseeing high cost cases

and getting ill or injured employees who have been hospitalized back home and to work in safe jobs. Within the realm of cost savings, the occupational health manager will need to target workers who are vulnerable to specific risks and recommend specific actions to reduce risks, including job reassignment and new or redesigned tools and work stations. Collaborative efforts will be required to achieve this purpose. The nurse will need to be able to communicate effectively and know what types of resources are readily available to provide for multidisciplinary collaboration. This includes the ability to demonstrate both efficient and effective employee health services through measuring outcomes of interventions. Quality improvement and quality assurance mechanisms, such as satisfaction surveys, audit tools, and peer reviews, will need to be implemented as a measure of accountability for cost-effective services. This may need to be company-specific, depending on the makeup of the workforce and concomitant health needs.

ORGANIZATION OF WORK

According to USDHHS/NIOSH (2002), in advanced industrialized countries such as the United States the organization of work has been subjected to sweeping changes that have been influenced by major forces that encompass, among others, the economic, technological, legal, and political realms. Manufacturing jobs continue to decline, giving way to work in service and information technology. Product and service demands are shifting rapidly amid pressure for higher quality and customized products. In many countries, these trends are occurring against the backdrop of an aging and increasingly diverse workforce and tightening labor markets.

Organizational practices have changed dramatically in this new economy. To compete more effectively, many large companies have restructured themselves by downsizing their workforces and outsourcing the affected functions. At the same time, nontraditional employment practices that depend on temporary workers and contract labor have grown steadily.

For many workers these trends have resulted in a variety of potentially stressful or hazardous circumstances, such as reduced job stability and increased workload. Data suggest, for example, that the average work year for prime age working couples has increased by nearly 700 hours in the last two decades (Bluestone & Rose, 1998; USDOL, 1999) and that high levels of emotional exhaustion at the end of the workday are the norm for 25% to 30% of the workforce (Bond et al., 1997). However, increased flexibility, responsibility, and learning opportunity in today's workplace may offer workers greater potential for self-direction, skill development, and career growth and lead to reduced stress and increased satisfaction and well-being. In reality, these revolutionary changes in the organization of work have far outpaced our understanding of their implications for work life quality and safety and health on the job.

Although the terms *work organization* or *organization of work* are increasingly used in discussions of worker safety and health, these terms have not been formally defined, and literature on this topic is still meager in the occupational safety and health field. As described by USDHHS/NIOSH (2002), organization of work refers to the work process (the way jobs are designed and performed) and to the organizational practices (management and production methods and accompanying human resources policies) that influence job design. Also included in this concept of organization of work are external factors, such as the legal and economic environment and technological factors that encourage or enable new organizational practices.

Box 20-1 depicts the multilevel concept of organization of work. How these factors work together will result in a positive or negative effect. For example, expanded employee training (a human resources function) is integral to the success of flexible production processes (an aspect of the work process). As an another example, studies of interplay between labor market and work process factors imply that increasing job demands or longer work hours may pose disproportionate risk for women because they bear a greater total workload than do men (Heyman, 2000; United Nations Development Programme, 1995).

Long work hours and staff reductions may increase the risk of overexertion injury. Increased public contact and alternative work schedules (e.g., night work), which are common in the growing service sector, may expose workers to heightened risk of violence in their jobs.

Box 20-1   Organization of Work

EXTERNAL CONTEXT

Economic, Legal, Political, Technological, and Demographic Forces at the National/International Level

- Economic developments (e.g., globalization of economy)
- Regulatory, trade, and economic policies (e.g., deregulation)
- Technological innovations (e.g., information/computer technology)
- Changing worker demographics and labor supply (e.g., aging population)

ORGANIZATIONAL CONTEXT

Management Structures, Supervisory Practices, Production Methods, and Human Resources Policies

- Organization restructuring (e.g., downsizing)
- New quality and process management initiatives (e.g., high performance work systems)

ORGANIZATIONAL CONTEXT — cont'd

- Alternative employment arrangements (e.g., contingent labor)
- Work/life/family programs and flexible work arrangements (e.g., telecommuting)
- Changes in benefits and compensation systems (e.g., gainsharing)

WORK CONTEXT

Job Characteristics

- Climate and culture
- Task attributes (e.g., temporal aspects, complexity, autonomy, physical and psychological demands)
- Social-relational aspects of work
- Worker roles
- Career development

From The *Changing Organization of Work and the Safety and Health of Working People* (NIOSH, Publication No. 2002-116), by Department of Health and Human Services, National Institute for Occupational Safety, and Health, 2002, Cincinnati, OH: Author.

In addition, worker safety and health might be threatened by more indirect effects of changing organizational practices. For example, worker access to occupational health services and programs might be adversely affected by organizational downsizing or by the growth of defined contribution or voucher-style health benefit programs. These multiple influences of organization of work on occupational safety and health are illustrated in Figure 20-1.

The limited understanding of risks posed by today's turbulent work environment illustrates the need for more information on the topic. In particular, nursing professionals need to better understand how emerging trends in organizational practices influence job demands, employee development, hazard exposures, health services, worker behaviors, balance between work and family, and other conditions that may influence risk of stress, illness, and injury in the workforce. Of primary significance is the need to examine positive and negative effects of changing organizational practices. Additional outcomes such as disability, utilization of health care and employee assistance programs, socioeconomic costs, and conflicts between work and family should be examined in order to portray more fully the difficulties of illness and injury associated with organizational stressors (Berg, 1999; Jackson and Martin, 1996; Jackson and Mullarky, 2000; Kaminski, 2001; Landsbergis et al., 1999; Smith, 1997; Sprigg et al., 2000).

WORKPLACE VIOLENCE

Workplace violence has emerged as an important safety and health issue in today's workplace. This includes violence perpetrated in the general workplace as well as terrorist attacks. Its most extreme form, the terrorist attacks of September 11, 2001, have demonstrated the need to be vigilant and well-prepared for these threats. This will be discussed later. Homicide is the second leading cause of fatal occupational injury in the United States. Nearly 1,000 workers are murdered and 1.5 million are assaulted in the workplace each year. According to the BLS *National Census of Fatal Occupational Injuries* (CFOI) (1999), there were 709 workplace homicides in 1998, accounting for 12% of the total 6,026 fatal work injuries in the United States. Each week, an average of 20 workers are murdered and 18,000 are assaulted while at work or on duty. Nonfatal assaults result in millions of lost workdays and cost workers millions of dollars in lost wages. Environmental conditions associated with workplace assaults have been identified and, environmental control strategies have been implemented in a number of work settings.

Workplace violence is clustered in certain occupational settings. For example, the retail trade and service industries account for more than half of workplace homicides and 85% of nonfatal workplace assaults. Taxicab drivers have the highest

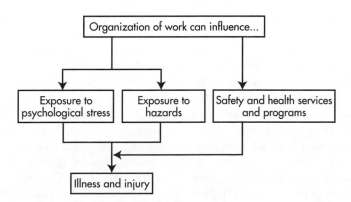

Figure 20-1   Pathways between organization of work and illness and injury. *(Modified from* The Changing Organization of Work and the Safety and Health of Working People *(NIOSH Publication No. 2002-116), by Department of Health and Human Services, National Institute for Occupational Safety and Health, Cincinnati, OH: National Institute for Occupational Safety and Health.)*

TABLE 20-1 Average Annual Number, Rate, and Percent of Workplace Victimization by Type of Crime, 1993-1999

CRIME	AVERAGE NUMBER OF VICTIMIZATIONS	RATE PER 1,000 WORKERS	PERCENT OF TOTAL
All violent crime	1,744,300	12.51	100%
Homicide	900	0.01	0.1
Rape/Sexual assault	36,500	0.30	2.1
Robbery	70,100	0.50	4.0
Aggravated assault	325,000	2.30	18.6
Simple assault	1,311,700	9.40	75.2

Homicide data from "National Census of Occupational Injuries, 1993," by Bureau of Labor Statistics, *BLS News* (USDL-94-384), Washington, DC: U.S. Department of Labor, Bureau of Labor Statistics. 1994; rape and sexual assault, robbery, aggravated assault, and simple assault data from *National Crime Victimization Survey: Violence in the Workplace, 1993-1999,* by U.S. Department of Justice, Washington, DC: Author. 2001.

risk of workplace homicides of any occupational group. Workers in health care, community services, and retail settings are at increased risk of nonfatal assaults (USDHHS/NIOSH, 1996).

Rape and sexual assault, robbery, and homicide accounted for a small percentage (6%) of all workplace violence crime occurring between 1993 and 1999 (Table 20-1). The majority of workplace violence incidents, almost 19 of every 20, were aggravated or simple assaults. Aggravated assault is a completed or attempted attack with a weapon, whether or not an injury occurred, or an attack without a weapon in which the victim is seriously injured. Simple assault is an attack without a weapon resulting in either no injury, minor injury (such as bruises, black eyes, cuts, scratches, or swelling), or an undetermined injury requiring less than 2 days of hospitalization. Simple assaults also include attempted assaults without a weapon (U.S. Department of Justice, 2001). Violent crime was experienced by persons at work or on duty at a rate of 13 per 1,000 people in the workforce. The simple assault rate (9 per 1,000 people in the workforce) was more than 3 times the rate of all other categories of violent workplace crime. Homicides were less than 1% of all workplace violence crimes.

People employed in law enforcement were victimized while at work or on duty at the highest rate of all occupations examined, followed by people working in the mental health field. Retail sales workers were victimized in the workplace at a somewhat higher rate (20 per 1,000 in the

workforce) than those employed in the teaching, transportation, or medical fields (Table 20-2).

The workplace violence victimization rate for nurses was not significantly different from that for physicians; however, nurses experienced workplace crime at a rate 72% higher than medical technicians (22 incidents versus 13 incidents per 1,000 workers) and at more than twice the rate of other medical field workers (22 versus 9 per 1,000). Professional (social worker/psychiatrist) and custodial care providers in the mental health care field were victimized at similar rates while at work or on duty (68 and 69 per 1,000, respectively), but at rates more than 3 times those in the medical field.

Almost 4 of every 10 robberies occurring while the victim was at work or on duty were committed against people in the retail sales or transportation field. Transportation workers were robbed at a higher rate than any other occupational field reported (3 per 1,000 in the workplace) (USDHHS/NIOSH, 1996).

The spectrum of workplace violence ranges from offensive language to homicide; however, NIOSH offers the following reasonable working definition of workplace violence: violent acts, including physical assaults and threats of assault, directed toward people at work or on duty (USDHHS/NIOSH, 1996).

The circumstances of workplace violence also vary and may include robbery-associated violence; violence by disgruntled clients, customers, patients, and inmates; violence by coworkers, employees, or employers; and domestic violence

| TABLE 20-2 | Average Annual Rate of Violent Victimization in the Workplace, by Occupation of the Victim, 1993-1999 |

OCCUPATION	AVERAGE NUMBER OF VICTIMIZATIONS	RATE PER 1,000 WORKERS	PERCENT OF TOTAL
TOTAL	12,328,000	12.6	100
Medical			
Physician	71,300	16.2	0.6
Nurse	429,100	21.9	3.5
Technician	97,600	12.7	0.8
Other	315,000	8.5	2.6
Mental Health			
Professional	290,900	68.2	2.4
Custodial	60,400	69.0	0.5
Other	186,700	40.7	1.5
Teaching			
Preschool	32,900	7.1	0.3
Elementary	262,700	16.8	2.1
Junior high	321,300	54.2	2.6
High school	314,500	38.1	2.6
College/university	41,600	1.6	0.3
Technical/industrial	7,400	12.2	0.1
Special education	102,000	68.4	0.8
Other	169,800	16.7	1.4
Law Enforcement			
Police	1,380,400	260.8	11.2
Corrections	277,100	155.7	2.3
Private security	369,300	86.6	3.0
Other	359,800	48.3	2.9
Retail Sales			
Convenience store	336,800	53.9	2.7
Gas station	86,900	68.3	0.7
Bartender	170,600	81.6	1.4
Other	1,383,100	15.3	11.2
Transportation			
Bus driver	105,800	38.2	0.9
Taxi cab driver	84,400	128.3	0.7
Other	350,500	11.7	2.8
Other	4,720,100	7.0	38.3

Note: Rates are calculated using population estimates from the National Crime Victimization Survey (NCVS) for occupations, 1993 to 1999. The total number of victimizations in this table and all other tables with detail for occupation differs from the total in tables without occupational detail because of the way teacher victimization was computed. Details may not add to total because of rounding.

that finds its way into the workplace. These circumstances all appear to be related to the level of violence in communities and in society in general. However, the following reasons exist for focusing specifically on workplace violence:

- Violence is a substantial contributor to death and injury on the job. NIOSH data indicate that homicide has become the second leading cause of occupational injury death, exceeded only by motor vehicle-related deaths (Jenkins, 1996). Estimates of nonfatal workplace assaults vary dramatically, but a reasonable estimate from the National Crime Victimization Survey (NCVS), (USDOJ, 2001) is that approximately 1 million people are assaulted while at work or on duty each year; this figure represents 15% of the acts of violence experienced by U.S. residents age 12 or older (Bachman, 1994).
- The circumstances of workplace violence differ significantly from those of all homicides (FBI, 1994). For example, 75% of all workplace homicides in 1993 were robbery-related; but in the general population, only 9% of homicides were robbery-related, and only 19% were committed in conjunction with any kind of felony (e.g., robbery, rape, arson). Furthermore, 47% of all murder victims in 1993 were related to or acquainted with their assailants, whereas the majority of workplace homicides (because they are robbery-related) are believed to occur between people who do not know one another. Only 17% of female victims of workplace homicides were killed by a spouse or former spouse (Windau and Toscano, 1994), whereas 29% of the female homicide victims in the general population were killed by a husband, ex-husband, boyfriend, or ex-boyfriend.
- Workplace violence is not distributed randomly across all workplaces but is clustered in particular occupational settings. More than half (56%) of workplace homicides occurred in retail trade and service industries. Homicide is the leading cause of death in these industries, as well as in finance, insurance, and real estate. Eighty-five percent of nonfatal assaults in the workplace occur in service and retail trade industries (BLS, 1994). As the U.S. economy continues to shift toward the service sectors, fatal and nonfatal workplace violence will be an increasingly important occupational safety and health issue.

- The risk of workplace violence is associated with specific workplace factors such as dealing with the public, exchanging money, and delivering services or goods. Consequently, great potential exists for workplace-specific prevention efforts such as bullet-resistant barriers and enclosures in taxicabs, convenience stores, gas stations, emergency departments, and other areas where workers come in direct contact with the public; locked drop safes and other cash-handling procedures in retail establishments; and threat assessment policies in all types of workplaces.

RISK FACTORS

A number of factors, including the following, may increase a worker's risk for workplace assault:

- Working with the public
- Exchanging money
- Delivering passengers, goods, or services
- Having a mobile workplace, such as a taxicab or police cruiser
- Working with unstable or volatile people in health care, social service, or criminal justice settings
- Working alone or in small numbers
- Working late at night or during early morning hours
- Working in high crime areas
- Guarding valuable property or possessions
- Working in community-based settings

PREVENTION STRATEGIES

Prevention strategies include environmental and administrative controls and behavioral strategies.

Environmental Controls

Commonly implemented cash-handling policies in retail settings include procedures such as using locked drop safes, carrying small amounts of cash, and posting signs and printing notices that limited cash is available. Cashless transactions in taxicabs and retail settings are also useful approaches that could be used in any setting where cash is currently exchanged between workers and customers. Other strategies include the following:

- The physical separation of workers from customers, clients, and the general public can be accomplished through the use of bullet-resistant barriers or enclosures for retail settings such as gas stations and convenience stores, hospital emergency departments, and social service agency claims areas.

- Making high risk areas visible to more people and installing good external lighting should decrease the risk of workplace assaults.
- Securing the number of entrances and exits through which nonemployees can gain access to work areas because doors are unlocked, as well as the number of areas where potential attackers can hide, also should decrease the risk of workplace violence.
- Use of numerous security devices may reduce the risk for assaults against workers. These security devices include closed-circuit cameras, alarms, two-way mirrors, card-key access systems, panic-bar doors locked from the outside only, and trouble lights or geographic locating devices in taxicabs and other mobile workplaces.
- Personal protective equipment such as body armor has been used effectively by public safety personnel to mitigate the effects of workplace violence. For example, the lives of more than 1,800 police officers have been saved by Kevlar vests (USDHHS/NIOSH, 1996).

Administrative Controls

Administrative controls include staffing plans and safe work practices, such as escorting patients and prohibiting unsupervised movement within and between clinic areas. Increasing the number of staff on duty, including security guards, may also be appropriate in any number of service and retail settings.

Policies and procedures for assessing and reporting threats allow employers to track and assess threats and violent incidents in the workplace. Such policies clearly indicate a zero tolerance of workplace violence and provide mechanisms by which incidents can be reported and handled. In addition, such information allows employers to assess whether prevention strategies are appropriate and effective. These policies should also include guidance on recognizing the potential for violence, methods for defusing or deescalating potentially violent situations, and instruction about the use of security devices and protective equipment. Procedures for obtaining medical care and psychological support following violent incidents also should be addressed. Training and education efforts are clearly needed to accompany such policies.

Behavioral Strategies

Training employees in nonviolent response and conflict resolution has been suggested to reduce the risk of volatile situations escalating to physical violence. Also critical is training that addresses hazards associated with specific tasks or worksites and relevant prevention strategies. Training should not be regarded as the sole prevention strategy but as a component in a comprehensive approach to reducing workplace violence. To increase vigilance and compliance with stated violence prevention policies, training should emphasize the appropriate use and maintenance of protective equipment, adherence to administrative controls, and increased knowledge and awareness of the risk of workplace violence (USDHHS, NIOSH, 1996).

Workplace Violence Prevention Programs

Developing and implementing a workplace violence prevention program and policy is vital. This includes establishing a system for documenting violent incidents in the workplace. Such data are essential for assessing the nature and magnitude of workplace violence in a given workplace and quantifying risk.

A written workplace violence policy should clearly indicate a zero tolerance of violence at work, whether the violence originates inside or outside the workplace. Just as workplaces have developed mechanisms for reporting and dealing with sexual harassment, they also must develop threat assessment teams to which threats and violent incidents can be reported. These teams should include representatives from human resources, security, employee assistance, unions, workers, management, and perhaps legal and public relations departments. The charge to this team is to assess threats of violence (e.g., to determine how specific a threat is and whether the person threatening the worker has the means for carrying out the threat) and determine what steps are necessary to prevent the threat from being carried out. This team should also be charged with periodic reviews of violent incidents to identify ways in which similar incidents can be prevented in the future. The violence prevention policy should explicitly state the consequences of making threats or committing acts of violence in the workplace.

A comprehensive workplace violence prevention policy and program also should include

TABLE 20-3 Number of Deaths* at World Trade Center, by Racial/Ethnic Group, Education, and Sex† — New York City, September 11, 2001

RACIAL/ETHNIC GROUP/ EDUCATION	SEX		
	MALE	FEMALE	TOTAL
HISPANIC			
Less than high school	9	2	11
High school	68	19	87
Some college	30	26	56
College or more	69	34	103
Unknown	1	—	1
Total	**177**	**81**	**258**
WHITE, NON-HISPANIC			
Less than high school	5	1	6
High school	246	100	346
Some college	199	36	235
College or more	1,195	267	1,462
Unknown	14	3	17
Total	**1,659**	**407**	**2,066**
BLACK, NON-HISPANIC			
Less than high school	3	—	3
High school	44	24	68
Some college	21	8	29
College or more	65	44	109
Unknown	3	3	6
Total	**136**	**79**	**215**

From "Deaths in World Trade Center Terrorist Attacks—New York City, 2001," by Centers for Disease Control and Prevention, *MMWR 51* (special issue), 15. 2002.
*Includes three deaths outside New York City.
†Preliminary data as of August 16, 2002.

procedures and responsibilities to be taken in the event of a violent incident in the workplace. This policy should explicitly state how the response team is to be assembled and who is responsible for the immediate care of the victim(s), the reestablishment of work areas and processes, and the organization and carrying out of stress debriefing sessions with victims, their coworkers, and perhaps the families of victims and coworkers. Employee assistance programs, human resources professionals, and local mental health and emergency service personnel can offer assistance in developing these strategies. For a situation that poses an immediate threat of workplace violence, all legal, human resources, employee assistance, community mental health, and law enforcement resources should be used to develop a response.

Much discussion has also centered on the role of stress in workplace violence. The most important thing to remember is that stress can be both a cause and an effect of workplace violence. That is, high levels of stress may lead to violence in the workplace, but a violent incident in the workplace will most certainly lead to stress, perhaps even to posttraumatic stress disorder. Referrals to employee assistance programs or other local mental health services may be appropriate for stress debriefing sessions after critical incidents.

TERRORISM

Everyone in the United States experienced profound changes in their lives, whether personal or professional, as a result of terrorist assaults on the nation and its citizens on September 11, 2001.

TABLE 20-3

Number of Deaths* at World Trade Center, by Racial/Ethnic Group, Education, and Sex†—New York City, September 11, 2001—cont'd

RACIAL/ETHNIC GROUP/ EDUCATION	SEX		
	MALE	FEMALE	TOTAL
ASIAN/PACIFIC ISLANDER			
Less than high school	—	—	—
High school	8	2	10
Some college	4	3	7
College or more	109	47	156
Unknown	1	2	3
Total	122	54	176
OTHER AND UNKNOWN			
Less than high school	—	—	—
High school	1	1	2
Some college	1	1	2
College or more	7	—	7
Unknown	—	—	—
Total	9	2	11
ALL RACIAL/ETHNIC GROUPS			
Less than high school	**17**	**3**	**20**
High school	**367**	**146**	**513**
Some college	**255**	**74**	**329**
College or more	**1,445**	**392**	**1,837**
Unknown	**19**	**8**	**27**
Total	**2,103**	**623**	**2,726**

Nearly 3,000 workers were killed in the course of their work as a result of these attacks (Table 20-3), and thousands more were injured physically, psychologically, and emotionally. As reported by the CDC (2002), the collapse of the World Trade Center (WTC) towers and several adjacent structures resulted in a vast, physically dangerous disaster zone. The height of the WTC towers produced extraordinary forces during their collapse, pulverizing considerable portions of the buildings' structural components and exposing first responders and civilians to substantial amounts of airborne particulate matter. Fires burned continuously under the debris until mid-December 2001. Because of ongoing fire activity and the large numbers of civilians and rescue workers who were killed during the attacks, approximately 11,000 New York City Fire Department (FDNY) firefighters and many emergency medical service (EMS) personnel worked on or directly adjacent to the rubble and incurred

substantial exposures (CDC, 2002). During the collapse 343 FDNY rescue workers died and, during the next 24 hours an additional 240 FDNY rescue workers sought emergency medical treatment (Table 20-4). Shortly thereafter, deaths due to anthrax exposure followed. Whether the terrorist threat is biological, chemical, or nuclear, immediate and long-term implications for occupational and environmental health must be addressed.

The Federal Bureau of Investigation (FBI) defines terrorism as "the unlawful use of force against persons or property to intimidate or coerce a government, the civilian population, or any segment thereof, in the furtherance of political or social objectives" (Code of Federal Regulations, 2001). This definition includes three elements:

1. Terrorist activities are illegal and involve the use of force.
2. The actions intend to intimidate or coerce.

TABLE 20-4 Number and Percentage of New York City Fire Department Rescue Workers Who Sought Emergency Medical Care During the 24 Hours After the Collapse of the World Trade Center Towers—New York City, September 11, 2001

DIAGNOSTIC CATEGORY	NUMBER	PERCENT*
RESPIRATORY		
Respiratory tract irritation	50	20.8
Chest pain without myocardial infarction or ischemia	8	3.3
Pneumothorax without rib fracture	I	0.4
Inhalation injury requiring emergent tracheostomy, pneumothorax, and prolonged mechanical ventilation for adult respiratory distress syndrome	I	0.4
Respiratory arrest with bronchospasm	I	0.4
Asthma exacerbation	I	0.4
TRAUMA		
Soft Tissue Trauma		
Concussions	8	3.3
Contusions	19	7.9
Puncture wounds	2	0.8
Lacerations	2	0.8
Back pain	10	4.2
Extremity strains and sprains	29	12.1
Meniscus tears	2	0.8
Fractures		
Upper extremity fractures	5	2.1
Lower extremity fractures	7	2.9
Pelvic fractures	I	0.4
Rib fractures without pneumothorax	I	0.4
Rib fractures with pneumothorax	2	0.8
Cervical spine fracture	I	0.4

From Injuries and Illnesses Among New York City Fire Department Rescue Workers After Responding to the World Trade Center Attacks, by Centers for Disease Control and Prevention, *MMWR, 51* (special issue), 4. 2002.
*Because each worker could have had more than one diagnosis, total percentage across all diagnostic categories could exceed 100%.

3. The actions are committed in support of political or social objectives.

Cangemi (2002) points out that it makes no difference to an occupational and environmental health nurse whether or not the incident is a terrorist act. If the act occurs at a workplace, the nurse may be among the first to arrive at the scene. However, the size and kind of terrorist action are key factors. It is important to note that an act of terrorism is essentially different from typical emergencies. Terrorist acts are geared to harm humans and destroy property. Occupational and environmental health nurses will have to address a new set of circumstances far different from the usual occupational emergencies for which companies have previously prepared. These emergencies can involve mass destruction of company property, widespread injury and death, unsafe conditions for caregivers, and the emotional stress brought forth by the intentional devastation (Cangemi, 2002, p. 190).

TABLE 20-4	Number and Percentage of New York City Fire Department Rescue Workers Who Sought Emergency Medical Care During the 24 Hours After the Collapse of the World Trade Center Towers—New York City, September 11, 2001—cont'd		
DIAGNOSTIC CATEGORY		**NUMBER**	**PERCENT***
TRAUMA—cont'd			
Burns			
Minor facial burns		3	1.2
OPHTHALMIC			
Eye irritation		25	10.4
SYSTEMIC			
Dehydration		5	2.1
Exposure†		70	29.2
PSYCHOLOGICAL			
Acute stress reaction		8	3.3
TOTAL		**240**	

†During the 24 hours following the collapse of the World Trade Center towers, documentation of this category was limited. Rescue workers sought medical care in emergency departments and were released without hospital admission after treatment for any combination of mild exhaustion, dehydration, and eye and/or respiratory tract irritations.

Occupational and environmental health nurses will need to become aware of the biological, chemical, nuclear, and incendiary devices that pose threats. Biological agents are typically odorless and colorless, so they are difficult to detect. The nurse will need to become familiar with signs and symptoms indicative of exposure, whether they be rapid or delayed effects. The CDC identifies biological agents of disease (Box 20-2), which are categorized into priority levels of A, B, and C.

Category A Diseases/Agents

The U.S. public health system and primary health care providers must be prepared to address various biological agents, including pathogens that are rarely seen in the United States. High priority agents include organisms that pose a risk to national security for the following reasons:

- The agents can be easily disseminated or transmitted from person to person;

- Exposure to the agents can result in high mortality rates and have the potential for major public health impact;
- The effects of the agents might cause public panic and social disruption;
- The agents and their effects require special action for public health preparedness.

Category B Diseases/Agents

Second highest priority agents include those that have the following qualities:

- Are moderately easy to disseminate
- Result in moderate morbidity rates and low mortality rates
- Require specific enhancements of the CDC's diagnostic capacity and enhanced disease surveillance

Category C Diseases/Agents

Third highest priority agents include emerging pathogens that could be engineered for mass dissemination in the future because of the following:

Box 20-2   Biological Diseases/Agents List

CATEGORY A

Anthrax *(Bacillus anthracis)*
Botulism *(Clostridium botulinum)*
Plague *(Yersinia pestis)*
Smallpox *(Variola major)*
Tularemia *(Francisella tularensis)*
Viral hemorrhagic fevers (filoviruses [e.g., Ebola, Marburg] and arenaviruses [e.g., Lassa, Machupo])

CATEGORY B

Brucellosis *(Brucella* species)
Epsilon toxin of *Clostridium perfringens*
Food safety threats (e.g., Salmonella species, *Escherichia coli* O157:H7, Shigella)
Glanders *(Burkholderia mallei)*
Melioidosis *(Burkholderia pseudomallei)*

CATEGORY B—cont'd

Psittacosis *(Chlamydia psittaci)*
Q fever *(Coxiella burnetii)*
Ricin toxin from *Ricinus communis* (castor beans)
Staphylococcal enterotoxin B
Typhus fever *(Rickettsia prowazekii)*
Viral encephalitis (alphaviruses [e.g., Venezuelan equine encephalitis, eastern equine encephalitis, western equine encephalitis])
Water safety threats (e.g., *Vibrio cholerae, Cryptosporidium parvum*)

CATEGORY C

Emerging infectious disease threats such as Nipah virus and hantavirus

From *Public Health Emergency Preparedness and Response,* by Centers for Disease Control and Prevention, 2002, http://www.bt.cdc.gov/Agent/agentlist.asp

---

- Availability
- Ease of production and dissemination
- Potential for high morbidity and mortality rates and major health impact

Occupational and environmental health nurses also will need to be prepared to suspect other types of threats as well, such as chemical nerve agent exposure. Because nerve agents are lethal, mass fatalities without other signs of trauma are common. Other outward signs of nerve agent release include the following (Khan, 2000):

- Hazardous materials or laboratory equipment that is not relevant to the occupancy
- Exposed individuals reporting unusual odors or tastes
- Explosions seeming only to destroy a package or bomb device
- Unscheduled dissemination of an unusual spray
- Abandoned spray devices
- Numerous dead animals, fish, or birds
- Absence of insect life in a warm climate
- Mass casualties without obvious trauma
- Distinct pattern of casualties and common symptoms
- Civilian panic in potential target areas (e.g., government buildings, public assemblies, subway systems) (Cangemi, 2002).

The purpose of a nuclear attack where nuclear materials are incorporated into a conventional explosive (e.g., radiological dispersal devices [RDDs]) is to spread radioactive materials around the bombsite. This would disrupt normal, day-to-day activities and raise the level of concern among occupational health professionals related to long-term health issues. It could be difficult to perform complete environmental decontamination (Cangemi, 2002).

Another possible scenario involving nuclear materials is detonation of a large device, such as a truck bomb (a large vehicle with high quantities of explosives) in the vicinity of a nuclear power plant or a radiological cargo transport. Such an attack could have widespread effects. All nuclear power plants have programs to protect against the potential threat that plant personnel may face, or that may aid, terrorists. New employees and contractor employees must pass stringent background checks related to employment, education, and criminal histories, as well as drug and alcohol screening tests and psychological evaluations. Anyone appearing to be under the influence of drugs or alcohol, or exhibiting erratic behavior, is immediately removed from the work area for evaluation (Cangemi, 2002). Again, the occupational and environmental health nurse will need to be familiar with the potential of nuclear threats and response approaches needed.

DIVERSITY

The U.S. population is becoming increasingly diverse. This diversity is reflected in workplaces throughout the country, and occupational and environmental health nurses will find they need to develop skills in assessing and managing the needs of multiple cultures. Culturally based norms, beliefs, and behaviors affect work practices and health-related values (Lusk & Holst, 2001). Occupational and environmental health nurses will need to have greater knowledge about and utilize transcultural approaches to health care. This includes demonstrating knowledge and understanding of the worker's culture, respecting cultural differences, and adapting care to meet the health care needs within the context of safe and quality health care delivery.

The nurse will need to recognize that in some cultures different treatment modalities such as herbal medicines may be the norm. However, it is still important to always emphasize health promotion and prevention of illnesses and injuries and incorporate ways to get this message across. In so doing, it is vital to involve diverse workers in health and safety discussions and decisions (Goode, 2000; Kerr et al., 2001) so health concepts can be shared and integrated appropriately.

Literacy is important in communicating in general, and it is important when interacting with the health professions community because low literacy is a risk factor for increased morbidity and mortality; those with low literacy have significant problems in accessing the health care system, understanding recommended treatments and appointment information, and comprehending medicine labels, consent forms, prescriptions, and health education materials (Baker et al., 1997; Baker et al., 1996; Perikh et al., 1996).

The magnitude of the literacy problem in the United States is significant. Results of a 1993 National Adult Literacy Survey indicated approximately 90 million individuals, about 47% of the U.S. adult population, were considered to have low or limited literacy skills. Approximately 25% of the 40 to 44 million adults who performed at the lowest level of literacy in the survey were immigrants from non-English language backgrounds (Kirch et al., 1993). Illiteracy and limited English skills affect health and safety training pro-grams. About 20% of the nation's work force is functionally illiterate and cannot read posted Occupational Safety and Health Administration instructions (Hays, 1999). Workplace illiteracy costs more than $60 billion annually as a result of lower productivity (Sunoo, 1999). Illiteracy also threatens healthy working relationships; illiterate workers may feel ashamed. In an effort to hide a literacy problem, they may seem aloof, angry, or anxious around coworkers (Tyler, 1996). Most training programs and teaching materials may be far above the learners' literacy or English speaking capacities. Thus, these programs and materials are ineffective in helping those illiterate workers (Bruening, 1989; Tyler, 1996).

To offset the effects of illiteracy, the occupational and environmental health nurse will need to explore a variety of options, including helping to establish programs for English competency skills; using a variety of teaching approaches (e.g., role play); and using multilinguistic teaching materials such as videotapes (Hong, 2001). It is crucial to establish a collaborative task force that includes health and safety educators, labor educators, English as a second language (ESL) and literacy instructors, union officials, and representatives of limited English proficiency workers. Active and ongoing involvement by the team members from project planning to implementation in this educational innovation process enhances the probability of a favorable outcome.

GENETICS

Over the past 10 years the definitions of health, disease and health care have been transformed by genetics. Detecting an inherited trait, diagnosing a hereditary condition, determining the likelihood that a hereditary condition will develop, and identifying genetic susceptibility to familial cancer are all possible now. These new directions are in large part the result of the Human Genome Project, an international 13-year effort begun in 1990 by the Department of Energy and the National Institutes of Health, which aimed to map and sequence the human genome in its entirety. The availability of genetic testing in health care has been one of the most immediate applications of the breakthrough. Improvements in disease prevention and treatment have resulted, leading to enhanced individual and public health (Lea, 2000). However, the complete mapping of the human genome has created for health care professionals, legislators, ethicists, and policy makers numerous ethical dimensions and considerations related to ethical, legal, and social implications of genetic testing. More than 6,500 disorders, including Huntington's disease, cystic fibrosis, and sickle cell anemia, are caused by single gene mutations, each of which may have numerous mutations themselves (Porth, 1998). Gene mutations also play a part in cancer, cardiovascular diseases, diabetes, and many other common disease of multifactorial origin (Schill, 2000). Although the field of genetic testing holds many promises through genetic identification of diseases, clinical treatment and preventive applications will likely take years to develop (Rogers, 2001).

Genetic testing extends beyond simply obtaining a sample; it involves informed consent, interpretations of results, and follow-up. The occupational and environmental health nurse will need to have a good understanding of the applications of genetic testing and genetic screening to educate and support workers and serve as better informed health care collaborators. Genetic testing refers to any procedure performed on chromosomes, genes, or gene products to determine whether a mutation is causing or may cause a specific condition. A variety of tests are performed including direct DNA/RNA testing, linkage testing involving family member explorations, biochemical assays on such materials as enzymes and proteins, and cytogenetic testing of chromosomes. Genetic screening is similar to genetic testing, except that screening is performed in populations known to have an increased risk of a specific genetic mutation or condition, independent of family history or symptomatology. Members of certain ethnic groups, pregnant women, and neonates often undergo such screening, which can be performed quickly but is not diagnostic (Lea & Williams, 2002).

The nurse will need to be prepared to answer important questions the worker may have about genetic testing and screening, questions such as the following:

- What will genetic testing tell me?
- Who else will have access to this information?
- Will the genetic test provide a cure?

- What will happen if my employer or insurance company finds out that I have had a genetic test?

Genetic testing and screening may be of concern to many people. Other questions related to having children, pregnancy termination, or new knowledge of genetic mutations may be disturbing. Counseling to address these concerns will clearly be needed. In addition, genetic testing involves the most private, confidential information about a person and should not be used to harm others. Improper use of genetic information includes any unauthorized disclosure to a third party or use of such information in any way that is discriminatory. Protection must be offered to individuals against increased health insurance premiums, denial of access to insurance coverage, loss of employment opportunities, and employment termination based on health status or genetic factors (Rogers, 2001).

Regardless of whether nurses specialize in genetics or a related area, they will be responsible for assisting individuals and families by answering questions and addressing concerns. This is the basic level of nursing, as defined by the *Statement of the Scope and Standards of Genetics Clinical Nursing Practice* (International Society of Nurses in Genetics, American Nurses Association, 1998), approved by the ANA in 1998. Nurses who do not specialize in genetics can participate in assessment of genetic risk, help individuals to understand genetic conditions and their management, support them in coping with a changing health status, and assist them in making decisions about genetic testing. The occupational and environmental health nurse will need to be prepared to address this new challenge.

CONTINUED COMPETENCY

To be well-prepared for the future, occupational and environmental health nurses will need to expand their knowledge base through academic and continuing education (Rogers, 1990). Knowledge, skills, and competencies need to be acquired for providing advanced clinical care, managing health care programs, and conducting research in the discipline. As occupational and environmental health nursing moves in this direction, individual nurses must consider alternative options for educational experiences, such as more independent and self-directed learning experiences and distance education; more flexibility in program scheduling to meet the needs of part-time students; and enhanced progression programs for individuals with diplomas or associate degrees who desire to obtain graduate degrees.

Occupational and environmental health nursing content within basic nursing school curricula must be upgraded. Only minimal content in occupational and environmental health nursing concepts, practice, and related fields of knowledge is included in undergraduate programs, with limited practicum experiences for students (Rogers, 1991). Well-prepared field preceptors are critically needed to work independently with undergraduate students to provide quality learning experiences based on achievement of objectives. At the graduate level more emphasis needs to be placed on the development of curricular content consistent with workplace trends and with emphasis on cost containment and effectiveness of health programs. Nursing faculty who have knowledge and expertise in the field of occupational and environmental health and safety and can engage in collaborative research to answer questions, evaluate interventions, and build knowledge are urgently needed.

The art of thinking, which enables a person to recognize and solve problems rather than learning through pedagogic lecturism, and multidisciplinary approaches for providing a broad and integrated knowledge base need to be enhanced. Educational content must include critical thinking, skills in collaboration, shared decision making, social epidemiological viewpoints, and analyses and interventions at the systems and aggregate levels (NLNAC, 2002). Analyses of ethical issues may be difficult and challenging but are important to successful outcomes.

Summary

The future is filled with exceptional challenges for occupational and environmental health nursing. This will require the occupational and environmental health nurse to have additional knowledge, skills, and abilities to recognize problems and develop strategies to address critical needs of workers. Health promotion and prevention will be key to successful health and safety achievements, and the occupational and environmental health nurse will be integral in developing and supporting initiatives for a safe and healthy workforce, workplace, and environment for all of us.

References

Bachman, R. (1994). Violence and theft in the workplace. In *U.S. Department of Justice Crime Data Brief* (NCJ-148199). Washington, DC: U.S. Government Printing Office.

Baker, D. W., Parker, R. M., Williams, M. V., Clark, W. S., & Nurss, J. (1997). The relationship of patient reading ability to self-reported health and use of health services. *American Journal of Public Health, 87*(6), 1027-1030.

Baker, D. W., Parker, R. M., Williams, M. V., Pitkin, K., Parikh, N. S., Coates, W., & Imara, M. (1996). The health care experience of patients with low literacy. *Archives of Family Medicine, 5*(6), 329-334.

Berg, P. (1999). The effects of high performance work practices on job satisfaction in the United States steel industry. *Industrial Relations 54*(1), 111-135.

Bluestone, B., & Rose, S. (1998). *Public policy brief: The unmeasured labor force—The growth of work hours.* Blithewood, Annandale-on-Hudson, NY: Jerome Levy Economics Institute of Bard College, Bard Publications Office, No. 39.

Bond, J. T., Galinsky, E., & Swanberg, J. E. (1997). *The 1997 national study of changing workforce.* New York: Families and Work Institute.

Bruening, J. C. (1989). Workplace illiteracy: The threat to worker safety. *Occupational Hazards, 51,* 118-122.

Bureau of Labor Statistics. (1994). *National census of fatal occupational injuries, 1993. BLS News* (USDL-94-384). Washington, DC: U.S. Department of Labor, Bureau of Labor Statistics.

Cangemi, C. W. (2002). Occupational response to terrorism. *AAOHN Journal, 50,* 190-196.

Centers for Disease Control and Prevention. (2002). Injuries and illnesses among NYC fire department rescue workers after responding to the World Trade Center attacks. *MMWR, 51* (special issue), 1-5, 16.

Code of Federal Regulations, Section 0.85. (August, 2001). (28 C.F.R.).

Federal Bureau of Investigation. (1994). *Uniform crime reports for the United States, 1993.* Washington, DC: U.S. Department of Justice, Federal Bureau of Investigation.

Goode, T. *Checklist—Culturally competent service delivery systems.* (2000). National Center for Cultural Competence. http://www.gucdc/georgetown.edu/cultural.html/

Hays, S. (1999). The ABCs of workplace literacy. *Workplace, 78*(4), 70-75.

Heyman, J. (2000). *The widening gap: Why America's working families are in jeopardy and what can be done about it.* New York: Basic Books.

Hong, O. S. (2001). Limited English proficiency workers: Health and safety education. *AAOHN Journal, 49,* 21-26.

International Society of Nurses in Genetics, American Nurses Association. (1998). *Statement on the scope and standards of genetic clinical nursing practice.* Washington, DC: American Nurses.

Jackson, P. R., & Martin, R. (1996). Impact of just-in-time on job content, employee attitudes and well-being: A longitudinal study. *Ergonomics 39*(1), 1-16.

Jackson, P. R., & Mullarkey, S. (2000). Lean production terms and health in garment manufacture. *Journal of Occupational Health Psychology, 5*(2), 231-245.

Jenkins, E. L. (1996). Workplace homicide: Industries and occupations at high risk. *Occupational Medicine: State of Art Reviews, 11*(2), 219-225.

Kaminski, M. (2001). Unintended consequences: organizational practices and their impact on workplace safety and productivity. *Journal of Occupational Health Psychology, 6*(2), 127-138.

Kerr, M. J., Struthers, R., & Huynh, W. C. (2001). Work force diversity: Implications for occupational health nursing. *AAOHN Journal, 49,* 14-20.

Kirch, I. S., Jungeblut, A., Jenkis, L., & Kolstad, A. (1993). *Adult literacy in America: A first look at the results of the National Adult Literacy Survey.* Washington, DC: U.S. Department of Education.

Landsbergis, P. A., Cahill, J., & Schnall, P. (1999). The impact of lean production and worker health. *Journal of Occupational Health Psychology, 4*(2), 108-130.

Lea, D. H., Williams, J. K., Jenkins, J., & Jones, S. (2000). Genetic health care: Creating interdisciplinary partnerships with nursing in clinical practice. *National Academy Practice Forum, 2*(3), 177-86.

Lea, D. H., & Williams, J. K. (2002). Genetic testing and screening. *American Journal of Nursing, 102,* 36-43.

Lusk, P., & Holst, P. (2001). Occupational health nursing with Navajo workers: Providing culturally competent care. *AAOHN Journal, 49,* 27-34.

Mastroianni, K. (1992). Child day care arrangements and employee health. *AAOHN Journal, 40*(2), 78-83.

McCloskey, J., Gardner, D., & Johnson, M. (1987). Costing out nursing services. *Nursing Economics, 5,* 45-253.

National Institute of Environmental Health Sciences. (1992). *Health through environmental research.* (Publication No. 992). Research Triangle Park, NC: Author.

National League for Nursing Accrediting Commission. (2003). *Accreditation manual and interpretive guidelines.* New York: Author.

Perikh, N. S., Parker, R. M., Nurss, J. R., Baker, D. W., & Williams, M. V. (1996). Shame and health literacy: The unspoken connection. *Patient Education & Counseling, 27*(1), 33-39.

Porth, C. M. (1998). *Pathophysiology: Concepts of altered health states* (5th ed.). New York: Lippincott.

Rogers, B. (1990). Occupational and environmental health nursing practice, education, and research: Challenges for the future. *AAOHN Journal, 38,* 536-543.

Rogers, B. (1991). Occupational and environmental health nursing education: Curricular content in baccalaureate programs. *AAOHN Journal, 39*(3), 101-108.

Rogers, B. (2001). Confidentiality and genetic information. *AAOHN Journal, 49,* 321-322.

Rogers, B., & Haynes, C. (1991). A study of hospital employee health programs. *AAOHN Journal, 39*(4), 157-166.

Schill, A. (2000). Genetic information in the workplace: Implications for occupational health surveillance. *AAOHN Journal, 48,* 80-91.

Smith, V. (1997). New forms of work organization. *Annual Review of Sociology, 23,* 315-339.

Sprigg, C. A., Jackson, P. R., & Parker, S. K. (2000). Production team-working: The importance of interdependence and autonomy for employee strain and satisfaction. *Human Relations 53*(11), 1519-1543.

Sunoo, B. P. (1999). Labor-management partnerships boost training. *Workforce, 78*(4), 80-84.

Tyler, K. (1996). Tips for structuring workplace literacy programs. *HR Magazine, 41*(10), 112-115.

U.S. Department of Health and Human Services, National Institute for Occupational Safety and Health. (1996). *Violence in the workplace* (Publication No. 96-100). Cincinnati, OH: Author.

U.S. Department of Health and Human Services, National Institute for Occupational Safety and Health. (2002). *The challenging organization of work and the safety and health of working people* (Publication No. 2002-116). Cincinnati, OH: NIOSH.

U.S. Department of Justice. (2001). *National crime victimization survey: Violence in the workplace, 1993-1999.* Washington, DC: Author.

U.S. Department of Labor. (1999). *Report on the American workforce.* Washington, DC: Author.

United Nations Development Programme. (1995). *Human development report, 1995.* New York: Oxford University Press, United Nations Development Programme.

Windau, J., & Toscano, G. (1994). *Workplace homicides in 1992: Compensation and working conditions, February 1994.* Washington, DC: U.S. Department of Labor, Bureau of Labor Statistics.

INDEX

A

AAIN. *See* American Association of Industrial Nurses.

AANP. *See* American Academy of Nurse Practitioners.

AAOHN. *See* American Association of Occupational Health Nurses.

AAPCC. *See* American Association of Poison Control Centers.

Abatement strategies in worksite assessment, 212-213

ABLES. *See* Adult Blood Lead Epidemiology and Surveillance Program.

ABOHN. *See* American Board for Occupational Health Nurses, Inc..

Abortion, spontaneous, chemical exposure and, 189t

Abrasion
    clinical nursing guidelines for, 342
    treated in emergency department, 19f

Abrasive blasting, hazards associated with, 196t

Absenteeism, behavioral health risks and, 405

Abuse
    child, federal information centers and clearinghouses related to, 453
    substance, 11-12
        in ages 11-24 years, 388b
        in ages 25-64 years, 391b
        in ages 65 and older, 393b
        birth to 10 years, 386b
        as leading health indicator, 381b
        national clearinghouse for, 451
        occupational safety and health objectives related to, 26t

Access to exposure and medical records, 558-559

Accident. *See Also* Injury; Safety.
    defined, 150
    in farming industry, 109-110
    investigation of by safety task group, 158-160

Accidental sampling, 646

Accountability, managerial creation of, 488

Acetaminophen, 146

Acetone, biologic monitoring for, 312t

Acetylsalicylic acid, 146

ACHE. *See* American Council for Headache Rehabilitation.

Achievement culture, 284b

ACOEM. *See* American College of Occupational Environmental Medicine.

Acquired immunodeficiency syndrome, 547. *See Also* Bloodborne Pathogens Standard.

Acrylonitrile, OSHA screening and surveillance of, 317

ACS. *See* American Cancer Society.

Actifed tablets, 146

Action
    in consulting process, 96t
    in Stages of Change Model, 408

Activated charcoal for traveler's diarrhea, 683

Active immunity, 107

Active sampling technique, 199

Activity limitations, 9. *See Also* Disability.

ADA. *See* Americans With Disabilities Act.

ADEAR. *See* Alzheimer Disease Education and Referral Center.

Administration. *See Also* Management.
    assessment of in PRECEDE-PROCEED Model, 402t, 403
    in ergonomic controls, 168-170, 171t
    in hazard control, 201, 309
    scope of practice, 60
    workplace violence prevention and, 705

Adolescent
    changing population of, 2
    disabilities among, 9
    Healthy People 2010 objectives for reduction of nonfatal injuries in, 22t
    periodic health examination chart for, 388b-390b

Adoption, clearinghouses and information centers on, 450

Adrenalin. *See* Epinephrine.

Adult Blood Lead Epidemiology and Surveillance Program, 124t

Adult learning, 425-428, 426t

Adverse effects, evaluation of in surveillance program, 309

Advisory committee, health promotion, 412-413

Advocacy
    in case management, 363
    as general environmental health competency, 257-259, 281-282

African American population, 2

Age factors
    in chemical toxicity, 187
    in death rates, 115-116, 116t
    epidemiologic, 105t, 108-109
    in health promotion program participation, 414

Figure is indicated by *f;* table is indicated by *t;* box is indicated by *b.*

715